Prentice Hall Health's
Q&A Review
Medical Technology/ Clinical Laboratory Science

Third Edition

Anna P. Ciulla, MCC, MT(ASCP)SC, CC(NRCC)
Associate Professor and Chair
Department of Medical Technology
College of Health and Nursing Sciences
University of Delaware
Newark, Delaware

Georganne K. Buescher, EdD, MS, SM(AAM)
Clinical Assistant Professor, Department of
Microbiology/Immunology, Jefferson Medical College
and Associate Dean, College of Graduate Studies,
Thomas Jefferson University
Philadelphia, Pennsylvania

D1611484

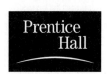

Prentice
Hall

Upper Saddle River, New Jersey 07458

Library of Congress Cataloging-in-Publication Data

Prentice Hall Health's question and answer review of medical technology/clinical
laboratory science   Anna P. Ciulla. Georganne K. Buescher [editors].—3rd ed.
    p. cm.
  Previously published: Medical technology examination review and study guide. 2nd ed.
  ISBN 0-8385-0340-3 (paper)
   1. Medical laboratory technology—Examinations, questions, etc. 2. Diagnosis,
Laboratory—Examination, questions, etc. I. Ciulla, Anna P. II. Buescher, Georganne K.
III. Medical technology examination review and study guide.

RB38.25 .M42 2001
616.07'56'076—dc21

2001051363

Publisher: Julie Levin Alexander
Editorial Assistant: Regina Bruno
Senior Acquisitions Editor: Mark Cohen
Assistant Editor: Melissa Kerian
Managing Editor for Development: Marilyn Meserve
Director of Production and Manufacturing : Bruce Johnson
Managing Editor for Production: Patrick Walsh
Production Editor: Alexander Ivchenko
Manufacturing Manager: Ilene Sanford
Manufacturing Buyer: Pat Brown
Creative Director: Cheryl Asherman
Cover Design Coordinator: Maria Guglielmo-Walsh
Formatting: Pine Tree Composition
Electronic Art Creation: ElectraGraphics, Inc.
Marketing Manager: David Hough
Product Information Manager: Rachele Triano
Printer/Binder: Banta Company, Harrisonburg, VA
Copy Editor: Terry Andrews
Proofreader: Marianne Peters Riordan
Cover Design: Janice Bielawa
Cover Printer: Banta Company, Harrisonburg, VA

Pearson Education LTD.
Pearson Education Australia PTY, Limited
Pearson Education Singapore, Pte. Ltd
Pearson Education North Asia Ltd
Pearson Education Canada, Ltd.
Pearson Educación de Mexico, S.A. de C.V.
Pearson Education -- Japan
Pearson Education Malaysia, Pte. Ltd

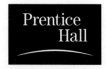

10 9 8 7 6 5 4 3 2
ISBN 0-8385-0340-3

Contents

Preface

Prentice Hall Health's Question & Answer Review of Medical Technology/Clinical Laboratory Science, Third Edition, has been designed to help examination candidates to prepare for national certification or state licensure examinations. It is also a useful tool for practicing clinical laboratory scientists as a source of "refresher" information. The excellent reception received by the first two editions of the book spurred the writing of this third edition. Educators and students alike have commented that the strength of the book is in the paragraph explanations that accompany each answer. In this way users of the book can more easily augment their knowledge or clear up misunderstandings.

To enhance the third edition and to make it even more valuable to users, new features have been added and some changes have been made. A color plate of 60 full-color pictures has been included to provide the user with experience in answering questions based on a color photo. Additionally, the 200-question self-assessment test has been revised and a 100-question self-assessment test for the CD-ROM has been developed as mechanisms for final evaluation of one's knowledge, thus allowing for the identification of one's strengths and weaknesses while there is still time to improve.

The book contains more than 2000 multiple choice questions that cover all the areas commonly tested on national certification examinations and state licensure examinations. The majority of questions have been revised or updated based on current clinical laboratory practice, terminology, and taxonomy. Additional case study questions have been incorporated into this edition. Many of the paragraph explanations have been revised, and matching puzzles have been added to the CD-ROM to further assess knowledge. Overall, this book provides the essential components needed in an effective medical technology examination review book. We hope that you find this book and the accompanying CD-ROM useful, and we wish you success with the examination and with your career as a clinical laboratory scientist.

Acknowledgments

This book is the end product of the labor and dedication of a number of outstanding professionals. The editors would like to acknowledge these individuals for their invaluable assistance in completing this project. The editors greatly appreciate the efforts of the contributing authors who worked so diligently to produce quality materials. We are also most grateful for the technical assistance of Raelene E. Maser, PhD, MT(ASCP), Associate Professor, Department of Medical Technology, University of Delaware, Newark, DE; and Cynthia Flickinger, BS, MT(ASCP)SBB, Assistant Professor, Department of Medical Technology, University of Delaware, Newark, DE. We also greatly appreciate the use of color slides from the private collection of Elmer W. Koneman MD, Professor Emeritus, University of Colorado School of Medicine and Medical Laboratory Director, Summit Medical Center, Frisco, Colorado. Lastly, we would like to thank our respective family members— mother, Josephine Ciulla, and husband, Jerome Buescher. We are eternally grateful for their understanding, support, and encouragement.

Certifying Agencies

Information pertaining to certification examinations, education and training requirements, and application forms may be obtained by contacting the certifying agency of your choice. The following is a list of the certification agencies that service clinical laboratory scientists.

American Society of Clinical Pathologists (ASCP)
Board of Registry
P.O. Box 12277
Chicago, IL 60612-0277
(312) 738-1336
E-mail: *bor@ascp.org*
Website: *http://www.ascp.org/bor*

National Credentialing Agency for Laboratory Personnel, Inc. (NCA)
P.O. Box 15945-289
Lenexa, KS 66285
(913) 438-5110, ext. 647
E-mail: *nca-info@goamp.com*
Website: *http://www.nca-info.org/*

American Medical Technologists (AMT)
710 Higgins Road
Park Ridge, IL 60068-5765
(847) 823-5169
E-mail: *amtmail@aol.com*
Website: *http://www.amt1.com/*

American Association of Bioanalysts (AAB)
Board of Registry
917 Locust Street
Suite 1100
St. Louis, MO 63101-1419
(314) 241-1445
E-mail: *aab@aab.org*
Website: *http://www.aab.org/*

Contributors

Georganne K. Buescher, EdD, MS, SM(AAM)
Clinical Assistant Professor,
Department of Microbiology/
Immunology, Jefferson Medical
College and Associate Dean, College
of Graduate Studies, Thomas
Jefferson University
Philadelphia, Pennsylvania 19107

Jerome G. Buescher, PhD
Adjunct Assistant Professor
Department of Microbiology
and Immunology
Jefferson Medical College
Thomas Jefferson University
Philadelphia, Pennsylvania 19107

Anna P. Ciulla, MCC, MT(ASCP)SC, CC(NRCC)
Associate Professor and Chair
Department of Medical Technology
College of Health and Nursing Sciences
University of Delaware
Newark, Delaware 19716

Deborah Costa, BS, MT(ASCP)
Instructor and Education Coordinator
Department of Medical Technology
College of Health and Nursing Sciences
University of Delaware
Newark, Delaware 19716

H. Jesse Guiles, EdD, MT(ASCP)SC, CLS(NCA)
Professor
Department of Clinical
Laboratory Sciences
School of Health Related Professions
University of Medicine & Dentistry
of New Jersey
Newark, New Jersey 07107

Karen A. Keller, BS, MT(ASCP)SH
Teaching Coordinator, Hematology
and Clinical Microscopy
Nebraska Health System—Clarkson
Hospital
Nebraska Medical Center
Omaha, Nebraska 68198-7549

Donald C. Lehman, MSc, MT(ASCP), SM(AAM)
Assistant Professor
Department of Medical Technology
College of Health and Nursing Sciences
University of Delaware
Newark, Delaware 19716

Mary Ann McLane, PhD, CLS(NCA)
Assistant Professor
Department of Medical Technology
College of Health and Nursing Sciences
University of Delaware
Newark, Delaware 19716

Mary E. Miele, PhD, MT(ASCP), RM(NRM)
Assistant Professor
Department of Medical Technology
College of Health and Nursing Sciences
University of Delaware
Newark, Delaware 19716

Joel E. Mortensen, PhD
Director of Microbiology and Virology
Children's Hospital Medical Center
Department of Pathology
and Laboratory Medicine
Cincinnati, Ohio 45229

Edward J. Peterson, Jr., MBA, MT(ASCP)
Administrative Director of Diagnostic Services
Department of Laboratory Medicine, Radiology,
and Radiation Oncology
Shore Memorial Hospital
Somers Point, New Jersey 08244

Susan Souder, MS, MT(ASCP)
Biological Safety Officer
Department of Environmental Health and Safety
Thomas Jefferson University
Philadelphia, Pennsylvania 19107

Mary Ann Spivey, MHS, MT(ASCP)SBB
Consultant
Department of Pathology and Laboratory
Medicine, Transfusion Medicine
Medical University of South Carolina
Charleston, South Carolina 29425

Linda Sykora, BS, MT(ASCP)SH
Hematology Teaching Coordinator
University of Nebraska Medical Center
Division of Medical Technology
Omaha, Nebraska 68198-1180

Sheryl A. Whitlock, MA, MT(ASCP)BB
Laboratory Coordinator
Student Health Services
University of Delaware
Newark, Delaware 19716

Reviewers

Cynthia Butler, EdD, MT(ASCP)
Program Director
Medical Laboratory Sciences
Florida Atlantic University
Boca Raton, Florida

Cheryl G. Davis, MS, CLS(NCA)
Assistant Professor
Program Director
Medical Technology
Tuskegee University
Tuskegee, Alabama

Dorothy J. Fike, MS, MT(ASCP)SBB
Associate Professor
Clinical Laboratory Sciences
Marshall University
Huntington, West Virginia

Cynthia Flickinger, BS, MT(ASCP)SBB
Assistant Professor
Department of Medical Technology
University of Delaware
Newark, Delaware

Mark Jaros, BS, MBA
Assistant Director
Rush Medical Laboratories
Chicago, Illinois

Johanna W. Laird, MS, MT(ASCP)
Program Director
Clinical Laboratory Science/Medical
Technology Program
Salisbury State University
Salisbury, Maryland

Raelene E. Maser, PhD, MT(ASCP)
Associate Professor
Department of Medical Technology
University of Delaware
Newark, Delaware

Phyllis Muellenberg, MA, MT(ASCP)
Chair and Program Director
Division of Medical Technology
University of Nebraska Medical Center
Omaha, Nebraska

**Lawrence R. Suddendorf, EdD, MT(ASCP),
CLS(NCAMLP)**
Clinical Laboratory Technology Program
Cincinnati State Technical and Community College
Cincinnati, Ohio

Robert J. Sullivan, PhD, MT(ASCP)
Associate Professor
Department of Medical Technology
Marist College
Poughkeepsie, New York

Jay Wilborn, MEd, MT(ASCP)
Program Director
Clinical Laboratory Technology Program
Garland County Community College
Hot Springs, Arkansas

Gail Williams, PhD, MT(ASCP)SBB
Assistant Professor
Clinical Laboratory Sciences Program
Northern Illinois University
DeKalb, Illinois

Introduction

If you are currently preparing for a Medical Technology Certification or Licensure Examination, or if you are a practicing clinical laboratory scientist who wants to "brush up" on medical technology information, then this is the review book for you. *Prentice Hall Health's Question & Answer Review of Medical Technology/Clinical Laboratory Science, Third Edition,* is a comprehensive text containing more than 2000 questions with paragraph explanations accompanying each answer. This format not only tests your knowledge of the subject matter but also facilitates additional study. Unique to this book is an enhanced color plate of 60 full-color pictures to help you prepare for national examinations in as realistic a manner as possible. In this edition are a revised 200-question self-assessment test and a new 100-question self-assessment test on the CD-ROM. Both formats will assist you in determining your mastery of the material, while allowing computer practice for those examinations that are offered as computerized testing and pencil-and-paper practice for those exams that are still available in written format. Also included on the CD-ROM is a new feature of matching puzzles to assess your knowledge in a less formal manner.

ORGANIZATION

The book is organized into 14 chapters corresponding to the areas tested on medical technology certification examinations. The chapters include:

1. Clinical Chemistry
2. Hematology
3. Hemostasis
4. Immunology
5. Immunohematology
6. Microbiology
7. Urinalysis and Body Fluids
8. Molecular Diagnostics
9. Laboratory Calculations
10. General Laboratory Principles and Safety
11. Laboratory Management
12. Education
13. Computers and Laboratory Informatics
14. Self-Assessment Test

As you can see, each chapter represents a specific discipline in the medical technology field. Some of the chapters are further divided into subsections to facilitate study of major topics within these disciplines. The chapters are separated between questions and answers, and a list of references is located at the end of each chapter for further review. The last chapter is a self-assessment test that should be used to determine overall competency upon completion of the previous chapters.

The CD-ROM located in the back of the book contains a 100-question self-assessment test to further assist you in preparing for computerized national examinations. In addition, the CD-ROM contains matching puzzles that will help you to review major points associated with each content area.

QUESTIONS

The style of the questions used adheres to that prevalent in most certification examinations. Each chapter contains questions in a multiple choice format with there being only one best answer (A-type question). In some cases, a group of two or more questions may be based on a case study or some other clinical situation. Questions are divided among three levels of difficulty: level 1 questions test recall of information, level 2 questions test understanding of information and application to new situations, and level 3 questions test problem-solving ability. Lastly, some of the questions are expressed in a negative manner (e.g., all the following *Except,* all are true *Except*). Each of the multiple choice questions is followed by four choices, with only one of the choices being completely correct. Although some choices may be partially correct, remember that there can only be one best answer.

HOW TO USE THIS BOOK

The best way to use *Prentice Hall Health's Question & Answer Review of Medical Technology/ Clinical Laboratory Science, Third Edition,* is to work through a small section at a time, reading the questions carefully and recording an answer for each. Then the correct answers should be consulted and the explanations read. It is important to read the paragraph explanations for both those questions answered correctly as well as for those missed, because very often additional information will be presented that will reinforce or clarify knowledge already present. If you answer a question incorrectly, it would be wise to consult the references listed at the end of the chapter. The inclusion of an expanded color plate in this book is an additional feature. It was enhanced so that you are not "surprised" on the day that you are examined. By preparing you to address questions based on color pictures during your study preparation, you should be better able to answer such types of questions on the actual examination. Lastly, you should take the self-assessment test as if it was the actual examination. Find a quiet place, free of interruptions and distractions, and allow yourself four hours to complete the 200-question self-assessment written test. For the 100-question self-assessment test on the CD-ROM, take two and one-half hours to complete the computerized test. These tests will give you a more realistic evaluation of your knowledge and your ability to function within a time constraint. It is important that you are comfortable taking a test that is computerized, since several of the certifying agencies now use either computer-administered or computer-adaptive testing. So be sure to practice on the computer using the CD-ROM that is included in the back of the book. By the time you have worked through the entire book and the two self-assessment tests, and the matching puzzles, you will have gained a solid base of knowledge.

For students of medical technology and practicing clinical laboratory scientists, this book has been designed both to test your knowledge and to explain unfamiliar information through use of the paragraph explanations that accompany each question. Working through the entire book will make you aware of the clinical areas in which you are strong or weak. This review will help you gauge your study time before taking any state licensure or national certification examination. Remember, there is no substitute for knowing the material.

TEST-TAKING TIPS

In addition to studying and reviewing the subject matter, you should also consider the following points:

1. Contact the Sponsoring Agency
Contact the agency that administers the examination and request general information about their test including:
    • The outline of the test content. Several agencies publish an outline of the test content areas.
    • The test question format.
    • Whether the test is computer-based or paper-and-pencil.
    • If computer-based, whether it is computer-administered or computer-adaptive.
    • The time allowed to complete the test and the number of questions on it.
    • The scoring policy.

    Note: Since certification examination requirements vary, it is important to read thoroughly all directions sent to you by the sponsoring agency and to read carefully the directions presented on the day of the examination. After completing the computerized examinations, most agencies permit you to return to previously answered questions and entered responses can be changed.

In some cases the sponsoring agency allows you to skip a question and return to it at the end of the exam, while other agencies require that you select an answer before being allowed to move to the next question. So know the rules! Checking your answers is a very important part of taking a major certification exam. During the exam, check the computer screen after an answer is entered to verify that the answer appears as it was entered.

2. Prepare before Examination Day
    • Study thoroughly prior to taking the exam. Set up a study schedule that allows sufficient time for review of each area.
    • Use this review book to help you to identify your strengths and weaknesses, to sharpen your test taking skills, and to be more successful with multiple choice examinations.
    • Know the locations of the test center and the parking facilities. If the area is unfamiliar to you, a visit to the site a week before the exam may help to prevent unnecessary anxiety on the morning of the test.
    • Check your calculator (if one is allowed) for proper function and worn batteries. Some agencies allow a nonprogrammable calculator to be used during the exam.
    • Get plenty of rest. Do not cram. A good night's sleep will prove to be more valuable than cramming the night before the exam.

3. Prepare on Examination Day
    • Eat a good breakfast.
    • Take your photo identification and your admission letter (if required by the agency).
    • Take at least two No. 2 soft-lead pencils with good erasers (if the test is paper-and-pencil format) and your nonprogrammable calculator (if one is allowed) to the test center.
    • Allow sufficient time to get to the test center without rushing. Most agencies require that you be at the test center 30 minutes prior to the start of the exam.

- Wear a wristwatch in order to budget your time properly.
- Read the directions thoroughly and carefully. Know what the directions are saying.
- Read each question carefully. Be sure to answer the question asked. Do not look for hidden meanings.
- Take particular note of such words as *except, least, not, best,* and *most.*
- Rapidly scan each choice to familiarize yourself with the possible responses.
- Reread each choice carefully, eliminating choices that are obviously incorrect.
- Select the one best answer.
- Enter in the computer the correct response, or mark your response next to the number on the answer sheet that corresponds to the number of the test question, being careful not to skip a number.
- Budget your time. If the test has, for example, 100 questions and 2 hours and 30 minutes are allowed for completion, you have approximately 1½ minutes for each question.
- Above all, Don't Panic! If you "draw a blank" on a particular question or set of questions skip it and go on unless directed to answer all questions. Return if you are permitted to any skipped questions at the end of the exam. Stay calm and do your best.

CHAPTER

1 Clinical Chemistry

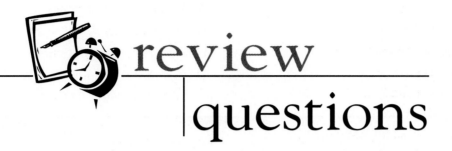

review questions

INSTRUCTIONS Each of the questions or incomplete statements that follow comprises four suggested responses. Select the *best* answer or completion statement in each case.

INSTRUMENTATION AND ANALYTICAL PRINCIPLES

1. Which of the following lamps provides a continuous spectrum of radiant energy in the visible, near IR, and UV regions of the spectrum?
   A. Tungsten-filament
   B. Hydrogen
   C. Deuterium
   D. Mercury vapor

2. Which of the following isolates light within a narrow region of the spectrum?
   A. Photomultiplier
   B. Monochromator
   C. Photovoltaic cell
   D. Detector

3. A photomultiplier tube may be described by all the following *except*
   A. Rapid response time
   B. Must be shielded from stray light
   C. Cannot be used with a chopper
   D. Amplifies current significantly

4. All the following statements about a photo-multiplier tube are true *except*
   A. Converts radiant energy (light) to electrical energy (current)

B. Amplifies the initial signal received
C. Has a very rapid response time
D. Is composed of an iron plate and a layer of selenium

5. Which type of photodetector has a linear array that allows it to respond to a specific wavelength resulting in complete UV/visible spectrum analysis?
   A. Photomultiplier tube
   B. Phototube
   C. Photodiode
   D. Photodiode array

6. When performing spectrophotometer quality control checks, what is the holmium oxide glass filter used to assess?
   A. Linearity
   B. Stray light
   C. Absorbance accuracy
   D. Wavelength accuracy

7. In spectrophotometric analysis, what is the purpose of the reagent blank?
   A. Correct for interfering chromogens
   B. Correct for lipemia
   C. Correct for protein
   D. Correct for color contribution of the reagents

8. All the following are true of bichromatic analysis *except*
   A. Absorbance measured at the peak using two wavelengths
   B. Eliminates background interferences
   C. Concentration determined from difference in two measured absorbances
   D. Functions as a reference blank for each sample

9. The bandpass of a spectrophotometer is 10 nm. If an instrument is set at 540 nm, the wavelengths that are permitted to impinge on the sample will be within what wavelength range?
   A. 530–540 nm
   B. 530–550 nm
   C. 535–545 nm
   D. 540–550 nm

10. Which of the following formulas is an expression of the Beer-Lambert law that is routinely applied to spectrophotometric analysis?
    A. $A_u \times \dfrac{C_s}{A_s} = C_u$

    B. $C_u \times \dfrac{C_s}{A_s} = A_u$

    C. $A_s \times \dfrac{C_s}{C_u} = A_u$

    D. $A = 2 - \log \% T$

11. In spectrophotometry, which of the following is a mathematical expression of the relationship between absorbance and transmittance?
    A. $A = abc$
    B. $\dfrac{A_u}{C_u} = \dfrac{A_s}{C_s}$
    C. $A = 2 - \log \% T$
    D. $A = \log \% T$

12. What feature distinguishes a double-beam spectrophotometer from a single-beam spectrophotometer?

    A. Has two light sources
    B. Has two recorders
    C. Has two beam splitters
    D. Compares sample and reagent blank absorbances simultaneously

13. Problems inherent in turbidimetry include all the following *except*
    A. Variation in particle size of samples
    B. Variation in particle size of standards
    C. Rate of aggregation or settling of particles
    D. Need to maintain a constant and specific temperature

14. Which of the following may be associated with reflectance spectrophotometry as it relates to the dry reagent slide technique?
    A. Light projected to the slide at 180-degree angle
    B. Dye concentration directly proportional to reflectance
    C. Photodetector positioned at 90-degree angle to reflected light
    D. Reflectance values linearly proportional to transmission values

15. Fluorometers are designed so that the path of the exciting light is at a right angle to the path of the emitted light. What is the purpose of this design?
    A. Prevent loss of emitted light
    B. Prevent loss of the excitation light
    C. Focus emitted and excitation light upon the detector
    D. Prevent excitation light from reaching the detector

16. Which of the following represents a primary advantage of performing fluorometric over absorption spectroscopic methods of analysis?
    A. Increased specificity and increased sensitivity
    B. Increased specificity and decreased sensitivity
    C. Purity of reagents used not as critical
    D. Ease of performing assays

17. Which of the following may be associated with fluorescence polarization?
    A. Plane-polarized light used for sample excitation
    B. Small molecular complexes show a greater amount of polarization
    C. Heterogeneous technique employed in fluorophore-ligand immunoassays
    D. Polarized light detected is directly proportional to concentration of ligand in sample

18. Which of the following may be associated with bioluminescence?
    A. Light emission produced with return of electron to ground state
    B. Less sensitive than direct fluorescent assays
    C. Electron excitation caused by radiant energy
    D. Employs a radioactive label

19. Nephelometry is based on the measurement of light that is
    A. Absorbed by particles in suspension
    B. Scattered by particles in suspension
    C. Produced by fluorescence
    D. Produced by excitation of ground state atoms

20. Which of the following instruments is used in the clinical laboratory to detect beta and gamma emissions?
    A. Fluorometer
    B. Nephelometer
    C. Scintillation counter
    D. Spectrophotometer

21. In flame emission photometry, a photon of light with a wavelength specific for a given element is emitted when
    A. An orbital electron is raised to a higher energy state.
    B. An excited orbital electron returns to the ground state.
    C. The element absorbs ultraviolet light.
    D. The bonds in the molecule vibrate.

22. In assaying an analyte with a single-beam atomic absorption spectrophotometer, what is the instrument actually measuring?
    A. Intensity of light emitted by the analyte on its return to the ground state
    B. Intensity of light that the analyte absorbs from the hollow cathode lamp
    C. Intensity of light that the analyte absorbs from the flame
    D. Intensity of the beam from the hollow cathode lamp after it has passed through the analyte-containing flame

23. Which of the following statements about atomic absorption spectrophotometry is *true*?
    A. It requires that the element to be measured be brought to a nonionized ground state.
    B. It uses a tungsten lamp as the light source.
    C. It uses a cathode made of the element lithium.
    D. It measures emission of light from excited atoms.

24. What is the function of the flame in atomic absorption spectroscopy?
    A. Absorb the energy emitted from the metal analyte in returning to ground state
    B. Supply the thermal energy needed to excite the metal analyte
    C. Bring the metal analyte to its ground state
    D. Supply the light that is absorbed by the metal analyte

25. Most atomic absorption spectrophotometers incorporate a beam chopper and a tuned amplifier. The purpose of these components is to avoid errors caused by
    A. Variations in flame temperature
    B. Deterioration of the hollow cathode lamp
    C. Stray light from the hollow cathode lamp
    D. Measurement of light of the specific wavelength emitted by the analyte

26. Which of the following lamps may be described as containing argon and having the element of interest coated on its cathode?
    A. Hollow cathode lamp
    B. Tungsten lamp
    C. Quartz-halogen lamp
    D. Deuterium lamp

27. In potentiometry, which of the following is considered the standard electrode?
    A. Hydrogen electrode
    B. Calcium electrode
    C. Potassium electrode
    D. Copper electrode

28. In an electrolytic cell, which of the following is the half-cell where reduction takes place?
    A. Anode
    B. Cathode
    C. Combination electrode
    D. Electrode response

29. Mercury covered by a layer of mercurous chloride in contact with saturated potassium chloride solution is a description of which of the following types of electrodes?
    A. Sodium
    B. Calomel
    C. Calcium
    D. Silver/silver chloride

30. When a pH-sensitive glass electrode is not actively in use, in what type of solution should it be kept?
    A. Tap water
    B. Physiologic saline solution
    C. The medium recommended by the manufacturer
    D. A buffer solution of alkaline pH

31. When measuring K^+ with an ion-selective electrode by means of a liquid ion-exchange membrane, what antibiotic will be incorporated into the membrane?
    A. Monactin
    B. Nonactin
    C. Streptomycin
    D. Valinomycin

32. All the following are true of ion-selective electrode analysis of sodium *except*
    A. Uses a glass membrane
    B. Errors occur from protein buildup on the membrane
    C. Membrane coated with valinomycin
    D. Principle based on potentiometry

33. What are the principles of operation for a chloride analyzer that generates silver ions as part of its reaction mechanism?
    A. Potentiometry and amperometry
    B. Amperometry and polarography
    C. Coulometry and potentiometry
    D. Amperometry and coulometry

34. When quantifying glucose using an amperometric glucose electrode system, all the following are components of the system *except*
    A. Product oxidation produces a current
    B. Hydrogen peroxide formed
    C. Hexokinase reacts with glucose
    D. Platinum electrode

35. To calibrate the pH electrode in a pH/blood gas analyzer, it is necessary that
    A. The barometric pressure be known and used for adjustments
    B. Calibrating gases of known high and low concentrations be used
    C. The calibration be performed at room temperature
    D. Two buffer solutions of known pH be used

36. The measurement of CO_2 in blood by means of a Pco_2 electrode is dependent on the
    A. Passage of H^+ ions through the membrane that separates the sample and the electrode
    B. Change in pH due to increased carbonic acid in the electrolyte surrounding the electrodes
    C. Movement of bicarbonate across the membrane that separates the sample and the electrode
    D. Linear relationship between Pco_2 in the sample and measured pH

37. The measurement of oxygen in blood by means of a Po_2 electrode involves which of the following?
    A. Wheatstone bridge arrangement of resistive elements sensitive to oxygen concentration
    B. Direct relationship between amount of oxygen in the sample and amount of current flowing in the measuring system
    C. Change in current resulting from an increase of free silver ions in solution
    D. Glass electrode sensitive to H^+ ions

38. All the following statements about anodic stripping voltammetry (ASV) are true *except*
    A. Based on potentiometry
    B. Occurs in an electrochemical cell
    C. Involves preconcentration of the analyte by electroplating
    D. Used to measure lead

39. Colligative properties of solutions include all the following *except*
    A. pH
    B. Freezing point
    C. Osmotic pressure
    D. Vapor pressure

40. Which of the following describes the basis for the freezing point osmometer?
    A. The freezing point depression is inversely proportional to the amount of solute in the solution.
    B. The freezing point depression varies as the logarithm of the concentration of solute.
    C. The freezing point is raised by an amount that is inversely proportional to the concentration of dissolved particles in the solution.
    D. The freezing point is lowered by an amount that is directly proportional to the concentration of dissolved particles in the solution.

41. Given the following information, calculate the plasma osmolality in milliosmoles per kilogram: sodium–142 mmol/L; glucose–130 mg/dL; urea nitrogen–18 mg/dL.
    A. 290
    B. 291
    C. 295
    D. 298

42. Which of the following may be associated with the colloid osmotic pressure (COP) osmometer?
    A. Utilizes a cooling bath set at $-7\,°C$
    B. Measures total serum osmolality
    C. Negative pressure on reference (saline) side equivalent to COP of sample
    D. Measures contribution of electrolytes to osmolality

43. Which of the following methods allows for the separation of charged particles based on their rates of migration in an electric field?
    A. Rheophoresis
    B. Electrophoresis
    C. Electroendosmosis
    D. Ion-exchange

44. Which of the following techniques is based on electro-osmotic flow?
    A. Capillary electrophoresis
    B. Zone electrophoresis
    C. Iontophoresis
    D. Isoelectric focusing

45. Which of the following is an electrophoretic technique employing a pH gradient that separates molecules with similar isoelectric points?
    A. Zone electrophoresis
    B. High-resolution electrophoresis
    C. Isoelectric focusing
    D. Immunoelectrophoresis

46. Given the following information on a particular compound that has been visualized by means of thin-layer chromatography, calculate the R_f of the compound.

    Distance from origin to spot
    center = 48 mm
    Distance from spot center to solvent
    front = 93 mm
    Distance from origin to solvent
    front = 141 mm

    A. 3
    B. 34
    C. 52
    D. 66

47. To achieve the best levels of sensitivity and specificity, to what type of detector system could a gas chromatograph be coupled?
    A. UV spectrophotometer
    B. Bichromatic spectrophotometer
    C. Mass spectrometer
    D. Fluorescence detector

48. Which of the following instruments has a sample-introduction system, solvent-delivery system, column, and detector as components?
    A. Atomic absorption spectrometer
    B. Mass spectrometer
    C. High-performance liquid chromatograph
    D. Nephelometer

49. Which type of elution technique may be used in high-performance liquid chromatography?
    A. Amphoteric
    B. Isoelectric
    C. Gradient
    D. Ion exchange

50. Which of the following statements best describes discrete analysis?
    A. Each sample-reagent mixture handled separately in its own reaction vessel
    B. Samples analyzed in a flowing stream of reagent
    C. Analyzer must be dedicated to measurement of only one analyte
    D. Does not have random access capability

51. Which of the following chromatography systems may be described as having a stationary phase that is liquid absorbed on particles packed in a column and a liquid moving phase that is pumped through a column?
    A. Thin-layer
    B. High-performance liquid
    C. Ion-exchange
    D. Gas-liquid

52. Which of the following chromatography systems is characterized by a stationary phase of silica gel on a piece of glass and a moving phase of liquid?
   A. Thin-layer
   B. Ion-exchange
   C. Gas-liquid
   D. Partition

53. All the following apply to gas-liquid chromatography *except*
   A. Separation depends on volatility of the sample.
   B. Separation depends on the sample's solubility in the liquid layer of the stationary phase.
   C. Stationary phase is a liquid layer adsorbed on the column packing.
   D. Mobile phase is a liquid pumped through the column.

54. Ion-exchange chromatography separates solutes in a sample based on the
   A. Solubility of the solutes
   B. Sign and magnitude of the ionic charge
   C. Adsorption ability of the solutes
   D. Molecular size

55. Which parameter is used in mass spectrometry to identify a compound?
   A. Molecular weight
   B. Molecular size
   C. Mobility
   D. Retention time

56. Which chromatography system is commonly used in conjunction with mass spectrometry?
   A. High-performance liquid
   B. Ion-exchange
   C. Partition
   D. Gas-liquid

57. Centrifugal force depends on all the following *except*
   A. Temperature of the centrifuge
   B. Mass of the material being centrifuged
   C. Speed of rotation
   D. Radius of the centrifuge

58. Which of the following is an advantage of the angle-head centrifuge over the horizontal-head centrifuge?
   A. Less air friction
   B. Smaller increase in sample temperature during centrifugation
   C. Can be operated at a higher speed
   D. All the above

59. What class of weights should be used to check the calibration of analytical balances?
   A. J
   B. M
   C. P
   D. S

60. Which of the following may be a sampling source of error for an automated instrument?
   A. Short sample
   B. Air bubble in bottom of cup
   C. Fibrin clot in sample probe
   D. All the above

61. Many chemical reactions require that an instrument maintain a specified incubation temperature. How frequently should the accuracy of the thermometer used to monitor the incubation temperature be verified?
   A. Daily
   B. Weekly
   C. Monthly
   D. Biannually

62. Checking instrument calibration, temperature accuracy, and electronic parameters are part of

A. Preventive maintenance

B. Quality control

C. Function verification

D. Precision verification

63. For which of the following laboratory instruments should preventive maintenance procedures be performed and recorded?

A. Analytical balance

B. Centrifuge

C. Chemistry analyzer

D. All the above

64. Preventive maintenance should include and be performed for all the following reasons *except* to

A. Clean instrument components

B. Replace worn parts

C. Extend the life of the equipment

D. Keep personnel busy when the laboratory work is slow

QUALITY ASSURANCE

65. What term applies to the sum of all the values in a set of numbers divided by the number of values in that set?

A. Median

B. Mode

C. Arithmetic mean

D. Geometric mean

66. Calculate the coefficient of variation (percent) for a set of data where the mean $(\overline{X}) = 89$ mg/dL and 2 standard deviations $(s) = 14$ mg/dL.

A. 7.8

B. 7.9

C. 15.7

D. 15.8

67. What does the preparation of a Levey-Jennings quality control chart for any single constituent of serum require?

A. Analysis of control serum over a period of 20 consecutive days

B. 20 to 30 analyses of the control serum, on 1 day, in one batch

C. Analyses consistently performed by one person

D. Weekly analyses of the control serum for 1 month

68. A batch of test results is out-of-control. What should you do first?

A. Report the results to the physician first, and then look for the trouble.

B. Follow the "out-of-control" procedure specified for the test method.

C. Repeat the tests with a new lot of standards (calibrators).

D. Repeat the tests with a new lot of reagents.

69. In addition to utilizing Levey-Jennings charts, what other criteria should be applied to interpret internal quality control data?

A. Westgard multirule

B. Cusum

C. Linear regression

D. Youden

70. A new standard (calibrator) has been prepared in error at a lower concentration than that required for the test. How would such an error appear on a quality control chart?

A. Upward trend

B. Downward trend

C. Upward shift

D. Downward shift

71. The ± 2 standard deviation ($\pm 2\ s$) range of acceptable values for a digoxin control is established as 2.0 to 2.6 ng/mL. On the average, the expectation that a value will be greater than 2.6 ng/mL is 1 in
   A. 10
   B. 20
   C. 40
   D. 100

72. While monitoring a quality control program, the laboratorian notices that the value of the control sample has been slowly drifting downward during the month. What is the most likely cause of this drift?
   A. Inadequate mixing of the control material
   B. Contamination of the standards (calibrators)
   C. Deterioration of reagent as a result of aging
   D. Recalibration error

73. What is the purpose of a Youden plot?
   A. Compares results on two control specimens, low and high controls, for the same analyte analyzed by several laboratories
   B. Evaluates the validity of daily results on a single control specimen over a period of 30 days
   C. Compares results on a single control specimen by two different methods for the same analyte
   D. Evaluates the validity of daily results of two control specimens within a single laboratory

74. If the therapeutic range for the gentamicin assay is a trough level of less than 2 µg/mL and a peak level of 5 to 8 µg/mL, what would be appropriate mean values for two control levels (in micrograms per milliliter) used to monitor the system?
   A. 1 and 2
   B. 1 and 3

   C. 1.5 and 6
   D. 5 and 6

75. Which of the following monitoring factors would *not* be included in a laboratory's quality assurance program?
   A. Scheduling of staff
   B. Specimen collection and identification
   C. Accuracy and precision of analyses
   D. Preventive maintenance of instruments

76. On a quality control chart, when would a statistical out-of-control situation requiring corrective action be suspected?
   A. Six successive plots fall above and below the mean within $\pm 1\ s$
   B. Six successive plots fall above and below the mean within $\pm 2\ s$
   C. One plot falls within the area of $\pm 2\ s$ to $3\ s$ within a 20 consecutive day span
   D. One plot falls outside the area of $\pm 3\ s$ within a 20 consecutive day span

77. Which of the following would result in a sudden shift in daily values on a quality control chart?
   A. Recalibrating the instrument when changing reagent lot numbers during an analytical run
   B. Replacing the instrument's sample aspiration probe
   C. Changing the spectrophotometer lamp in the middle of a sample run
   D. Changing the operating technologist

78. What assistance does an external quality assurance program provide for a laboratory?
   A. Means to correlate tests performed by different departments within the same laboratory
   B. Delta checks with previous tests on the same patient
   C. Evaluation of its performance by comparison with other laboratories using the same method
   D. Limits for reference intervals

79. Which of the following terms refers to the measure of scatter of experimental data around the mean of a Gaussian (normal) distribution curve?
    A. Median
    B. Mode
    C. Coefficient of variation
    D. Standard deviation

80. What term describes the extent of agreement between repeated analyses?
    A. Random error
    B. Precision
    C. Accuracy
    D. Reliability

81. Which combination best describes a Gaussian (normal) distribution?
    A. Median > mean
    B. Median < mean
    C. Mean = median = mode
    D. Mode > mean

82. Which of the following terms refers to deviation from the true value caused by indeterminate errors inherent in every laboratory measurement?
    A. Random error
    B. Standard error of the mean
    C. Parametric analysis
    D. Nonparametric analysis

83. What is the following formula used to calculate?

$$\sqrt{\frac{\Sigma(x - \overline{x})^2}{n - 1}}$$

    A. Coefficient of variation
    B. Variance
    C. Confidence limits
    D. Standard deviation

84. Which of the following terms refers to the closeness with which the measured value agrees with the true value?
    A. Random error
    B. Precision
    C. Accuracy
    D. Variance

85. What percentage of values will fall between $\pm 2\,s$ in a Gaussian (normal) distribution?
    A. 34.13%
    B. 68.26%
    C. 95.45%
    D. 99.74%

86. Which of the following terms refers to a measure of dispersion or spread of values around a central value?
    A. Range
    B. Validity
    C. Variance
    D. Coefficient of variation

87. Which of the following is the range of values described as the mean plus or minus some number of standard deviations, forming the basis of statistical rules for acceptance and rejection of quality control values?
    A. Variance
    B. Degrees of freedom
    C. Coefficient of variation
    D. Confidence interval

88. Which of the following describes the ability of an analytical method to maintain both accuracy and precision over an extended period of time?
    A. Reliability
    B. Validity
    C. Probability
    D. Sensitivity

89. What is the following formula used to calculate?

$$\frac{\Sigma(x - \bar{x})^2}{n - 1}$$

   A. Coefficient of variation
   B. Variance
   C. Confidence limits
   D. Standard deviation

90. All the following pertain to the characteristics and use of control material *except*
   A. Has physical and chemical properties resembling test specimen
   B. Contains preanalyzed concentrations of analytes being measured
   C. Can be interchanged in terms of use with primary standards or calibrators
   D. Concentrations of analytes should be in normal and abnormal ranges

91. Which of the following is material of known composition available in a highly purified form?
   A. Standard
   B. Control
   C. Technical reagent
   D. Test analyte

92. A group of physicians consistently complains that they are not receiving STAT patient results quickly enough. The supervisor is likely to refer to which quality assurance variable?
   A. Specimen separation and aliquoting
   B. Test utilization
   C. Analytical methodology
   D. Turnaround time

93. To provide independent validation of internal quality control programs, external surveys have been developed. Which of the following is a representative survey program?

   A. ISCLT (International Society for Clinical Laboratory Technology)
   B. ASCLS (American Society for Clinical Laboratory Science)
   C. ASCP (American Society of Clinical Pathologists)
   D. CAP (College of American Pathologists)

94. A tech is scheduled to perform a specialized test that she/he is familiar with, but is not *exactly* certain of the steps required. What is the best course of action to take?
   A. Ask another tech to perform the test.
   B. Consult the procedure manual and notify the supervisor.
   C. Run the test as best as possible, being careful to note control values.
   D. Reject the specimen.

95. A tech has completed the first run of morning specimens. She/he notices that the one control being used is outside $\pm 3\ s$. What course of action should be taken?
   A. Release the results.
   B. Repeat the control only, and if it comes in, release results.
   C. Check equipment and reagents to determine source of error; repeat the entire analysis including the control and patients; if the control value is within $\pm 2\ s$ release results.
   D. Repeat the control; if the same thing happens, attribute the cause to random error; release results.

96. Which of the following describes the Westgard multirule 2_{2s}?
   A. Two control data points are within $\pm 2\ s$.
   B. One control data point falls outside $+2\ s$ and a second point falls outside $-2\ s$.
   C. Two consecutive data points fall outside $+2\ s$ or fall outside $-2\ s$.

D. Two consecutive data points fall outside $+2\ s$.

97. Which Westgard multirule applies to a situation where one control point exceeds the mean by $+2\ s$ and a second control point exceeds the mean by $-2\ s$?
   A. 1_{2s}
   B. 2_{2s}
   C. 4_{1s}
   D. R_{4s}

98. Upon admission to the hospital, a chemistry profile is performed on a patient. The patient has a total bilirubin of 2.0 mg/dL. The next day a second chemistry profile is done, and the patient's total bilirubin is 6.2 mg/dL. What should be done in regard to these results since the normal and abnormal controls are within acceptable limits?
   A. Immediately call the physician to alert him/her to the second abnormal result.
   B. Immediately send the second result to the patient's floor for charting.
   C. Repeat the entire second run of patient specimens since there must be an error.
   D. Perform a delta check and, if warranted, look for possible sources of error.

99. When comparing a potential new test with a comparative method in order to bring a new method into the laboratory, one observes error that is consistently affecting results in one direction. What is this type of error known as?
   A. Systematic error
   B. Random error
   C. Constant systematic error
   D. Proportional systematic error

100. When establishing a reference interval for a new test being introduced into the laboratory, what is the preferred number of subjects that should participate?

   A. 30
   B. 50
   C. 75
   D. 120

101. A small laboratory has collected blood samples from 20 individuals as part of a reference interval study for a new test being introduced into the laboratory. Of the test results, four are outside the reference interval published by the manufacturer. How should you proceed?
   A. Delete the four results and only use the 16 within the range to establish the lab's reference interval.
   B. Use all 20 results when calculating the $\pm 2\ s$ range since outliers are to be expected.
   C. Run four additional samples and if within the manufacturer's range, add them to the original 16 for statistical analysis.
   D. Obtain an additional 20 samples for testing, and if two or less are outside the suggested range, then the manufacturer's reference interval can be accepted.

102. To determine the predictive value of a positive test, all the following parameters must be known *except*
   A. Sensitivity
   B. Specificity
   C. Disease prevalence
   D. Precision

103. Which of the following must be known in order to determine the sensitivity of a test?
   A. True positives and false negatives
   B. True negatives and false positives
   C. True positives and false positives
   D. True negatives and false negatives

104. A new test to assess for the presence of malignancy has been developed. By testing a group of benign individuals, it is determined that 45 of 50 subjects test negative for the new marker. What is the specificity of this new assay?
    A. 10%
    B. 11%
    C. 90%
    D. 100%

105. Which of the following must be known in order to determine the predictive value of a negative test, that is, the percentage of individuals who test negative and are not diseased?
    A. True negatives and false negatives
    B. True positives and false positives
    C. True positives and false negatives
    D. True negatives and false positives

106. All the following statements are true about proficiency-testing programs *except*
    A. Participation mandated by HCFA under CLIA-88
    B. College of American Pathologists and the American Association of Bioanalysts are two major providers of these programs
    C. Samples of unknown concentrations are periodically sent to labs participating in the program
    D. Acceptable ranges are provided with the samples so labs can determine if repeating the assay is necessary

107. Which of the following has as its purpose to promote the incorporation of principles of quality management and quality assurance into daily work routines?
    A. ISO 9000
    B. NCCLS
    C. CAP
    D. NIST

CARBOHYDRATES

108. What does hydrolysis of sucrose yield?
    A. Glucose only
    B. Galactose and glucose
    C. Maltose and glucose
    D. Fructose and glucose

109. In what form is glucose stored in muscle and liver?
    A. Glycogen
    B. Maltose
    C. Lactose
    D. Starch

110. Which of the following carbohydrates is a polysaccharide?
    A. Starch
    B. Sucrose
    C. Lactose
    D. Glucose

111. Which of the following defines the term glycolysis?
    A. Conversion of hexoses into lactate or pyruvate
    B. Conversion of glucose to glycogen
    C. Breakdown of glycogen to form glucose
    D. Breakdown of lipids to form glucose

112. What is the glucose concentration in fasting whole blood?
    A. Less than the concentration in plasma or serum
    B. Greater than the concentration in plasma or serum
    C. Equal to the concentration in plasma or serum
    D. Meaningless because it is not stable

113. Of the following blood glucose levels, which would you expect to result in glucose in the urine?
    A. 60 mg/dL
    B. 120 mg/dL

C. 150 mg/dL

D. 225 mg/dL

114. Which test may be performed to assess the average plasma glucose level that an individual maintained during a previous 6- to 8-week period?

A. Plasma glucose

B. Two-hour postprandial glucose

C. Oral glucose tolerance

D. Glycated hemoglobin

115. An individual has blood drawn for glucose analysis as part of an oral glucose tolerance test (OGTT), and the following serum glucose results are obtained. These results are indicative of what state?

Fasting serum glucose 120 mg/dL

2-hour postload serum glucose 227 mg/dL

A. Normal

B. Diabetes mellitus

C. Addison's disease

D. Hyperinsulinism

116. A 30-year-old pregnant woman has a gestational diabetes mellitus screening test performed at 26 weeks of gestation. Her serum glucose level is 150 mg/dL at 1 hour. What should occur next?

A. This confirms diabetes, give insulin.

B. This confirms diabetes, dietary intake of carbohydrates should be lessened.

C. This is suspicious of diabetes, an oral glucose tolerance test should be performed.

D. This is an expected glucose level in a pregnant woman.

117. A sample of blood is collected for glucose in a sodium fluoride tube before the patient has had breakfast. The physician calls 2 hours later and requests that determination

of blood urea nitrogen (BUN) be performed on the same sample rather than obtaining another specimen. The automated analyzer in your laboratory utilizes the urease method to quantify BUN. What should you tell the physician?

A. Will gladly do the test if sufficient specimen remains

B. Could do the test using a micromethod

C. Can do the BUN determination on the automated analyzer

D. Cannot perform the procedure

118. Type 1 diabetes mellitus may be described by all the following except

A. Insulin deficiency

B. Associated with autoimmune destruction of pancreatic β-cells

C. Ketoacidosis prone

D. Occurs more frequently in adults

119. Insulin may be described by all the following except

A. Synthesized from proinsulin

B. Synthesized by beta-cells in the pancreas

C. C-peptide is active form

D. Two-chain polypeptide

120. Which of the following statements may be associated with the activity of insulin?

A. Increases blood glucose levels

B. Decreases glucose uptake by muscle and fat cells

C. Stimulates release of hepatic glucose into the blood

D. Stimulates glycogenesis in the liver

121. All the following are characteristic of severe hyperglycemia except

A. Polyuria

B. Ketonuria

C. Glycosuria

D. Hypoglucagonemia

122. Which of the following statements applies to the preferred use of plasma or serum, rather than whole blood, for glucose determination?
    A. Glucose is more stable in separated plasma or serum.
    B. Specificity for glucose is higher with most methods when plasma or serum is used.
    C. It is convenient to use serum or plasma with automated instruments because whole blood requires mixing immediately before sampling.
    D. All the above.

123. In monitoring complications of diabetes, all the following analytes would commonly be measured *except*
    A. Serum urea nitrogen
    B. Urinary albumin
    C. Serum creatinine
    D. Serum bilirubin

124. Ingestion of which of the following drugs may cause hypoglycemia?
    A. Ethanol
    B. Propranolol
    C. Salicylate
    D. All the above

125. All the following may be associated with hypoglycemia *except*
    A. Neuroglycopenia
    B. Symptoms occur with plasma glucose levels less than 70 mg/dL
    C. Decreased hepatic glucose production
    D. Diagnostic test is 72-hour fast

126. Which glucose method can employ a polarographic oxygen electrode?
    A. Hexokinase
    B. Glucose oxidase
    C. Glucose dehydrogenase
    D. *o*-Toluidine

127. Which glucose method catalyzes the phosphorylation of glucose by adenosine triphosphate, forming glucose-6-phosphate and adenosine diphosphate with the absorbance of the NADPH product read at 340 nm?
    A. *o*-Toluidine
    B. Glucose oxidase
    C. Hexokinase
    D. Glucose dehydrogenase

128. An enzymatic serum glucose method requires all the following reagents *except*
    A. NAD^+
    B. Glucose oxidase
    C. Peroxidase
    D. *o*-Dianisidine

129. Which of the following glucose methods should *not* be used during the administration of an oral xylose absorption test?
    A. Glucose oxidase—colorimetric
    B. Glucose oxidase—polarographic
    C. Glucose dehydrogenase
    D. Hexokinase

130. Which glucose method is considered to be the reference method?
    A. Glucose oxidase
    B. *o*-Toluidine
    C. Hexokinase
    D. Glucose dehydrogenase

131. An individual has a serum glucose level of 110 mg/dL. What would be the approximate glucose concentration in this patient's cerebrospinal fluid?
    A. 33 mg/dL
    B. 55 mg/dL
    C. 66 mg/dL
    D. 110 mg/dL

132. What is the reference interval for fasting serum glucose in an adult expressed in SI units?
    A. 1.7–3.3 mmol/L
    B. 3.3–5.6 mmol/L
    C. 4.1–5.9 mmol/L
    D. 6.7–8.3 mmol/L

133. When measuring glycated hemoglobin levels, which of the following methods should *not* be used to avoid interference from hemoglobin F?
    A. Immunoassay
    B. Ion-exchange chromatography
    C. High-performance liquid chromatography
    D. Isoelectric focusing

134. All the following hormones promote an increase in the blood glucose level *except*
    A. Growth hormone
    B. Cortisol
    C. Glucagon
    D. Insulin

135. What effect if any would be expected when the secretion of epinephrine is stimulated by physical or emotional stress?
    A. Decreased blood glucose level
    B. Increased blood glucose level
    C. Increased glycogen storage
    D. No effect on blood glucose or glycogen levels

136. What would an individual with Cushing's syndrome tend to exhibit?
    A. Hyperglycemia
    B. Hypoglycemia
    C. Normal blood glucose level
    D. Decreased 2-hour postprandial glucose

137. What is the expected glucose value of a normal 2-hour postprandial serum specimen as compared to the reference interval for a fasting serum glucose?

A. Significantly greater in the 200 mg/dL range
B. Moderately greater in the 160 mg/dL range
C. Significantly lower in the 50 mg/dL range
D. Approximately the same in the 120 mg/dL or less range

138. A cerebrospinal fluid specimen is sent to the lab at 9:00 P.M. for glucose analysis. The specimen is cloudy and appears to contain red blood cells. Which of the following statements is *true*?
    A. Glucose testing cannot be performed on the specimen.
    B. Specimen should be centrifuged and the glucose test run immediately.
    C. Specimen can be refrigerated as received and the glucose run the next day.
    D. Specimen can be frozen as received and the glucose run the next day.

139. A patient has a urine uric acid level of 1575 mg/day. What effect will this have on the measured urine glucose level when the glucose oxidase/peroxidase method is employed?
    A. Urine glucose level will be falsely low.
    B. Urine glucose level will be falsely high.
    C. Urine glucose level will be accurate.
    D. Urine glucose level will exceed the linearity of the method.

140. Laboratory tests are performed on a postmenopausal, 57-year-old female as part of an annual physical examination. The patient's random serum glucose is 220 mg/dL, and the glycated hemoglobin (Hb A_{1c}) is 11%. Based on this information, how should the patient be classified?
    A. Normal glucose tolerance
    B. Impaired glucose tolerance
    C. Gestational diabetes mellitus
    D. Type 2 diabetes mellitus

141. Which of the following is characterized by a deficiency of glucose-6-phosphatase resulting in hepatomegaly, lactic acidosis, and severe fasting hypoglycemia?
    A. Type I—von Gierke's disease
    B. Type II—Pompe's disease
    C. Type III—Forbes' disease
    D. Type IV—Andersen's disease

LIPIDS AND LIPOPROTEINS

142. Bile acids that are synthesized in the liver are derived from what substance?
    A. Bilirubin
    B. Fatty acids
    C. Cholesterol
    D. Triglycerides

143. The turbid, or milky, appearance of serum after fat ingestion is termed postprandial lipemia. This lipemic appearance is caused by the presence of what substance?
    A. Bilirubin
    B. Cholesterol
    C. Chylomicrons
    D. Phospholipids

144. Cholesterol ester is formed through the esterification of the alcohol cholesterol with what substance?
    A. Protein
    B. Triglyceride
    C. Fatty acids
    D. Digitonin

145. Which of the following tests would most likely be included in a routine lipid profile?
    A. Triglycerides, fatty acids, chylomicrons
    B. Cholesterol, triglyerides, phospholipids
    C. HDL cholesterol, LDL cholesterol, chylomicrons
    D. Cholesterol, triglycerides, HDL cholesterol

146. To produce reliable results, when should blood specimens for lipid studies be drawn?
    A. Immediately after eating
    B. A random specimen may be drawn any time during the day
    C. In the fasting state, approximately 2 to 4 hours after eating
    D. In the fasting state, approximately 12 to 14 hours after eating

147. Which of the following lipid tests is *least* affected by the fasting status of the patient?
    A. Cholesterol
    B. Triglycerides
    C. Fatty acids
    D. Lipoproteins

148. What compound is a crucial intermediary in the metabolism of triglycerides to form energy?
    A. Bile
    B. Acetyl-coenzyme A
    C. Acetoacetate
    D. Pyruvate

149. The more current kinetic methods for quantifying serum triglycerides employ enzymatic hydrolysis. The hydrolysis of triglycerides may be accomplished by what enzyme?
    A. Amylase
    B. Leucine aminopeptidase
    C. Lactate dehydrogenase
    D. Lipase

150. Enzymatic methods for the determination of total cholesterol in serum utilize a cholesterol oxidase-peroxidase method. In this method, cholesterol oxidase reacts specifically with what?
    A. Free cholesterol and cholesterol esters
    B. Free cholesterol and fatty acids
    C. Free cholesterol only
    D. Cholesterol esters only

151. Exogenous triglycerides are transported in the plasma in what form?
    A. Phospholipids
    B. Cholesteryl esters
    C. Chylomicrons
    D. Free fatty acids

152. Ketone bodies are formed because of an excessive breakdown of fatty acids. Of the following metabolites, which may be classified as a ketone body?
    A. Pyruvic acid
    B. Beta-hydroxybutyric acid
    C. Lactic acid
    D. Oxaloacetic acid

153. Which of the following is most associated with the membrane structure of nerve tissue?
    A. Cholesterol
    B. Triglycerides
    C. Phospholipids
    D. Sphingolipids

154. Each lipoprotein fraction is composed of varying amounts of lipid and protein components. The beta-lipoprotein fraction consists primarily of which lipid?
    A. Fatty acids
    B. Cholesterol
    C. Phospholipids
    D. Triglycerides

155. What substance is the precursor to all steroid hormones?
    A. Fatty acids
    B. Cholesterol
    C. Triglycerides
    D. Phospholipids

156. The term "lipid storage diseases" is used to denote a group of lipid disorders, the majority of which are inherited as autosomal recessive mutations. What is the cause of these diseases?

    A. Excessive dietary fat ingestion
    B. Excessive synthesis of chylomicrons
    C. A specific enzyme deficiency or nonfunctional enzyme form
    D. An inability of adipose tissue to store lipid materials

157. Several malabsorption problems are characterized by a condition known as steatorrhea. Steatorrhea is caused by an abnormal accumulation of what substance in the feces?
    A. Proteins
    B. Lipids
    C. Carbohydrates
    D. Vitamins

158. When lipoprotein electrophoresis is performed at pH 8.6 with the use of agarose gel, which fraction migrates the fastest toward the anode?
    A. Chylomicron
    B. LDL
    C. VLDL
    D. HDL

159. The quantification of the high-density lipoprotein cholesterol level is thought to be significant in the risk assessment of what disease?
    A. Pancreatitis
    B. Cirrhosis
    C. Coronary artery disease
    D. Hyperlipidemia

160. The surfactant/albumin ratio by fluorescence polarization is performed to assess what physiological state?
    A. Hyperlipidemia
    B. Coronary artery disease
    C. Hemolytic disease of the newborn
    D. Fetal lung maturity

161. The very low density lipoprotein (VLDL) fraction primarily transports what substance?
    A. Cholesterol
    B. Chylomicrons
    C. Triglyceride
    D. Phospholipids

162. What is the sedimentation nomenclature associated with alpha-lipoprotein?
    A. Very low density lipoproteins (VLDL)
    B. High-density lipoproteins (HDL)
    C. Low-density lipoproteins (LDL)
    D. Chylomicrons

163. Name a commonly used precipitating reagent to separate high-density lipoprotein cholesterol from other lipoprotein cholesterol fractions.
    A. Zinc sulfate
    B. Trichloroacetic acid
    C. Heparin-manganese
    D. Isopropanol

164. What is the principle of the "direct" or "homogeneous" HDL cholesterol automated method, which requires no intervention by the technologist/ technician? The Direct HDL method
    A. Quantifies only the cholesterol in HDL, whereas the precipitation HDL method quantifies the entire lipoprotein
    B. Utilizes polymers and detergents that make the HDL cholesterol soluble while keeping the other lipoproteins insoluble
    C. Uses a nonenzymatic method to measure cholesterol, whereas the other methods use enzymes to measure cholesterol
    D. Uses a column chromatography step to separate HDL from the other lipoproteins, whereas the other methods use a precipitation step

165. Which of the following results would be the most consistent with high risk for coronary heart disease?
    A. 20 mg/dL HDL cholesterol and 250 mg/dL total cholesterol
    B. 50 mg/dL HDL cholesterol and 190 mg/dL total cholesterol
    C. 55 mg/dL HDL cholesterol and 180 mg/dL total cholesterol
    D. 60 mg/dL HDL cholesterol and 170 mg/dL total cholesterol

166. A patient's total cholesterol is 300 mg/dL, his HDL cholesterol is 50 mg/dL, his triglyceride is 200 mg/dL. What is this patient's calculated LDL cholesterol?
    A. 200
    B. 210
    C. 290
    D. 350

167. A patient's Total Cholesterol/HDL Cholesterol ratio is 10.0. What level of risk for coronary heart disease does this result indicate?
    A. No risk
    B. Half average risk
    C. Average risk
    D. Twice average risk

168. Which of the following techniques can be used to quantify apolipoproteins?
    A. Gas chromatography
    B. Ion-selective electrode
    C. Enzyme-linked immunosorbent assay
    D. Refractometry

169. Which of the following may be described as a variant form of LDL, associated with increased risk of atherosclerotic cardiovascular disease?
    A. Lp(a)
    B. HDL
    C. Apo A-I
    D. Apo A-II

170. In what way is the "normal" population reference interval for cholesterol in America different than that of other clinical chemistry parameters (i.e., protein, sodium, BUN, creatinine, etc.)?
   A. Established units for cholesterol are mg/dL; no other chemistry test has these units.
   B. Reference interval is artificially set to reflect good health even though Americans as a group have "normally" higher cholesterol levels.
   C. Total cholesterol reference interval must be interpreted in line with triglyceride, phospholipid and sphingolipid values.
   D. Cholesterol reference interval is based on a manual procedure, whereas all other chemistry parameters are based on automated procedures.

171. Your lab routinely uses a precipitation method to separate HDL cholesterol. You receive a slightly lipemic specimen for HDL cholesterol. The total cholesterol and triglyceride for the specimen were 450 mg/dL and 520 mg/dL, respectively. After adding the precipitating reagents and centrifuging, you notice that the supernatant still looks slightly cloudy. What is your next course of action in analyzing this specimen?
   A. Perform the cholesterol test; there is nothing wrong with this specimen.
   B. Take off the supernatant and recentrifuge.
   C. Take off the supernatant and add another portion of the precipitating reagent to it and recentrifuge.
   D. Send specimen to a lab that offers other techniques to separate more effectively the HDL cholesterol.

172. A 46-year-old known alcoholic with liver damage is brought into the ER unconscious. One would expect his lipid values to be affected in what way?
   A. Increased
   B. Decreased
   C. Normal
   D. Unaffected by the alcoholism

173. A healthy, active 10-year-old boy with no prior history of illness comes to the lab after school for a routine chemistry screen in order to meet requirements for summer camp. After centrifugation, the serum looks cloudy or creamy. The specimen had the following results: blood glucose = 240 mg/dL, cholesterol = 285 mg/dL, triglyceride = 420 mg/dL. What would be the most probable explanation of these findings? The boy
   A. Has a high risk for coronary artery disease
   B. Is a diabetic
   C. Has an inherited genetic disease causing a lipid imbalance
   D. Was not fasting when the specimen was drawn

174. A mother brings her obese, four-year-old child who is a known Type I diabetic to the laboratory for a blood workup. She states that the boy has followed his diet and has been fasting for the past 12 hours. After centrifugation the tech notes that the serum looks creamy. The specimen had the following results: blood glucose = 180 mg/dL, cholesterol = 410 mg/dL, total cholesterol/HDL cholesterol ratio = 16.50, triglyceride = 550 mg/dL. What best explains these findings? The boy
   A. Is a low risk for coronary artery disease
   B. Is a good candidate for a 3-hour glucose tolerance test
   C. Has secondary hyperlipidemia due to the diabetes
   D. Was not fasting when the specimen was drawn

PROTEINS, ELECTROPHORESIS, AND TUMOR MARKERS

175. Proteins, carbohydrates, and lipids are the three major biochemical compounds of human metabolism. What is the element that distinguishes proteins from carbohydrate and lipid compounds?
    A. Carbon
    B. Hydrogen
    C. Oxygen
    D. Nitrogen

176. Proteins may become denatured when subjected to mechanical agitation, heat, or extreme chemical treatment. How are proteins affected by denaturation?
    A. Alteration in primary structure
    B. Alteration in secondary structure
    C. Alteration in tertiary structure
    D. Increase in solubility

177. What is the basis for the Kjeldahl technique for the determination of serum total protein?
    A. Quantification of peptide bonds
    B. Determination of the refractive index of proteins
    C. Ultraviolet light absorption by aromatic rings at 280 nm
    D. Quantification of the nitrogen content of protein

178. When quantifying serum total proteins, upon what is the intensity of the color produced in the biuret reaction dependent?
    A. Molecular weight of the protein
    B. Acidity of the medium
    C. Number of peptide bonds
    D. Nitrogen content of the protein

179. Which of the following reagents can be used to measure protein in cerebrospinal fluid?
    A. Biuret
    B. Coomassie brilliant blue
    C. Ponceau S
    D. Bromcresol green

180. An elevated protein level in cerebrospinal fluid may be indicative of all the following disorders except
    A. Bacterial meningitis
    B. Multiple sclerosis
    C. Cerebral infarction
    D. Hyperthyroidism

181. Which term describes a congenital disorder that is characterized by a split in the albumin band when serum is subjected to electrophoresis?
    A. Analbuminemia
    B. Anodic albuminemia
    C. Prealbuminemia
    D. Bisalbuminemia

182. In what condition would an increased level of serum albumin be expected?
    A. Malnutrition
    B. Acute inflammation
    C. Dehydration
    D. Renal disease

183. Identification of which of the following is useful in early stages of glomerular dysfunction?
    A. Microalbuminuria
    B. Ketonuria
    C. Hematuria
    D. Urinary light chains

184. Myoglobin will be elevated in the serum in all the following disorders except
    A. Renal failure
    B. Vigorous exercise
    C. Acute myocardial infarction
    D. Hepatitis

185. All the following are true of cardiac troponin I (cTnI) as it relates to acute myocardial infarction (AMI) *except*
    A. Increase above reference interval seen in 4 to 8 hours
    B. Measure initially and serially in 3- to 6-hour intervals
    C. Remains elevated 3 to 5 days
    D. Expressed in regenerating and diseased skeletal muscle and cardiac muscle disorders

186. Which of the following is a low weight protein that is found on the cell surfaces of nucleated cells?
    A. C-reactive protein
    B. β_2-Microglobulin
    C. Ceruloplasmin
    D. α_2-Macroglobulin

187. Which glycoprotein binds with hemoglobin to facilitate the removal of hemoglobin by the reticuloendothelial system?
    A. Haptoglobin
    B. Ceruloplasmin
    C. Alpha$_1$-antitrypsin
    D. Fibrinogen

188. In a healthy individual, which protein fraction has the greatest concentration in serum?
    A. Alpha$_1$-globulin
    B. Beta-globulin
    C. Gamma-globulin
    D. Albumin

189. Which of the following is an anionic dye that binds selectively with albumin?
    A. Amido black
    B. Ponceau S
    C. Bromcresol green
    D. Coomassie brilliant blue

190. Which total protein method requires copper sulfate, potassium iodide in sodium hydroxide, and potassium sodium tartrate in its reagent system?
    A. Kjeldahl
    B. Biuret
    C. Folin-Ciocalteu
    D. Ultraviolet absorption

191. All the following plasma proteins are manufactured by the liver *except*
    A. Albumin
    B. Haptoglobin
    C. Fibrinogen
    D. IgG

192. There are five immunoglobulin classes: IgG, IgA, IgM, IgD, and IgE. With which globulin fraction do these immunoglobulins migrate electrophoretically?
    A. Alpha$_1$-globulins
    B. Alpha$_2$-globulins
    C. Beta$_1$-globulins
    D. Gamma-globulins

193. Of the five immunoglobulin classes, IgG is the simplest, consisting of how many light chains/heavy chains, respectively?
    A. 5/2
    B. 1/1
    C. 2/5
    D. 2/2

194. Which immunoglobulin class, characterized by its possession of a secretory component, is found in saliva, tears, and body secretions?
    A. IgA
    B. IgD
    C. IgG
    D. IgM

195. Which immunoglobulin class is able to cross the placenta from the mother to the fetus?
    A. IgA
    B. IgD
    C. IgE
    D. IgG

196. Which of the following is an acute phase reactant protein, that is able to inhibit enzymatic proteolysis and has the highest concentration of any of the plasma proteolytic inhibitors?
    A. C-reactive protein
    B. Haptoglobin
    C. Alpha$_2$-macroglobulin
    D. Alpha$_1$-antitrypsin

197. Which of the following is a copper transport protein that migrates as an alpha$_2$-globulin?
    A. Ceruloplasmin
    B. Haptoglobin
    C. Transferrin
    D. Fibrinogen

198. Which of the following proteins is normally produced by the fetus but found in increased amounts in the amniotic fluid in cases of spina bifida?
    A. Alpha$_1$-antitrypsin
    B. Alpha$_1$-acid glycoprotein
    C. Alpha$_1$-fetoprotein
    D. Alpha$_2$-macroglobulin

199. The thermal method used to identify the presence of Bence Jones protein in urine is based on the solubility characteristics of this protein at varying temperatures. Bence Jones protein may be differentiated from other proteins because of its precipitation or redissolving at what temperatures respectively?

A. 56–70 °C and 40–60 °C
B. 56–70 °C and 85–100 °C
C. 50–60 °C and 90–100 °C
D. 40–60 °C and 56–70 °C

200. Bence Jones proteinuria is a condition characterized by the urinary excretion of what type of light chain?
    A. Kappa light chains
    B. Lambda light chains
    C. Both kappa and lambda light chains
    D. Either kappa or lambda light chains

201. Multiple myeloma, a plasma cell dyscrasia that usually affects persons over the age of 40 years, may be characterized by all the following *except*
    A. Monoclonal band in the gamma region
    B. Hypercalcemia
    C. Hyperalbuminemia
    D. Hyperglobulinemia

202. What technique is used to quantify specific immunoglobulin classes?
    A. Immunonephelometry
    B. Serum protein electrophoresis
    C. Isoelectric focusing
    D. Immunoelectrophoresis

203. Portal cirrhosis is a chronic disease of the liver. As observed on an electrophoretic serum protein pattern, what is a predominant characteristic of this disease?
    A. Monoclonal band in the gamma-globulin region
    B. Polyclonal band in the gamma-globulin region
    C. Bridging effect between the beta and gamma-globulin bands
    D. Increase in the alpha$_2$-globulin band

204. The abnormal metabolism of several of the amino acids has been linked with disorders

classified as inborn errors of metabolism. What technique is commonly used to differentiate among several different amino acids?

A. Electrophoresis
B. Microbiological analysis
C. Enzyme immunoassay
D. Chromatography

205. Which of the following characteristics will a protein have at its isoelectric point?

A. Net negative charge
B. Net positive charge
C. Net zero charge
D. Mobility at pH 7.0

206. In serum protein electrophoresis when a buffer solution of pH 8.6 is used, which of the following characterizes the proteins?

A. Exhibit net negative charge
B. Exhibit net positive charge
C. Exhibit charge neutrality
D. Migrate toward the cathode

207. Serum protein electrophoresis is routinely performed on the serum obtained from a clotted blood specimen. If a plasma specimen is substituted for serum, how will the electrophoresis be affected?

A. Electrophoresis cannot be performed because the anticoagulant will retard the mobilities of the protein fractions.
B. Electrophoresis cannot be performed because the anticoagulant will cause migration of the protein fractions in the direction of the cathode.
C. Electrophoresis will show an extra fraction in the beta-gamma region.
D. Electrophoresis will show an extra fraction in the prealbumin area.

208. In serum protein electrophoresis when a barbital buffer of pH 8.6 is employed, what protein fraction will migrate the fastest toward the anode?

A. Albumin
B. Alpha$_1$-globulin
C. Beta-globulin
D. Gamma-globulin

209. All the following are types of support media used today for serum protein electrophoresis *except*

A. Agarose gel
B. Cellulose acetate
C. Acrylamide
D. Paper

210. What dye may be used for staining protein bands following electrophoresis?

A. Fat red 7B
B. Sudan black B
C. Ponceau S
D. Oil red O

211. When electrophoresis is performed, holes appear in the staining pattern, giving the stained protein band a doughnut-like appearance. What is the probable cause of this problem?

A. Protein denatured and will not stain properly
B. Ionic strength of the buffer was too high
C. Protein reached its isoelectric point and precipitated out
D. Protein concentration was too high

212. What is the purpose of using ampholytes in isoelectric focusing?

A. Maintain the polyacrylamide gel in a solid state
B. Maintain the protein sample in a charged state
C. Maintain the pH of the buffer solution
D. Establish a pH gradient in the gel

213. All the following may be associated with silver stains *except*
    A. Reactive to nanogram concentrations of proteins
    B. Polypeptides stain a variety of colors
    C. Not as sensitive as Coomassie brilliant blue
    D. Preconcentration of CSF not necessary

214. All the following may be associated with isoelectric focusing *except*
    A. Continuous pH gradient
    B. Migration of proteins with net charge of zero
    C. Separation dependent on isoelectric point
    D. Zone electrophoresis

215. All the following may be associated with carcinoembryonic antigen *except*
    A. Increased levels seen with malignancies of the lungs
    B. Quantified by using capillary electrophoresis
    C. Used to monitor treatment of colon cancer
    D. Glycoprotein in nature

216. In cases of hepatoma, which protein not normally found in adult serum is synthesized by liver cells?
    A. Alpha$_1$-acid glycoprotein
    B. Alpha$_1$-fetoprotein
    C. Alpha$_2$-macroglobulin
    D. Carcinoembryonic antigen

217. All the following are true of prostate-specific antigen *except*
    A. Serum quantified using immunoassays
    B. Single-chain glycoprotein
    C. Used as a tumor marker
    D. Not elevated in benign prostatic hyperplasia

218. Which of the following is an oncofetal antigen that is elevated in nonmucinous epithelial ovarian cancer?
    A. CA 549
    B. CA 125
    C. CA 19-9
    D. CA 15-3

219. Which of the following is an asialylated Lewis blood group antigen associated with colorectal carcinoma?
    A. CA 19-9
    B. CA 15-3
    C. CA 549
    D. CEA

220. Elevations of serum levels of alpha-fetoprotein are associated with all the following disorders *except*
    A. Testicular germ cell tumors
    B. Prostatic carcinoma
    C. Pancreatic carcinoma
    D. Gastric carcinoma

221. All the following may be associated with chorionic gonadotropin *except*
    A. β subunit confers immunogenic specificity
    B. Used to confirm pregnancy
    C. Used as a tumor marker
    D. Found in hepatoma

222. While serum elevations are not generally seen in early stages, which of the following tumor markers are elevated in more advanced stages of breast cancer?
    A. CEA and AFP
    B. AFP and CA 125
    C. PSA and CA 15-3
    D. CA 15-3 and CA 549

NONPROTEIN NITROGENOUS SUBSTANCES

223. What is the compound that comprises the majority of the nonprotein-nitrogen fractions in serum?
    A. Uric acid
    B. Creatinine
    C. Ammonia
    D. Urea

224. Express 30 mg/dL of urea nitrogen as urea.
    A. 14 mg/dL
    B. 20 mg/dL
    C. 50 mg/dL
    D. 64 mg/dL

225. In the urea method, the enzymatic action of urease is inhibited when blood for analysis is drawn in a tube containing what anticoagulant?
    A. Sodium heparin
    B. Sodium fluoride
    C. Sodium oxalate
    D. Ethylenediaminetetraacetic acid

226. In the diacetyl method, what does diacetyl react with to form a yellow product?
    A. Ammonia
    B. Urea
    C. Uric acid
    D. Nitrogen

227. What endogenous substance may cause a positive interference in the urease/glutamate dehydrogenase assay?
    A. Ammonia
    B. Creatinine
    C. Glucose
    D. Cholesterol

228. Which of the following methods utilizes urease and glutamate dehydrogenase for the quantification of serum urea?
    A. Berthelot
    B. Coupled enzymatic
    C. Conductimetric
    D. Indicator dye

229. In the Berthelot reaction, what contaminant will cause the urea level to be falsely elevated?
    A. Sodium fluoride
    B. Protein
    C. Ammonia
    D. Bacteria

230. To maintain acid-base balance, it is necessary that the blood ammonia level be kept within narrow limits. This is accomplished primarily by which of the following?
    A. Synthesis of urea from ammonia
    B. Synthesis of glutamine from ammonia
    C. Excretion of ammonia in the bile
    D. Excretion of ammonia in the stools

231. When a blood ammonia determination is performed, the blood specimen must be treated in a manner that will ensure that
    A. The deamination process continues *in vitro*
    B. Glutamine formation *in vitro* is avoided
    C. The transamination process continues *in vitro*
    D. Ammonia formation *in vitro* is avoided

232. What analyte may be quantified by first adsorbing it onto a strongly acidic cation-exchange resin and then eluting it off for participation in a colorimetric reaction?
    A. Urea
    B. Ammonia
    C. Uric acid
    D. Creatinine

233. All the following precautions should be exercised in the collection, handling, and use of a specimen for ammonia analysis *except*
    A. Avoid use of a hemolyzed specimen
    B. Collect blood in EDTA or heparin evacuated tubes
    C. Place specimen in a 37 °C water bath immediately
    D. Prohibit patient from smoking for 8 hours before blood collection

234. Which of the following statements can be associated with the enzymatic assay of ammonia?
    A. Increase in absorbance monitored at 340 nm
    B. NAD required as a cofactor
    C. Ammonium ion isolated from specimen before the enzymatic step
    D. Reaction catalyzed by glutamate dehydrogenase

235. Elevated blood levels of ammonia occur in all the following disorders *except*
    A. Reye's syndrome
    B. Renal failure
    C. Chronic liver failure
    D. Diabetes mellitus

236. An increased serum level of which of the following analytes is most commonly associated with decreased glomerular filtration?
    A. Creatinine
    B. Uric acid
    C. Urea
    D. Ammonia

237. A serum creatinine was found to be 6.0 mg/dL. Which of the following urea nitrogen serum results would support the same pathological condition?
    A. 6 mg/dL
    B. 20 mg/dL

C. 35 mg/dL
D. 70 mg/dL

238. From what precursor is creatinine formed?
    A. Urea
    B. Glucose
    C. Creatine
    D. Uric acid

239. What analyte is measured using the Jaffe reaction?
    A. Urea
    B. Uric acid
    C. Ammonia
    D. Creatinine

240. When the Jaffe reaction is employed as a kinetic assay to quantify serum creatinine, which of the following is used in the analysis?
    A. Serum sample used directly
    B. Folin-Wu filtrate
    C. Somogyi-Nelson filtrate
    D. Trichloroacetic acid filtrate

241. The creatinine clearance test is routinely used to assess the glomerular filtration rate. Given the following information for an average size adult, calculate a creatinine clearance.

    Urine creatinine—120 mg/dL
    Plasma creatinine—1.2 mg/dL
    Urine volume for 24 hours—1520 mL

    A. 11 mL/min
    B. 63 mL/min
    C. 95 mL/min
    D. 106 mL/min

242. When it is not possible to perform a creatinine assay on a fresh urine specimen, to what pH level should the urine be adjusted?
    A. 3.0
    B. 5.0
    C. 7.0
    D. 9.0

243. What compound normally found in urine may be used to assess the completeness of a 24-hour urine collection?
    A. Urea
    B. Uric acid
    C. Creatine
    D. Creatinine

244. When coupled enzymatic reactions are employed to quantify serum creatinine, all the following reagents are required *except*
    A. Picric acid
    B. Chromogenic dye
    C. Creatinine amidohydrolase
    D. Sarcosine oxidase

245. An endogenous substance assayed to assess the glomerular filtration rate may be described as being filtered by the glomeruli, not reabsorbed by the tubules, and only secreted by the tubules when plasma levels become elevated. What is this frequently assayed substance?
    A. Inulin
    B. Uric acid
    C. Creatinine
    D. Urea

246. What is the end product of purine catabolism in man?
    A. Urea
    B. Uric acid
    C. Allantoin
    D. Ammonia

247. When mixed with phosphotungstic acid, what compound causes the reduction of the former to a tungsten blue complex?
    A. Urea
    B. Ammonia
    C. Creatinine
    D. Uric acid

248. In the ultraviolet procedure for quantifying uric acid, what does the reaction between uric acid and uricase cause?
    A. Production of NADH
    B. The formation of allantoin
    C. An increase in absorbance
    D. A reduction of phosphotungstic acid

249. Which of the following disorders is best characterized by laboratory findings that include increased serum levels of inorganic phosphorus, magnesium, potassium, uric acid, urea, and creatinine and decreased serum calcium and erythropoietin levels?
    A. Chronic renal failure
    B. Renal tubular disease
    C. Nephrotic syndrome
    D. Acute glomerulonephritis

250. In gout, what analyte deposits in joints and other body tissues?
    A. Calcium
    B. Creatinine
    C. Urea
    D. Uric acid

251. During chemotherapy for leukemia, which of the following analytes would most likely be elevated in the blood?
    A. Uric acid
    B. Urea
    C. Creatinine
    D. Ammonia

HEMOGLOBIN, HEME DERIVATIVES, AND LIVER FUNCTION

252. Which compounds originally condense to form aminolevulinic acid?
    A. Oxoglutarate and aspartate
    B. Isocitrate and coenzyme II
    C. Oxalacetate and malate
    D. Succinyl coenzyme A and glycine

253. What compound chelates iron and is the immediate precursor of heme formation?
    A. Porphobilinogen
    B. Protoporphyrinogen IX
    C. Uroporphyrinogen III
    D. Protoporphyrin IX

254. Which of the following is a qualitative screening test for porphobilinogen that may be performed to aid in the diagnosis of the porphyrias?
    A. Caraway test
    B. Gutman test
    C. Jendrassik-Grof test
    D. Watson-Schwartz test

255. What compound may be detected by observing its orange-red fluorescence in acid solution?
    A. Porphobilinogen
    B. Uroporphyrinogen
    C. Aminolevulinic acid
    D. Coproporphyrin

256. The laboratory receives a request that assays for urinary aminolevulinic acid, porphobilinogen, uroporphyrin, and coproporphyrin be performed on a patient. All the following will contribute to the integrity of the sample, when these assays are to be performed on the same urine specimen *except*
    A. Refrigeration
    B. Addition of hydrochloric acid
    C. 24-hour urine collection
    D. Use of a brown bottle

257. Which globin chains compose hemoglobin A?
    A. Two alpha chains and two beta chains
    B. Two alpha chains and two delta chains
    C. Two alpha chains and two gamma chains
    D. Two beta chains and two delta chains

258. Which hemoglobin may be differentiated from other hemoglobins on the basis of its resistance to denature in alkaline solution?
    A. A
    B. A_2
    C. C
    D. F

259. Hemoglobin S is an abnormal hemoglobin that is characterized by a substitution of which amino acid?
    A. Valine for glutamic acid in position 6 on the beta chain
    B. Valine for glutamic acid in position 6 on the alpha chain
    C. Lysine for glutamic acid in position 6 on the beta chain
    D. Lysine for glutamic acid in position 6 on the alpha chain

260. When performing electrophoresis at pH 8.6, which hemoglobin molecule migrates the fastest on cellulose acetate toward the anode?
    A. A
    B. A_2
    C. F
    D. S

261. Because of similar electrophoretic mobilities, several hemoglobins cannot be differentiated on cellulose acetate medium. Electrophoresis of hemoglobins at pH 6.2 on agar gel may be useful in differentiating which hemoglobins?
    A. A from A_2
    B. A from D
    C. A from E
    D. C from A_2

262. In addition to performing hemoglobin electrophoresis, a solubility test may be performed to detect the presence of what hemoglobin?
    A. A
    B. C

C. F

D. S

263. What is the immediate precursor of bilirubin formation?

A. Mesobilirubinogen

B. Verdohemoglobin

C. Urobilinogen

D. Biliverdin

264. To quantify serum bilirubin levels, it is necessary that bilirubin couples with diazotized sulfanilic acid to form what complex?

A. Verdobilirubin

B. Azobilirubin

C. Azobilirubinogen

D. Bilirubin glucuronide

265. What enzyme system catalyzes the conjugation of bilirubin?

A. Leucine amino peptidase

B. Glucose-6-phosphate dehydrogenase

C. Uridine diphosphate glucuronyltransferase

D. Carbamoyl phosphate synthetase

266. What breakdown product of bilirubin metabolism is produced in the colon from the oxidation of urobilinogen by microorganisms?

A. Porphobilinogen

B. Urobilin

C. Stercobilinogen

D. Protoporphyrin

267. Which of the following functions as a transport protein for bilirubin in the blood?

A. Alpha$_1$-globulin

B. Beta-globulin

C. Gamma-globulin

D. Albumin

268. What condition is characterized by yellow pigmentation of the skin?

A. Jaundice

B. Hemolysis

C. Cholestasis

D. Kernicterus

269. In the condition kernicterus, the abnormal accumulation of bilirubin occurs in what tissue?

A. Brain

B. Liver

C. Kidney

D. Blood

270. As a reduction product of bilirubin catabolism, this compound is partially reabsorbed from the intestine through the portal circulation for reexcretion by the liver. What is this compound?

A. Verdohemoglobin

B. Urobilinogen

C. Urobilin

D. Biliverdin

271. All the following factors may adversely affect the accurate quantification of bilirubin in serum except

A. Lipemia

B. Hemolysis

C. Exposure to light

D. Specimen refrigeration

272. Which bilirubin fraction is unconjugated and covalently bound to albumin?

A. Alpha

B. Beta

C. Delta

D. Gamma

273. As the red blood cells disintegrate, hemoglobin is released and converted to the pigment bilirubin. Which organ is primarily responsible for this function?

A. Spleen

B. Kidneys

C. Intestines

D. Liver

274. All the following methods have been used for the quantification of serum bilirubin concentrations *except*
    A. Bilirubinometer
    B. Jendrassik and Grof
    C. Zimmerman
    D. Bilirubin oxidase

275. All the following describe the direct bilirubin component *except*
    A. Insoluble in water
    B. Conjugated in the liver
    C. Conjugated with glucuronic acid
    D. Excreted in the urine of jaundiced patients

276. Which of the following reagent systems contains the components sulfanilic acid, hydrochloric acid, and sodium nitrite?
    A. Jaffe
    B. Zimmerman
    C. Diazo
    D. Lowry

277. Indirect-reacting bilirubin may be quantified by reacting it initially in which reagent?
    A. Dilute hydrochloric acid
    B. Dilute sulfuric acid
    C. Caffeine-sodium benzoate
    D. Sodium hydroxide

278. Which of the following methods employs a reaction where bilirubin is oxidized to colorless biliverdin?
    A. Bilirubinometer
    B. Bilirubin oxidase
    C. High-performance liquid chromatography
    D. Jendrassik-Grof

279. What collective term encompasses the reduction products stercobilinogen, urobilinogen, and mesobilirubinogen?

    A. Urobilinogen
    B. Mesobilirubinogen
    C. Urobilin
    D. Bilirubin

280. What condition is characterized by an elevation of total bilirubin primarily due to an increase in the conjugated bilirubin fraction?
    A. Hemolytic jaundice
    B. Neonatal jaundice
    C. Crigler-Najjar syndrome
    D. Obstructive jaundice

281. Which of the following is characteristic of hemolytic jaundice?
    A. Unconjugated serum bilirubin level increased
    B. Urinary bilirubin level increased
    C. Urinary urobilinogen level decreased
    D. Fecal urobilin level decreased

282. What may be the cause of neonatal physio-logical jaundice of the hepatic type?
    A. Hemolytic episode caused by an ABO incompatibility
    B. Stricture of the common bile duct
    C. Hemolytic episode caused by a Rh in-compatibility
    D. Deficiency in the bilirubin conjugation enzyme system

283. A complete obstruction of the common bile duct would be characterized by all the following laboratory results *except*
    A. Negative urine urobilinogen
    B. Negative fecal urobilinogen and urobilin
    C. Negative urine bilirubin
    D. Excretion of a pale-colored stool

284. Which of the following characterizes hepatic dysfunction in the early stage of viral hepatitis?

A. Elevation in urobilinogen and urobilin excretion in the feces
B. Elevation in the serum unconjugated bilirubin fraction
C. Depression in the serum conjugated bilirubin fraction
D. Depression in urinary urobilinogen excretion

285. Which of the following characterizes Crigler-Najjar disease?
A. Inability to transport bilirubin from the sinusoidal membrane to the microsomal region
B. Deficiency of the enzyme system required for conjugation of bilirubin
C. Inability to transport bilirubin glucuronides to the bile canaliculi
D. Severe liver cell damage accompanied by necrosis

286. Which of the following disorders is characterized by an inability to transport bilirubin from the sinusoidal membrane into the hepatocyte?
A. Carcinoma of the common bile duct
B. Crigler-Najjar syndrome
C. Dubin-Johnson syndrome
D. Gilbert's syndrome

287. Dubin-Johnson syndrome is characterized by all the following except
A. Impaired excretion of bilirubin into the bile
B. Hepatic uptake of bilirubin is normal
C. Inability to conjugate bilirubin
D. Increased level of bilirubin in urine

288. All the following disorders represent types of hepatic jaundice except
A. Cirrhosis
B. Crigler-Najjar syndrome

C. Hepatitis
D. Neoplasm of common bile duct

289. Which of the following disorders can be classified as a form of prehepatic jaundice?
A. Acute hemolytic anemia
B. Cirrhosis
C. Dubin-Johnson syndrome
D. Neoplasm of common bile duct

290. The following laboratory results are determined on a patient with a suggested diagnosis of biliary obstruction:

Serum total bilirubin—increased
Serum conjugated bilirubin—normal
Urine bilirubin—increased
Fecal urobilin—decreased

Which laboratory result is the *least* consistent with such a diagnosis?
A. Serum total bilirubin
B. Serum conjugated bilirubin
C. Urine bilirubin
D. Fecal urobilin

ELECTROLYTES

291. What is the normal renal threshold of sodium (measured in millimoles per liter)?
A. 80–85
B. 90–110
C. 110–130
D. 135–148

292. Of the total serum osmolality, sodium, chloride and bicarbonate ions normally contribute approximately what percent?
A. 8
B. 45
C. 75
D. 92

293. The presence of only slightly visible hemolysis will significantly increase the serum level of which of the following electrolytes?
    A. Sodium
    B. Potassium
    C. Chloride
    D. Bicarbonate

294. All the following contribute to the total anion content of serum *except*
    A. Acetoacetate
    B. Protein
    C. Lactate
    D. Iron

295. All the following describe potassium *except*
    A. Has no renal threshold
    B. Increased serum level in acidosis
    C. Hemolysis causes false increase in serum levels
    D. Major anion of intracellular fluid

296. Which of the following is a spectrophotometric method for quantifying serum chloride?
    A. Ferric perchlorate
    B. Ammonium molybdate
    C. Bathophenanthroline
    D. Cresolphthalein complexone

297. All the following statements about the electrolyte chloride are true *except*
    A. Main anion of the extracellular fluid
    B. Can shift from the extracellular plasma to the intracellular fluid of red blood cells
    C. Unable to be reabsorbed by active transport
    D. Measured in serum, urine, and sweat

298. Using the following data: $Na^+ =$ 143 mmol/L; $K^+ = 4.9$ mmol/L; $Cl^- =$ 105 mmol/L; and $HCO_3^- = 25$ mmol/L, all the following statements are correct *except*

A. Patient results are not acceptable
B. Anion gap is useful in detecting some disease states
C. Anion gap equals 18 mmol/L
D. Anion gap is useful for checking analytical error

299. A patient presents with Addison's disease. Serum sodium and potassium analyses are done. What would the results reveal?
    A. Normal sodium, low potassium levels
    B. Low sodium, low potassium levels
    C. Low sodium, high potassium levels
    D. High sodium, low potassium levels

300. Primary aldosteronism results from a tumor of the adrenal cortex. How would the extracellular fluid be affected?
    A. Normal sodium, decreased potassium levels
    B. Decreased sodium, decreased potassium levels
    C. Decreased sodium, increased potassium levels
    D. Increased sodium, decreased potassium levels

301. Hyponatremia may be found in all the following conditions *except*
    A. Addison's disease
    B. Diarrhea
    C. Diuretic therapy
    D. Cushing's syndrome

302. Of the total serum calcium, free ionized calcium normally represents approximately what percent?
    A. 10
    B. 40
    C. 50
    D. 90

303. Measuring the tubular reabsorption of phosphate is useful in diagnosing diseases that affect which of the following organs?
   A. Liver
   B. Adrenal gland
   C. Thyroid gland
   D. Parathyroid gland

304. Plasma calcium levels may be influenced by all the following *except*
   A. Parathyroid hormone
   B. Vitamin D
   C. Calcitonin
   D. Aldosterone

305. Which of the following is an effect of increased parathyroid hormone secretion?
   A. Decreased blood calcium levels
   B. Increased renal reabsorption of phosphate
   C. Decreased bone resorption
   D. Increased intestinal absorption of calcium

306. The following laboratory results are obtained on a 60-year-old woman who is complaining of anorexia, constipation, abdominal pain, nausea, and vomiting:

   Ionized serum calcium elevated
   Serum inorganic phosphate decreased
   Urine calcium elevated
   Urine phosphate elevated

   What do these results suggest?
   A. Primary hyperparathyroidism
   B. Vitamin D deficiency
   C. Hypoparathyroidism
   D. Paget's disease

307. Secondary hyperparathyroidism is often the result of
   A. Vitamin C deficiency
   B. Liver disease
   C. Renal disease
   D. Thyroid disease

308. Which of the following reagents is used to determine the concentration of serum inorganic phosphate?
   A. Ehrlich's reagent
   B. Ammonium molybdate
   C. 8-Hydroxyquinoline
   D. Bathophenanthroline

309. Which of the following reagents is used in a colorimetric method to quantify the concentration of serum calcium?
   A. Cresolphthalein complexone
   B. Lanthanum
   C. Malachite green
   D. Amino-naphthol-sulfonic acid

310. Which of the following has an effect on plasma calcium levels?
   A. Sodium
   B. Inorganic phosphate
   C. Potassium
   D. Iron

311. A patient's serum inorganic phosphate level is found to be elevated but the physician cannot determine a physiological basis for this abnormal result. What could possibly have caused an erroneous result to be reported?
   A. Patient not fasting when blood was drawn
   B. Specimen was hemolyzed
   C. Effect of diurnal variation
   D. Patient receiving intravenous glucose therapy

312. To what metal does ceruloplasmin firmly bind?
   A. Chromium
   B. Copper
   C. Zinc
   D. Iron

313. In iron-deficiency anemia, what would be the expected percent saturation of transferrin with iron?
    A. Less than 15
    B. Between 30 and 40
    C. Between 40 and 50
    D. Greater than 55

314. What is the primary storage form of iron?
    A. Apotransferrin
    B. Myoglobin
    C. Ferritin
    D. Hemosiderin

315. A serum ferritin level may not be a useful indicator of iron deficiency anemia in patients with what type of disorder?
    A. Chronic infection
    B. Malignancy
    C. Viral hepatitis
    D. All the above

316. All the following chromogens will produce a colored complex with iron that can be measured spectrophotometrically *except*
    A. Bathophenanthroline
    B. 8-Hydroxyquinoline
    C. Tripyridyl triazine
    D. Ferrozine

317. In what disorder would an increased percent saturation of transferrin be expected?
    A. Hemochromatosis
    B. Iron deficiency anemia
    C. Myocardial infarction
    D. Malignancy

318. Which of the following disorders is best characterized by these laboratory results?

    Serum iron—decreased
    Total iron binding capacity—increased
    Transferrin saturation—decreased
    Serum ferritin—decreased

    Free erythrocyte protoporphyrin—increased
    A. Anemia of chronic disease
    B. Thalassemia
    C. Iron-deficiency anemia
    D. Hemochromatosis

319. In magnesium deficiency tetany typical findings include all the following *except*
    A. High serum phosphate level
    B. Normal serum calcium level
    C. Normal blood pH value
    D. Low serum potassium level

320. Which of the following constituents normally present in serum must be chemically eliminated so that it will not interfere with the measurement of serum magnesium?
    A. Calcium
    B. Chloride
    C. Iron
    D. Potassium

321. In the collection of plasma specimens for lactate determinations, which of the following anticoagulants would be more appropriate?
    A. Sodium heparin
    B. Sodium citrate
    C. EDTA
    D. Oxalate plus fluoride

322. Which of the following disorders is characterized by increased production of chloride in sweat?
    A. Multiple myeloma
    B. Hypoparathyroidism
    C. Cystic fibrosis
    D. Wilson's disease

ACID-BASE BALANCE: BLOOD GASES

323. Which is the most predominant buffer system in the body?

A. Bicarbonate/carbonic acid

B. Acetate/acetic acid

C. Phosphate/phosphorous acid

D. Hemoglobin

324. The measurement of the pressure of dissolved CO_2 ($P\text{co}_2$) in the blood is most closely associated with the concentration of what substance?

A. pH

B. Bicarbonate (HCO_3^-)

C. Carbonic acid (H_2CO_3)

D. $P\text{o}_2$

325. What is the term that describes the sum of carbonic acid and bicarbonate in plasma?

A. Total CO_2

B. Standard bicarbonate

C. Buffer base

D. Base excess

326. To maintain a pH of 7.4 in plasma, it is necessary to maintain a

A. 10:1 ratio of bicarbonate to carbonic acid

B. 20:1 ratio of bicarbonate to carbonic acid

C. 1:20 ratio of bicarbonate to carbonic acid

D. 20:1 ratio of carbonic acid to bicarbonate

327. In the plasma, an excess in the concentration of bicarbonate without a change in $P\text{co}_2$ from normal will result in what metabolic state?

A. Respiratory acidosis

B. Respiratory alkalosis

C. Metabolic acidosis

D. Metabolic alkalosis

328. Which of the following characterizes respiratory acidosis?

A. Excess of bicarbonate

B. Deficit of bicarbonate

C. Excess of dissolved carbon dioxide ($P\text{co}_2$)

D. Deficit of dissolved carbon dioxide ($P\text{co}_2$)

329. What is the specimen of choice for analysis of acid-base disturbances involving pulmonary dysfunction in an adult?

A. Venous blood

B. Arterial blood

C. Capillary blood

D. Urine

330. What is the anticoagulant of choice for blood gas analysis?

A. EDTA

B. Heparin

C. Sodium fluoride

D. Citrate

331. If a blood gas specimen is left exposed to air, which of the following changes will occur?

A. $P\text{o}_2$ and pH increase; $P\text{co}_2$ decreases

B. $P\text{o}_2$ and pH decrease; $P\text{co}_2$ increases

C. $P\text{o}_2$ increases; pH and $P\text{co}_2$ decrease

D. $P\text{o}_2$ decreases; $P\text{co}_2$ and pH increase

332. How would blood gas parameters change if a sealed specimen is left at room temperature for 2 or more hours?

A. $P\text{o}_2$ increases, $P\text{co}_2$ increases, pH increases

B. $P\text{o}_2$ decreases, $P\text{co}_2$ decreases, pH decreases

C. $P\text{o}_2$ decreases, $P\text{co}_2$ increases, pH decreases

D. $P\text{o}_2$ increases, $P\text{co}_2$ increases, pH decreases

333. The bicarbonate ion concentration may be calculated from the total CO_2 and $P\text{co}_2$ blood levels by using which of the following formulas?

A. $0.03 \times (P\text{co}_2 - \text{total } CO_2)$

B. $(\text{total } CO_2 + 0.03) \times P\text{co}_2$

C. $0.03 \times (\text{total } CO_2 - P\text{o}_2)$

D. $\text{total } CO_2 - (0.03 \times P\text{co}_2)$

334. Which of the following blood gas parameters are measured directly by the blood gas analyzer electrochemically as opposed to being calculated by the instrument?
   A. pH, HCO_3^-, total CO_2
   B. Pco_2, HCO_3^-, Po_2
   C. pH, Pco_2, Po_2
   D. Po_2, HCO_3^-, total CO_2

335. In order to maintain electrical neutrality in the red blood cell, bicarbonate leaves the red blood cell and enters the plasma through an exchange mechanism with what electrolyte?
   A. Sodium
   B. Potassium
   C. Chloride
   D. Phosphate

336. In acute diabetic ketoacidosis, which of the following laboratory findings would be expected?
   A. Fasting blood glucose elevated, pH elevated, ketone bodies present
   B. Fasting blood glucose elevated, pH low, ketone bodies present
   C. Fasting blood glucose elevated, pH normal, ketone bodies absent
   D. Fasting blood glucose decreased, pH low, ketone bodies absent

337. Which of the following is a cause of metabolic alkalosis?
   A. Late stage of salicylate poisoning
   B. Uncontrolled diabetes mellitus
   C. Renal failure
   D. Excessive vomiting

338. Which of the following statements is true about partially compensated respiratory alkalosis?
   A. Pco_2 is higher than normal
   B. HCO_3^- is higher than normal

C. More CO_2 is eliminated through the lungs by hyperventilation
   D. Renal reabsorption of HCO_3^- is decreased

339. Which is a compensatory mechanism in respiratory acidosis?
   A. Hypoventilation
   B. Decreased reabsorption of bicarbonate by the kidneys
   C. Increased Na^+/H^+ exchange by the kidneys
   D. Decreased ammonia formation by the kidneys

340. Which of the following will cause a shift of the oxygen dissociation curve to the right, resulting in a decreased affinity of hemoglobin for O_2?
   A. Low plasma pH level
   B. Low Pco_2 level
   C. Low concentration of 2,3-diphosphoglycerate
   D. Low temperature

341. Which of the following statements about carbonic anhydrase (CA) is true?
   A. Catalyzes conversion of CO_2 and H_2O to $HHCO_3$ in red blood cells
   B. Causes shift to the left in oxygen dissociation curve
   C. Catalyzes formation of H_2CO_3 from CO_2 and H_2O in the tissues
   D. Inactive in renal tubular cells

342. Which of the following statements best describes "base excess"?
   A. Primarily refers to carbonic acid concentration
   B. Positive values reflect metabolic alkalosis
   C. Created through metabolism of carbohydrates

D. Negative values represent a respiratory imbalance

343. Given the following information, calculate the blood pH.

Pco_2 = 44 mm Hg
Total CO_2 = 29 mmol/L

A. 6.28
B. 6.76
C. 7.42
D. 7.44

344. A 75-year-old woman comes to her physician complaining of abdominal pain. She says she has had a sore stomach for the last three weeks and has been taking increasing doses of anti-acid pills to control it. Until now she is taking a box of pills a day. Blood gases are drawn with the following results: pH = 7.49, Pco_2 = 59 mm Hg, HCO_3^- = 38 mmol/L. What do these data indicate?

A. Metabolic alkalosis, partially compensated
B. Respiratory acidosis, uncompensated
C. A dual problem of acidosis
D. An error in one of the blood gas measurements

345. A 24-year-old drug abuser is brought into the ER unconscious. He has shallow breaths, looks pale, and is "clammy." Blood gases show the following results: pH = 7.29, Pco_2 = 50 mm Hg, HCO_3^- = 25 mmol/L. What condition is indicated by these results?

A. Metabolic alkalosis, partially compensated
B. Respiratory acidosis, uncompensated
C. A dual problem of acidosis
D. An error in one of the blood gas measurements

346. Blood gases are drawn on a 68-year-old asthmatic who was recently admitted for treatment of a kidney infection. Blood gas results are as follows: pH = 7.25, Pco_2 = 56 mm Hg, HCO_3^- = 16 mmol/L. What condition is indicated by these results?

A. Metabolic alkalosis, partially compensated
B. Respiratory acidosis, uncompensated
C. A dual problem of acidosis
D. An error in one of the blood gas measurements

347. A mother brings her daughter, a 22-year-old medical technology student, to her physician. The patient is hyperventilating and has glossy eyes. The mother explains that her daughter is scheduled to take her final course exam the next morning. She has been running around frantically all day in a worried state and then started to breathe heavily. Blood gases are drawn in the office with the following results: pH = 7.58, Pco_2 = 55 mm Hg, HCO_3^- = 18 mmol/L. What do these data indicate?

A. Metabolic alkalosis, partially compensated
B. Respiratory acidosis, uncompensated
C. A dual problem of acidosis
D. An error in one of the blood gas measurements

ENZYMES

348. What does an increase in the serum enzyme levels indicate?

A. Decreased enzyme catabolism
B. Accelerated enzyme production
C. Tissue damage and necrosis
D. Increased glomerular filtration rate

349. In the assay of an enzyme, zero order kinetics are best described by which of the following statements?
    A. Enzyme is present in excess; rate of reaction is variable with time and dependent only on the concentration of the enzyme in the system.
    B. Substrate is present in excess; rate of reaction is constant with time and dependent only on the concentration of enzyme in the system.
    C. Substrate is present in excess; rate of reaction is constant with enzyme concentration and dependent only on the time in which the reaction is run.
    D. Enzyme is present in excess; rate of reaction is independent of both time and concentration of the enzyme in the system.

350. Based on the following graph of velocity of an enzyme reaction *vs.* substrate concentration, you are designing a new method to measure the activity of an enzyme of clinical interest. To formulate the new methodology so that enzyme activity is assessed using zero order kinetics, which concentration of substrate should you first determine experimentally?

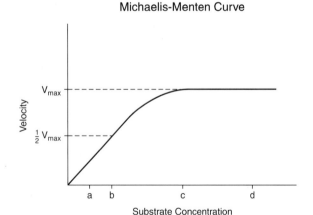

Michaelis-Menten Curve

    A. *a*
    B. *b*
    C. *c*
    D. *d*

351. When measuring enzyme activity, if the instrument is operating 5 °C lower than the temperature prescribed for the method, how will the results be effected?
    A. Lower than expected
    B. Higher than expected
    C. Varied, showing no particular pattern
    D. All will be clinically abnormal

352. Given the following information for a rate reaction, calculate the activity of a serum specimen for alanine aminotransferase in international units per liter.

Time	Absorbance	
1 min	1.104	Specimen volume = 20 μL
2 min	1.025	Reagent volume = 3.0 mL
3 min	0.950	Molar absorptivity for
4 min	0.873	NADH at 340 nm =
		6.22 × 10³ L/mol·cm
		Light path = 1 cm

    A. 186
    B. 198
    C. 1857
    D. 1869

353. The properties of enzymes are correctly described by which of the following statements?
    A. Enzymes are stable proteins.
    B. Enzymes are protein catalysts of biological origin.
    C. Enzymes affect the rate of a chemical reaction by raising the activation energy needed for the reaction to take place.
    D. Enzyme activity is not altered by heat denaturation.

354. Which of the following is a true statement concerning serum enzymes?

A. The presence of hemolyzed red cells is of no significance for an accurate assay of most serum enzymes.

B. Serum asparate transaminase (AST), but not serum lactate dehydrogenase (LD), is usually elevated in acute myocardial infarction.

C. Increased serum alkaline phosphatase may be found in bone disease.

D. Aspartate transaminase was formerly known as glutamate pyruvate transaminase.

355. Enzymes that catalyze the transfer of groups between compounds are classified as belonging to which enzyme class?
    A. Hydrolases
    B. Lyases
    C. Oxidoreductases
    D. Transferases

356. Which of the following enzymes does *not* belong to the class of enzymes known as the hydrolases?
    A. Alkaline phosphatase
    B. Aldolase
    C. Amylase
    D. Lipase

357. To what class of enzymes does lactate dehydrogenase belong?
    A. Isomerases
    B. Ligases
    C. Oxidoreductases
    D. Transferases

358. Which of the following enzymes catalyzes the transfer of amino groups causing the inter-conversion of amino acids and α-oxoacids?
    A. Amylase
    B. Aspartate transaminase
    C. Alkaline phosphatase
    D. Lactate dehydrogenase

359. What abbreviation has been used in the past to designate alanine aminotransferase?
    A. AST
    B. AAT
    C. GOT
    D. GPT

360. Although a total lactate dehydrogenase (LD) determination performed alone yields little information as to the area of tissue destruction, an electrophoretic separation of the LD isoenzymes may be useful. With what disorder is an increase in LD-5 and LD-4 associated?
    A. Acute hepatic disease
    B. Acute myocardial infarction
    C. Pulmonary infarction
    D. Pancreatitis

361. All the following accurately describe properties associated with lactate dehydrogenase *except*
    A. Optimum pH for the catalysis of lactate to pyruvate is 7.4–7.8
    B. Increased in a hemolyzed serum specimen
    C. Catalyzes the oxidation of lactate to pyruvate with mediation of nicoti-namide adenine dinucleotide
    D. LD-4 and LD-5 are labile in the cold

362. When separated by electrophoresis, the most anodic (fastest-moving) fraction of the lactate dehydrogenase isoenzymes is elevated in the presence of which of the following conditions?
    A. Acute viral hepatitis
    B. Pernicious anemia
    C. Intramuscular injections
    D. Skeletal muscle injury

363. Lactate dehydrogenase (LD) catalyzes the following reaction:

$$\text{Lactate} + \text{NAD}^+ \overset{\text{LD}}{\rightleftharpoons} \text{pyruvate} + \text{NADH}$$

As the reaction is written, which of the following techniques can be used to assess LD activity?
   A. Measure the colorimetric product pyruvate.
   B. Measure the colorimetric product NADH.
   C. Measure the increase in absorbance at 340 nm as NADH is produced.
   D. Measure the decrease in absorbance at 340 nm as NADH is produced.

364. All the following are true of myoglobin as it relates to acute myocardial infarction (AMI) *except*
   A. Measure serially
   B. Cardiac specific
   C. Initial increase occurs in 1–3 hours
   D. Doubling of initial value within 1–2 hours suggestive of AMI

365. Elevation of serum creatine kinase may be associated with all the following disorders *except*
   A. Cerebrovascular accidents
   B. Hypothyroidism
   C. Bone disease
   D. Intramuscular injection

366. All the following statements concerning creatine kinase are true *except*
   A. Rises early after acute myocardial infarction
   B. Catalyzes the phosphorylation of creatine by ATP
   C. Requires Ca^{++} for activity
   D. Found mainly in skeletal and cardiac muscles and in brain tissue

367. Which enzyme is measured by methodologies that use small oligosaccharides and 4-nitrophenyl-glycoside for substrates?

A. Lipase
B. Amylase
C. Creatine kinase
D. Cholinesterase

368. True statements concerning gamma-glutamyltransferase include all the following *except*
   A. Present in almost all cells of the body
   B. Elevated in liver and some pancreatic diseases
   C. Elevated in chronic alcoholism
   D. Elevated in bone disease

369. Which of the following statements correctly describes alkaline phosphatase?
   A. Decreased in Paget's disease
   B. Decreased in third trimester of a normal pregnancy
   C. Increased in obstructive jaundice
   D. Primarily found in cardiac muscle

370. Enzymes frequently assayed that aid in the assessment of liver function include all the following *except*
   A. Alanine aminotransferase
   B. Creatine kinase
   C. Alkaline phosphatase
   D. Gamma-glutamyltransferase

371. In acute pancreatitis, a significant increase in which serum enzyme would be expected diagnostically?
   A. Creatine kinase
   B. Amylase
   C. Alkaline phosphatase
   D. Aspartate aminotransferase

372. For assessing carcinoma of the prostate, quantification of prostate-specific antigen has virtually replaced the measurement of which of the following enzymes?
   A. Alkaline phosphatase
   B. Acid phosphatase

C. Alanine aminotransferase

D. Trypsin

373. All the following statements may be associ-
ated with serum cholinesterase *except*
A. Inhibited by organic insecticides
B. Referred to as "true" cholinesterase
C. Decreased level causes prolonged apnea
after administration of succinyldicholine
D. Acts on the substrate propionylthiocholine

374. Which of the following sets of tests would
be the most useful in diagnosing an acute
myocardial infarction?
A. AST, LD, CK-MB
B. LD, CK-MB, troponin
C. CK-MB, troponin, myoglobin
D. LD, troponin, myoglobin

375. A physician orders several laboratory tests
on a 55-year-old male patient who is complaining of pain, stiffness, fatigue, and
headaches. Based on the following serum
test results, what is the most likely
diagnosis?

Alkaline phosphatase—significantly
increased
Gamma-glutamyltransferase—normal

A. Biliary obstruction
B. Cirrhosis
C. Hepatitis
D. Osteitis deformans

376. A 53-year-old female presents with fatigue,
pruritus, and an enlarged, nontender liver.
The physician orders a series of blood tests.
Based on the following serum test results,
what is the most likely diagnosis?

Alkaline phosphatase—markedly
elevated
Alanine aminotransferase—slightly
elevated

Lactate dehydrogenase—slightly
elevated
Gamma-glutamyltransferase—markedly
elevated
Total bilirubin—slightly elevated

A. Alcoholic cirrhosis
B. Infectious mononucleosis
C. Intrahepatic cholestasis
D. Viral hepatitis

377. A 42-year-old male presents with anorexia,
nausea, fever, and icterus of the skin and
mucous membranes. He noticed that his
urine had appeared dark for the past several
days. The physician orders a series of biochemical tests. Based on the following test
results, what is the most likely diagnosis?

Serum alkaline phosphatase—slightly
elevated
Serum alanine aminotransferase—
markedly elevated
Serum aspartate aminotransferase—
markedly elevated
Serum gamma-glutamyltransferase—
slightly elevated
Serum total bilirubin—moderately
elevated
Urine bilirubin—positive
Fecal urobilinogen—decreased

A. Acute hepatitis
B. Alcoholic cirrhosis
C. Metastatic carcinoma of the pancreas
D. Obstructive jaundice

378. To aid in the diagnosis of skeletal muscle
disease, which of the following serum en-
zyme measurements would be of most use?
A. Creatine kinase
B. Alkaline phosphatase
C. Aspartate aminotransferase
D. Alanine aminotransferase

379. When an acute myocardial infarction occurs, in what order (list first to last) will
the enzymes aspartate aminotransferase
(AST), creatine kinase (CK), and lactate
dehydrogenase (LD) become elevated in
the serum?
    A. AST, LD, CK
    B. CK, LD, AST
    C. CK, AST, LD
    D. LD, CK, AST

380. All the following characterize the assessment of acute myocardial infarction *except*
    A. Elevated serum cTnI level
    B. Elevated serum CK-2 level
    C. Abnormal serum alkaline phosphatase
       isoenzyme pattern
    D. Blood collected upon presentation and
       serially in 3- to 6-hour intervals

381. A 10-year-old female presents with varicella.
The child has been experiencing fever, nausea, vomiting, lethargy, and disorientation. A
diagnosis of Reye's syndrome is determined.
All the following laboratory results are consistent with the diagnosis *except*
    A. Elevated serum AST
    B. Elevated serum ALT
    C. Elevated plasma ammonia
    D. Elevated serum bilirubin

382. Which of the following enzyme activities
can be determined by utilizing a dilute olive
oil emulsion substrate, whose hydrolyzed
product is monitored as a decrease in
turbidity or light scatter?
    A. Alkaline phosphatase
    B. Amylase
    C. Lipase
    D. Trypsin

383. Cystic fibrosis can be characterized by all
the following *except*
    A. Decreased bicarbonate concentration in
       duodenal fluid
    B. Decreased lipase activity in duodenal
       fluid
    C. Decreased amylase activity in duodenal
       fluid
    D. Increased trypsin in feces

ENDOCRINOLOGY

384. Secretion of hormones by the anterior
pituitary may be controlled by the
circulating levels of hormones from the
respective target gland as well as hormones
secreted by what organ?
    A. Posterior lobe of the pituitary gland
    B. Intermediate lobe of the pituitary gland
    C. Hypothalamus
    D. Adrenal medulla

385. An elevated level of which of the following hormones will inhibit pituitary secretion of adrenocorticotropic hormone
(ACTH)?
    A. Aldosterone
    B. Cortisol
    C. 17β-Estradiol
    D. Progesterone

386. Which of the following is the major
mineralocorticoid?
    A. Aldosterone
    B. Cortisol
    C. Corticosterone
    D. Testosterone

387. Plasma renin activity (PRA) measurements
are usually made by measuring which of the
following using radioimmunoassay?
    A. Angiotensinogen
    B. Angiotensin I

C. Angiotensin II

D. Angiotensin-converting enzyme

388. What effect would a low-salt diet, upright position, and diuretics have on the following results?

A. Renin ↑, aldosterone ↑, hypernatremia, hypokalemia

B. Renin ↑, aldosterone ↓, hypernatremia, hypokalemia

C. Renin ↓, aldosterone ↓, hyponatremia, hyperkalemia

D. Renin ↓, aldosterone ↑, hyponatremia, hyperkalemia

389. As a screening test for Cushing's syndrome, the physician wishes to see whether a patient exhibits normal diurnal rhythm in his or her cortisol secretion. At what time should the specimens be drawn for plasma cortisol determination?

A. 6 A.M., 2 P.M.

B. 8 A.M., 4 P.M.

C. 12 noon, 6 P.M.

D. 12 noon, 12 midnight

390. A patient is suspected of having Addison's disease. His symptoms are weakness, fatigue, loss of weight, skin pigmentation, and hypoglycemia. His laboratory tests show low serum sodium and chloride, elevated serum potassium, and elevated urine sodium and chloride levels. The serum cortisol level is decreased and the plasma ACTH is increased. To make a definitive diagnosis, the physician orders an adrenocorticotropin hormone (ACTH) stimulation test and serum cortisol levels are measured.

If the patient has primary hypoadrenocortical function (Addison's disease), what would be the expected level of serum cortisol? If the patient has hypopi-

tuitarism, secondary hypoadrenocortical function, what would be the expected level of serum cortisol?

A. Increase from baseline; decrease from baseline

B. Decrease from baseline; increase from baseline

C. Slight increase from baseline; no change from baseline

D. No change from baseline; slight increase from baseline

391. What does the concentration of urinary free cortisol mainly reflect?

A. Total serum cortisol

B. Conjugated cortisol

C. Unbound serum cortisol

D. Protein-bound serum cortisol

392. A 30-year-old woman is admitted to the hospital. She has truncal obesity, buffalo humpback, moon face, purple striae, hypertension, hyperglycemia, increased facial hair, acne, and amenorrhea. The physician orders endocrine testing. The results are as follows:

Urine free cortisol—increased

Serum cortisol (8 A.M.)—increased

Plasma ACTH—decreased

Dexamethasone suppression test

Overnight low-dose—no suppression of serum cortisol

High dose—no suppression of serum cortisol

What is the most probable diagnosis?

A. Pituitary adenoma

B. Ectopic ACTH lung cancer

C. Adrenocortical carcinoma

D. Addison's disease

393. Which of the following is the most common cause of the adrenogenital syndrome, congenital adrenal hyperplasia, and which test is used for its diagnosis?
    A. 17α-Hydroxylase deficiency; progesterone assay
    B. 21-Hydroxylase deficiency; 17α-hydroxyprogesterone assay
    C. 3β-Hydroxysteroid dehydrogenase-isomerase deficiency; 17α-hydroxypregnenolone assay
    D. 11β-Hydroxylase deficiency; 11-deoxycortisol assay

394. Which of the following is the most potent androgen?
    A. Androstenedione
    B. Dehydroepiandrosterone
    C. Androsterone
    D. Testosterone

395. All the following tissues secrete steroid hormones *except*
    A. Ovaries
    B. Pituitary gland
    C. Testes
    D. Adrenal cortex

396. Which of the following is the most potent estrogen and considered to be the true ovarian hormone?
    A. Estriol (E_3)
    B. Estrone (E_1)
    C. 17β-Estradiol (E_2)
    D. 16α-Hydroxyestrone

397. During pregnancy in the second trimester, chorionic gonadotropin (CG) levels _____ and progesterone and estriol levels _____.
    A. Increase, increase
    B. Increase, decrease
    C. Decrease, increase
    D. Decrease, decrease

398. The triple test for Down's syndrome includes quantification of all the following *except*
    A. α-Fetoprotein
    B. Unconjugated estriol
    C. Progesterone
    D. Chorionic gonadotropin

399. Because of infertility problems, a physician would like to determine when a woman ovulates. The physician orders serial assays of plasma progesterone. From these assays, how can the physician recognize when ovulation occurs?
    A. After ovulation progesterone rapidly increases.
    B. After ovulation progesterone rapidly decreases.
    C. Right before ovulation progesterone rapidly increases.
    D. There is a gradual, steady increase in progesterone throughout the menstrual cycle.

400. The placenta secretes numerous hormones both protein and steroid. Which of the following hormones is not secreted by the placenta?
    A. Chorionic gonadotropin (CG)
    B. Estrogen
    C. Human placental lactogen (HPL)
    D. Luteinizing hormone (LH)

401. During pregnancy estriol is synthesized in the placenta from _____ formed in the _____.
    A. Estradiol, mother
    B. Estradiol, fetus
    C. 16α-hydroxy-DHEA-S, mother
    D. 16α-hydroxy-DHEA-S, fetus

402. What percentage decrease in plasma or urinary estriol, in comparison with the

previous day's level, is considered significant during pregnancy?

A. 5

B. 10

C. 25

D. 40

403. Which of the following compounds is a precursor of the estrogens?

A. Progesterone

B. Testosterone

C. Cholesterol

D. Aldosterone

404. When do the highest levels of gonadotropins occur?

A. During the follicular phase of the menstrual cycle

B. During the luteal phase of the menstrual cycle

C. At the midpoint of the menstrual cycle

D. Several days prior to ovulation

405. What would be an example of ectopic hormone production?

A. Prolactin production by pituitary tumors

B. Calcitonin production by thyroid tumors

C. Growth hormone production by lung tumors

D. Cortisol production by adrenal tumors

406. Which of the following hormones initiates its response by binding to cytoplasmic receptors?

A. Estradiol

B. Epinephrine

C. Growth hormone

D. Follicle-stimulating hormone

407. The adrenal medulla secretes which of the following in the greatest quantity?

A. Metanephrine

B. Norepinephrine

C. Epinephrine

D. Dopamine

408. In a patient who is suspected of having pheochromocytoma, measurement of which of the following would be most useful?

A. Metanephrine

B. Homovanillic acid

C. 5-Hydroxyindoleacetic acid

D. Homogentisic acid

409. Diabetes insipidus is associated with depressed secretion of which of the following hormones?

A. Prolactin

B. Antidiuretic hormone

C. Growth hormone

D. Oxytocin

410. Measurement of C-peptide may be useful in all the following *except*

A. Diagnosis of diabetic ketoacidosis

B. Diagnosis of insulinoma

C. Identification of surreptitious insulin injection

D. Follow-up assessment of total pancreatectomy

411. Of which of the following is 5-hydroxyindoleacetic acid (5-HIAA) the primary metabolite?

A. Epinephrine

B. Norepinephrine

C. Serotonin

D. Prolactin

412. Which of the following functions as an inhibiting factor for somatotropin release?

A. Gonadotropin-releasing hormone

B. Growth hormone-releasing hormone

C. Somatomedin

D. Somatostatin

413. All the following are associated with growth hormone *except*
    A. Somatotropin
    B. Secreted by posterior pituitary
    C. Hypersecretion results in acromegaly
    D. Effects lipid, carbohydrate, and protein metabolism

414. The secretion of which of the following is controlled by growth hormone?
    A. Growth hormone-releasing hormone
    B. Corticotropin-releasing hormone
    C. Somatomedin
    D. Somatostatin

415. Which of the following would be elevated in the blood in medullary carcinoma of the thyroid?
    A. Calcitonin
    B. Thyroxine
    C. Catecholamines
    D. Secretin

416. What is the predominant form of thyroid hormone in the circulation?
    A. Thyroxine
    B. Triiodothyronine
    C. Diiodotyrosine
    D. Monoiodotyrosine

417. Once synthesized, the thyroid hormones are stored as thyroglobulin in what area of the thyroid gland?
    A. Epithelial cell wall of the follicle
    B. Colloid in the follicle
    C. Isthmus of the thyroid gland
    D. Extracellular space of the thyroid gland

418. How is the majority of reverse T_3 (rT_3) made?
    A. Peripheral deiodination of T_4
    B. Peripheral deiodination of T_3
    C. From T_3 in the thyroid gland
    D. From thyroglobulin in the thyroid gland

419. Which of the following is an autoantibody that binds to TSH receptor sites on thyroid cell membranes preventing thyroid-stimulating hormone from binding?
    A. Antithyroglobulins
    B. Antimicrosomal antibodies
    C. Thyroid-stimulating immunoglobulins
    D. Thyroxine-binding globulins

420. In a patient with suspected primary hyper-thyroidism associated with Graves' disease, one would expect the following laboratory serum results: free thyroxine (FT_4) _____, thyroid hormone binding ratio (THBR) _____, and thyroid-stimulating hormone (TSH) _____.
    A. Increased, decreased, increased
    B. Increased, decreased, decreased
    C. Increased, increased, decreased
    D. Decreased, decreased, increased

421. In a patient suspected of having primary myxedema, one would expect the following serum results: free thyroxine (FT_4) _____, thyroid hormone binding ratio (THBR) _____, and thyroid-stimulating hormone (TSH) _____.
    A. Decreased, increased, decreased
    B. Increased, increased, decreased
    C. Decreased, decreased, increased
    D. Increased, decreased, increased

422. Thyroid-releasing hormone (TRH) is given to a patient. Serum thyroid-stimulating hormone (TSH) levels are taken before and after the injection, and the values are the same—low. This patient probably has which of the following disorders?
    A. Primary hypothyroidism
    B. Secondary hypothyroidism

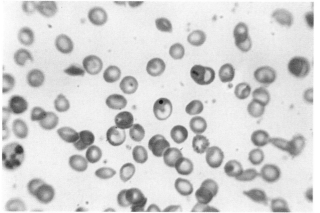

Color Plate 1

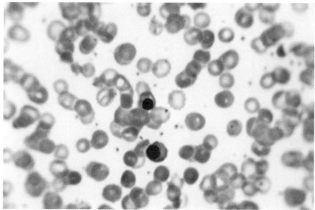

Color Plate 2

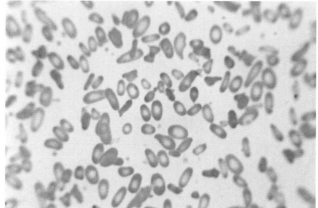

Color Plate 3

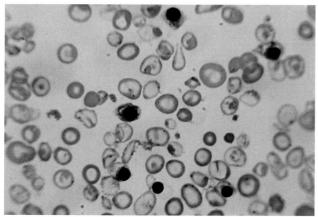

Color Plate 4

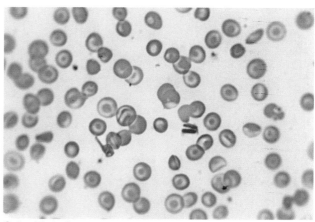

Color Plate 5

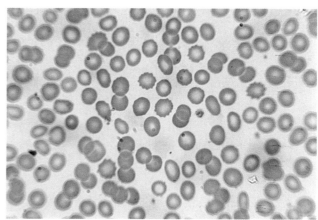

Color Plate 6

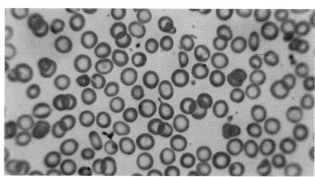

Color Plate 7

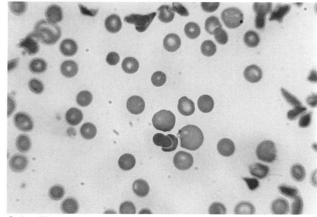

Color Plate 8

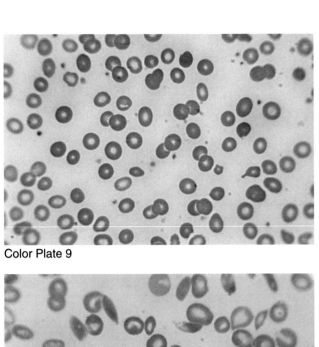

Color Plate 9

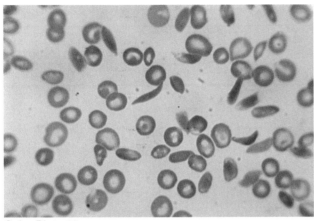

Color Plate 10

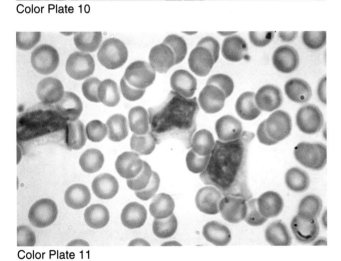

Color Plate 11

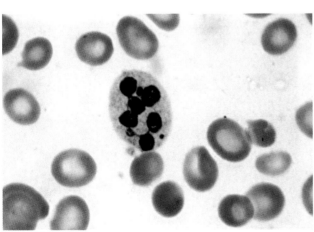
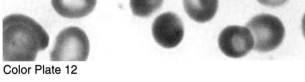

Color Plate 12

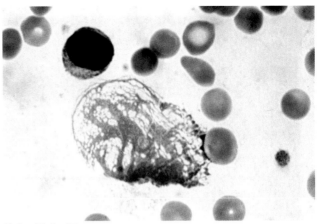

Color Plate 13

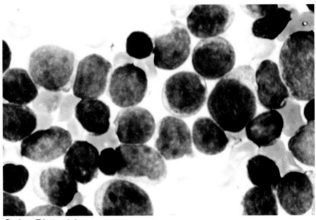

Color Plate 14

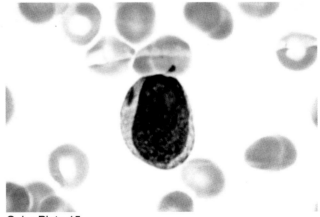

Color Plate 15

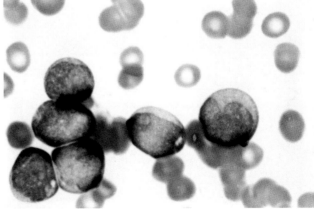

Color Plate 16

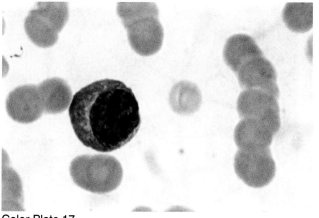
Color Plate 17

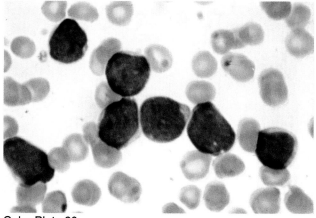
Color Plate 20

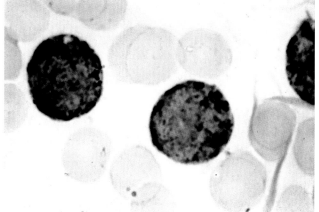
Color Plate 18

Immunoglobulin Molecule

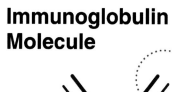
Color Plate 21

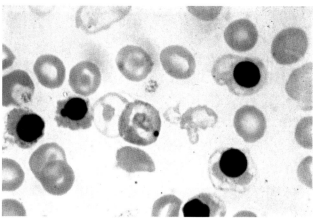
Color Plate 19

Dimeric IgA Molecule

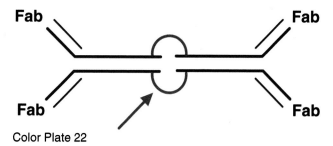
Color Plate 22

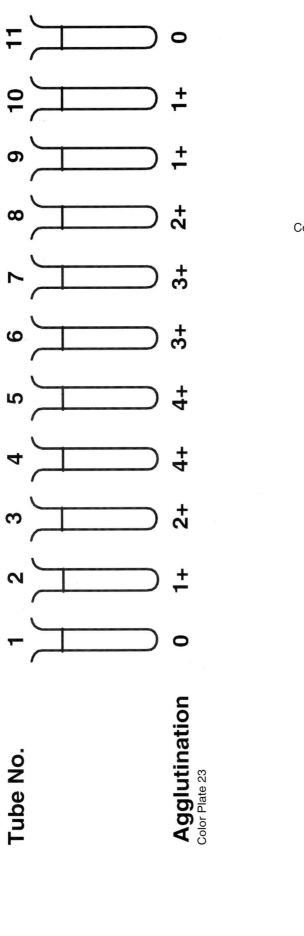

Tube No.

1	2	3	4	5	6	7	8	9	10	11

Agglutination

0	1+	2+	4+	4+	3+	3+	2+	1+	1+	0

Color Plate 23

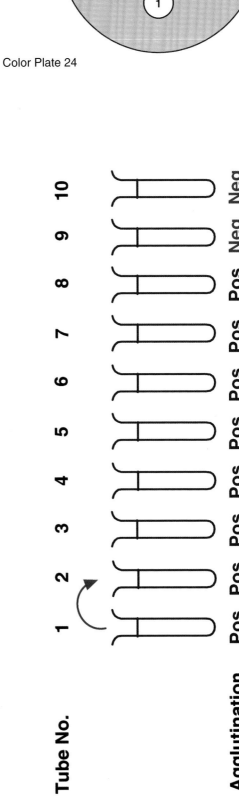

Color Plate 24

Tube No.

1	2	3	4	5	6	7	8	9	10

Agglutination

Pos	Pos	Pos	Pos	Pos	Pos	Pos	Pos	Neg	Neg

Color Plate 25

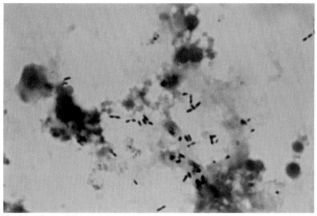
Color Plate 26

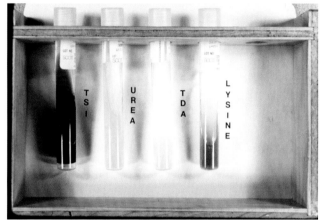
Color Plate 27

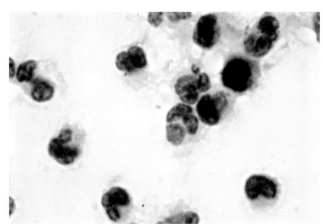
Color Plate 28

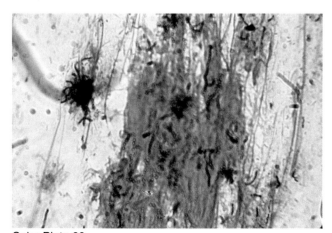
Color Plate 29

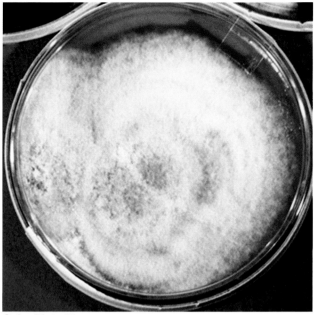
Color Plate 30

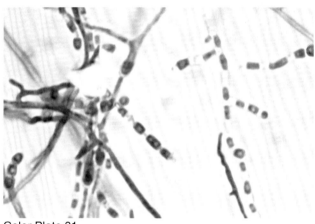
Color Plate 31

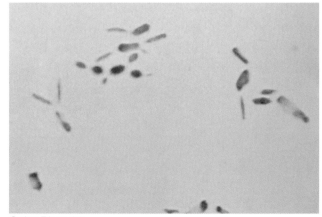
Color Plate 32

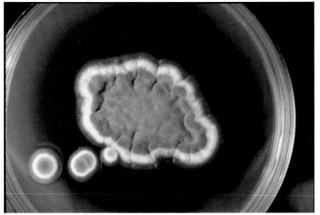

Color Plate 33

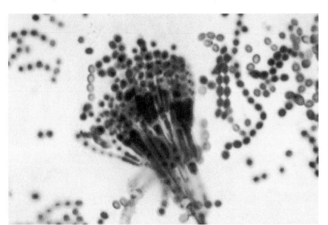

Color Plate 34

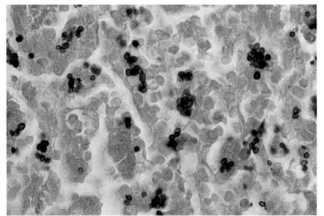

Color Plate 35

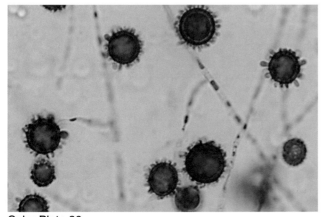

Color Plate 36

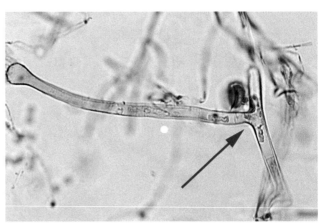

Color Plate 37

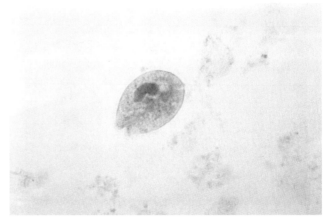

Color Plate 38

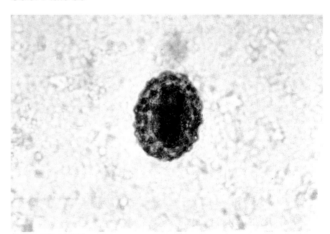

Color Plate 39

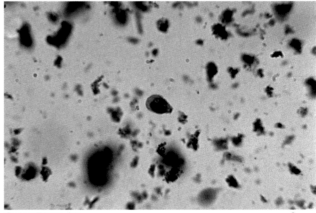

Color Plate 40

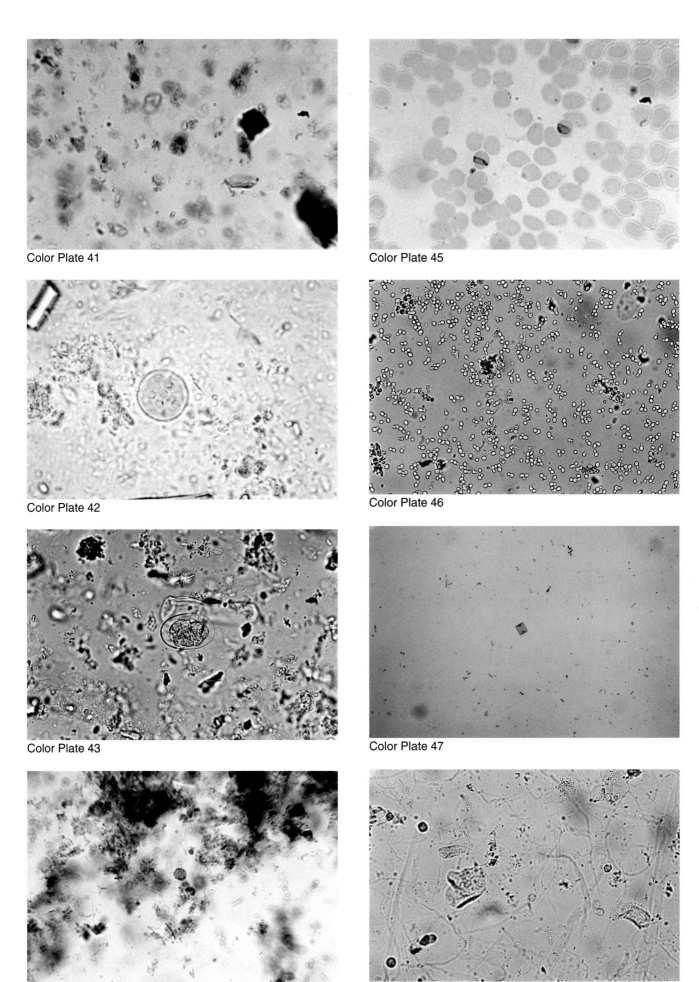

Color Plate 41

Color Plate 42

Color Plate 43

Color Plate 44

Color Plate 45

Color Plate 46

Color Plate 47

Color Plate 48

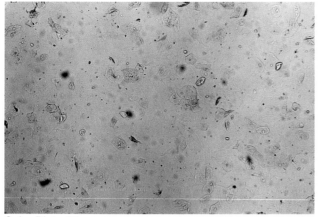

Color Plate 49

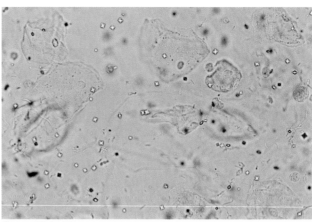

Color Plate 53

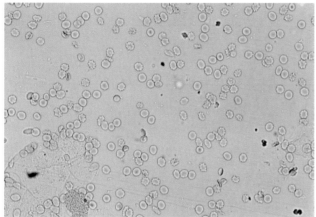

Color Plate 50

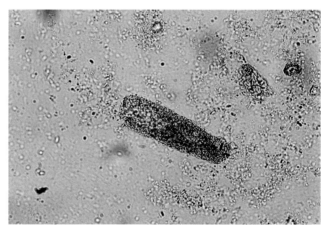

Color Plate 54

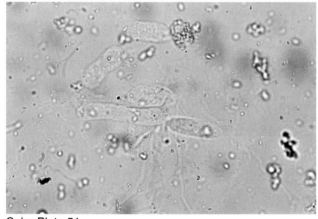

Color Plate 51

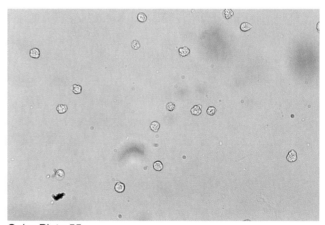

Color Plate 55

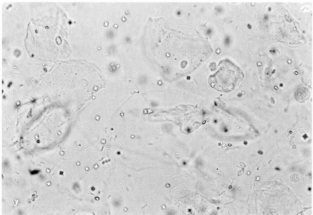

Color Plate 52

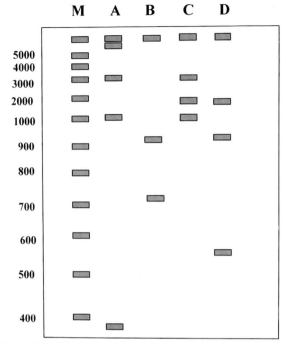

M A B C D

5000
4000
3000
2000
1000
900
800
700
600
500
400

Color Plate 56

Digest DNA with restriction enzyme
Separate by electrophoresis

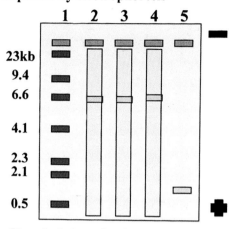

1 2 3 4 5

23kb
9.4
6.6
4.1
2.3
2.1
0.5

Chemical depurination
Denaturation
Neutralization

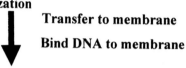

Transfer to membrane

Bind DNA to membrane

Hybridize membrane with ³²P labeled probe
Wash off excess probe
Expose to X-ray film
Develop autoradiogram

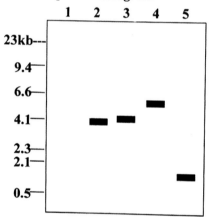

1 2 3 4 5

23kb---
9.4-
6.6-
4.1-
2.3-
2.1-
0.5-

Color Plate 57

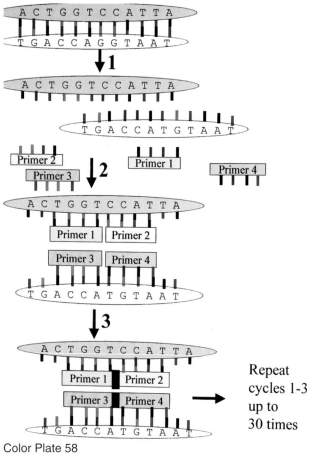

Color Plate 58

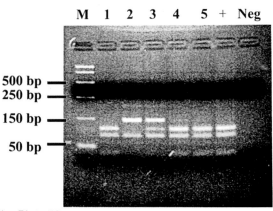

Color Plate 59

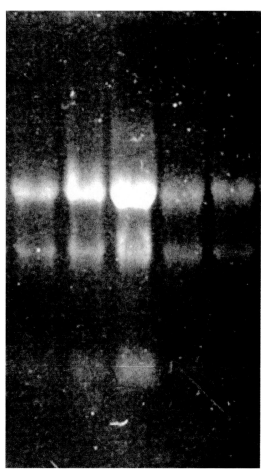

Color Plate 60

C. Tertiary hypothyroidism

D. Iodine deficiency

423. The presence of a very high titer for antithyroglobulin antibodies and the detection of antimicrosomal antibodies is highly suggestive of what disorder?

A. Pernicious anemia

B. Hashimoto's thyroiditis

C. Multinodular goiter

D. Thyroid adenoma

424. What is the major carrier protein of the thyroid hormones in the blood?

A. Albumin

B. Thyroxine-binding globulin

C. Thyroxine-binding prealbumin

D. Thyroglobulin

425. Why are the total thyroxine (T_4) levels increased in pregnant women and those who take oral contraceptives?

A. Inappropriate iodine metabolism

B. Changes in tissue use

C. Changes in concentration of thyroxine-binding globulin (TBG)

D. Changes in thyroglobulin synthesis

426. Which of the following is the Hollander insulin test used to confirm?

A. Hyperglycemia

B. Vagotomy

C. Pancreatectomy

D. Insulinoma

427. Zollinger-Ellison syndrome is characterized by an elevated blood level of which of the following?

A. Trypsin

B. Pepsin

C. Gastrin

D. Cholecystokinin-pancreozymin

428. The separation of the bound from the free labeled species is the basis for all the following techniques *except*

A. Radioimmunoassay

B. Enzyme-linked immunosorbent assay

C. Immunoradiometric assay

D. Enzyme-multiplied immunoassay technique

429. The substance to be measured reacts with a specific macromolecule of limited binding capacity. This is the principle involved in all the following assays *except*

A. Radioimmunoassay (RIA)

B. Enzyme-multiplied immunoassay technique (EMIT)

C. Fluorescence polarization immunoassay (FPI)

D. High-performance liquid chromatography (HPLC)

430. In a radioimmunoassay, the less unlabeled antigen that is present in the assay mixture

A. The greater the amount of labeled antigen that binds to antibody

B. The lesser the number of counts per minute in the bound fraction

C. The greater the amount of unlabeled antigen that binds to antibody

D. The greater the number of counts per minute in the free fraction

TOXICOLOGY AND THERAPEUTIC DRUG MONITORING

431. Levels of 8–9% carboxyhemoglobin saturation of whole blood are commonly found in which of the following situations?

A. Fatal carbon monoxide poisoning

B. Acute carbon monoxide poisoning

C. Nonsmoking residents of rural areas

D. Cigarette smokers

432. Which of the following methods would yield reliable quantification of ethanol in the presence of isopropanol?
    A. Reaction with permanganate and chromotropic acid
    B. Conway diffusion followed by dichromate reaction
    C. Alcohol dehydrogenase reaction
    D. Gas-liquid chromatography

433. Which of the following tests would be particularly useful in determining isopropanol exposure?
    A. Serum osmolality and urine acetone
    B. Urine osmolality and serum osmolality
    C. Urine acetone and urine osmolality
    D. Serum sodium and serum acetone

434. Reinsch's test is used in screening urine for toxic concentrations of all the following *except*
    A. Bismuth
    B. Arsenic
    C. Mercury
    D. Cyanide

435. Heroin is synthesized from what drug?
    A. Diazepam
    B. Morphine
    C. Ecgonine
    D. Chlorpromazine

436. After absorption, codeine is rapidly metabolized to what compound?
    A. Phencyclidine
    B. Morphine
    C. Methadone
    D. Propoxyphene

437. THC (Δ^9-tetrahydrocannabinol) is the principal active component of what drug?
    A. Benzodiazepine
    B. Marijuana
    C. Morphine

    D. Codeine

438. Identification of the urinary metabolite ecgonine would be useful in determining exposure to which of the following drugs?
    A. Codeine
    B. Cocaine
    C. Amphetamine
    D. Propoxyphene

439. Of the following specimens, which would be appropriate for determining exposure to lead?
    A. EDTA plasma
    B. Serum
    C. Whole blood
    D. Cerebrospinal fluid

440. Free erythrocyte protoporphyrin (FEP) levels are useful as a screening method for exposure to which of the following metals?
    A. Zinc
    B. Lead
    C. Iron
    D. Mercury

441. Anticoagulated whole blood is the preferred specimen in determining exposure to what compound?
    A. Methanol
    B. Mercury
    C. Acetaminophen
    D. Carbon monoxide

442. What are the approximate number of half-life periods required for a serum drug concentration to reach 97–99% of the steady state?
    A. 1–3
    B. 2–4
    C. 5–7
    D. 7–9

443. For what colorimetric determination is the Trinder reaction widely used?

A. Acetaminophen

B. Propoxyphene

C. Salicylate

D. Barbiturate

444. Acetaminophen is particularly toxic to what organ?

A. Heart

B. Kidney

C. Spleen

D. Liver

445. Which of the following is an example of a long-acting barbiturate?

A. Phenobarbital

B. Amobarbital

C. Secobarbital

D. Pentobarbital

446. Increased trough levels of aminoglycosides in the serum are often associated with toxic effects to what organ?

A. Heart

B. Kidney

C. Pancreas

D. Liver

447. Which of the following is an example of an antiarrhythmic drug that has a metabolite with the same action?

A. Quinidine

B. Digoxin

C. Procainamide

D. Nortriptyline

448. In what form must a drug be in order to elicit a pharmacologic response?

A. Free

B. Bound to albumin

C. Bound to globulins

D. Bound to fatty acids

449. An epileptic patient receiving phenytoin develops acute glomerulonephritis. What

change, if any, would be expected in the patient's circulating drug level?

A. Decrease in free drug

B. Increase in free drug

C. Increase in protein-bound drug

D. No change in circulating drug level

450. Free drug levels can generally be determined by analyzing what body fluid?

A. Whole blood

B. Ultrafiltrate of plasma

C. Urine

D. Protein-free filtrate of plasma

451. Which of the following drugs is used as an immunosuppressant in organ transplantation, especially in liver transplants?

A. Methotrexate

B. Amiodarone

C. Tacrolimus

D. Paroxetine

452. Which of the following is a commonly encountered xanthine that could potentially interfere with the determination of theophylline?

A. Nicotine

B. Caffeine

C. Amphetamine

D. Procainamide

453. What is the major active metabolite of the anticonvulsant drug primidone?

A. Phenytoin

B. Acetazolamide

C. NAPA

D. Phenobarbital

454. Nortriptyline is the active metabolite of which of the following drugs?

A. Amitriptyline

B. Desipramine

C. Imipramine

D. Doxepin

455. Which of the following is used in the treatment of manic depression?
    A. Potassium
    B. Lithium
    C. Calcium
    D. Chloride

456. When is a blood sample for determination of the trough level of a drug appropriately drawn?
    A. During the absorption phase of the drug
    B. During the distribution phase of the drug
    C. Shortly before drug administration
    D. Two hours after drug administration

457. All the following statements are true concerning drug distribution patterns *except*
    A. Drug metabolism is slower in newborns than adults.
    B. Drug metabolism is more rapid for 6-year-old children than for adults.
    C. Renal clearance of drugs is faster in newborns than adults.
    D. Drug metabolism often changes during pubescence.

458. Which of the following serum components is able to alter the free drug level in plasma?
    A. Creatinine
    B. Urea
    C. Albumin
    D. Calcium

459. Which of the following is an example of a phenothiazine drug?
    A. Cyclosporine
    B. Theophylline
    C. Phenytoin
    D. Chlorpromazine

460. What is the recommended name for diphenylhydantoin?
    A. Phenytoin
    B. Nalorphine

    C. Primidone
    D. Carbamazepine

461. Which of the following classes of compounds has a sedative effect and as such is used to treat anxiety?
    A. Amphetamines
    B. Opiates
    C. Cannabinoids
    D. Benzodiazepines

462. What is the active metabolite of the antiarrhythmic drug procainamide?
    A. Pronestyl
    B. Disopyramide
    C. PEMA
    D. NAPA

463. Which of the following drugs is used as a bronchodilator?
    A. Theophylline
    B. Phenytoin
    C. Amikacin
    D. Clozapine

464. All the following are associated with the enzyme-multiplied immunoassay technique (EMIT) *except*
    A. Is a homogeneous enzyme immunoassay
    B. Determines antigen concentration
    C. Employs a labeled reactant
    D. Enzyme reacts with drug in serum sample

465. In the enzyme-multiplied immunoassay technique (EMIT), the enzyme is coupled to
    A. Antibody
    B. Antigen
    C. Substrate
    D. Coenzyme

466. The enzyme activity measured in the EMIT is the result of the reaction between the substrate and coenzyme with
    A. Free antibody
    B. Free unlabeled antigen

C. Free labeled antigen

D. Labeled antigen-antibody complexes

467. Radioimmunoassay methods are available for quantifying all the following *except*

A. Vitamins

B. Hormones

C. Electrolytes

D. Drugs

VITAMINS

468. Which of the following techniques is more commonly used to measure vitamins?

A. High-performance liquid chromatography

B. Spectrophotometry

C. Nephelometry

D. Microbiological

469. In the United States, most cases of scurvy occur in children between the ages of 7 months to 2 years. Scurvy is a disease caused by a deficiency in which of the following?

A. Vitamin A

B. Vitamin C

C. Vitamin D

D. Vitamin K

470. The term *lipid* encompasses a wide variety of compounds characterized as being insoluble in water but soluble in nonpolar solvents. All the following vitamins are lipid in nature and classified as fat-soluble *except*

A. Vitamin A

B. Vitamin C

C. Vitamin D

D. Vitamin E

471. Measuring which of the following compounds is useful in the diagnosis of steatorrhea?

A. Vitamin B_{12}

B. Vitamin C

C. Carotenoids

D. Folic acid

472. Which of the following is another name for vitamin B_{12}?

A. Retinol

B. Pyridoxine

C. Cyanocobalamin

D. Riboflavin

473. Vitamin B_{12} is associated with all the following items *except*

A. Insoluble in water

B. Intrinsic factor

C. Schilling test

D. Pernicious anemia

474. Which of the following tissues is important in vitamin D metabolism?

A. Skin

B. Spleen

C. Pancreas

D. Thyroid

475. A deficiency in which of these vitamins leads to increased clotting time and may result in hemorrhagic disease in infancy?

A. Riboflavin

B. Pyridoxine

C. Tocopherols

D. Menaquinone

476. Which vitamin is a constituent of two redox coenzymes?

A. Vitamin A

B. Vitamin B_2

C. Vitamin B_6

D. Vitamin C

477. Which disorder is associated with thiamin deficiency?

A. Beriberi

B. Pellagra

C. Rickets

D. Dermatitis

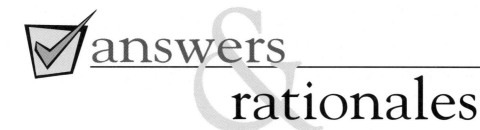

answers & rationales

INSTRUMENTATION AND ANALYTICAL PRINCIPLES

1.

A. A tungsten-filament lamp is the most common light source for photometry in the visible region. It provides a continuous spectrum (360–800 nm) from the near infrared (IR) through the visible to the near ultraviolet (UV) region. Most of the radiant energy is in the near IR. Only about 15% is in the visible region—the region usually used. Because of the large emission in the near IR, tungsten lamps generate a significant amount of heat. Hydrogen and deuterium lamps are used for work in the 200–375 nm range. The mercury vapor lamp does not provide a continuous spectrum, emitting radiation at specific wavelengths.

2.

B. Photometric methods are based on the use of Beer's law, which is applicable only for monochromatic light. A monochromator is a device for selecting a narrow band of wavelengths from a continuous spectrum. The three kinds of monochromators are filters, prisms, and diffraction gratings.

3.

C. A photomultiplier tube responds to the radiant energy (light) it absorbs by emitting electrons in a proportional amount to the initial light absorbed. These electrons then go through a series of stages where amplification occurs. The cascade effect, as the electrons go through 10 to 15 stages, results in

a final current that may be one million times the initial current. The photomultiplier tube exhibits rapid response time and sensitivity. These qualities also dictate that this type of detector be shielded from stray light and room light to prevent burnout. The rapid response time of a photomultiplier tube makes it able to monitor interrupted light beams produced by a chopper.

4.

D. A photomultiplier (PM) tube has two functions: (1) it is a transducer that converts light to electricity; (2) it amplifies the signal within the tube. Amplification can be as great as 1 million times. The emission of electrons by a light-sensitive surface, that is, the conversion of light energy to electrical energy, is virtually instantaneous. Hence, PM tubes have a very rapid response time. An iron plate and a layer of selenium are partial descriptions of the composition of a photocell or barrier layer cell.

5.

D. Photodiode array detectors are designed with 256 to 2048 photodiodes that are arranged in a linear fashion. This arrangement allows each photodiode to respond to a specific wavelength that results in a continuous UV/visible spectrum. Resolution is generally 1 to 2 nm.

6.

D. Wavelength calibration of a spectrophotometer is performed to verify that the radiant energy emitted from the monochromator through the exit slit is the same as the wavelength selector indicates. The glass filters holmium oxide, used in the ultraviolet (UV) and visible ranges, and didymium, used in the visible and near infrared (IR) regions, are employed to check wavelength accuracy. Solutions of stable chromogens such as nickel sulfate may be used. Source lamps may be replaced with mercury-vapor or deuterium lamps. These lamps have strong emission lines and provide the most accurate method of wavelength calibration.

7.

D. The reagent blank contains the same reagents as those used for assaying the specimen. By adjusting the spectrophotometer to $100\%T$ (or 0 absorbance) with the reagent blank, the instrument automatically subtracts the color contributed by the reagents from each succeeding reading of specimens, controls, and standards. This technique is used both in manual procedures and automated instruments. Since the reagent blank does not contain sample, there is no correction for interfering chromogens or lipemia.

8.

A. Measurement of an assay at two different wavelengths is termed bichromatic. The wavelengths chosen for absorbance readings will represent the peak and base of the spectral absorbance curve for the particular assay. By determining the difference between the two measured absorbances, the sample's concentration can be calculated with elimination of background interference from such substances as bilirubin and hemoglobin. Thus, bichromatic analysis functions as a reference blank for each individual sample.

9.

C. The bandpass or bandwidth is the range of wavelengths that are passed by a monochromator. In the example given, the bandpass will permit a 10 nm range of wavelengths to pass through the monochromator and impinge on the sample solution in the cuvet. Thus, 540 nm ± 5 nm (10 nm bandpass) will be equivalent to a wavelength range of 535–545 nm.

10.

A. When the absorbance of a sample in solution varies directly with the concentration of the sample, Beer's law is followed. In turn, when the absorbance increases exponentially with an increase in the light path, the Lambert law is followed. In-

corporation of these two laws may be stated as $A = abc$ where A = absorbance, a = absorptivity of the substance being measured, b = light path in cm, and c = concentration of the measured substance. When the Beer-Lambert law is applied to spectrophotometric analyses of standards and unknown samples that are being measured, the following equation is derived: $A_u \times \dfrac{C_s}{A_s} = C_u$ where A_u = absorbance of unknown, C_u = concentration of unknown, A_s = absorbance of standard, and A_u = absorbance of unknown. This formula is applied to assays that exhibit linear relationships between changes in absorbance with changes in concentration to calculate the concentration of the unknown sample.

11.

C. In spectrophotometry, molecules in solution will cause incident light to be absorbed while the remaining light energy will be transmitted. Absorbance is the term used to describe the monochromatic light that is absorbed by the sample, and transmittance describes the light that passes through the sample. The mathematical relationship between absorbance and transmittance is expressed by $A = 2 - \log \%T$.

12.

D. A single-beam spectrophotometer has only one light source and one detector. Its optical path is designed as a single alignment between the light source and the detector, and as such a single-beam instrument cannot read the absorbances of a sample and reagent blank simultaneously. In contrast, a double-beam spectrophotometer will be equipped with a vibrating or rotating mirror to direct the light path from one source in two directions. Light from each beam will strike the detector alternately or the system may be designed with two detectors, thus allowing a sample and a reagent blank to be read simultaneously. A double-beam-in-time spectrophotometer has as part of its general components: one light source, one monochromator, a beam splitter, a sample cuvette holder, and a reference cuvette holder. A double-beam-in-time spectrophotometer also has a chopper and a single detector system. The chopper is an important component, because its function is to alternately focus the beams from the sample cuvette and the reagent blank (reference) cuvette on the detector. The distinguishing feature of a double-beam-in-space spectrophotometer is that it has two detectors, one for the sample cuvette and the other for the reference (reagent blank) cuvette. Systems are designed with a beam splitter that divides the light coming from the light source into two beams. One beam passes through the sample cuvette and the other passes through the reference cuvette. The beams then fall on their respective detectors, with the absorbances being compared by a ratio recorder.

13.

D. Turbidimetry is the measurement of the amount of light blocked by particulate matter in passing through a turbid solution. The amount of light blocked depends on the number and the size of the particles. Hence the particle size in samples and standards must be comparable. Consistent timing of sample preparation and assay helps to avoid errors resulting from aggregation or settling of particles. The procedure is usually carried out at room temperature. Slight variations in temperature are not critical.

14.

C. In the dry reagent slide technique, as light from a radiant energy source passes through an interference filter, it is projected to the slide at a 45-degree angle. The light then follows a path through the clear support material and reagent layer and hits a white spreading layer; the unabsorbed light is then reflected back through the reagent and support layers. This reflected light impinges on the photodetector, which is positioned at a 90-degree angle to the slide. Since reflectance values are neither linearly proportional to transmission values nor consequently to dye concentration, the microcomputer utilizes an algorithm as a linearizing transformation of reflectance values to transmission values so that concentration may be calculated.

15.

D. In a fluorometer, light from the excitation lamp travels in a straight line, whereas the fluorescent light is radiated in all directions. If the detector for the emitted fluorescent light is placed at a right angle to the path of the excitation light, the excitation light will not fall on the detector. In addition, baffles can be placed around the cuvet to avoid reflection of the exciting light from the surface of the cuvet to the detector. The right-angle configu-

ration does not prevent loss of the exciting or the emitted light.

16.

A. Fluorescence occurs when a molecule absorbs light of a particular wavelength and is thereby stimulated to emit light of a longer wavelength. The emitted light has a characteristic spectrum, the emission spectrum, that is unique for each fluorescing molecule. Hence, fluorometric methods are extremely sensitive and highly specific. Because of this extreme sensitivity, reagents used must be of a higher degree of purity than is required for spectroscopy, since even slight traces of impurities may fluoresce.

17.

A. Instrumentation employing fluorescence polarization is used for measuring therapeutic drug levels and for fetal lung maturity testing. In these immunologic assays, plane-polarized light excites fluorophors in the sample cuvet. The free fluorophore-labeled ligands rotate freely because of their small size and primarily emit depolarized light. The labeled ligand-antibody complexes rotate slower because of their large size and emit polarized fluorescent light. Because of the differences in emitted light, it is not necessary to separate free from bound fluorophore-labeled ligands, allowing for use of the homogeneous assay technique. The emitted fluorescence intensity is measured by a polarization analyzer in the vertical plane, followed by its 90-degree movement for measurement in the horizontal plane. The amount of polarized light detected is inversely proportional to the concentration of ligand in the serum sample.

18.

A. Bioluminescence is a type of chemiluminescence in which the excitation energy is supplied by a chemical reaction rather than by radiant energy, as in fluorescence and phosphorescence. Bioluminescence assays may employ either an NADH:FMN oxidoreductase-bacterial luciferase or an adenosine triphosphate-firefly luciferase system. Bioluminescence assays are nonradioactive, having sensitivity levels in the attomole (10^{-18}) to zeptomole (10^{-21}) ranges, which makes them more sensitive than direct fluorescence assays. Bioluminescence has been applied in the development of immunoassays.

19.

B. Nephelometry is the measurement of the amount of light scattered by particles in suspension. The amount of light scattered depends on the size and shape of the particles and on the wavelength of the incident light. Ultraviolet light should not be used because it might produce some fluorescence, which would lead to erroneously high results.

20.

C. Radionuclides are quantified by measuring the amount of energy that they emit. This can be in the form of alpha emission ($^4_2He^{+2}$), beta emission (electrons ejected from the nucleus of a radioisotope during radioactive decay), or gamma emission (electromagnetic radiation emitted during radioactive decay). Beta and gamma emissions can be detected by scintillation counters. The sensing element of a scintillation counter is a fluor, a substance capable of converting radiation energy to light energy. The light energy is converted to electrical energy and amplified by a photomultiplier tube. A fluor commonly employed in solid scintillation counters is a large crystal of sodium iodide containing a small amount of thallium as an activator; it is used for gamma counting. Beta emission is counted by liquid scintillation counters using fluors dissolved in organic solvents. Alpha emission has very low penetrating power and is not measured in the clinical laboratory.

21.

B. Many metallic elements can absorb energy in the form of hcat. This moves their orbital electrons from the ground state to a higher energy level that is unstable. As the excited electrons drop back to the ground state, they give off their energy in the form of light at specific wavelengths unique for each element. The amount of light given off can be correlated to the amount of element present. This phenomenon provides the basis for flame emission photometry. Flame photometry is still used to some degree for determination of Li^+. However, the quantification of Na^+, K^+, and Li^+ is primarily accomplished by use of ion-selective electrodes.

22.

D. In a single-beam atomic absorption spectrophotometer, the amount of light that the analyte absorbs from the hollow cathode lamp is what we wish to know. However, what is actually measured is the intensity of the beam after it has passed through the flame. This measurement is made with and without sample in the flame. In this way the instrument calculates the amount of light absorbed because of the presence of the analyte in the flame.

23.

A. Atomic absorption spectrophotometry (AAS) is based on the principle that atoms in a basic ground state are capable of absorbing energy in the form of light at a specific wavelength. Since most samples usually have the analyte in the form of a compound or an ion, the analyte must first be converted to nonionized atoms. This is achieved by heating in a flame. About 99% of the atoms of analyte in the flame are in the ground state and, therefore, are capable of absorbing energy at the appropriate wavelength. Hence, light absorbed is essentially proportional to the concentration of the analyte. The light source in AAS is a hollow cathode lamp in which the cathode contains the element that is to be measured.

24.

C. The basis of AAS is the measurement of light, at a specific wavelength, that is absorbed by an element whose atoms are in a ground state. The flame in AAS serves two functions—to accept the sample, thus serving as a cuvet, and to supply heat for converting the element, which is usually present in the sample in molecular form, into its atomic form at ground state energy level. The hollow cathode lamp supplies the emission line of light required for the analysis.

25.

D. A beam chopper is a device for interrupting a beam of light so that a pulsed beam is produced. In an atomic absorption spectrophotometer, if the light entering the flame from the hollow cathode lamp is pulsed, then the light leaving the flame will consist of unabsorbed pulsed light and unpulsed light from the flame and from a small amount of emission by excited atoms of the analyte. The detector has an amplifier that is tuned to recognize and amplify only the pulsed signal. Thus errors caused by light from the flame and light emitted by the analyte are avoided. However, the beam chopper and tuned amplifier do not compensate for errors introduced by variations in flame temperature or deterioration of the hollow cathode lamp.

26.

A. The hollow cathode lamp is used in atomic absorption spectroscopy. The metal element of interest is coated on the cathode. When the inert gas, either argon or neon, becomes ionized, it is drawn toward the cathode. The impact excites the metal element coated on the cathode, resulting in the emission of spectral lines specific for the element. This light emission is then absorbed by the metal element in the sample.

27.

A. A half-cell, also called an electrode, is composed of a single metallic conductor surrounded by a solution of electrolyte. An electrochemical cell consists of two half-cells. If two different kinds of half-cells are connected in such a way as to make a complete circuit, a current will flow because of the potential difference between the two electrodes. The connection must be between the two metallic conductors and also between the two electrolyte solutions, usually by means of a salt bridge. In the analytical technique of potentiometry, a comparison is made between the voltage of one half-cell connected to another half-cell. It is customary that all half-cell potentials be compared to the potential generated by a standard electrode. The universally accepted standard half-cell with which all other half-cells are compared is the standard hydrogen electrode, arbitrarily assigned a potential E° of 0.000 volt.

28.

B. Oxidation involves the loss of electrons, and reduction the gain of electrons. In an electrolytic cell composed of two different half-cells—for example, zinc in zinc sulfate and copper in copper sulfate—electrons will flow from the anode to the cathode. Thus reduction takes place at the cathode, while oxidation occurs at the anode. Combination electrode refers to the combining of indicator and reference electrodes into a single unit. Electrode response refers to the ability of an ion-selective electrode to respond to a change in concentration of the ion being measured by exhibiting a change in potential.

29.

B. In practical applications of potentiometry, it is desirable to use one half-cell with a known and constant potential that is not sensitive to the composition of the material to be analyzed. This is called the reference electrode. One type of reference electrode is the calomel electrode, which consists of mercury covered by a layer of mercurous chloride in contact with a saturated solution of potassium chloride. The other half-cell, called the indicator electrode, is selected on the basis of the change in its potential with change in the concentration of the analyte of interest. The silver-silver chloride electrode is a commonly used type of reference electrode. The sodium and calcium electrodes are types of ion-selective electrodes.

30.

C. For optimum performance, pH-sensitive glass electrodes that are not actively in use should be kept immersed in an aqueous medium. Since the exact composition of the pH-sensitive glass varies from one manufacturer to another, the glass electrode should be maintained in the medium recommended by the manufacturer. Usual media are deionized water, dilute HCl, and buffer with a pH near the pH of the solution to be measured. The functioning of a glass electrode depends on the properties of the pH-sensitive glass. A typical glass electrode is made by sealing a thin piece of pH-sensitive glass at the end of a piece of glass tubing and filling the tube with a solution of hydrochloric acid saturated with silver chloride. A silver wire is immersed in the solution in the tube with one end extending outside the tube for external connection. This is essentially a silver/silver chloride reference electrode sealed within the tube with the pH-sensitive glass tip. This pH-sensitive glass functions appropriately only when it is saturated with water. Then each surface of the glass develops a hydrated lattice, where exchange of alkaline metal ions in the lattice for hydrogen ions in the test solution can occur.

31.

D. The ion-exchange electrode is a type of potentiometric, ion-selective electrode that consists of a liquid ion-exchange membrane that is made of an inert solvent and an ion-selective neutral carrier material. A collodion membrane may be used to separate the membrane solution from the sample solution being analyzed. Because of its ability to bind K^+, the antibiotic valinomycin is used as the neutral carrier for the K^+-selective membrane. The antibiotics nonactin and monactin are used in combination as the neutral carrier for the NH_4^+-selective membrane.

32.

C. Ion-selective electrodes for the measurement of sodium are glass membrane electrodes with selective capability. They are constructed from glass that consists of silicon dioxide, sodium oxide, and aluminum oxide. This type of electrode is based on the principle of potentiometry. Measurement errors may occur from protein buildup on the membrane surface. Potassium is measured using an ion-exchange electrode where the liquid ion-exchange membrane consists of valinomycin as the ion-selective carrier.

33.

D. A chloride coulometer employs a coulometric system based on Faraday's law, which states that in an electrochemical system, the number of equivalent weights of a reactant oxidized or reduced is directly proportional to the quantity of electricity used in the reaction. The quantity of electricity is measured in coulombs. The coulomb is the unit of electrical quantity; 1 coulomb of electricity flowing per minute constitutes a current of 1 ampere. Thus, if the current is constant, the number of equivalent weights of reactant oxidized or reduced depends only on the duration of the current. In the chloride coulometer, the electrochemical reaction is the generation of Ag^+ ions by the passage of a direct current across a pair of silver electrodes immersed in a conducting solution containing the sample to be assayed for chloride. As the Ag^+ ions are generated, they are immediately removed from solution by combining with chloride to form insoluble silver chloride. When all the chloride is precipitated, further generation of Ag^+ ions causes an increase in conductivity of the solution. Thus the instrument provides an electrometric titration, in which the titrant is Ag^+ ions and the end point of the titration is indicated by the increase in conductivity of the solution. Amperometry is used to measure the increase in conductivity. The amperometric circuit includes a second pair of silver elec-

trodes that are immersed in the solution. They are provided with a small, steady constant voltage. The appearance of free Ag^+ ions in the solution generates a sharp increase in conductivity, which, in turn, causes a sudden rise in the current between the electrodes in the amperometric circuit. This increase in current activates a relay that stops the further generation of Ag^+ ions and also stops an automatic timer placed in the circuit to measure the total duration of current in the coulometric circuit. While this system is no longer used for routine analysis, it is still employed for sweat chloride analysis.

34.

C. In an amperometric glucose electrode system, glucose oxidase reacts with glucose to produce hydrogen peroxide and gluconic acid. The platinum electrode that operates at a positive potential oxidizes the hydrogen peroxide to oxygen. The oxidation of hydrogen peroxide produces a current that is directly proportional to the glucose level in the sample.

35.

D. A pH/blood gas analyzer contains a pH-sensitive glass electrode, a P_{CO_2} electrode, and a P_{O_2} electrode. The glass electrode is calibrated by comparison with two primary standard buffers of known pH. Since pH readings are temperature sensitive, the calibration must be carried out at a constant temperature of 37 °C. pH readings are not appreciably sensitive to changes in barometric pressure. Note that if the P_{CO_2} and P_{O_2} electrodes were also to be calibrated, then it would be essential to know the barometric pressure, since that affects the P_{CO_2} and P_{O_2} calibrating gases.

36.

B. In a blood gas analyzer, the P_{CO_2} electrode is actually a pH electrode immersed in a bicarbonate solution. The bicarbonate solution is separated from the sample by a membrane that is permeable to gaseous CO_2 but not to ionized substances such as H^+ ions. When CO_2 from the sample diffuses across the membrane, it dissolves, forming carbonic acid and thus lowering the pH. The pH is inversely proportional to the log of the P_{CO_2}. Hence the scale of the meter can be calibrated directly in terms of P_{CO_2}. It should be noted that whereas pH refers to the negative logarithm of the H^+ ion concentration, Pco_2 refers to the partial pressure of CO_2.

37.

B. In a blood gas analyzer, the electrode for measuring the partial pressure of oxygen (Po_2) in the blood is an electrochemical cell consisting of a platinum cathode and a Ag/AgCl anode connected to an external voltage source. The cathode and anode are immersed in buffer. A polypropylene membrane selectively permeable to gases separates the buffer from the blood sample. When there is no oxygen diffusing into the buffer, there is practically no current flowing between the cathode and the anode because they are polarized. When oxygen diffuses into the buffer from a sample, it is reduced at the cathode. The electrons necessary for this reduction are produced at the anode. Hence a current flows; the current is directly proportional to the Po_2 in the sample.

38.

A. In polarography, an electrochemical cell is used. A gradually increasing voltage is applied between the two electrodes of the cell that are in contact with a solution containing the analyte. The current flowing in the system is measured. Plotting the voltage change *vs.* current change gives a polarogram. The voltage at which the sharp rise in current occurs is characteristic of the electrochemical reaction involved, that is, characteristic of the analyte. The amount of increase in current (i.e., the wave height) is proportional to the concentration of analyte. In anodic stripping voltammetry, a negative potential is applied to one of the electrodes. Trace metal ions in the solution are thereby reduced and plated onto the anodic electrode. This is a preconcentrating step. The plated electrode is then used as the anode in a polarographic cell. The metal is thereby stripped off the anode. The current flow during the stripping provides a polarogram that both identifies and quantifies the trace metals. The method is particularly appropriate for assaying heavy metals such as lead in blood.

39.

A. Colligative properties of a solution are those properties that depend only on the number of particles in solution, not on the nature of the particles. The colligative properties are boiling point, freezing point, osmotic pressure, and vapor pressure. Terms used to describe the concentration of particles in

solution are osmole (the number of particles, 6.0224×10^{23}, that lowers the freezing point 1.86 °C) and osmolal (a concentration of 1 Osm of solute per kilogram of water). One mole of an unionized solute dissolved in 1 kg of water lowers the freezing point 1.86 °C. Thus it is an osmolal solution. For un-ionized substances such as glucose, 1 mol equals 1 Osm. For substances that ionize, such as sodium chloride, wherein each molecule in solution becomes two ions and thus two particles, 1 mol of sodium chloride theoretically equals 2 Osm. In reality, however, this is not always the case; an osmotic activity coefficient factor is used to correct for the deviation. In practice, three types of osmometers are available. They are the freezing point, vapor pressure, and colloid osmotic pressure osmometers.

40.

D. The freezing point of an aqueous solution is lowered 1.86 °C for every osmole of dissolved particles per kilogram of water. These particles may be ions, for example Na^+ and Cl^-, or undissociated molecules such as glucose. The freezing point osmometer is an instrument designed to measure the freezing point of solutions. It uses a thermistor that is capable of measuring very small changes in temperature.

41.

D. When the osmolality has been both measured in the laboratory and calculated, the osmolal gap may then be determined by subtracting the calculated osmolality from the measured. Plasma osmolality may be calculated when the plasma sodium, glucose, and urea nitrogen values are known. The equation for calculating osmolality expresses Na^+, glucose, and urea nitrogen in mmol/L (SI units). To convert glucose and urea nitrogen from mg/dL to mmol/L, the conversion factors 0.056 and 0.36 are used respectively. For sodium, the factor 2 is used to count the cation (sodium) once and its corresponding anion once. Since glucose and urea nitrogen are undissociated molecules, they are each counted once. Use the following equation. Calculated osmolality (mOsm/kg) =

$$2.0 \text{ Na}^+ \text{ (mmol/L)} + \text{Glucose (mmol/L)} + \text{Urea nitrogen (mmol/L)}$$

$$2.0 \text{ (142 mmol/L)} + (0.056 \times 130 \text{ mg/dL}) + (0.36 \times 18 \text{ mg/dL}) = \text{mOsm/kg}$$

$$284 + 7.3 + 6.5 = 298 \text{ mOsm/kg}$$

42.

C. The colloid osmotic pressure (COP) osmometer is composed of a semipermeable membrane that separates two chambers, a mercury manometer, a pressure transducer, and a meter. When a serum sample is introduced into the sample chamber, saline solution from the reference chamber moves across the membrane by osmosis. This causes the development of a negative pressure on the saline side that is equivalent to the COP, which represents the amount of protein in the serum sample. COP osmometers measure the serum protein contribution to the total osmolality in terms of millimeters of mercury. COP levels are helpful in monitoring intravenous fluid therapy.

43.

B. Electrophoresis is a method of separating charged particles by their rates of migration in an electric field. An electrophoretic chamber consists of two reservoirs to hold buffer, a means of supporting a strip in the chamber so that the ends are dipping into the reservoirs, and a means of applying an electric current to the strip. The whole chamber is sealed to make it vaporproof.

44.

A. Capillary electrophoresis is based on electroosmotic flow (EOF). When an electric field is applied, the flow of liquid is in the direction of the cathode. Thus, EOF regulates the speed at which solutes move through the capillary. Cations migrate the fastest, since EOF and electrophoretic attraction are in the direction of the cathode.

45.

C. Protein molecules can exist as anions, cations, or zwitterions, depending on the pH of the solution in which they are placed. The pH at which they exist in the form of zwitterions and hence have no net charge is called the isoelectric point. The principle of isoelectric focusing is based on the ability to separate proteins due to differences in their isoelectric points. Aliphatic polyamino polycarboxylic acids, known as ampholytes, are used to produce the pH gradient.

46.

B. In thin-layer chromatography (TLC), the R_f describes the distance traveled by the solute (compound of interest) in relation to the distance traveled by the solvent (mobile phase). Measurements of the TLC plate are made from the origin or point of sample application to the center of the developed spot and from the origin to the solvent front. An R_f may be calculated by means of the following formula:

$$R_f = \frac{\text{Distance from origin to spot center}}{\text{Distance from origin to solvent front}} \times 100$$

$$R_f = \frac{48 \text{ mm}}{141 \text{ mm}} \times 100 = 34$$

The R_f of the compound of interest, along with chromogenic spray characteristics, may then be compared with standards for identification of the unknown compound.

47.

C. The column and carrier gas flow rate used in gas chromatography are important aspects of the separation and resolving power of the system. When the column eluent is introduced into a mass spectrometer, additional information pertaining to elemental composition, position of functional groups, and molecular weight may be determined for the purpose of identifying compounds, e.g., drugs in biological samples. Mass spectrometers consist of a vacuum system, ion source, mass filter, and detector.

48.

C. High-performance liquid chromatography (HPLC) systems are composed of four basic units: sample-introduction system, solvent-delivery system, column, and detector. The sample-introduction system is generally a fixed-loop injection valve, which allows the sample to be injected into a stainless steel external loop for flushing onto the column by the solvent. The solvent-delivery system may be composed of one or two pumps for the purpose of forcing the mobile phase and sample through the column. Photometric, fluorometric, and electrochemical detectors are available for monitoring the eluate as it emerges from the column.

49.

C. In HPLC, the technique used for the mobile phase may be isocratic or gradient elution. With isocratic elution the strength of the solvent remains constant during the separation. With gradient elution the strength of the solvent is continually increased (percent per minute) during the separation process. The gradient elution technique is sometimes employed to improve HPLC resolution and sensitivity.

50.

A. Discrete analyzers are designed so that each specimen-reagent mixture is analyzed separately in its own vessel. While a discrete analyzer may be designed to measure only one analyte, most discrete analyzers are very versatile and are able to run multiple tests on each sample. In addition, some discrete analyzers also have random access capability that allows STAT samples to be easily accessed.

51.

B. High-performance liquid chromatography (HPLC) is also called high-pressure liquid chromatography. It is a form of column chromatography in which a liquid moving phase is actively pumped through the column, thus speeding the separation process considerably. HPLC is used in therapeutic drug monitoring and in assaying vitamin and hormone concentrations.

52.

A. Chromatography provides a variety of means of separating mixtures of substances on the basis of their physicochemical properties, primarily their solubility in a variety of solvents. Chromatographic methods always involve a stationary phase and a mobile phase. The sample containing the substances to be separated is carried in the mobile phase; the mobile phase passes over the stationary phase at different rates depending on their relative solubilities in the two phases. The amount of separation depends on (1) the rate of diffusion, (2) the solubility of the substances being separated, and (3) the nature of the solvent. In thin-layer chromatography (TLC), the stationary phase is a thin layer of some sorbent such as silica gel uniformly spread on a piece of glass or plastic.

53.

D. In gas-liquid chromatography (GLC), the stationary phase is a liquid adsorbed on particles packed in a column. The mobile phase is a gas that passes through the column. Since the sample is carried in the mobile phase, it must be volatile at the temperature of the column so that it can be carried by the gas. In addition, separation is dependent on the

solubility of the solute in the liquid layer of the stationary phase.

54.

B. Ion-exchange chromatography utilizes synthetic ion-exchange resins. They may be cation- or anion-exchange resins. They can be used in either a column or a thin layer. Separation of mixtures of substances by ion-exchange chromatography depends primarily on the sign and the ionic charge density of the substances being separated.

55.

A. Mass spectrometry identifies a compound based on the compound's molecular weight. It also identifies the positioning of functional groups of the compound. This technique is useful in the clinical laboratory for drug identification.

56.

D. Mass spectrometry is used in the clinical laboratory in conjunction with gas or liquid chromatography (GC-MS). In gas chromatography a compound is identified by its retention time. If two compounds have very similar retention times, the compound may be misidentified. Gas chromatography complements mass spectrometry in that the eluted peak is subjected to mass spectrometric analysis for molecular weight determination. Use of the two systems in tandem allows for more accurate identification of compounds.

57.

A. Centrifugal force depends on the mass and on the speed and radius of rotation. Since most materials being centrifuged in the clinical laboratory have specific gravity close to 1.00, only the speed and radius need be considered. The relative centrifugal force (RCF) is calculated by the formula:

$$RCF = 1.118 \times 10^{-5} \times r \times (rpm)^2$$

where r = radius in centimeters and rpm = the number of revolutions per minute. The RCF is expressed as a number times the force of gravity (or the number × g). The radius is measured from the center of the centrifuge shaft to the inside bottom of the centrifuge cup. The number of revolutions per minute (rpm) is measured by a tachometer. The centrifugal force is not influenced by temperature.

58.

D. In an angle-head centrifuge, the cups are rigidly supported in the head at a fixed angle to the shaft, and they are fully enclosed within the head. In a horizontal-head centrifuge, the cups hang down in a vertical position when the centrifuge is at rest and swing out to a horizontal position when the centrifuge is rotating. Because cups in the angle-head centrifuge are enclosed in a head specifically designed to reduce wind resistance, there is less air friction and, consequently, less of an increase in sample temperature during centrifugation. Because of the reduced wind resistance, angle-head centrifuges can provide a force of over $9000 \times g$, whereas horizontal-head centrifuges provide about $1650 \times g$.

59.

D. The National Institute of Standards and Technology (NIST) recognizes the use of five specific types of calibrating weights. Analytical balances should be checked monthly and prior to accurate analytical work for proper calibration using Class S weights. To calibrate the weights themselves, Class M weights are used to check other weights, since their quality is that of a primary standard. Class P weights are allowed greater tolerance levels than Class S-1, with the latter being used for routine analytical work. Class J weights are used for microanalytical work.

60.

D. With automated instruments the quality of the specimen and its handling are critical to producing accurate test results. Sampling errors can occur that cause falsely low results to be generated. These errors include short sampling, air pocket in the bottom of the sample cup, and fibrin clots in the sample probe.

61.

D. The accuracy of the thermometer used to monitor the incubation temperature of an instrument should be verified every 6 to 12 months. Thermometers certified by the NIST should be used to check all thermometers used in the laboratory. For the monitoring of enzymatic reactions, thermometers should agree within 0.1 °C with the NIST reference thermometer. Thermometers used to check refrigerator and freezer temperatures should agree within 1.0 °C with the reference thermometer.

Thermometers should be discarded if they differ by more than 1 °C from the reference thermometer. On a daily basis the operation temperature of the incubation area should be checked, and the thermometer itself should be observed for splits in the mercury column.

62.

C. As part of a good quality assurance program, a laboratory should perform function verification, performance verification, and preventive maintenance for all instrument systems. Function verification is the monitoring of specific instrument functions, and the correcting of these functions when necessary to assure reliable operation. Function verification includes the monitoring and recording of temperature, electronic parameters, instrument calibration, and the analysis of quality control material.

63.

D. It is imperative that preventive maintenance procedures be performed and the results recorded for all laboratory instrumentation. This includes maintenance of analytical balances, refrigerators, freezers, centrifuges, ovens, water baths, heating blocks, thermometers, pipetters, dilutors, automated analyzers, and all other laboratory equipment used for analyzing specimens. Preventive maintenance is performed at scheduled times such as per shift, daily, weekly, monthly, or yearly.

64.

D. In order to prevent excessive downtime and costly repairs, a preventive maintenance schedule should be devised, implemented, and recorded for all laboratory equipment. Preventive maintenance procedures include the cleaning of instrument components, the replacing of worn parts, and the adjusting of certain parts or parameters. Following a preventive maintenance schedule will help to extend the life of the equipment. It is important that all laboratory personnel recognize the need for routine maintenance and follow prescribed maintenance schedules.

QUALITY ASSURANCE

65.

C. The arithmetic mean of a set of numbers is obtained by adding all the numbers in the set and dividing the sum by the number of values in that set.

It is a precise way of expressing what is often called the average. It is not to be confused with the mode, which is the value that occurs most frequently in the set. The geometric mean is the antilogarithm of the sum of the logarithms of all the values divided by the number of values. The median is the middle value in a set of numbers that are arranged according to their magnitude.

66.

B. The coefficient of variation is calculated from the formula

$$CV = \frac{s}{\overline{X}} \times 100\%$$

where CV = coefficient of variation, s = standard deviation, and $\overline{X}$ = mean. Given that the mean = 89 mg/dL and 2 s = 14 mg/dL,

$$CV = \frac{7}{89} \times 100\% = 7.86\%$$

Since there are only two significant figures in each of the given numbers, there can be only two figures in the answer. Therefore the answer, rounded to the nearest tenth, is 7.9, not 7.8.

67.

A. Any analytical result has some degree of uncertainty because of unavoidable random errors in the procedure. A Levey-Jennings quality control chart is a graphic representation of the acceptable limits of variation in the results of an analytical method. To prepare such a chart, it is first necessary to obtain a large-enough batch of normal and abnormal pooled serum to last for a minimum of 12 months. Analyses of aliquots of the pools are done in duplicate over a period of 20 days, preferably by all workers who will subsequently be using the controls. The data thus collected are statistically analyzed to determine the mean and standard deviation. Any results falling above or below the mean ±3 s are discarded. The mean and standard deviation are then recalculated. The acceptable range is assigned, usually the mean ±2 s. The data thus developed are used to prepare the Levey-Jennings quality control chart.

68.

B. The purpose of a quality control chart is to facilitate the identification of analytical problems that are not otherwise apparent. A quality control program must include clearly written instructions for the steps that

are to be taken when a control serum value is out-of-control. These instructions must be used whenever a set of test results is out of the established control limits. Usually the procedures will include a visual inspection of the equipment, reagents, and instruments used, and a check of calculations. The next step might be to rerun the batch of tests with a fresh aliquot of control serum. Additional steps to take include preparing newly reconstituted controls, recalibration of the instrument, and using a fresh bottle of reagent. Out-of-control results should never be reported to the physician.

69.

A. When assessing daily, internal quality control, the Westgard multirule procedure aids in interpretation of control data. A chart similar to the Levey-Jennings chart is constructed with control limits drawn at the mean as well as ±1 s, ±2 s, ±3 s and even ±4 s. The Westgard multirules are then applied to the graphical representation, giving a more structured approach to data interpretation.

70.

C. On a quality control chart, when the control values change abruptly and on several consecutive days are consistently on one side of the mean, although within the ±2 s limits, this is called a shift. An upward shift could be produced by changing to a new standard (calibrator) that was prepared in error at a lower concentration than specified. A downward shift could be caused by the use of too concentrated a standard (calibrator) than what is specified. A gradual change observed over the course of several days is called a trend. It may be upward or downward. Its presence suggests gradual deterioration of one of the reagents or instrument components.

71.

C. If the range of acceptable values for a quality control material is based on the ±2 s intervals on either side of the expected mean value for the control, then about 19 of every 20 values obtained for the control are expected to fall within the acceptable range. Conversely, about 1 of every 20 values obtained are expected to fall outside the ±2 s range with about 1 of every 40 values above the upper acceptable limit and the same number below the acceptable limit. For example, if a digoxin control is established to have an acceptable range from 2.0 to 2.6 ng/mL, about 1 value in 40 would be expected above 2.6 ng/mL.

72.

C. When the values on a quality control chart show a gradual downward drift during the month, possible causes are deterioration of reagents because of aging or concentration of standards (calibrators) because of evaporation. Other considerations such as inadequate mixing of control material, contamination of standards (calibrators) and faulty recalibration are all sources of error that will affect the quality control data, but they would not be expressed as a drift. The system is out-of-control, even though the control values lie within the $\pm 2\,s$ range.

73.

A. A Youden plot is a type of quality control chart that is used to compare results obtained on a high and low control serum by several different laboratories. It is particularly useful for interlaboratory quality control programs. The Youden plot displays the results of the analyses by plotting the mean values for one specimen on the ordinate and the other specimen on the abscissa. It is desirable for a laboratory to have its point fall at the center of the plot.

74.

C. The choice of appropriate concentrations for control materials is important in implementing a quality control program. The concentrations chosen should be sensitive to assay variability in the clinically significant region of the particular compound being measured. For instance, the therapeutic range for the drug gentamicin in many laboratories is a trough level of less than 2 µg/mL and a peak level of 5 to 8 µg/mL. Control levels of 1.5 and 6 µg/mL would appropriately monitor both trough and peak regions of the standard curve. If both controls are above 5 or below 4 µg/mL, only one region of the curve would be monitored.

75.

A. Scheduling of staff is not involved in quality assurance programs. Quality assurance in a broad sense includes monitoring every aspect of laboratory work from collection and identification of specimens to delivery of valid results to the physician. Laboratory protocol should include procedures that ensure that the correct specimen is collected and that the specimen is correctly labeled. The quality of the laboratory supplies, including the deionized water and reagents, should meet the specifications of the appropriate professional or governmental agency (i.e., the College of American Pathologists, the American Chemical Society, or the National Institute of Standards and Technology). The accuracy and precision of the analyses should be ensured through the use of appropriate standards (calibrators) and controls. Also, quality control charts that define the acceptable range of results for control specimens and participation in external proficiency testing programs are part of any quality assurance program. Since most analyses are done with instruments, the performance of the instruments must be monitored. Establishment of a regularly scheduled preventive maintenance program provides for optimum performance of the instruments as well as continuous monitoring of their performance.

76.

D. On a quality control chart the acceptable range generally encompasses the mean $\pm 2\,s$. The control values should occur randomly in this area, falling to both sides of the mean. If more than five successive plots occur at a constant level in one area, e.g., near the $\pm 2\,s$ line, an out-of-control situation should be considered. One plot falling outside the mean $\pm 2\,s$ in 20 successive days is expected statistically. While one should be alert to the possibility of a potential problem, it does not necessarily imply an out-of-control situation. However, the occurrence of a value outside the area of $\pm 3\,s$ would require corrective action.

77.

C. When a quality control chart shows a sudden shift in daily values, there are several possible causes. Use of a new batch of reagents or reference standards (calibrators) that have been improperly made can cause such a shift. Another cause for a sudden shift in daily values might be a change in one of the components of the instrument used, such as a new lamp in a spectrophotometer. Whenever an instrument component is changed, the instrument must be recalibrated. A change in operating personnel should not cause any change in quality control values.

78.

C. An external quality assurance procedure involves analyzing specimens that are provided by some external agency to all laboratories participating in the program. The results are sent to the agency, which then provides a statistical analysis of all results to each participating laboratory. This allows a laboratory to evaluate its performance by comparing the mean, the standard deviation, and the coefficient of variation for each of its methods with those of other laboratories that are using the same method. In addition, a comparison of results obtained by different methods for the same analyte based on a comparison of their standard deviations and coefficients of variation can be used to select the most reliable methods for a particular laboratory. A consistent bias, either positive or negative, would be apparent from the results generated in an external quality assurance procedure, as would a totally out-of-control situation.

79.

D. The standard deviation reflects how much the data values vary around the mean. The mean is the arithmetic average of the data and is a measure of the location of the distribution. The median describes the middle value; half of the observations are greater than the median, half are less than the median. The mode is the most frequently obtained value. The coefficient of variation expresses random variation of analytical methods in units independent of methodology, because it is a percentage comparison of the standard deviation divided by the mean.

80.

B. Precision defines the reproducibility of an analytical method. Accuracy describes the ability of an analytical method to obtain a "true" value. Random errors are deviations from the true value caused by indeterminate and, therefore, unavoidable errors inherent in every laboratory analysis.

81.

C. A Gaussian (normal) distribution is a population probability distribution that is symmetric about the mean. The mean, median, and mode are the same value when the data fit this type of distribution. The parametric analysis is the statistical method of choice.

82.

A. Random errors are deviations from the true value caused by unavoidable errors inherent in laboratory measurements. The standard error of the mean is a statistical concept reflecting sampling variation. It is the standard deviation of the entire population. Parametric statistics refer to a Gaussian (normal) distribution of data. Nonparametric statistics are more general and require no assumptions.

83.

D. To determine the standard deviation, compute the difference between each value and the mean $(x - \overline{x})$, square the differences, and add all the squared differences $[\Sigma (x - \overline{x})^2]$. Then divide the sum by one less than the number of values $(n - 1)$ and take the square root. The standard deviation is the estimated random error.

84.

C. The accuracy of an analytical result is the closeness with which the measured value agrees with the true value. Precision is reproducibility. Accuracy and precision are independent, but it is the goal of the clinical laboratory to design methods that are both precise and accurate.

85.

C. The normal distribution is a symmetric distribution about the mean. In a normal distribution, 95.45% of the values will be within an area enclosed by the mean $\pm 2\ s$ and approximately 5% will normally fall outside; 68.26% will lie within $\pm 1\ s$; 99.74% will lie within $\pm 3\ s$. The $\pm 2\ s$ (95.45%) interval forms the basis of statistical quality control in the laboratory.

86.

C. Variance is one way in which members of a group are dispersed about the mean. It is a square of the standard deviation (s^2). Both standard deviation and variance are measures that describe how observed values vary.

87.

D. Confidence intervals are regions within a Gaussian curve that reflect on the percentage of data that will normally fall within the stated region. The usual confidence limit used to evaluate data in the clinical laboratory is the mean $\pm 2\ s$ (in actuality, it is the mean $\pm 1.96\ s$) at a 95% confidence limit. This means that one can be confident that 95% of the data will normally fall within $\pm 2\ s$ of the mean.

88.

A. The reliability of an analytical procedure is its ability to maintain accuracy and precision over an extended period of time during which supplies, equipment, and personnel in the laboratory may change. It is often used interchangeably with the term consistency. It is the goal of every clinical laboratory to produce reliable results.

89.

B. The variance is the measure of dispersion, which is the square of the standard deviation. To determine the variance, find the difference between each value and the mean, square this difference, add the differences, and divide by one less than the number of values. The variance reflects scattering about the mean.

90.

C. A control is a specimen of known concentration with physical and chemical properties closely resembling the test specimen. The control is generally composed of the same matrix as the sample. The concentrations of analytes in different control materials should be in the normal and abnormal ranges. Both primary standards and calibrators are used to calculate the concentration of specimens being analyzed. Calibrators are considered secondary standards and must meet specific criteria as outlined by NCCLS. These criteria need not be met for controls and thus their uses cannot be interchanged.

91.

A. A standard is a material of known composition and a stated high degree of purity. Standards of particular interest to the clinical laboratory scientist are available from the National Institute of Standards and Technology. Because each standard reference material is described with regard to certain chemical or physical properties, it can be used to characterize other materials. The concentration of secondary standards is determined by testing using a reference method calibrated with a primary standard. Calibrators should meet the criteria of secondary standards.

92.

D. Maintaining quality assurance includes control of pre-analytical, analytical and post-analytical factors. One variable to assess is turnaround time. It is the total amount of time required to procure the specimen, prepare the specimen, run the test, and relate the results. The supervisor should refer to the turnaround time of the stated procedure and relate to the techs the need to work within the stated limits.

93.

D. The College of American Pathologists (CAP) comprehensive survey involves thousands of participating clinical chemistry laboratories. This survey and others have been established to provide independent validation of quality control programs. A CAP survey provides unknown samples for analysis. The program, when properly used, gives valid estimation of the inherent accuracy of a system. ISCLT, ASCLS, and ASCP are all organizations to which medical laboratory personnel may apply for professional membership.

94.

B. Whenever one needs to review the details of a procedure, she/he should review the procedure manual and notify the supervisor so that guidance can be received. The procedure manual is one way in which a laboratory can document analytical protocols. This leads to consistency in test results regardless of which person is performing the analysis.

95.

C. When checking control results that fall outside acceptable limits, one can apply the Westgard Multirule procedure, specifically 1_{3s}. Anytime only one control is used and it exceeds the mean $\pm 3\ s$, you must reject the test run. You should check out the instrument and reagent system to locate the problem if possible. A new control along with the patient specimens should be analyzed. No results should be reported until the control is within the limits of $\pm 2\ s$ from the mean.

96.

C. Westgard multirule 2_{2s} describes an out-of-control situation where two consecutive data points fall outside the same mean $+2\ s$ or fall outside the same mean $-2\ s$. This is an example of systematic error. The test run would be rejected, and all samples would need to be retested.

97.

D. When one control point exceeds the mean by $+2\,s$ and a second control point exceeds the mean by $-2\,s$, the R_{4s} multirule will apply. In this case the out-of-control problem is most likely due to random error. The test run would be rejected, and all samples would need to be retested.

98.

D. When the same test is ordered on a patient more than once, a delta check can be performed to compare consecutive test results. Bilirubin results obtained on two consecutive days on an adult should not vary by more than 50%. If the results vary by greater than 50%, it is most likely that an error has occurred or that an acute change has taken place. One of the first things to check is proper identification of the patient's specimen. As part of a quality assurance program, one should also check patient results based on the clinical correlation of laboratory test results.

99.

A. When comparing a potential new test with a comparative method in order to bring a new method into the laboratory, linear regression analysis should be performed using the results of the two methods. By calculating the slope and y intercept, the presence of systematic error can be identified. Unlike random error that is due to chance and can occur in either direction, systematic error consistently affects results in only one direction. Specific types of systematic error are termed constant and proportional, but the stated question did not give sufficient information to differentiate between the types.

100.

D. While some laboratories may use the reference interval recommended by the manufacturer or ranges published in medical books, it is preferred that laboratories establish their own limits. When subjects are not easily available, a laboratory should use at least 20 individuals to verify a published range. Whenever possible a minimum of 120 subjects from each age and sex group should be included in the reference interval study.

101.

D. When the population served by a laboratory is similar to that described by a manufacturer, then the reference interval published by the manufacturer can be adopted provided the laboratory successfully completes a small study. Such a study need only include 20 individuals. If two or less subjects tested have test values that fall outside the suggested range, then the manufacturer's reference interval can be used. If three or more subjects have test values that fall outside the range, then an additional 20 subjects need to be tested. Provided that two or less are outside the range on this second attempt, then the manufacturer's reference interval can be accepted. In the event that this second attempt fails, the laboratory should assess what differences there may be between their population and that of the manufacturer. If differences cannot be determined, then a complete reference interval study using 120 subjects should be completed by the laboratory.

102.

D. To determine the percent of individuals with a positive test result who actually have the disease, the predictive value of a positive test is calculated. The sensitivity, specificity, and disease prevalence must be known to calculate the predictive value. Sensitivity in this case refers to the percent of individuals having the disease who test positively. Specificity refers to the percent of individuals who do not have the disease and test negatively.

103.

A. The *sensitivity* of a test is the percentage of individuals with a specific disease that are correctly identified or predicted by the test as having the disease. To determine the sensitivity of an assay, the true positives, represented by the number of individuals correctly identified by the test as having the disease, and the false negatives, represented by the number of diseased individuals not correctly identified by the test, must be established for the assay in question. The formula for determining sensitivity follows, where TP = true positives and FN = false negatives.

$$\text{Sensitivity} = \frac{\text{TP}}{\text{TP} + \text{FN}} \times 100$$

104.

C. The *specificity* of a test is the percentage of individuals without the specific disease that are correctly identified or predicted by the test as not having the disease. To determine the specificity of an assay, the true negatives, represented by the number of individuals correctly identified by the test as not having the disuse, and the false positives, represented by the number of nondiseased individuals not correctly identified by the test, must be established for the assay in question. The formula for determining specificity follows, where TN = true negatives and FP = false positives.

$$\text{Specificity} = \frac{TN}{FP + TN} \times 100$$

$$= \frac{45}{5 + 45} \times 100$$

$$= \frac{45}{50} \times 100$$

$$\text{Specificity} = 90\%$$

105.

A. The predictive value of a test utilizes the parameters of test sensitivity and specificity as well as disease prevalence. The predictive value of a negative test, i.e., the percentage of individuals who test negative and are not diseased, may be determined by knowing the number of true negatives and false negatives. The formula for determining the predictive value of a negative test (PV⁻) follows, where TN = true negatives and FN = false negatives.

$$PV^- = \frac{TN}{TN + FN} \times 100$$

106.

D. A proficiency testing program is part of external quality control that aids a lab in assessing the quality of its testing methods. Samples of unknown concentrations are purchased through a recognized professional agency such as the College of American Pathologists or the American Association of Bioanalysts. Following analysis of the samples, the lab sends its results to the agency for review. If significant problems are detected, the laboratory needs to take corrective action.

107.

A. ISO 9000 is a group of four standards with the general purpose of promoting principles of quality

management and quality assurance into the manufacturing and service industries. The International Organization for Standardization (ISO) is an international federation. Clinical laboratories interested in certification would adopt ISO 9002 standards. To date, the main impact of ISO 9000 has been on transfusion laboratories in the U.S. who have begun to follow the standards.

CARBOHYDRATES

108.

D. When two monosaccharides condense with loss of a molecule of water, a disaccharide is formed. Disaccharides, therefore, can be hydrolyzed into two monosaccharides. The most important disaccharides are maltose, lactose, and sucrose. On hydrolysis, sucrose will yield one molecule of glucose and one molecule of fructose. Maltose can be hydrolyzed into two molecules of glucose. Lactose can be hydrolyzed into glucose and galactose.

109.

A. Glycogen is a polysaccharide composed of many glucose molecules. In contrast to the amylopectin molecule, a glycogen molecule is more highly branched and more compact. Glycogen is found in a variety of animal tissues, particularly in the liver, providing the storage form for carbohydrates in the body. When energy requirements warrant it, glycogen may be broken down to glucose by a series of phosphorylating and related enzymes.

110.

A. There are three major classifications of carbohydrates: monosaccharides, disaccharides, and polysaccharides. Starch is classified as a polysaccharide because its structure is composed of many molecules of glucose (a monosaccharide) condensed together. Monosaccharides (e.g., glucose) are carbohydrates with the general molecular formula $C_n(H_2O)_n$ that cannot be broken down to simpler substances by acid hydrolysis. Disaccharides (e.g., sucrose, lactose) are condensation products of two molecules of monosaccharides with loss of one molecule of water.

111.

A. The level of glucose in the blood is a result of a variety of metabolic processes. Processes that increase the blood glucose include ingestion of sugar, synthesis of glucose from noncarbohydrate sources, and breakdown of glycogen. Processes that decrease blood glucose include metabolizing glucose to produce energy and converting glucose to glycogen or fat. Glycogen is a polysaccharide, which is the storage form of carbohydrates in animals. *Glycogenesis* refers to the formation of glycogen in the liver from blood glucose. This occurs in response to increased blood glucose levels. In response to decreasing blood glucose levels, glycogen in the liver is broken down to glucose. This process is called *glycogenolysis*. When glucose is metabolized, for example, to produce energy, it is converted to lactate or pyruvate. This process is called *glycolysis*. When the body synthesizes glucose from noncarbohydrate sources, that is, amino acids, glycerol, or lactate, the process is called *gluconeogenesis*. When the body uses glucose to synthesize fat, this process is called *lipogenesis*.

112.

A. When highly specific analytical methods are used, the glucose concentration in fasting whole blood is approximately 12–15% lower than in plasma or serum. While glucose diffuses freely between the water phase of plasma and red blood cells, there is a higher concentration of water in plasma (approximately 12%) than in whole blood, accounting for the increased glucose concentration in plasma. The water content of whole blood depends on the hematocrit.

113.

D. Renal threshold is defined as the plasma level that must be exceeded in order for the substance to appear in the urine. The renal threshold for glucose is 180 mg/dL. This means that the blood glucose level must exceed 180 mg/dL in order for glucose to be excreted in the urine.

114.

D. Glycated hemoglobin, also known as fast hemoglobin (because of its electrophoretic mobility), is a collective term encompassing the three glycated hemoglobin fractions—hemoglobin A_{1a}, hemoglobin A_{1b}, and hemoglobin A_{1c}. Hb A_{1c} is the fraction of Hb A_1 that is present in the greatest concentration. Some commercially available column chromatography methods measure the three fractions collectively. Glycated hemoglobin refers to the specific red cell hemoglobin A types to which a

glucose molecule becomes irreversibly attached. The greater the glucose concentration in the plasma, the greater the number of hemoglobin molecules that will become glycated. Since red blood cells have an average life span of 120 days and the glycation is irreversible, measurement of glycated hemoglobin reflects the average plasma glucose level of an individual during the previous 6- to 8-week period. This test is used as a monitor of diabetic control.

115.

B. The American Diabetes Association has published new criteria (1997) for the classification and diagnosis of diabetes mellitus. Three criteria have been defined with only one needing to be present to establish the diagnosis of diabetes mellitus. The three criteria include: classic diabetic symptoms and a random serum glucose of ≥200 mg/dL, a fasting serum glucose of ≥126 mg/dL, and a 2-hour postload serum glucose (part of OGTT) of ≥200 mg/dL.

116.

C. Increased insulin resistance is commonly seen in the late second and third trimesters of pregnancy. Most women are able to compensate by secreting additional insulin and, thus, are able to maintain normal blood glucose levels. In cases of gestational diabetes mellitus, women are unable to make sufficient insulin to meet their needs. In the screening test, serum glucose is assessed at 1 hour following the ingestion of a 50-gram glucose load. If the serum glucose is ≥140 mg/dL, the next step is to perform an oral glucose tolerance test.

117.

D. Sodium fluoride is a weak anticoagulant that acts as a preservative for glucose. It functions as a glucose preservative by inhibiting glycolysis. However, it is not suitable for use with many enzyme procedures. In the determination of BUN, where urease activity is utilized, the high concentration of fluoride in the plasma acts as an enzyme inhibitor, preventing the necessary chemical reaction.

118.

D. Based on the biochemistry of the disease, diabetes mellitus has been classified as Type 1 and Type 2. Since Type 1 occurs more commonly in individuals under 20 years of age, it was formerly called juvenile diabetes. Studies suggest that Type 1 is associated with autoimmune destruction of β-cells, and it is characterized by insulin deficiency and thus a dependency on injection of insulin. Unlike people afflicted with Type 2, Type 1 individuals are prone to ketoacidosis and to such complications as angiopathy, cataracts, nephropathy, and neuropathy.

119.

C. The protein hormone insulin is synthesized in the pancreas by the β-cells of the islets of Langerhans. Insulin, a two-chain polypeptide, consists of 51 amino acids. A single-chain preproinsulin is cleaved to proinsulin, which is the immediate precursor of insulin. Proinsulin is hydrolyzed to form insulin, a two-chain polypeptide, and inactive C-peptide. Insulin promotes the entry of glucose into tissue cells.

120.

D. Insulin may be described as an anabolic, polypeptide hormone. Insulin stimulates glucose uptake by muscle cells (which increases protein synthesis), by fat cells (which increases triglyceride synthesis), and by liver cells (which increases lipid synthesis and glycogenesis). If cellular uptake of glucose is stimulated, the glucose concentration in the circulation decreases.

121.

D. In uncontrolled diabetes mellitus, the blood glucose level exceeds the renal threshold of approximately 180 mg/dL for glucose, leading to glycosuria and polyuria. The excess secretion of glucagon stimulates lipolysis, with increased formation of acetoacetic acid. In the blood, the ketoacids dissociate, with the hydrogen ions being buffered by bicarbonate. This causes the bicarbonate to become depleted and leads to metabolic acidosis.

122.

D. Glucose determinations are generally performed on serum or plasma rather than whole blood. Serum or plasma is more convenient to use than whole blood in most automated systems because serum does not require mixing before sampling. Glucose stability is greater in separated plasma than in whole blood because glycolysis is minimized. Specificity for glucose is higher when plasma or serum is used because variations attrib-

utable to interfering substances in the red cells are avoided.

123.

D. Research has demonstrated that there is a correlation between blood glucose levels in diabetes and the development of long-term complications. These complications may include such disorders as retinopathy, neuropathy, atherosclerosis, and renal failure. Thus, quantifying such blood analytes as urea, creatinine, and lipids as well as urinary albumin can aid in monitoring diabetics.

124.

D. There are greater than 100 causes of hypoglycemia. Among the causes is the ingestion of certain drugs. Use of ethanol, propranolol, and salicylate has been linked to the occurrence of hypoglycemia.

125.

B. The diagnostic test for hypoglycemia is the 72-hour fast, which requires the analysis of glucose, insulin, C-peptide, and proinsulin at 6-hour intervals. The test should be concluded when plasma glucose levels drop to ≤45 mg/dL, hypoglycemic symptoms appear, or after 72 hours have elapsed. In general, hypoglycemic symptoms occur when the plasma glucose level falls below 55 mg/dL. Such symptoms may include headache, confusion, blurred vision, dizziness, and seizures. The term neuroglycopenia has been applied to these central nervous system disorders. While decreased hepatic glucose production and increased glucose utilization may cause hypoglycemia, there are over 100 causes of this disorder.

126.

B. Glucose in the presence of oxygen is oxidized to gluconic acid and hydrogen peroxide. This reaction is catalyzed by glucose oxidase. By using a polarographic oxygen electrode, the rate of oxygen consumption is measured and related to the concentration of glucose in the sample.

127.

C. The hexokinase method for quantifying glucose employs two coupled enzymatic reactions. In the first reaction, which is catalyzed by hexokinase, glucose is phosphorylated by adenosine triphosphate, forming glucose-6-phosphate and adenosine diphosphate. In the second reaction, glucose-6-

phosphate dehydrogenase (derived from yeast) catalyzes the oxidation of glucose-6-phosphate and the reduction of nicotinamide adenine dinucleotide phosphate. The amount of reduced NADPH formed is proportional to the glucose concentration in the sample. Thus, the greater the absorbance reading of NADPH at 340 nm, the greater the glucose concentration. If bacterial G-6-PD is used, the cofactor is NAD^+ with the production of NADH.

128.

A. The glucose oxidase method for quantifying glucose employs two coupled enzymatic reactions. In the first reaction, which is catalyzed by glucose oxidase, glucose in the presence of oxygen is oxidized to gluconic acid and hydrogen peroxide. In the second reaction, peroxidase catalyzes a reaction between hydrogen peroxide and the reduced form of a chromogenic oxygen acceptor, o-dianisidine, forming an oxidized colored product that is read spectrophotometrically.

129.

C. The glucose dehydrogenase method employs only one enzymatic reaction for the measurement of glucose in a sample. Glucose dehydrogenase catalyzes the oxidation of glucose and the reduction of nicotinamide adenine dinucleotide. The amount of reduced NADH formed is proportional to the glucose concentration in the sample. When measuring blood glucose levels during the administration of an oral xylose tolerance test, the glucose dehydrogenase method should not be used, since the relative rate of reaction of D-xylose as compared to glucose is 15% with this method. In contrast, D-xylose will not react in the hexokinase and glucose oxidase methods, thus allowing glucose to be measured accurately.

The D-xylose absorption test is useful in distinguishing two types of malabsorption: intestinal malabsorption and malabsorption resulting from pancreatic insufficiency. When D-xylose is administered orally, it is absorbed by passive diffusion into the portal vein from the proximal portion of the small intestine. Since D-xylose is not metabolized by the liver, it is excreted unchanged by the kidneys. In intestinal malabsorption, the amount of D-xylose excreted, as measured in a 5-hour urine specimen, is less than normal because of decreased absorption of D-xylose. In malabsorption caused by pancreatic insufficiency, the absorption of D-xylose is normal.

130.

C. Although there are several reliable enzymatic glucose methods available, the hexokinase method is the reference method for quantifying glucose. The reference method requires that a protein-free filtrate be made using barium hydroxide and zinc sulfate. The clear supernatant is then used as the sample in the hexokinase/glucose-6-phosphate dehydrogenase coupled enzyme reactions. For routine clinical use, serum is used directly in the hexokinase method because deproteinization is too time-consuming.

131.

C. The reference interval for CSF is 60% of the normal plasma value. For a serum glucose of 110 mg/dL, the expected CSF glucose level would be 66 mg/dL. The equilibration of CSF with plasma glucose takes several hours. The reference interval for the CSF glucose level is 40–70 mg/dL as compared with a normal fasting plasma glucose level. Low levels of CSF glucose are associated with a number of diseases including bacterial meningitis and tuberculous meningitis, while viral disease generally presents with a normal level of CSF glucose.

132.

C. The reference interval for fasting serum glucose in an adult expressed in conventional units is 74–106 mg/dL. To convert conventional units to SI units (Système International d'Unites), multiply the conventional units in mg/dL by the 0.0555 conversion factor to obtain SI units in mmol/L. Thus, 74 mg/dL $\times$ 0.0555 = 4.1 mmol/L and 106 mg/dL $\times$ 0.0555 = 5.9 mmol/L. While conventional units are used commonly in the United States, many scientific journals require the use of SI units in their publications and many foreign countries use SI units routinely in clinical practice. To identify additional conversion factors for other analytes, consult the appendix of a clinical chemistry textbook.

133.

B. Hemoglobin A_{1c} is the major component of the glycated hemoglobins. When measuring glycated hemoglobin levels, Hb A_{1c} is best separated from other hemoglobins, including Hb F, by use of high-performance liquid chromatography, isoelectric focusing, and immunoassay techniques. When using ion-exchange chromatography, Hb F will elute with Hb A_1, causing falsely increased results.

134.

D. Regulation of the blood glucose concentration depends on a number of hormones. These include insulin, glucagon, cortisol, epinephrine, growth hormone, adrenocorticotropic hormone, and thyroxine. Of these hormones, *insulin* is the only one that decreases the blood glucose level. *Glucagon* is produced in the pancreas by the alpha cells. Glucagon promotes an increase in the blood glucose concentration by its stimulatory effect on glycogenolysis in the liver. *Cortisol* is produced by the adrenal cortex. It stimulates gluconeogenesis, thus increasing the blood level of glucose. *Epinephrine* is produced by the adrenal medulla. It promotes glycogenolysis, thus increasing blood glucose. *Growth hormone* and *adrenocorticotropic hormone* are produced by the anterior pituitary gland. Both hormones are antagonistic to insulin and hence increase blood glucose. *Thyroxine* is produced by the thyroid gland. It not only stimulates glycogenolysis but also increases the intestinal absorption rate of glucose.

135.

B. Epinephrine is produced by the adrenal medulla. It promotes glycogenolysis, thus increasing the blood glucose level. Epinephrine also inhibits the secretion of insulin and stimulates the secretion of glucagon.

136.

A. In Cushing's syndrome the adrenal cortex secretes an excessive amount of the hormone cortisol. Since cortisol has a stimulatory effect on gluconeogenesis, hyperglycemia commonly occurs as a secondary disorder. Hypoglycemia frequently characterizes Addison's disease in which there is decreased production of cortisol.

137.

D. When a 2-hour postprandial glucose test is performed, the individual either consumes a test meal high in carbohydrates or a 75-g glucose test solution. Normally following carbohydrate ingestion, blood glucose levels peak within 60 to 90 minutes and return to fasting levels by 2 hours. Plasma glucose values less than 120 mg/dL are normal, values above 140 mg/dL are abnormal, and values between 120 and 140 mg/dL are questionable and additional testing may be needed.

138.

B. Due to the critical reasons for aspirating a cerebrospinal fluid (CSF) specimen, the testing is performed as soon as possible upon receipt of the specimen in the laboratory. In this case, the cloudy appearance would be most likely due to the presence of bacteria. Both bacteria and red blood cells can utilize glucose in vitro. Thus any delay in glucose testing could result in a falsely low result. The CSF specimen should be centrifuged to remove cellular material and assayed immediately.

139.

A. In the glucose oxidase/peroxidase method, the second coupled enzyme reaction involves peroxidase catalyzing the reaction between hydrogen peroxide and a chromogenic oxygen acceptor, which is oxidized to its colored form. Several blood constituents, including uric acid, ascorbic acid, bilirubin, tetracycline, hemoglobin, and glutathione, when present in increased concentrations can interfere with the assay by competing for the hydrogen peroxide produced in the first coupled enzyme reaction. This loss of hydrogen peroxide would result in falsely low plasma glucose results. Owing to the high levels of uric acid normally found in urine, the glucose oxidase/peroxidase method would not be suitable for measuring urine glucose.

140.

D. A random serum glucose should be less than 200 mg/dL. The reference range for glycated hemoglobin (Hb A_{1c}) is 4.5–8.5%. Since the individual is a postmenopausal, 57-year-old female, with abnormal test results being found as part of an annual physical examination, the most likely diagnosis is Type 2 diabetes mellitus.

141.

A. Carbohydrate is stored in the body in the form of glycogen. There are many enzymes involved in the metabolism of glycogen. A deficiency of any one of the enzymes involved will result in what are called glycogen storage diseases or glycogenoses. There are at least 10 distinct types of glycogen storage diseases, and all of them are rare. All are hereditary. Diagnosis of each type can be made by the assay of the deficient enzymes from the appropriate tissue and by microscopic study of the affected tissues.

- Type I—von Gierke's disease is clinically characterized by severe fasting hypoglycemia and lactic acidosis. This is due to a deficiency of the enzyme glucose-6-phosphatase. Glucose cannot be transported from the liver as glucose-6-phosphate during the breakdown of glycogen. It is metabolized to lactic acid and thus results in lactic acidosis.
- Type II—Pompe's disease is caused by a deficiency of lysosomal alpha-1,4-glucosidase. This results in an increase of glycogen in all organs and abnormally large lysosomes. The glycogen cannot be degraded because of the deficiency of alpha-1,4-glucosidase.
- Type III—Forbes' disease is caused by the absence of a debrancher enzyme. This disease is characterized by hypoglycemia, hepatomegaly, seizures, and growth retardation.
- Type IV—Andersen's disease is caused by a deficiency of brancher enzyme. It is a rare disease characterized by progressive liver enlargement or cirrhosis and muscular weakness by the age of 2 months. Storage glycogen is not usually found, but unbranched amylopectin accumulates in this disease.

LIPIDS AND LIPOPROTEINS

142.

C. Bile acids are synthesized in the hepatocytes of the liver. They are C_{24} steroids that are derived from cholesterol. With fat ingestion, the bile salts are released into the intestines, where they aid in the emulsification of dietary fats. Thus bile acids also serve as a vehicle for cholesterol excretion. A majority of the bile acids, however, are reabsorbed from the intestines into the enterohepatic circulation for reexcretion into the bile. The two principal bile acids are cholic acid and chenodeoxycholic acid. These acids are conjugated with one of two amino acids, glycine or taurine. Measurement of bile acids is possible via immuno-techniques and may aid in the diagnosis of some liver disorders such as obstructive jaundice, primary biliary cirrhosis, and viral hepatitis.

143.

C. After fat ingestion, lipids are first degraded, then reformed, and finally incorporated by the intestinal mucosal cells into absorbable complexes known as chylomicrons. These chylomicrons enter the blood through the lymphatic system, where they impart a turbid appearance to serum. Such lipemic plasma specimens frequently interfere with absorbance or change in absorbance measurements, causing invalid results.

144.

C. Total cholesterol consists of two fractions, free cholesterol and cholesterol ester. In the plasma, cholesterol exists mostly in the cholesterol ester form. Approximately 70% of total plasma cholesterol is esterfied with fatty acids. The formation of cholesterol esters is such that a transferase enzyme catalyzes the transfer of fatty acids from phosphatidylcholine to the carbon-3 alcohol function position of the free cholesterol molecule. Laboratories routinely measure total cholesterol by first using the reagent cholesterol esterase to break the ester bonds with the fatty acids.

145.

D. A "routine" lipid profile would most likely consist of a measurement of total cholesterol, triglycerides, and HDL cholesterol. These measurements are most easily adapted to today's multichannel chemistry analyzers. Both cholesterol and triglycerides use an enzymatic technique to drive the reaction to completion. HDL cholesterol is a commonly requested test to help determine patient risk for coronary heart disease. The HDL is separated from other lipoproteins using a precipitation technique, immuno-techniques, and/or polymers and detergents. The latter techniques are preferred because they can give better precision, be adapted to an automated chemistry analyzer, and be run without personnel intervention.

146.

D. Blood specimens for lipid studies should be drawn in the fasting state at least 12 to 14 hours after eating. Although fat ingestion only slightly affects cholesterol levels, both the triglyceride and lipoprotein electrophoresis results are greatly affected. Triglycerides peak at about 4 to 6 hours after a meal, and these exogenous lipids should be cleared from the plasma before analysis. The detection of chylomicrons by electrophoresis is always indicative of hyperlipidemia; therefore the presence of chylomicrons as a result of an inadequate fasting period must be avoided.

147.

A. Cholesterol is only slightly affected by the fasting status of the patient whereas triglycerides, fatty acids, and lipoproteins are greatly affected. This is because chylomicrons are rich in triglycerides and fatty acids and contain very little cholesterol. The majority of cholesterol is produced by the liver and other tissues. High levels of exogenous triglycerides and/or fatty acids will interfere with the measurement of lipoproteins. Chylomicrons are normally cleared from the body after 6 hours.

148.

B. The long chain fatty acids of triglycerides can be broken down to form energy through the process of beta-oxidation, also known as the Fatty Acid Cycle. In this process, two carbons at a time are cleaved from long chain fatty acids to form acetyl-coenzyme A. Acetyl-coenzyme A, in turn, can enter the Krebs cycle to be converted to energy or be converted to acetoacetyl-Co-A and converted to energy by an alternate pathway leaving behind the acidic by-product ketones composed of beta-hydroxybutyrate, acetoacetate, and acetone. Under proper conditions, pyruvate can be converted to acetyl-coenzyme A at the end of glycolysis of glucose. Bile is a breakdown product of cholesterol used in the digestion of dietary cholesterol.

149.

D. The kinetic methods used today for quantifying serum triglycerides employ a reaction system of coupling enzymes. It is first necessary to hydrolyze the triglycerides to free fatty acids and glycerol. This hydrolysis step is catalyzed by the enzyme lipase. The glycerol is then free to react in the enzyme-coupled reaction system that includes glycerokinase, pyruvate kinase, and lactate dehydrogenase or in the enzyme-coupled system that includes glycerokinase, glycerophosphate oxidase, and peroxidase.

150.

C. In the enzymatic method for quantifying total cholesterol in serum, it is necessary that the serum specimen initially be treated with cholesteryl ester hydrolase. This enzyme hydrolyzes the cholesterol esters into free cholesterol and fatty acids. Both the free cholesterol, derived from the cholesterol ester fraction, and any free cholesterol normally present in serum may react in the cholesterol oxidase-peroxidase reactions for total cholesterol. The hydrolysis of the cholesterol ester fraction is necessary because cholesterol oxidase reacts only with free cholesterol.

151.

C. Chylomicrons are protein-lipid complexes composed primarily of triglycerides and containing only small amounts of cholesterol, phospholipids, and protein. After food ingestion, the chylomicron complexes are formed in the epithelial cells of the intestines. From the epithelial cells, the chylomicrons are released into the lymphatic system, which transports chylomicrons to the blood. The chylomicrons may then carry the triglycerides to adipose tissue for storage, to organs for catabolism, or to the liver for incorporation of the triglycerides into very low density lipoproteins. Chylomicrons are normally cleared from plasma within 6 hours after a meal.

152.

B. Beta-hydroxybutyric acid, acetoacetic acid, and acetone are collectively referred to as ketone bodies. They are formed as a result of the process of beta-oxidation in which liver cells degrade fatty acids with a resultant excess accumulation of acetyl-coenzyme A (CoA). The acetyl-CoA is the parent compound from which ketone bodies are synthesized through a series of reactions.

153.

D. Sphingolipids, most notably sphingomyelin, are the major lipids of the cell membranes of the central nervous system (i.e., the myelin sheath). Like phospholipids, sphingolipids are amphipathic containing a polar, hydrophilic head and a nonpolar, hydrophobic tail making them excellent membrane formers. Although sometimes considered a subgroup of phospholipids, sphingomyelin is derived from the amino alcohol sphingosine instead of glycerol.

154.

B. All the lipoproteins contain some amount of triglyceride, cholesterol, phospholipid, and protein. Each of the lipoprotein fractions is distinguished by its unique concentration of these substances. The beta-lipoprotein fraction is composed of approximately 50% cholesterol, 6% triglycerides, 22% phospholipids, and 22% protein. The beta-lipoproteins, which are also known as the low-density lipoproteins, are the principal transport vehicle for cholesterol in the plasma. Both the chylomicrons and the prebeta-lipoproteins are composed primarily of triglycerides. The chylomicrons are considered transport vehicles for exogenous triglycerides. In other words, dietary fat is absorbed through the intestine in the form of chylomicrons. After a meal, the liver will clear the chylomicrons from the blood and use the triglyceride component to form the prebeta-lipoproteins. Therefore in the fasting state triglycerides are transported in the blood primarily by the prebeta-lipoproteins. The prebeta-lipoproteins are composed of approximately 55% triglycerides.

155.

B. The 27 carbon ringed structure of cholesterol is the backbone of steroid hormones. The nucleus is called the cyclopentanoperhydrophenanthrene ring. The steroid hormones containing this ring include estrogens (18 carbons), androgens (19 carbons), glucocorticoids (21 carbons), and mineralocorticoids (21 carbons).

156.

C. The majority of the lipid (lysosomal) storage diseases are inherited as autosomal recessive mutations. This group of diseases is characterized by an accumulation of sphingolipids in the central nervous system or some other organ. Such lipid accumulation frequently leads to mental retardation or progressive loss of central nervous system functions. The cause of such lipid accumulation has been attributed either to specific enzyme deficiencies or to nonfunctional enzyme forms that inhibit the normal catabolism of the sphingolipids.

157.

B. Pancreatic insufficiency, Whipple's disease, cystic fibrosis, and tropical sprue are diseases that are characterized by the malabsorption of lipids from the intestines. This malabsorption results in an excess lipid accumulation in the feces that is known as steatorrhea. When steatorrhea is suspected, the amount of lipid material present in the feces may be quantified. A 24- or 72-hour fecal specimen should be collected, the latter being the specimen of choice. The lipids are extracted from the fecal specimen and analyzed by gravimetric or titrimetric methods.

158.

D. In lipoprotein electrophoresis, the major fractions that may be distinguished at pH 8.6 on agarose gel are the chylomicron, beta-, prebeta-, and alpha-lipoproteins. Alpha-lipoprotein (HDL) is the fastest band, migrating the closest to the anode, followed by prebeta- (VLDL) and beta-lipoproteins (LDL). The chylomicrons remain at the origin and are the closest to the cathode. While difficult to identify visually with electrophoresis, there is an intermediate-density lipoprotein (IDL) that migrates between beta- and prebeta-lipoproteins. To characterize visually or to scan optically the lipoprotein fractions after electrophoresis, it is necessary to stain the fractions with a dye that has an affinity for the lipoproteins. Fat red 7B and oil red O are two dyes frequently used for staining lipoproteins.

159.

C. The quantification of the high-density lipoprotein (HDL) cholesterol level is thought to contribute in assessing the risk that an individual may develop coronary artery disease (CAD). There appears to be an inverse relationship between HDL cholesterol and CAD. With low levels of HDL cholesterol, the risk of CAD increases. It is thought that the HDL facilitates the removal of cholesterol from the arterial wall, therefore decreasing the risk of atherosclerosis. In addition, LDL cholesterol may be assessed, since increased LDL cholesterol and decreased HDL cholesterol are associated with increased risk of CAD.

160.

D. Respiratory distress syndrome (RDS), also referred to as hyaline membrane disease, is commonly seen in preterm infants. A deficiency of pulmonary surfactant causes the infant's alveoli to collapse during expiration, resulting in improper oxygenation of capillary blood in the alveoli. Currently, the surfactant/albumin ratio by fluorescence polarization is performed using amniotic fluid to assess fetal lung maturity. The amniotic fluid is mixed with a fluorescent dye. When the dye binds to albumin there is a high polarization, and when the dye binds to surfactant there is a low polarization. Thus the surfactant/albumin ratio is determined. The units are expressed as milligrams of surfactant per gram of albumin, with fetal lung maturity being sufficient with values greater than 50 mg/g. Older methodologies have employed the determinations of phosphatidylglycerol, foam stability, and lecithin/sphingomyelin (L/S) ratio. The L/S ratio is based on the physiological levels of lecithin and sphingomyelin. Lecithin is a surfactant, which prepares lungs to expand and take in air. Sphingomyelin is incorporated into the myelin sheath of the central nervous system of the fetus. The amounts of lecithin and sphingomyelin produced during the first 34 weeks of gestation are approximately equal; however, after the 34th week, the amount of lecithin synthesized greatly exceeds that of sphingomyelin. At birth, an L/S ratio of 2:1 or greater would indicate sufficient lung maturity.

161.

C. The very low density lipoprotein (VLDL) fraction is primarily composed of triglycerides and lesser amounts of cholesterol and phospholipids. Protein components of VLDL are mostly apoprotein C and apoprotein B-100. VLDL migrates electrophoretically in the prebeta region.

162.

B. A double nomenclature exists for the five principal lipoprotein fractions. The nomenclature is such that the various fractions have been named on the basis of both the electrophoretic mobilities and the ultracentrifugal sedimentation rates. The chylomicrons are known as chylomicrons by both methods. The chylomicrons are the least dense fraction, exhibiting a solvent density for isolation of less than 0.95 g/mL, and have the slowest electrophoretic mobility. The HDLs, also known as the alpha-lipoproteins, have the greatest density of 1.063–1.210 g/mL and move the fastest electrophoretically toward the anode. The VLDLs, also known as the prebeta-lipoproteins, move slightly slower electrophoretically than the alpha fraction. The VLDLs have a density of 0.95–1.006 g/mL. The IDLs, intermediate-density lipoproteins, have a density of 1.006–1.019 g/mL and migrate as a broad band between beta- and prebeta-lipoproteins. The LDLs, also known as the beta-lipoproteins, have an electrophoretic mobility that is slightly slower than that of the IDL fraction. The LDLs have an intermediate density of 1.019–1.063 g/mL, which is between the IDLs and the HDLs. To summarize the electrophoretic mo-

bilities, the alpha-lipoprotein fraction migrates the farthest toward the anode from the origin, followed in order of decreasing mobility by the prebeta-lipoprotein, broad band between beta- and prebeta-lipoprotein, beta-lipoprotein, and chylomicron fractions. The chylomicrons remain more cathodic near the point of serum application.

163.

C. Either a magnesium-phosphotungstate mixture or a heparin-manganese mixture may be used to precipitate the low-density lipoprotein (LDL) and very low-density lipoprotein (VLDL) cholesterol fractions. This allows the high-density lipoprotein (HDL) cholesterol fraction to remain in the supernatant. An aliquot of the supernatant may then be used in a total cholesterol procedure for the quantification of the HDL cholesterol level.

164.

B. Both the direct and the heparin-manganese precipitation methods measure HDL cholesterol. The direct or homogeneous method for HDL cholesterol uses a mixture of polyanions and polymers that bind to LDL and VLDL and chylomicrons causing them to become stabilized. The polyanions neutralize ionic charges on the surface of the lipoproteins that enhances their binding to the polymer. When a detergent is added, HDL goes into solution, whereas the other lipoproteins remain attached to the polymer/polyanion complexes. The HDL cholesterol then reacts with added cholesterol enzyme reagents while the other lipoproteins remain inactive. The reagents, polymer/polyanions and detergent can be added to the specimen in an automated way without the need for any manual pretreatment step. Furthermore, the direct HDL cholesterol procedure has the capacity for better precision than the manual precipitation methods. Both the adaptability to automated instruments and the better precision make the direct method a preferred choice for quantifying HDL cholesterol.

165.

A. A number of risk factors are associated with developing coronary heart disease. Notable among these factors are increased total cholesterol and decreased HDL cholesterol levels. Although the reference ranges for total cholesterol and HDL cholesterol vary with age and sex, reasonable generalizations can be made: the mean HDL cholesterol for men is 45 mg/dL and for women it is 55 mg/dL; total cholesterol values of less than 200 mg/dL are desirable, values between 200 and 239 mg/dL are borderline/high risk, and values of 240 mg/dL or greater are high risk.

166.

B. Once the total cholesterol, triglyceride, and HDL cholesterol are known, LDL cholesterol can be quantified by using the Friedewald equation.

$$\text{LDL cholesterol} = \text{Total cholesterol} - (\text{HDL cholesterol} + \text{Triglyceride}/5)$$

In this example all results are in mg/dL:

$$
\begin{aligned}
\text{LDL cholesterol} &= 300 - (50 + 200/5) \\
&= 300 - (90) \\
&= 210 \text{ mg/dL}
\end{aligned}
$$

This estimation of LDL cholesterol has been widely accepted in routine clinical laboratories and can be easily programmed into laboratory computers. However, direct LDL methods are now under study, which may make the formula obsolete. *Note*: the equation should not be used with triglyceride values exceeding 400 mg/dL because the VLDL composition is abnormal, making the [triglyceride/5] factor inapplicable.

167.

D. Both total cholesterol and HDL cholesterol are independent measurable indicators of risk of coronary heart disease (CHD). By relating total and HDL cholesterol in a mathematical way, physicians can obtain valuable additional information in predicting risk for CHD. Risk of CHD can be quantified by ratio: Total cholesterol/HDL cholesterol along the following lines

Ratio	Risk CHD
3.43	half average
4.97	average
9.55	two times average
24.39	three times average

Thus this patient shows approximately twice the average risk for CHD. Risk ratios for CHD can easily be calculated by instrument and/or laboratory computers given the total and HDL cholesterol values. Reports indicating level of risk based on these results can be programmed by the laboratory and/or manufacturer.

168.

C. A number of immunochemical assays can be used to quantify the apolipoproteins. Some of the techniques that can be used include radial immunodiffusion (RID), radioimmunoassay (RIA), immunonephelometric assay, enzyme-linked immunosorbent assay (ELISA), and immunoturbidimetric assay. Several commercial kits are available for the quantification of Apo A-I and Apo B-100. Measuring the apolipoproteins can be of use in assessing increased risk for coronary heart disease.

169.

A. Lipoprotein (a) is an apolipoprotein that is more commonly referred to as Lp(a). It is a variant form of LDL, with an electrophoretic mobility generally in the prebeta region. The reference range for Lp(a) is 0.05–1.90 mmol/L (20–760 mg/L). Lp(a) is believed to interfere with the lysis of clots by competing with plasminogen in the coagulation cascade, thus increasing the likelihood of atherosclerotic cardiovascular disease.

170.

B. Historically, cholesterol levels of Americans have been below 300 mg/dL. Other countries, however, have relatively lower population cholesterol levels. The prevalent diet of these countries, however, may be vegetarian or fish, as opposed to meat, oriented. Higher cholesterol resulting from a meat diet has been established. Clinical studies have also shown an increased risk of CAD in individuals with cholesterol greater than 200 mg/dL. Thus, the upper reference interval of acceptable cholesterol was artificially lowered to 200 mg/dL to reflect the lower risk of CAD associated with it.

171.

D. The Abell-Kendall assay is commonly used to separate HDL cholesterol from other lipoproteins. In this precipitation technique a heparin-manganese mixture is used to precipitate the low-density lipoprotein (LDL) and very low-density lipoprotein (VLDL) cholesterol fractions. This technique works well as long as there is no significant amount of chylomicrons or lipemia in the specimen and/or the triglyceride is under 400 mg/dL. Incomplete sedimentation is seen as cloudiness or turbidity in the supernatant after centrifugation. It indicates the presence of other lipoproteins and leads to over estimation of HDL cholesterol. The lipemic specimens may be cleared and the HDL cholesterol separated more effectively by using ultrafiltration, extraction, latex immobilized antibodies and/or ultracentrifugation. These techniques are usually not available in a routine laboratory.

172.

A. Hyperlipoproteinemia can be genetically inherited or secondary to certain diseases such as diabetes mellitus, hypothyroidism, or alcoholism. If the alcoholism has advanced to the state where there is liver damage, the liver can become inefficient in its metabolism of fats leading to an increase of cholesterol, triglyceride, LDL, and/or VLDL in the bloodstream. The elevation of these lipids along with the previous liver damage (e.g., cirrhosis) leads to a poor prognosis for the patient.

173.

D. In evaluating lipid profile results it is important to start with the integrity of the sample. From the case history, it is doubtful that a 10-year-old healthy, active boy would be suffering from a lipid or glucose disorder manifesting these kinds of results. Furthermore, the boy came in for testing after school. It is improbable that a 10-year-old boy would be able to maintain a 12–14 hour fast during the school day. In this case, the boy should have been thoroughly interviewed by the laboratory staff prior to the blood test to determine if he was truly fasting. Specimen integrity is the first thing that must be ensured before running any lipid tests.

174.

C. In this case the child fits the description of a suspected hyperlipemic patient. He is known to have diabetes mellitus, and the mother has assured the laboratory that the boy has followed the proper fasting protocol before the test. Hyperlipoproteinemia can be secondary to diabetes mellitus. He has a relatively high risk to develop CAD, and as a known diabetic, should never undergo a 3-hour glucose tolerance test.

PROTEINS, ELECTROPHORESIS, AND TUMOR MARKERS

175.

D. The three major biochemical compounds that exert primary roles in human intermediary metab-

olism are proteins, carbohydrates, and lipids. The presence of nitrogen in all protein compounds distinguishes proteins from carbohydrates and lipids. Protein compounds contain approximately 16% nitrogen. Although there are only 20 common alpha-amino acids that are found in all proteins and a total of 40 known amino acids, a protein compound may contain from 50 to thousands of amino acids. The uniqueness of any protein is dictated by the number, type, and sequencing of the alpha-amino acids that compose it. The alpha-amino acids are linked to each other through peptide bonds. A peptide bond is formed through the linkage of the amino group of one amino acid to the carboxyl group of another amino acid.

176.

C. A variety of external factors such as mechanical agitation, application of heat, and extreme chemical treatment with acids or salts may cause the denaturation of proteins. When proteins are denatured, they undergo a change in their tertiary structure. Tertiary structure describes the appearance of the protein in its folded, globular form. When the covalent, hydrogen, or disulfide bonds are broken, the protein loses its shape as its polypeptide chain unfolds. With the loss of this tertiary structure, there is also a loss in some of the characteristic properties of the protein. In general, proteins will become less soluble, and enzymes will lose catalytic activity. Denaturation by use of chemicals has been a useful laboratory tool. The mixing of serum proteins with sulfosalicylic acid or trichloroacetic acid causes the precipitation of both the albumin and globulin fractions. When albumin is placed in water, dilute salt solutions, or moderately concentrated salt solutions, it remains soluble. However, the globulins are insoluble in water but soluble in weak salt solutions. Both the albumins and globulins are insoluble in concentrated salt solutions. Primary structure refers to the joining of the amino acids through peptide bonds to form polypeptide chains. Secondary structure refers to the twisting of more than one polypeptide chain into coils or helices.

177.

D. Although the Kjeldahl technique for the determination of protein nitrogen is too cumbersome for use in routine testing, it is considered to be the reference method of choice to validate materials used with the biuret method. The Kjeldahl technique is based on the quantification of the nitrogen content of protein. It is estimated that the average nitrogen content of protein is 16% of the total weight. In the Kjeldahl technique, protein undergoes a digestion process with sulfuric acid through which the nitrogen content of the protein is converted to ammonium ion. The ammonium ion in turn may be reacted with Nessler's reagent, forming a colored product that is read spectrophotometrically, or the ammonium ion may undergo distillation, liberating ammonia that is titrated.

178.

C. A commonly used method to quantify serum total proteins is the biuret procedure. The biuret reaction is based on the complexing of cupric ions in an alkaline solution with the peptide linkages of protein molecules. Since the amino acids of all proteins are joined together by peptide bonds, this method provides an accurate quantification of the total protein content of serum. The greater the amount of protein in a specimen, the greater will be the number of available peptide bonds for reaction and the more intense the colored reaction will be. In the biuret reaction, the intensity of the reddish violet color produced is proportional to the number of peptide bonds present. Generally, one cupric ion complexes with four to six peptide linkages. However, a colored product may be formed when the cupric ion links through coordinate bonds with at least two peptide linkages, with the smallest compound able to react being the tripeptide. Therefore, not only will proteins contribute to the formation of the colored product, but so, too, will any tripeptides and polypeptides present in a serum sample.

179.

B. The concentration of total protein in cerebrospinal fluid (CSF) is 15–45 mg/dL. Such a low level of protein requires a method with sufficient sensitivity such as Coomassie brilliant blue. Turbidimetric methods can also be used to quantify protein in CSF. Neither biuret nor Ponceau S has the sensitivity needed, and bromcresol green measures only albumin and does not react with the globulins.

180.

D. Cerebrospinal fluid (CSF), an ultrafiltrate of blood plasma, is made in the choroid plexus of the ventricles of the brain. Protein quantification is among the tests generally ordered on CSF; other

tests include glucose, culture and sensitivity, and differential cell count. The reference range for CSF protein is 15–45 mg/dL. CSF protein may be quantified using turbidimetric (e.g., sulfosalicylic acid and benzethonium chloride) or dye-binding methods (e.g., Coomassie brilliant blue). Elevated levels of CSF protein are found in such disorders as bacterial, viral, and fungal meningitis, multiple sclerosis, neoplasm, disk herniation, and cerebral infarction. Low levels of CSF protein are found in hyperthyroidism and in CSF leakage from the central nervous system.

181.

D. Bisalbuminemia is a congenital disorder that does not exhibit any clinical manifestations. The only sign of this disorder is the splitting of albumin into two distinct bands when serum is subjected to electrophoresis. The extra albumin band may occur either anodically or cathodically to the normal albumin band depending on its speed of migration. The intensity of the two bands when quantified by densitometry may show that the two forms are of equal concentration. In a less common variation the abnormal albumin band may represent only 10–15% of the total albumin concentration.

182.

C. There are no physiological diseases that cause increased production of albumin by the liver. Elevated serum albumin is only associated with dehydration. It is a relative increase that will return to normal when fluids are administered to alleviate the dehydration. Disorders such as malnutrition, acute inflammation, and renal disease are characterized by decreased serum albumin levels.

183.

A. In renal disease, glomerular or tubular malfunction results in proteinuria. In early stages of glomerular dysfunction small quantities of albumin will appear in the urine. Since the concentration is so low, urine dipstick assays are unable to detect the presence of such a small quantity of albumin; hence the term microalbuminuria. Annual testing of diabetics for microalbuminuria is recommended, since identification of these low levels of albumin that precede nephropathy would allow for clinical intervention to control blood glucose levels and blood pressure. The reference interval for urinary albumin is less than 30 mg/day. Microalbuminuria may be quantified using radioimmunoassay, immunonephelometry, and enzyme immunoassay.

184.

D. The heme protein myoglobin can bind oxygen reversibly and is found in cardiac and striated muscles. In cases of acute myocardial infarction, myoglobin increases within 1–3 hours of the infarct. Since myoglobin is not cardiac specific, increased serum levels occur in vigorous exercise, intramuscular injections, rhabdomyolysis, and muscular dystrophy. Since myoglobin is a relatively small protein and able to be excreted by the kidneys, elevated serum levels occur in renal failure.

185.

D. Troponin is a group of three proteins that function in muscle contraction by binding to the thin filaments of cardiac and skeletal striated muscle. The three proteins are known as troponin T (TnT), troponin I (TnI), and troponin C (TnC). With acute myocardial infarction, the cardiac-specific isoforms of troponin are released into the blood; the two of clinical interest are cTnI and cTnT. Cardiac troponin I (cTnI) will show an increase that exceeds the reference interval in approximately 4–8 hours following an acute myocardial infarction (AMI). Quantification should be done serially starting with an initial measurement at presentation followed by testing at 3–6 hours, 6–9 hours, and 12–24 hours. cTnI will remain elevated for 3 5 days. Unlike cTnT, which is expressed in small quantities in regenerating and diseased skeletal muscle, cTnI is not which makes it specific for cardiac muscle.

186.

B. β_2-Microglobulin is a single polypeptide chain that is the light chain component of human leukocyte antigens (HLA). It is found on the surface of nucleated cells and is notably present on lymphocytes. Increased plasma levels of β_2-microglobulin are associated with renal failure, lymphocytosis, rheumatoid arthritis, and systemic lupus erythematosus.

187.

A. Haptoglobin is a glycoprotein produced mainly by the liver that migrates electrophoretically as an alpha$_2$-globulin. Increased serum concentrations of haptoglobin are seen in inflammatory conditions and tissue necrosis, whereas decreased levels are seen in hemolytic situations in which there is extensive red blood cell destruction. In the latter situation, haptoglobin binds with free hemoglobin to form a stable complex that may then be removed by the reticuloendothelial system. Because of the size of the haptoglobin-hemoglobin complex, urinary excretion of hemoglobin by the kidney is avoided, thereby preventing the loss of iron by the kidney.

188.

D. The serum proteins are divided into five principal fractions based on their electrophoretic mobilities. The five fractions are albumin, alpha$_1$-globulin, alpha$_2$-globulin, beta-globulin, and gamma-globulin. Albumin constitutes the largest individual fraction of the serum proteins. The reference concentration of albumin in serum ranges between 3.5 and 5.2 g/dL, and the total globulin concentration is between 2.3 and 3.5 g/dL.

189.

C. Bromcresol green (BCG) and bromcresol purple (BCP) are anionic dyes that bind selectively with albumin without preliminary extraction of the globulins. The nature of the dyes is such that the color of the free dye is different from the color of the albumin-dye complex so that the color change is directly proportional to the concentration of albumin in the specimen. Although amido black, Ponceau S and Coomassie brilliant blue are able to bind albumin, they also react with the globulins, thus prohibiting their use in a direct procedure for quantification of serum albumin.

190.

B. Biuret reagent is a combination of copper sulfate, potassium iodide in sodium hydroxide, and potassium sodium tartrate. The copper sulfate is the key to the reaction because it is the cupric ion that complexes with the peptide bonds of protein. To keep the copper in solution until its use, potassium sodium tartrate is employed as a complexing agent, whereas the autoreduction of copper is prevented by potassium iodide.

191.

D. The majority of the plasma proteins are manufactured by the liver. Albumin, fibrinogen, and most of the alpha- and beta-globulins are produced by the liver. The immunoglobulins, including IgG, IgA, IgM, IgD, and IgE, are produced by the lymphoid cells.

192.
D. The immunoglobulins, IgG, IgA, IgM, IgD, and IgE, migrate electrophoretically with the gamma-globulin fraction. The normal serum levels of the IgD and IgE classes are so low that these two immunoglobulins do not normally contribute to the intensity of the stained gamma-globulin electrophoretic fraction. The primary component of the gamma fraction consists of IgG, with IgA and IgM contributing to the intensity of the stained fraction to a lesser degree. In disease states the concentration relationship between the immunoglobulins may be significantly altered from the normal.

193.
D. All the immunoglobulins consist of heavy- and light-chain polypeptides. The heavy chains are designated as gamma γ, alpha α, mu μ, delta δ, and epsilon ε and are specific for the immunoglobulins IgG, IgA, IgM, IgD, and IgE, respectively. The light chains are designated as kappa κ and lambda λ, with both types being found in each of the immunoglobulin classes, although the two light chains attached to a particular set of heavy chains must be of the same type. Therefore, IgG consists of two heavy chains of the gamma type and two light chains of either the kappa or lambda type. The immunoglobulins IgA, IgD, and IgE have a structure similar to that of IgG in that they consist of two light chains and two heavy chains of the respective type. IgM is a macromolecule with a pentamer type of structure. IgM consists of five sets of two heavy-chain and two light-chain units, with the basic units being linked to each other by peptide fragments.

194.
A. The immunoglobulin class IgA is found in both plasma and body secretions, with the two types being differentiated by their sedimentation coefficients. Plasma IgA has an average sedimentation coefficient of 7S, and secretory IgA has a sedimentation coefficient of 11S. Secretory IgA is present in saliva, tears, and secretions of nasal, gastrointestinal, and tracheolbronchial origin. Secretory IgA is dimeric in structure and possesses a glycoprotein secretory component attached to its heavy chains and a J polypeptide. The principal immunoglobulin found in secretions is IgA, with only trace amounts of IgG being present. The presence of IgM, IgD, or IgE in secretions has not been detected.

195.
D. The only immunoglobulin class that is able to cross the placenta from the mother's circulation to the fetus is IgG. Therefore, at birth there is very little immunoglobulin present in the infant except for the maternal IgG. After birth, as the infant comes in contact with antigens, the levels of IgG, IgA, and IgM slowly increase.

196.
D. Alpha$_1$-antitrypsin is an acute-phase reactant protein whose concentration increases in response to inflammation. Alpha$_1$-antitrypsin inhibits the self-destruction of one's own tissue by forming inactive complexes with proteolytic enzymes. In this way the enzymes are inhibited, and tissue destruction through self-digestion is avoided. Alpha$_1$-antitrypsin has been found to have the highest concentration in serum of any of the plasma proteolytic inhibitors. It is an effective inhibitor of the enzymes chymotrypsin, plasmin, thrombin, collagenase, and elastase. The primary effect of alpha$_1$-antitrypsin may be seen in the respiratory tract and the closed spaces of the body where physiological pH values are maintained. Alpha$_1$-antitrypsin is least effective in the stomach and intestines.

197.
A. Ceruloplasmin, a metalloprotein, is the principal transport protein of copper in the plasma. In the plasma, copper is primarily bound to ceruloplasmin, with only very small amounts of copper bound to albumin or in a dialyzable free state. When subjected to an electric field, ceruloplasmin migrates as an alpha$_2$-globulin.

198.
C. The liver of a fetus and the yolk sac produce a protein known as alpha$_1$-fetoprotein (AFP). The concentration of AFP in the blood of a fetus reaches a maximum concentration at approximately 16 to 18 weeks gestation. Blood levels decline from this point and finally disappear approximately 5 weeks after birth. In cases of open spina bifida or anencephaly, the fetus leaks large amounts of AFP into

the amniotic fluid. By means of an amniocentesis, the amount of AFP present in the amniotic fluid may be quantified by enzyme labeled immunoassay or radioimmunoassay techniques.

199.

C. Although the thermal method for the detection of Bence Jones protein in urine has been replaced by the more reliable immunofixation electrophoresis methods, the thermal method warrants mention because it illustrates a major difference in the reaction of Bence Jones protein to temperature changes in comparison with the serum globulins and albumin. In the thermal method, an aliquot of urine is mixed with a 2 M acetate buffer, pH 4.9. The mixture is then heated to approximately 56 °C. In the presence of Bence Jones protein, precipitation of the protein will occur between 50 °C and 60 °C. The water temperature is then increased to 100 °C. If Bence Jones protein had precipitated at the lower temperature, it would then redissolve between 90 °C and 100 °C. This is unlike the serum globulins and albumin, which would precipitate out of a solution at 100 °C.

200.

D. The immunoglobulins are composed of both heavy and light chains. In Bence Jones proteinuria, there is an overproduction of one type of light chain by a single clone of plasma cells. Therefore, the plasma cells produce either an excessive amount of kappa light chains or an excessive amount of lambda light chains. The light-chain type produced is in such abundance that the renal threshold is exceeded, resulting in the excretion of free light chains of the kappa or lambda type in the urine. The type of light chain excreted in the urine may be identified by performing immunoelectrophoresis on a concentrated urine specimen. In addition, immunoturbidimetric and immunonephelometric methods may also be used.

201.

C. In multiple myeloma there is an abnormal proliferation of plasma cells. These plasma cells produce a homogeneous immunoglobulin protein that stains as a well-defined peak in the gamma region. Because of the presence of this monoclonal protein, the serum total protein will be elevated. Bone destruction is commonly seen in this disorder, with the plasma cells forming densely packed

groups in the lytic areas. Hypercalcemia is primarily the result of bone destruction.

202.

A. Immunonephelometric and immunoturbidimetric techniques are used to quantify specific immunoglobulin classes. Nephelometric techniques used to quantify the immunoglobulins are based on the measurement of light scatter by the antigen-antibody complexes formed. This method also calls for the comparison of unknowns with standards. While radial immunodiffusion can be used to quantify the immunoglobulins, it is not a method of choice. Serum protein electrophoresis, immunoelectrophoresis, and isoelectric focusing cannot be used to quantify the immunoglobulins.

203.

C. Portal cirrhosis is a chronic disease of the liver in which fibrosis occurs as a result of tissue necrosis and diffuse small nodules form as liver cells regenerate with a concomitant distortion of liver structure. The cause of this disorder may include alcoholism, malnutrition, or submassive hepatic necrosis. When a serum protein electrophoresis is performed, the characteristic pattern seen in portal cirrhosis is an elevation of both the gamma- and beta-globulin regions, with these two regions showing a bridging or fusing appearance. This beta-gamma bridging effect is due to an increased level of IgA, which migrates with beta mobility. It should also be noted that the albumin level is depressed.

204.

D. Although microbiological analysis and chemical analysis may be employed to detect and quantify a specific amino acid, chromatographic analysis is preferred as a screening technique for amino acid abnormalities or when differentiation among several amino acids is necessary. Thin-layer chromatography, either one- or two-dimensional, is being used in conjunction with a mixture of ninhydrin-collidine for color development. To quantify amino acids high-performance liquid chromatography, ion-exchange chromatography, and tandem mass spectrometry are used.

205.

C. Proteins are dipolar or zwitterion compounds because they contain amino acids that exhibit both negative and positive charges. The isoelectric point (pI) of a protein refers to the pH at which the number of positive charges on the protein molecule equals the number of negative charges, causing the protein to have a net charge of zero. Since the protein exhibits electrical neutrality at its isoelectric point, it is unable to migrate in an electrical field.

206.

A. Buffer solutions used for serum protein electrophoresis usually have a pH of approximately 8.6. At this alkaline pH, the serum proteins have a net negative charge. Therefore, the negative charged serum proteins migrate toward the anode. This is true for all the proteins except the gamma-globulins, which tend to show the phenomenon of endosmosis.

207.

C. Protein electrophoresis is performed on a serum specimen. If plasma is substituted for serum, the electrophoresis will show an extra fraction in the beta-gamma region, since fibrinogen is a $beta_2$-globulin. This extra fraction represents the protein fibrinogen that is present in a plasma specimen. Fibrinogen contributes approximately 0.2–0.4 g/dL to the total protein concentration.

208.

A. When serum proteins are exposed to a buffer solution of pH 8.6, the proteins take on a net negative charge. The negative charged proteins will migrate toward the anode (+) when exposed to an electrical field. Albumin migrates the fastest toward the anode while the gamma-globulins remain close to the point of application and actually move slightly in a cathodic (−) direction because of the effects of endosmosis. The order of migration of the serum proteins, starting at the anode with the fastest-moving fraction, is albumin, $alpha_1$-globulin, $alpha_2$-globulin, beta-globulin, and gamma-globulin.

209.

D. When serum is applied to a support medium placed in a buffer solution of alkaline pH and subjected to an electrical field, the serum proteins will be separated into fractions for identification and quantification. Support media that may be used for electrophoretic separations include agarose gel, starch gel, cellulose acetate, and acrylamide. The pore size of the agarose gel and cellulose acetate is large enough that the protein molecules are able to move freely through the

media with the resolution of between five and seven fractions. Since the pore size of starch gel and acrylamide is somewhat smaller, the resolution of approximately 20 fractions is possible with this type of medium. Agarose gel and cellulose acetate are the more commonly used media in the routine clinical laboratory.

210.

C. Amido black 10B, Coomassie brilliant blue, and Ponceau S are dyes that are used to stain serum proteins after electrophoresis. Once the serum protein bands are stained, they may be quantified by scanning the support media at the appropriate wavelength with a densitometer. Oil red O and fat red 7B are dyes that are used to stain lipoproteins following electrophoresis.

211.

D. In electrophoresis, each band in the stained protein pattern should be uniformly colored; that is, no holes should appear within an individual band. Such a doughnut-like appearance occurs when the protein is present in too high a concentration, thus exceeding the complexing ability of the stain. This problem is sometimes seen with high concentrations of lactate dehydrogenase isoenzymes when the linearity of the color reaction is exceeded. To overcome this problem, dilute elevated specimens before rerunning the electrophoresis.

212.

D. Ampholytes are mixtures of polyanions and polycations used to establish a pH gradient within the gel media in isoelectric focusing. When an electrical field is applied to the gel, ampholytes seek their own isoelectric point where they become stationary, establishing a pH gradient. Similarly, proteins will migrate within the gel-gradient until they reach the pH of their isoelectric point, thus becoming stationary or focused. This system is most useful in separating proteins that have close isoelectric points.

213.

C. Silver stains react with nanogram concentrations of proteins and nucleic acids, staining them shades of green, yellow, blue, and red. Silver stains are approximately 30 times more sensitive than Coomassie blue stains. Because of their sensitivity, silver stains are being used in electrophoretic methods to identify cerebrospinal fluid and urine proteins without preconcentration of the specimens.

214.

B. Isoelectric focusing is a type of zone electrophoresis. It requires the establishment of a pH gradient, within the agarose or polyacrylamide gel medium, to obtain the separation of charged proteins. Under constant power the proteins migrate to the pH that corresponds to the isoelectric point of the particular protein.

215.

B. Carcinoembryonic antigen (CEA), a glycoprotein, is found in increased amounts in serum when malignant tumors of the colon, lung, pancreas, stomach, and breast are present. Care must be exercised in treating CEA as a diagnostic test, since elevated values are also seen in smokers, hepatitis patients, and patients with several other nonmalignant disorders. Clinically, CEA is more valuable in prognosis and treatment monitoring. Radioimmunoassay and enzyme immunoassay are available for the quantification of CEA.

216.

B. Alpha$_1$-fetoprotein is normally produced only by the fetus, with blood levels disappearing shortly after birth. However, in the adult, such conditions as hepatoma or teratoma stimulate the production of this primitive protein by the tumor cells. The quantification of alpha-fetoprotein may be used both diagnostically and as a monitor of chemotherapy.

217.

D. Prostate-specific antigen (PSA) is a single-chain glycoprotein whose function aids in the liquefaction of seminal coagulum. PSA is found specifically in the prostate gland, and elevated levels are associated with prostate cancer and benign prostatic hyperplasia (BPH). Thus, combining the quantification of PSA with the performance of the digital rectal examination is more beneficial for prostate cancer detection. In addition to radioimmunoassays, immunoassays using enzyme, fluorescent and chemiluminescent labels are available to quantify PSA.

218.

B. CA 125 is an oncofetal antigen, glycoprotein in nature, that is produced by ovarian epithelial cells.

The majority of individuals with nonmucinous epithelial ovarian cancer exhibit elevated levels of CA 125. It is also increased in other malignancies including endometrial, breast, colon, pancreas, and lung cancers. Several benign disorders also exhibit CA 125 elevated levels. It appears that the primary usefulness of CA 125 is in monitoring the success of therapy in treating ovarian carcinoma.

219.

A. CA 19-9 is an oncofetal protein that is an asialylated Lewis blood group antigen. It is found in increased levels in colorectal carcinoma as well as in gastric, hepatobiliary, and pancreatic cancers. CA 19-9 is also elevated in several benign disorders including pancreatitis, extrahepatic cholestasis, and cirrhosis. The combination use of CA 19-9 and CEA (carcinoembryonic antigen) is helpful in monitoring the recurrence of colorectal cancer.

220.

B. Elevations of serum levels of alpha-fetoprotein (AFP) are found in a number of malignant as well as benign disorders. While AFP is considered the most specific laboratory test for hepatocellular carcinoma, increased levels are also found in benign liver disease including viral hepatitis, chronic active hepatitis, and cirrhosis. Other malignant disorders associated with increased levels of AFP include testicular and ovarian germ cell tumors, pancreatic carcinoma, gastric carcinoma, and colonic carcinoma. Thus, AFP is not a tissue specific tumor marker. AFP is not elevated in prostatic cancer, which is characterized by an elevation in prostate-specific antigen (PSA). The use of AFP in conjunction with chorionic gonadotropin (CG) is effective in monitoring treatment and identifying recurrence of testicular cancer.

221.

D. Chorionic gonadotropin (CG) is a dimer consisting of alpha and beta polypeptide chains, with the β subunit conferring immunogenic specificity. While CG is more commonly associated with testing to confirm pregnancy, it is also associated with certain forms of cancer. β-CG is used as a tumor marker for hydatidiform mole, gestational choriocarcinoma, and placental-site trophoblastic tumor. CG's utility also extends to monitoring the success of therapy in testicular and ovarian germ cell tumors. In addition, increased levels of CG have been identified in hematopoietic malignancy, melanoma, gastrointestinal tract neoplasms, sarcoma, and lung, breast, and renal cancers.

222.

D. CA 15-3 and CA 549 are oncofetal antigens that are glycoprotein in nature. CA 15-3 is found on mammary epithelium. Increased serum levels of CA 15-3 are found in breast, pancreatic, lung, colorectal, and liver cancers. CA 549 is found in the cell membrane and luminal surface of breast tissue. Increased serum levels of CA 549 are found in breast, lung, prostate, and colon cancers. While both CA 15-3 and CA 549 are elevated in more advanced stages of breast cancer, neither is helpful in detecting early stages of breast cancer.

NONPROTEIN NITROGENOUS SUBSTANCES

223.

D. Constituents in the plasma that contain the element nitrogen are categorized as being protein- or nonprotein-nitrogen compounds. The principal substances included among the nonprotein-nitrogen compounds are urea, amino acids, uric acid, creatinine, creatine, and ammonia. Of these compounds, urea is present in the plasma in the greatest concentration, comprising approximately 45% of the nonprotein-nitrogen fraction.

224.

D. Since the group of substances classified as nonprotein-nitrogen (NPN) compounds were quantified by assaying for their nitrogen content, it became customary to express urea as urea nitrogen. When urea was expressed as urea nitrogen, a comparison could be made between the concentration of urea and the concentration of other NPN compounds. This type of comparison is not necessary today because the NPN determination has been replaced by individualized procedures for each of the NPN compounds. When it is necessary to convert urea nitrogen values to urea, the concentration may be calculated easily by multiplying the urea nitrogen value by 2.14. This factor is derived from the molecular mass of urea (60 daltons) and the molecular weight of its two nitrogen atoms (28):

$$\frac{60}{28} = 2.14$$

225.

B. In addition to the fact that sodium fluoride is a weak anticoagulant, it also functions as an antiglycolytic agent and is used as a preservative for glucose in blood specimens. With the urease reagent systems for the quantification of urea, the use of sodium fluoride must be avoided because of its inhibitory effect on this system. Additionally, contamination from the use of ammonium oxalate and ammonium heparin must be avoided, since urease catalyzes the production of ammonium carbonate from urea. In several methods, the ammonium ion formed reacts proportionally to the amount of urea originally present in the sample. Anticoagulants containing ammonium would contribute falsely to the urea result.

226.

B. In the diacetyl method, acidic diacetyl reacts directly with urea to form a yellow-diazine derivative. Thiosemicarbazide and ferric ions are reagents used to intensify the color of the reaction. Since urea is quantified directly, the method does not suffer from interferences from ammonia contamination as do some of the urea methods.

227.

A. Adequate specificity is generally obtained when using the urease/glutamate dehydrogenase method. Since urease hydrolyzes urea to ammonia and water, a positive interference from endogenous ammonia will occur with elevated blood levels of ammonia. Such interference may occur from use of aged blood specimens and in certain metabolic diseases.

228.

B. A more current method for quantifying urea employs urease and glutamate dehydrogenase (GLDH) in a coupled enzymatic reaction. Urease catalyzes the production of ammonium carbonate from urea. The ammonium ion produced reacts with 2-oxoglutarate and NADH in the presence of GLDH with the formation of NAD^+ and glutamate. The decrease in absorbance, as NADH is oxidized to NAD^+, is followed kinetically at 340 nm using a spectrophotometer. In the conductimetric method, the formation of ammonium ions and carbonate ions, from the ammonium carbonate, cause a change in conductivity that is related to the amount of urea present in the sample.

229.

C. The Berthelot reaction is based on the production of a blue-indophenol compound when ammonia reacts in an alkaline medium with phenol and sodium hypochlorite. This basic colorimetric reaction can be used to quantify both urea and blood ammonia levels. Therefore, any ammonia contamination (i.e., in the distilled water used to make reagents for the urea procedure and on glassware) must be avoided so that falsely elevated urea values will not be obtained.

230.

A. The catabolism of some amino acids involves a transamination reaction in which the alpha-amino group of the amino acid is enzymatically removed. After its removal, the alpha-amino group is transferred to an alpha-keto acid (alpha-ketoglutarate) with the formation of L-glutamate. Glutamate, which is the common product formed by most transaminase reactions, then may undergo oxidative deamination in the liver mitochondria with the formation of ammonia. The ammonia thus formed leaves the mitochondria as the amino group of citrulline. Citrulline, in turn, condenses with aspartate, which contains the second amino group needed for urea synthesis, forming argininosuccinate, which ultimately leads to the formation of urea. Therefore, the formation of urea and its excretion in the urine provide the principal means by which the body is able to free itself of excess ammonia.

231.

D. It is necessary that certain precautions in specimen handling be exercised because the enzymatic process of deamination of amides continues at room temperature after a blood sample is drawn. When blood is drawn for ammonia analysis, it is critical that any in vitro ammonia formation be prevented. It is recommended that the tube containing the blood specimen be placed in an ice bath immediately after the blood is drawn, since the cold environment will help retard metabolic processes. It is also important that the chemical analysis of the specimen be started within 20 minutes of drawing the specimen.

232.

B. The ammonia concentration in blood may be quantified by use of a cation exchange resin technique. In this procedure, plasma is mixed with a strongly acidic cation exchange resin of the sodium form. The ammonium ion formed is adsorbed onto the resin by an exchange process between the ammonium ion in the plasma and the sodium ion of the resin. After the resin is washed with ammonia-free water, sodium chloride is used to elute the ammonium ion from the resin. The eluted mixture is then reacted with sodium phenoxide in the presence of hypochlorite and nitroprusside. This reaction, known as the indophenol reaction, yields a stable blue coloration that may be read spectrophotometrically and compared with a standard curve.

233.

C. Plasma is the specimen of choice for ammonia analysis. Ethylenediaminetetraacetic acid (EDTA) and heparin (not the ammonium salt) are acceptable anticoagulants. Since exposure of blood to air is contraindicated, the evacuated tube should be filled completely. The blood specimen should be placed on ice immediately and centrifuged as soon as possible to inhibit deamination of amino acids. Since the concentration of ammonia in red blood cells is approximately three times greater than in plasma, the analysis should be performed on a nonhemolyzed specimen. Because of the false increase in ammonia levels caused by smoking, patients should be instructed to refrain from smoking for 8 hours before blood collection.

234.

D. Ion-exchange, ion-selective electrode, and enzymatic methods have been employed for the analysis of ammonia in plasma specimens. Since the enzymatic method is a direct assay, prior separation of ammonium ions is not required. The enzymatic reaction catalyzed by glutamate dehydrogenase follows:

$$2\text{-Oxoglutarate} + NH_4^+ + NADPH \rightleftarrows$$
$$Glutamate + NADP^+ + H_2O$$

The rate of oxidation of NADPH to $NADP^+$ is followed as a decreasing change in absorbance at 340 nm.

235.

D. The gastrointestinal tract is the primary source of blood ammonia. With normal liver function, ammonia is metabolized to urea for urinary excretion. When blood ammonia levels become elevated, toxicity of the central nervous system occurs. Diseases associated with elevated blood ammonia levels include Reye's syndrome, renal failure, chronic liver failure, cirrhosis, and hepatic encephalopathy.

236.

A. Creatinine is a waste product of muscle metabolism and as such its production is rather constant on a daily basis. Creatinine is freely filtered by the glomerulus with only a very small amount secreted by the proximal tubule. Thus, measurement of creatinine is a reflection of glomerular filtration. An increase in the serum creatinine level would be indicative of decreased glomerular filtration. While uric acid, urea, and ammonia levels may be increased with decreased glomerular filtration, increased levels of these analytes are associated with a number of specific metabolic diseases and, therefore, they are not used as indicators of the glomerular filtration rate.

237.

D. Serum urea nitrogen and creatinine levels are frequently requested together so that their ratio can be evaluated. The normal ratio of serum urea nitrogen to creatinine ranges between 10:1 and 20:1. Abnormal values obtained when kidney function tests are performed may be the result of a prerenal, renal, or postrenal malfunction. The ratio of urea nitrogen to creatinine is sometimes used as an index in the assessment of kidney function and as a means of differentiating the source of the malfunction.

238.

C. Creatine is synthesized from the amino acids arginine, glycine, and methionine. In tissues that include the kidneys, small intestinal mucosa, pancreas, and liver, arginine and glycine form guanidoacetate through a transaminidase reaction. The guanidoacetate is transported in the blood to the liver, where it reacts with *S*-adenosylmethionine through a transmethylase reaction to form creatine. Creatine is transported in the blood to muscle tissue. Creatine in the form of phosphocreatine is a high-energy storage compound that provides the phosphate needed to produce adenosine triphosphate (ATP) for muscle metabolism. When ATP is formed from phosphocreatine, free creatine is also released. Creatine, through a spontaneous and irreversible reaction, forms creatinine. Creatinine

serves no functional metabolic role. It is excreted in the urine as a waste product of creatine.

239.

D. The Jaffe reaction, which was described in 1886, remains the basis for most creatinine methods. The Jaffe reaction employs the use of an alkaline picrate solution that reacts with creatinine to form a bright orange-red complex. A drawback to this procedure is its lack of specificity for creatinine, since noncreatinine chromogens, glucose, and proteins are also able to react with alkaline picrate. The specificity of this procedure may be improved by using Lloyd's reagent, an aluminum silicate that adsorbs creatinine and separates it from interfering chromogens before color development.

240.

A. Since protein will interfere with the Jaffe reaction, serum for a manual creatinine analysis is treated with sodium tungstate and sulfuric acid to precipitate the proteins. The use of tungstic acid to make a protein-free filtrate is known as the Folin-Wu method. The protein-free filtrate, which still contains creatinine and other reducing substances, is then mixed with alkaline picrate reagent to yield the characteristic Jaffe reaction. Automated methods have replaced manual methods. These kinetic methods employing the alkaline picrate reagent system have been adapted to use small volumes of serum and have readings taken within a short interval of 25–60 seconds following initiation of the reaction. Because of the speed at which the analysis is performed and the small serum sample requirement, serum may be used directly, alleviating the need for a protein-free filtrate.

241.

D. The creatinine clearance test is used to assess the glomerular filtration rate. An accurately timed 24-hour urine specimen and a blood sample, drawn in the middle of the 24-hour urine collection, are required. The creatinine concentrations of the urine specimen and the plasma are determined, and these values, along with the urine volume, are used to determine the creatinine clearance. The body surface area will not be used in the calculation because the clearance is being done on an average-size adult. The following general mathematical formula is used to calculate creatinine clearance:

$$\frac{U}{P} \times V = \text{Creatinine clearance (mL/min)}$$

where U = urine creatinine concentration in milligrams per deciliter, P = plasma creatinine concentration in milligrams per deciliter, and V = volume of urine per minute, with volume expressed in milliliters and 24 hours expressed as 1440 minutes. Applying this formula to the problem presented in the question:

$$\frac{120 \text{ mg/dL}}{1.2 \text{ mg/dL}} \times \frac{1520 \text{ mL/24 hr}}{1440 \text{ min/24 hr}} = 106 \text{ mL/min}$$

It should be noted that both the size of the kidney and the body surface area of an individual influence the creatinine clearance rate. Since normal values for creatinine clearance are based on the average adult body surface area, it is necessary that the clearance rate be adjusted when the body surface area of the individual being tested differs significantly from the average adult area. This type of adjustment is especially critical if the individual is an infant, a young child, or an adolescent. The body surface area may be calculated from an individual's height and weight, or it may be determined from a nomogram. The average body surface area is accepted as being 1.73 m². The mathematical formula used to calculate a creatinine clearance when the body surface area of the individual is required follows:

$$\frac{U}{P} \times V \times \frac{1.73}{A} = \begin{array}{l}\text{Creatinine clearance} \\ \text{(mL/min/standard surface area)}\end{array}$$

where 1.73 = standard adult surface area in square meters and A = body surface area of the individual in square meters.

242.

C. Creatinine assays are preferably performed on fresh urine specimens. If an acid urine specimen is kept for a time, any creatine in the urine will be converted to creatinine. In alkaline urine, an equilibrium situation will occur between the creatine and creatinine present in the specimen. To avoid either of these situations, it is recommended that the urine be adjusted to pH 7.0 and that the specimen be frozen. It is thought that at a neutral pH, the integrity of the urine specimen will be maintained because it will require days or even weeks for equilibrium to occur between the two compounds.

243.

D. Creatine is predominantly found in muscle cells where the quantity of creatine is proportional to muscle mass. As muscle metabolism proceeds, creatine is freed from its high-energy phosphate form, and the creatine, thus liberated, forms the anhydride creatinine. The quantity of creatinine formed daily is a relatively constant amount because it is related to muscle mass. Therefore, it has been customary to quantify the creatinine present in a 24-hour urine specimen as an index of the completeness of the collection.

244.

A. In addition to the end-point and kinetic methods, which utilize the Jaffe reaction (picric acid), several methods have been developed that employ coupled enzymatic reactions for the quantification of creatinine. In one such method, creatinine amidohydrolase (creatininase) catalyzes the conversion of creatinine to creatine and subsequently to sarcosine and urea. Sarcosine oxidase catalyzes the oxidation of sarcosine to glycine, formaldehyde, and hydrogen peroxide. The hydrogen peroxide reacts with the reduced form of a chromogenic dye in the presence of peroxidase to form an oxidized colored dye product that is read spectrophotometrically.

245.

C. Creatinine is an endogenous substance that is filtered by the glomeruli and normally is neither reabsorbed nor secreted by the tubules. When plasma levels of creatinine rise, some secretion of creatinine by the tubules will occur. The filtration properties of creatinine and the fact that it is a substance normally present in blood make the creatinine clearance test the method of choice for assessing the glomerular filtration rate.

246.

B. Through a sequence of enzymatic reactions, the purine nucleosides, adenosine and guanosine, are catabolized to the waste product uric acid. The catabolism of purines occurs primarily in the liver, with the majority of uric acid being excreted as a urinary waste product. The remaining amount of uric acid is excreted in the biliary, pancreatic, and gastrointestinal secretions through the gastrointestinal tract. In the large intestine, uric acid is further degraded by bacteria and excreted in the stool.

247.

D. Uric acid may be quantified by reacting it with phosphotungstic acid reagent in alkaline solution. In this reaction, uric acid is oxidized to allantoin and the phosphotungstic acid is reduced, forming a tungsten blue complex. The intensity of the tungsten blue complex is proportional to the concentration of uric acid in the specimen.

248.

B. Uric acid absorbs light in the ultraviolet region of 290–293 nm. When uricase is added to a uric acid mixture, uricase destroys uric acid by catalyzing its degradation to allantoin and carbon dioxide. On the basis of these two characteristics, differential spectrophotometry has been applied to the quantification of uric acid. This type of method is used on analyzers that are capable of monitoring the decrease in absorbance as uric acid is destroyed by uricase. The decrease in absorbance is proportional to the concentration of uric acid in the specimen.

249.

A. As renal function continues to be lost over time, chronic renal failure develops. Chronic renal failure is manifested by loss of excretory function, inability to regulate water and electrolyte balance, and increased production of parathyroid hormone, all of which contribute to the abnormal laboratory findings. The decreased production of erythropoietin causes anemia to develop.

250.

D. Gout is a pathological condition that may be caused by a malfunction of purine metabolism or a depression in the renal excretion of uric acid. Two of the major characteristics of gout are hyperuricemia and a deposition of uric acid as monosodium urate crystals in joints, periarticular cartilage, bone, bursae, and subcutaneous tissue. Such a deposition of urate crystals causes inflammation of the affected area and precipitates an arthritic attack.

251.

A. An increase in serum uric acid levels may be seen during chemotherapy for leukemia. The cause of this is the accelerated breakdown of cell nuclei in response to the chemotherapy. Other proliferative disorders that may respond similarly are lymphoma, multiple myeloma, and polycythemia. It is important that serum uric acid be monitored during chemotherapy to avoid nephrotoxicity.

HEMOGLOBIN, HEME DERIVATIVES, AND LIVER FUNCTION

252.

D. The biochemical synthesis of the porphyrins consists of a series of reactions. Succinyl coenzyme A and glycine are the two compounds that originally condense to form aminolevulinic acid (ALA). Through a second condensation reaction, two molecules of ALA condense and cyclize to form porphobilinogen. Porphobilinogen is a monopyrrole structure and the precursor of porphyrin synthesis.

253.

D. Heme is derived from a series of biochemical reactions that begin with the formation of porphobilinogen from succinyl coenzyme A and glycine. Since porphobilinogen is a monopyrrole, four molecules of porphobilinogen condense and cyclize to form the porphyrinogen precursors of protoporphyrin IX. It is protoporphyrin IX that chelates iron to form heme and is, therefore, the immediate precursor of heme formation.

254.

D. Porphobilinogen is a precursor compound in the biosynthesis of heme. In acute intermittent porphyria, excess amounts of porphobilinogen are excreted in the urine. The Watson-Schwartz test employs *p*-dimethylaminobenzaldehyde reagent (also known as Ehrlich's aldehyde reagent) to form a red condensation product with porphobilinogen.

255.

D. The porphyrins that are of clinical significance include uroporphyrin, coproporphyrin, and protoporphyrin. These three porphyrin compounds may be detected in acid solution by irradiating the solution with long-wave ultraviolet light, which causes the porphyrins to fluoresce. The intense orange-red fluorescence of the porphyrins is due to the conjugated unsaturation of the tetrapyrrole ring structure.

256.

B. When measurement of aminolevulinic acid, porphobilinogen, uroporphyrin, and coproporphyrin are requested, a 24-hour urine specimen should be collected. The urine should be refrigerated during collection and stored in a brown bottle to protect light-sensitive compounds. Since porphobilinogen is more stable under alkaline conditions and aminolevulinic acid is more stable under acid conditions, sodium bicarbonate should be added as a compromise to maintain the pH near 7.

257.

A. Hemoglobin is a tetramer composed of four globin chains, four heme groups, and four iron atoms. In adult hemoglobin, or hemoglobin A, there are two alpha chains and two beta chains. Hemoglobin A₂, which comprises less than 4% of the normal adult hemoglobin, is composed of two alpha chains and two delta chains. Hemoglobin F, or fetal hemoglobin, is composed of two alpha chains and two gamma chains.

258.

D. Although hemoglobin differentiation is best achieved by use of electrophoresis, hemoglobin F may be differentiated from the majority of human hemoglobins because of its alkali resistance. Hemoglobin F is able to resist denaturation and remain soluble when added to an alkaline solution. In contrast to hemoglobin F, most hemoglobins will denature in alkaline solution and precipitate on the addition of ammonium sulfate. After 1 year of age, the normal concentration of hemoglobin F is less than 1% of the total hemoglobin. However, hemoglobin F may be present in elevated concentrations in disorders that include thalassemia, sickle cell disease, and aplastic anemia.

259.

A. A number of hemoglobinopathies exist where a substitution of one amino acid on either the alpha chain or the beta chain causes the formation of an abnormal hemoglobin molecule. Hemoglobin S is an abnormal hemoglobin that is characterized by the substitution of valine for glutamic acid in position 6 of the beta chain. Hemoglobin C is an abnormal hemoglobin in which lysine replaces glutamic acid in position 6 of the beta chain. The structural changes that are seen in hemoglobin S and C disorders are inherited as autosomal recessive traits.

260.

A. At pH 8.6, hemoglobins have a net negative charge and migrate from the point of application toward the anode. When hemoglobin electrophoresis is performed on cellulose acetate at pH 8.6, hemoglobin A migrates the fastest toward the anode, followed respectively by hemoglobins F and S. Hemoglobins A₂ and C have the same electrophoretic mobility and migrate slightly slower than hemoglobin S. Since hemoglobins A₂ and C exhibit nearly the same mobility, they cannot be differentiated on cellulose acetate.

261.

D. At pH 6.2 on agar gel, hemoglobins exhibit different electrophoretic mobilities in comparison with hemoglobins electrophoresed at pH 8.6 on cellulose acetate. The order of migration of hemoglobins on cellulose acetate, proceeding from the most anodal hemoglobin to the most cathodal hemoglobin, is respectively A and F, followed by G, D, and S, which migrate with the same mobility, followed by the group A₂, C, O, and E, which migrate the most slowly with the same mobility. This migration pattern is in contrast to agar gel electrophoresis at pH 6.2 in which the order of migration, from the most anodal hemoglobin to the most cathodal hemoglobin, is, respectively, C and S, followed by the group A, A₂, D, E, and G, which migrate with the same mobility, followed by F. The different migration patterns seen with these two media systems are useful in differentiating hemoglobins that migrate with the same electrophoretic mobility. In the case of hemoglobins A₂ and C, which migrate with the same mobility on cellulose acetate, it is not possible to discern which hemoglobin is present in a particular blood specimen. By electrophoresing this specimen on agar gel at pH 6.2, hemoglobin A₂ may be differentiated from hemoglobin C because hemoglobin A₂ exhibits mobility similar to that of hemoglobin A, whereas hemoglobin C migrates alone closest to the anode.

262.

D. Although hemoglobin electrophoresis is the recommended method for hemoglobin identification, solubility testing may be warranted for large-scale screening for hemoglobin S. Solubility testing is possible because the solubility properties of most hemoglobins differ enough from those of hemoglobin S. In this method, sodium hydrosulfite acts as a reducing agent to deoxygenate hemoglobin. In the presence of hemoglobin S, the concentrated phosphate buffer test solution will become turbid because deoxygenated hemoglobin S is insoluble in the buffer solution. Hemoglobins A, C, D, and F, when present, will remain soluble in the phosphate buffer solution and show no visible signs of turbidity. Therefore, the detection of turbidity is associated with the presence of hemoglobin S.

263.

D. In the catabolic process of hemoglobin degradation, the alpha-carbon methene bridge of the tetrapyrrole ring structure of heme opens oxidatively to form verdohemoglobin. Verdohemoglobin is a complex composed of biliverdin, iron, and the protein globin. This complex then undergoes degradation in which iron is removed and returned to the body iron stores, the globin portion is returned to the amino acid pool, and the biliverdin undergoes reduction to form bilirubin. It is biliverdin, therefore, that is the immediate precursor of bilirubin formation. Mesobilirubinogen and urobilinogen represent intestinal breakdown products of bilirubin catabolism.

264.

B. Diazo reagent is a mixture of sulfanilic acid, sodium nitrite, and hydrochloric acid. The mixing of sodium nitrite with hydrochloric acid forms nitrous acid, which in turn reacts with sulfanilic acid to form a diazonium salt. This diazotized sulfanilic acid mixture, when mixed with solubilized bilirubin, forms a red azobilirubin complex. The azobilirubin complexes are isomeric structures formed from the splitting of the bilirubin compound in half. Each half then reacts with the diazo reagent to form two isomeric azobilirubin complexes.

265.

C. In order for the bilirubin-albumin complex to reach the parenchymal cells of the liver, the complex must be transported from the sinusoids to the sinusoidal microvilli and into the parenchymal cell. The microsomal fraction of the parenchymal cell is responsible for the conjugation of bilirubin. It is here that bilirubin reacts with uridine diphosphate glucuronate in the presence of the enzyme system uridine diphosphate glucuronyltransferase to form bilirubin diglucuronide.

266.

B. Bilirubin that has been secreted through the bile into the small intestine is reduced by anaerobic microorganisms to urobilinogen. One of the possible fates of urobilinogen is its conversion to urobilin. In the colon, a portion of the urobilinogen is oxidized by the action of microorganisms to urobilin, which is excreted in the feces as an orange-brown pigment.

267.

D. The cells of the reticuloendothelial system are able to phagocytize aged red blood cells and convert the hemoglobin to the excretory product bilirubin. It is then necessary for the bilirubin to be transported to the liver, where it is conjugated for excretion in the bile. Albumin acts as the transport vehicle for unconjugated bilirubin in the blood, with each mole of albumin capable of binding two moles of bilirubin.

268.

A. When total bilirubin levels exceed 2.5 mg/dL, the clinical manifestation of jaundice develops. Characteristically, such body areas as the skin and sclera develop a yellow-pigmented appearance. Jaundice may be caused by an increase in either the unconjugated or conjugated form of bilirubin. Such increases in bilirubin levels may be caused by prehepatic, hepatic, or posthepatic disorders.

269.

A. An abnormal accumulation of bilirubin in the body may be due to increased production or decreased excretion of bilirubin. Terms frequently associated with a buildup of bilirubin include jaundice, kernicterus, and icterus. Both jaundice and icterus are characterized by the yellow coloration of the skin, sclera, and mucous membranes that results from increased plasma concentrations of either conjugated or unconjugated bilirubin or both. This yellow coloration is also visible in serum and plasma specimens in vitro. Kernicterus refers to the accumulation of bilirubin in brain tissue that occurs with elevated levels of unconjugated bilirubin. This condition is most commonly seen in newborns with hemolytic disease resulting from maternal-fetal Rh incompatibility. Newborns afflicted with kernicterus will exhibit severe neural symptoms.

270.

B. In the small intestine, urobilinogen is formed through the enzymatic reduction process of anaerobic bacteria on bilirubin. The fate of urobilinogen is such that some of the urobilinogen will be excreted unchanged in the stool, a portion will be oxidized to urobilin for excretion in the stool, and up to 20% will be absorbed from the intestine into the portal circulation. This circulating urobilinogen is almost completely picked up by the liver, with only a small amount excreted in the urine. The liver oxidizes a small part of the recycled urobilinogen to bilirubin. This newly formed bilirubin and any unchanged urobilinogen are transported through the bile canaliculi into the bile for reexcretion by the intestines. This recycling of urobilinogen is part of the enterohepatic circulation.

271.

D. Bilirubin will deteriorate when exposed to either white or UV light. This deterioration is also temperature sensitive. Thus specimens for bilirubin analysis should be stored in the dark at refrigerator temperature until the assay can be performed. Lipemia should be avoided, due to its interference with spectrophotometric analyses. Since hemoglobin reacts with diazo reagent, use of hemolyzed specimens should be avoided. Hemolysis will cause bilirubin results to be falsely low.

272.

C. Four bilirubin fractions represented by Greek letters have been identified: unconjugated (alpha), monoconjugated (beta), diconjugated (gamma), and unconjugated bilirubin covalently bound to albumin (delta). Delta-bilirubin is normally present in low concentration in the blood, and it is known to react directly with diazotized sulfanilic acid. Increased serum levels of delta-bilirubin are associated with liver-biliary disease.

273.

A. The cells of the reticuloendothelial system are responsible for the removal of old red blood cells from the peripheral circulation. As the red blood cells reach the end of their 120-day life span, the specialized cells mainly of the spleen phagocytize the aged cells and convert the released hemoglobin into the excretory pigment bilirubin. The bone marrow is also responsible for the destruction of a small number of red blood cells that have not completed the maturation process. The bilirubin produced by the reticuloendothelial cells is indirect bilirubin, which, as a protein-bound compound, is transported to the liver for conjugation into direct bilirubin.

274.

C. Bilirubinometer, bilirubin oxidase and Jendrassik-Grof are methods that have been used to quantify serum bilirubin concentrations. The bilirubinometer is used for direct spectrophotometric assay in which the bilirubin concentration is read directly at 454 nm. In the bilirubin oxidase method, bilirubin is oxidized to biliverdin and the reaction is followed at 405–460 nm. The Jendrassik-Grof method utilizes a caffeine-sodium benzoate mixture to accelerate the coupling reaction of unconjugated bilirubin with diazo reagent to form an azobilirubin complex. Because of a high recovery rate, the Jendrassik-Grof method is considered to be the method of choice for bilirubin analysis.

275.

A. Direct bilirubin was so named because of its ability in the van den Bergh method to react directly with diazotized sulfanilic acid without the addition of alcohol. Such a direct reaction is possible because direct bilirubin is conjugated in the liver with glucuronic acid, thereby making it a polar, water-soluble compound. Since conjugated bilirubin is both water soluble and not protein bound, it may be filtered through the glomerulus and excreted in the urine of jaundiced patients. Indirect bilirubin is a protein-bound unconjugated compound that is soluble in alcohol but not in water, and because of these properties, it is unable to be excreted in the urine.

276.

C. Ehrlich's diazo reagent consists of sulfanilic acid, hydrochloric acid, and sodium nitrite. Sulfanilic acid is dissolved in hydrochloric acid and diluted to volume with deionized water. Sodium nitrite is dissolved in deionized water and diluted to volume. Aliquots of these two reagent mixtures are combined to prepare Ehrlich's diazo reagent, which must be prepared fresh before use because of its unstable nature.

277.

C. Unlike direct bilirubin, indirect-reacting bilirubin is insoluble in deionized water and dilute hydrochloric acid. Indirect-reacting bilirubin must first be mixed with methanol or caffeine-sodium benzoate to solubilize it before one can proceed with the diazo reaction. Because of these properties, total bilirubin and direct bilirubin are usually chemically analyzed, and the indirect, or unconjugated, fraction is calculated from the difference between the total and direct values. The total value represents the reaction of both conjugated and unconjugated bilirubin, whereas the direct value represents only the reaction of conjugated bilirubin.

278.

B. In the bilirubin oxidase method, the enzyme bilirubin oxidase catalyzes the oxidation of bilirubin to the product biliverdin, which is colorless. This is seen as a decrease in absorbance and is monitored between 405 and 460 nm. Although the method is not widely used, it has an advantage over diazo methods in that hemoglobin does not interfere in the assay and cause falsely low results.

279.

A. Conjugated bilirubin and a small amount of unconjugated bilirubin will pass from the bile into the small intestine. In the small intestine, enzyme systems of anaerobic bacteria are able to reduce bilirubin to the reduction products mesobilirubinogen, stercobilinogen, and urobilinogen. These three reduction products of bilirubin catabolism are collectively referred to as urobilinogen.

280.

D. Obstructive jaundice is a term applied to conditions in which the common bile duct is obstructed because of gallstone formation, spasm, or neoplasm. Such an obstruction blocks the flow of bile from the gallbladder into the small intestine. This impedance of bile flow will result in a backflow of bile from the gallbladder into the sinusoids of the liver and ultimately into the peripheral circulation. Since the liver is not initially involved and the disorder is of posthepatic origin, the increased levels of bilirubin in the blood are caused by the backflow of conjugated bilirubin. If the disorder is allowed to progress, the continued backflow of bile will cause parenchymal cell destruction. Such cellular necrosis will result in a depression of the conjugating ability of the liver, and an elevation of unconjugated bilirubin levels in the blood will ensue.

281.

A. Hemolytic jaundice is also referred to as prehepatic jaundice. It is caused by excessive destruction of erythrocytes at a rate that exceeds the conjugating ability of the liver. As a result, increased levels

of unconjugated bilirubin appear in the blood. The amount of conjugated bilirubin being formed in the liver is proportionately greater than normal; this is reflected in the increased levels of urobilinogen and urobilin found in the stool. Because of the enterohepatic circulation, the increased urobilinogen levels in the small intestines are reflected by an increase in the circulating blood levels of urobilinogen. Since the liver is unable to pick up all the circulating urobilinogen, the urinary levels of urobilinogen are increased. Urinary bilirubin levels are negative because the blood level of conjugated bilirubin is usually normal.

282.

D. The enzyme system uridine diphosphate glucuronyltransferase catalyzes the conjugation of bilirubin with glucuronic acid. In newborns, especially premature infants, this liver enzyme system is not fully developed or functional. Because of this deficiency in the enzyme system, the concentration of unconjugated bilirubin rises in the blood, since only the conjugated form may be excreted through the bile and urine. The increased levels of unconjugated bilirubin will cause the infant to appear jaundiced. Generally, this condition persists for only a short period because the enzyme system usually becomes functional within several days after birth. Neonatal physiological jaundice resulting from an enzyme deficiency is hepatic in origin. Hemolytic jaundice resulting from either Rh or ABO incompatibility is a prehepatic type of jaundice, whereas a stricture of the common bile duct is classified as posthepatic jaundice.

283.

C. With complete obstruction of the common bile duct, bilirubin diglucuronide would be unable to pass from the bile into the intestines. Such obstruction to the flow of bile will cause the conjugated bilirubin to be regurgitated into the sinusoids and the general circulation. Since conjugated bilirubin is water soluble, it will be excreted in the urine. However, because of the lack of bile flow into the intestines, neither urobilinogen nor urobilin will be present in the feces. The lack of urobilin in the feces will be apparent from the light brown to chalky-white coloration of the stools. Since there is no urobilinogen in the intestines to be picked up by the enterohepatic circulation, the urinary excretion of urobilinogen will be negative. Since the obstruction may sometimes be only partial, then this description would be somewhat altered. Provided that some bile was able to flow into the intestines, the fecal urobilinogen and urobilin concentrations would be present but depressed, the urinary urobilinogen excretion would be below normal, and the urinary bilirubin level would be increased.

284.

B. In disorders such as viral hepatitis, toxic hepatitis, and cirrhosis, hepatocellular damage occurs. The damaged parenchymal cells lose their ability either to conjugate bilirubin or to transport the bilirubin that is conjugated into the bile. Because of loss of conjugating ability by some parenchymal cells, the early stage of viral hepatitis is characterized by an increase in the unconjugated bilirubin fraction in the blood. An increase of lesser magnitude in the conjugated fraction is also demonstrated. The increase in conjugated bilirubin is due to the fact that some cells are able to conjugate but are damaged in such a way that there is leakage of conjugated bilirubin into the sinusoids and the general circulation. Because of this increase in the conjugated fraction, urinary bilirubin excretion is positive. Since the amount of conjugated bilirubin reaching the intestines is less than normal, it follows that the fecal urobilinogen and urobilin levels will also be less than normal. However, the urinary urobilinogen levels will be greater than normal because the urobilinogen that does reach the enterohepatic circulation is not efficiently removed by the liver but, rather, is excreted by the urinary system.

285.

B. Both Crigler-Najjar syndrome and neonatal jaundice, a physiological disorder, are due to a deficiency in the enzyme-conjugating system. With a deficiency in uridine diphosphate glucuronyltransferase, the liver is unable to conjugate bilirubin, and both of these conditions are characterized by increased levels of unconjugated bilirubin. Unlike Crigler-Najjar syndrome, which is a hereditary disorder, neonatal physiological jaundice is a temporary situation that usually corrects itself within a few days after birth.

286.

D. Gilbert's syndrome is a preconjugation transport disturbance. In this disorder the hepatic uptake of bilirubin is defective because the transportation of bilirubin from the sinusoidal membrane to the microsomal region is impaired. Gilbert's syndrome is inherited as an autosomal dominant trait characterized by increased levels of unconjugated bilirubin.

287.

C. In Dubin-Johnson syndrome the transport of conjugated (direct) bilirubin from the microsomal region to the bile canaliculi is impaired. In this rare familial disorder, plasma conjugated bilirubin levels are increased because of defective excretion of bilirubin in the bile. Since conjugated bilirubin is water soluble, increased amounts of bilirubin are found in the urine.

288.

D. Abnormal conditions characterized by jaundice may be classified according to their type of liver involvement. The three types of jaundice are prehepatic, hepatic, and posthepatic. Hepatic jaundice may be subdivided into two groups on the basis of the type of excessive bilirubin: conjugated bilirubin or unconjugated bilirubin. Gilbert's syndrome and Dubin-Johnson syndrome are disorders in which the process of bilirubin transport is malfunctioning. Both Crigler-Najjar syndrome and neonatal jaundice, a physiological disorder, are due to a deficiency in the enzyme-conjugating system. Disorders such as viral hepatitis, toxic hepatitis, and cirrhosis cause damage and destruction of liver cells so that the ability of the liver to remove unconjugated bilirubin from the blood and to conjugate it with glucuronic acid becomes impaired. As these disorders progress, the level of unconjugated bilirubin in the blood rises. There is also an increase, although not as great as that of unconjugated bilirubin, in blood levels of conjugated bilirubin. The cause is a leakage of conjugated bilirubin from damaged parenchymal cells into the sinusoids. Neoplasm of the common bile duct is a form of posthepatic jaundice.

289.

A. Prehepatic jaundice is also known as hemolytic jaundice, a term that is descriptive of the cause of the disorder. Any disorder that causes the destruction of erythrocytes at a faster rate than the liver is able to conjugate the bilirubin being formed by the reticuloendothelial system will exhibit hyperbilirubinemia. The increased concentration of bilirubin and the ensuing jaundice is not due to any hepatic malfunction but only to the inability of the liver to handle the conjugation of such a bilirubin overload. Therefore, the jaundice is caused by an increased concentration of unconjugated bilirubin. Disorders that follow this type of course are acute hemolytic anemia, chronic hemolytic anemia, and neonatal jaundice. Causes of hemolytic anemia may be genetic or acquired and include hereditary spherocytosis, sickle-cell anemia, and blood transfusion reactions. Neonatal jaundice may be due to an ABO or a Rh incompatibility, as seen in erythroblastosis fetalis.

290.

B. Posthepatic jaundice is caused by an obstruction in the common bile duct, extrahepatic ducts, or the ampulla of Vater. Such an obstruction may be caused by gallstones, neoplasms, or strictures. In this type of jaundice, the liver is functioning properly in its conjugation of bilirubin, but the obstruction causes a blockage so that the conjugated bilirubin is unable to be excreted through the intestines. Therefore, there is a backup of bile into the sinusoids and an overflow into the blood. The circulating blood will characteristically contain excessive amounts of conjugated bilirubin, which will cause increased amounts of bilirubin to be excreted in the urine. Since the blockage prevents proper excretion of bilirubin into the intestines, the formation of urobilinogen and urobilin is impeded. This pattern will continue until the regurgitation of bile causes hepatocellular damage. With destruction of the parenchymal cells, conjugation of bilirubin will be depressed and the blood levels of unconjugated bilirubin will also rise.

ELECTROLYTES

291.

C. Sodium is the principal cation found in the plasma. The normal serum sodium level is 136–146 mmol/L, whereas in urine the sodium concentration ranges between 40–220 mmol/day, being dependent on dietary intake. Since sodium is a threshold substance, it is normally excreted in the urine when the serum sodium concentration exceeds 110–130 mmol/L. When serum levels fall below 110 mmol/L, all the sodium in the glomerular filtrate is virtually reabsorbed in the proximal and distal tubules. This reabsorption process is influenced by the hormone aldosterone.

292.

D. Osmolality is a measure of the total number of solute particles per unit weight of solution and is expressed as milliosmoles per kilogram of water. The normal osmolality of serum is in the range of 275–295 mOsm/kg water. For monovalent cations or anions the contribution to osmolality is approximately 92%. Other serum electrolytes, serum proteins, glucose, and urea contribute to the remaining 8%.

293.

B. Hemolysis of blood specimens because of physiological factors is often difficult to differentiate from hemolysis produced by the blood collection itself. In either case, the concentration of potassium will be increased in the serum because of the release of the very high level of intracellular potassium from the erythrocytes into the plasma. When hemolysis is present, the serum concentrations of sodium, bicarbonate, chloride, and calcium will be decreased because their concentrations are lower in erythrocytes than in plasma.

294.

D. The largest fractions of the anion content of serum are normally provided by chloride and bicarbonate. The third largest anion fraction is contributed by the proteins that are negatively charged at physiological pH and that provide about 16 mmol ion charge per liter. Of the remaining organic anions, the largest contribution is generally from lactate, which ranges normally from 1 mmol/L up to 25 mmol/L in lactic acidosis. The ketone bodies, including acetoacetate, normally constitute only a small fraction of the total anions, but their total contribution may increase to 20 mmol/L in diabetic acidosis. Iron is present in the serum as a cation and does not contribute.

295.

D. In contrast to sodium, which is the principal plasma cation, potassium is the principal cellular cation. After absorption in the intestinal tract, potassium is partially filtered from the plasma by the kidneys. It is then almost completely reabsorbed from the glomerular filtrate by the proximal tubules and subsequently reexcreted by the distal tubules. Unlike sodium, potassium exhibits no renal threshold, being excreted into the urine even in K^+-depleted states. In acidotic states, as in renal tubular acidosis in which the exchange of Na^+ for H^+ is impaired, the resulting retention of potassium causes an elevation in serum K^+ levels. Hemolysis must be avoided in blood specimens that are to be used for K^+ analysis because erythrocytes contain a potassium concentration 23 times greater than serum K^+ levels. If the red blood cells are hemolyzed, a significant increase in serum K^+ will result.

296.

A. Chloride can be quantified by the spectrophotometric ferric perchlorate method. The reagent reacts with chloride to form a colored complex. Other methods employed are the spectrophotometric mercuric thiocyanate method, the coulometric-amperometric titration method, and ion-selective electrode method.

297.

C. Chloride is the principal plasma anion. The average concentration of chloride in plasma is 103 mmol/L. In the kidneys, chloride ions are removed from the blood through the glomerulus and then passively reabsorbed by the proximal tubules. The chloride pump actively reabsorbs chloride in the thick ascending limb of the loop of Henle. In the lungs, chloride ions participate in buffering the blood by shifting from the plasma to the red blood cells to compensate for ionic changes that occur in the alveoli when the HCO_3^- from the red blood cells enters the plasma. This is termed the chloride shift. Chloride can be measured in a variety of body fluids including serum, plasma, urine, and sweat.

298.

A. The calculation of the anion gap may be used both to assess instrument performance and as a quality assurance tool for electrolyte analyses. The following is one of several equations that may be used to calculate the anion-gap: anion gap (mmol/L) = $(Na^+ + K^+) - (Cl^- + HCO_3^-)$. The acceptable reference range for this method of calculation is 10–20 mmol/L. If the values of a particular patient fall within this acceptable level, it is presumed that there are no gross problems with the electrolyte measurements. In this case, the anion gap is 18 mmol/L and within the reference range. When using the anion gap it is important to remember that values are affected not only by measurement

errors but also by such disease processes as renal failure, ketoacidosis, and salicylate poisoning. Therefore, it is important to differentiate between laboratory errors and true disease states.

299.

C. Addison's disease is characterized by the hyposecretion of the adrenocortical hormones by the adrenal cortex. Both aldosterone, a mineralocorticoid, and cortisol, a glucocorticoid, are inadequately secreted in this disorder. The decreased secretion of aldosterone will affect body electrolyte balance and extracellular fluid volume. The decrease in sodium reabsorption by the renal tubules will be accompanied by decreased chloride and water retention. This loss of sodium, chloride, and water into the urine will cause the extracellular fluid volume to be decreased. Additionally, the decreased reabsorption of sodium will interfere with the secretion of potassium and hydrogen ions in the renal tubules, causing an increase in the serum potassium ion and hydrogen ion (acidosis) concentrations.

300.

D. Primary aldosteronism is characterized by the hypersecretion of aldosterone, a mineralocorticoid, by the zona glomerulosa cells of the adrenal cortex. Excessive secretion of aldosterone will increase renal tubular reabsorption of sodium resulting in a decrease in the loss of sodium in the urine. The net result of this mechanism is increased sodium in the extracellular fluid. Additionally, there will be increased renal excretion of potassium, causing a decrease of potassium in the extracellular fluid.

301.

D. A decreased serum sodium concentration, or hyponatremia, is associated with a variety of disorders, including (1) *Addison's disease*, which involves the inadequate secretion of aldosterone, resulting in decreased reabsorption of sodium by the renal tubules; (2) *diarrhea*, which involves the impaired absorption from the gastrointestinal tract of dietary sodium and of sodium from the pancreatic juice, causing an excessive quantity of sodium to be excreted in the feces; (3) *diuretic therapy*, which causes a loss of water with concurrent loss of electrolytes including sodium; and (4) *renal tubular disease*, which involves either the insufficient reabsorption of sodium in the tubules or a defect in the Na^+-H^+ tubular exchange mechanism. A diagnosis of Cushing's syndrome is incorrect because the disorder is associated with hypernatremia.

302.

C. Free ionized calcium normally accounts for about 50% of total serum calcium, with the remainder being made up of complexed calcium (about 10%) and calcium bound to proteins (about 40%). The main factors that affect the free ionized calcium fraction are the protein concentration and the pH of the blood. Calcium ions are bound mainly to albumin, but they also bind to globulins. Since the binding is reversible, factors that decrease the protein concentration will increase the free ionized fraction of calcium in the blood. A decrease in blood pH will also increase the fraction of free ionized calcium.

303.

D. The renal tubular reabsorption of phosphate is controlled by the action of parathyroid hormone (PTH) on the kidney. Increased PTH secretion from any cause will lead to a decreased tubular reabsorption of phosphate (increased urine phosphate and decreased serum phosphate). The test is useful in distinguishing serum hypercalcemia that is a result of excess PTH production by the parathyroid glands from hypercalcemia due to other causes (e.g., bone disease).

304.

D. Parathyroid hormone (PTH), calcitonin, vitamin D, plasma proteins, and plasma phosphates are factors that influence plasma calcium levels. *PTH* is a hormone important in maintaining plasma calcium levels. It mobilizes calcium from bones. It increases the synthesis of one of the vitamin D derivatives, thereby causing an increase in bone resorption and intestinal absorption of calcium. When normal calcium levels are restored, PTH secretion is cut off (negative-feedback mechanism). *Calcitonin* (thyrocalcitonin) is a hormone secreted by the thyroid in response to elevated levels of plasma calcium. It acts by inhibiting bone resorption of calcium, thereby preventing significant variations in plasma calcium concentrations. Hydroxylation of *vitamin D* gives a derivative that will increase the intestinal absorption of calcium and phosphates.

305.

D. PTH has physiological actions on bone, kidney, and intestine. Its overall effect is to raise serum ionized calcium levels and lower serum phosphorus levels. Its actions on various organs are the result of a combination of both direct and indirect effects. In bones, PTH directly acts to increase bone resorption, thereby increasing both calcium and phosphorus in the blood. In the kidneys, PTH directly acts on the renal tubules to decrease phosphate reabsorption. In combination with the effect on bone, the overall result is a decrease in blood phosphorus levels. In the intestines, PTH acts to increase absorption of calcium by its action in increasing 1,25-dihydroxyvitamin D_3 synthesis in the kidneys, which in turn stimulates intestinal absorption of calcium.

306.

A. Primary hyperparathyroidism is a disorder characterized by increased secretion of PTH into the blood without the stimulus on the parathyroid gland of a decreased level of ionized calcium. The increase in PTH produces increased blood calcium and vitamin D_3 levels, along with a decreased blood phosphorus level. The hypersecretion is most often caused by a single parathyroid adenoma. PTH secretion can usually, but not in all cases, be suppressed by calcium infusion. The decreased blood phosphate level is a result of the action of PTH on the kidneys, which decreases tubular reabsorption of phosphate ions. The increased blood level of 1,25-dihydroxyvitamin D_3 is also caused by PTH action on the kidneys in that PTH stimulates increased renal synthesis of this compound.

307.

C. Secondary hyperparathyroidism is a disorder that represents the response of a normally functioning parathyroid gland to chronic hypocalcemia. In most patients the hypocalcemia is the result of renal disease or vitamin D deficiency. Vitamin D deficiency decreases intestinal calcium absorption, resulting in hypocalcemia. The hypocalcemia resulting from renal disease is more complex. It can result either from the increased serum phosphate level caused by decreased glomerular filtration or from the decreased synthesis of 1,25-dihydroxyvitamin D_3 in kidney disease.

308.

B. Serum inorganic phosphate concentrations are determined most commonly by reacting with ammonium molybdate reagent. The molybdenum-phosphate complexes can be quantified at 340 nm. Alternately, treatment of the phosphomolybdate compound formed with a reducing agent leads to the formation of molybdenum blue, which can be measured spectrophotometrically. Use of the anticoagulants EDTA, oxalate, and citrate should be avoided, since they interfere with the formation of phosphomolybdate.

309.

A. Total serum calcium concentration is often determined by the spectrophotometric quantification of the color complex formed with cresolphthalein complexone. Magnesium will also form a color complex and, therefore, is removed by reacting the serum with 8-hydroxyquinoline. Calcium concentration is determined with the use of a variety of other reagents and most reliably by means of atomic absorption spectrophotometry.

310.

B. Plasma phosphates influence plasma calcium levels. Case studies show that there is a reciprocal relationship between calcium and phosphorus. A decrease in plasma calcium will be accompanied by an increase in plasma inorganic phosphate.

311.

B. Similarly to potassium, which is a major intracellular cation, phosphate is a major intracellular anion. Therefore, when blood is drawn for serum inorganic phosphate measurement, hemolysis of the specimen must be avoided. Also, serum should be removed from the clot as soon after collection as possible to avoid leakage of phosphate into the serum. Both of these situations would contribute to falsely increased serum phosphate levels. Conversely, serum phosphate levels will be depressed following meals, during the menstrual period, and during intravenous glucose and fructose therapy.

312.

B. Copper is found in the plasma mainly in two forms, a minor fraction loosely bound to albumin and the majority, representing about 80–95%, firmly bound to the enzyme ceruloplasmin, an α2-globulin, which is important in the oxidation of iron from the ferrous to the ferric state. Copper is also an essential constituent of a variety of other enzymes found in erythrocytes and in other sites throughout the body. The major clinical usefulness of determining serum copper or ceruloplasmin levels is that the decreased level of both is associated with Wilson's disease. Decreased levels of copper are also found in protein malnutrition and malabsorption and in nephrosis.

313.

A. Transferrin is a glycoprotein that reversibly binds serum iron that is not combined with other proteins such as hemoglobin and ferritin. Transferrin concentration in serum is rarely determined directly but, rather, in terms of the serum iron content after saturation with iron. This is the total iron binding capacity (TIBC). The percent saturation of transferrin is determined by dividing the serum iron level by the serum TIBC and expressing this value as a percentage. Normally in adults the percent saturation of transferrin is in the range of 20–50%, whereas in iron deficiency anemia the saturation is expected to be less than 15%. In iron deficiency anemia complicated by other disorders that either increase serum iron concentration or decrease the TIBC, the percent saturation may remain within the reference range.

314.

C. In adults the total body iron content averages 3–4 g. The majority of this iron is found in the active pool as an essential constituent of hemoglobin, with a much lesser amount being an integral component of myoglobin and a number of enzymes. Approximately 25% of the body iron is found in inactive storage forms. The major storage form of iron is ferritin, with a lesser amount being stored as hemosiderin. Ferritin may be found in most body cells but especially in reticuloendothelial cells of the liver, spleen, and bone marrow.

315.

D. In cases of iron deficiency anemia uncomplicated by other diseases, serum ferritin levels correlate well with the evidence of iron deficiency obtained by marrow examination for stainable iron. This indicates that ferritin is released into the serum in direct proportion to the amount stored in tissues.

In iron deficiency, serum ferritin levels fall early in the disease process. However, in certain disorders there is a disproportionate increase in serum ferritin in relation to iron stores. Examples include chronic infections, chronic inflammation, malignancies, and liver disease. For individuals who have these chronic disorders or iron deficiency, it is common for their serum ferritin levels to appear normal.

316.

B. Serum iron concentrations are most often determined by the colorimetric reaction with ferrozine, bathophenanthroline, tripyridyltriazine, or terosite. The same reagent is usually used in the determination of serum total iron binding capacity (TIBC) by saturating the transferrin in the serum with an excess of iron, removing any unbound iron, and measuring the iron bound to transferrin. This measurement of TIBC provides a measure of transferrin concentration. Several magnesium methods require the precipitation of magnesium as part of the analysis, and 8-hydroxyquinoline effectively precipitates magnesium.

317.

A. Transferrin is the iron transport protein in serum and is normally saturated with iron to the extent of approximately 20–50%. An increased percent saturation of transferrin is expected in patients with hemochromatosis, an iron overload disease, and iron poisoning. The increased saturation is due to the increased iron concentration in the serum. In patients with chronic infections and malignancies, there is impairment of iron release from body storage sites leading to a decreased percent saturation of transferrin. In myocardial infarction the serum iron levels are depressed, but the TIBC levels are normal. Iron deficiency anemia because of poor absorption, poor diet, or chronic loss results in decreased serum iron, increased transferrin, and decreased percent saturation of transferrin in most cases.

318.

C. In order to differentiate between diseases, it is necessary to perform several laboratory determinations to properly assess iron metabolism. In iron deficiency anemia, the serum iron is decreased while the total iron binding capacity (TIBC) is increased. Thus it follows that the transferrin saturation is decreased. The serum ferritin level, which represents stored

body iron, is depressed, and the free erythrocyte protoporphyrin (FEP) level is increased. FEP is not a specific test for iron deficiency anemia, but it can function as a screening test.

319.

A. A low ionized serum magnesium level is characteristic of a magnesium deficiency tetany. The serum magnesium level usually ranges between 0.15 and 0.5 mmol/L when tetany occurs. In addition, the serum calcium level and blood pH are normal, while the serum potassium level is decreased. This type of tetany is treated with $MgSO_4$ to increase the level of serum magnesium, thus alleviating the tetany and convulsions that accompany this disorder.

320.

A. Magnesium measurements are commonly done spectrophotometrically using reagent systems such as calmagite, methylthymol blue, and chlorophosphonazo III. Calcium will interfere and is eliminated by complexing with a chelator that binds calcium and not magnesium. Atomic absorption is a specific and sensitive method for analysis of magnesium, with the only significant interference being phosphate ions, which are removed by complexing with a lanthanum salt.

321.

D. Plasma lactate concentrations are increased in cases of lactic acidosis. The accumulation of lactate in the blood results from any mechanism that produces oxygen deprivation of tissues and thereby anaerobic metabolism. Lactate concentrations in whole blood are extremely unstable because of the rapid production and release of lactate by erythrocytes as a result of glycolysis. One method of stabilizing blood lactate levels in specimen collection is to add an enzyme inhibitor such as fluoride or iodoacetate to the collection tubes. Heparin, ethylenediaminetetraacetic acid (EDTA), and oxalate will act as anticoagulants but will not prevent glycolysis in the blood sample.

322.

C. Measuring the concentration of chloride in sweat is a commonly used diagnostic procedure for determining the disorder of cystic fibrosis (CF). The majority of patients with CF will present with increased concentrations of sodium and chloride in their sweat. Generally, children with CF will manifest sweat chloride levels that are two to five times the reference interval. In sweat testing, sweat production is stimulated by iontophoresis with pilocarpine. Then the sweat is either collected and analyzed for chloride or an ion-selective electrode is applied to the skin surface to quantify chloride. It has been established that the gene abnormality causing CF is located on chromosome 7.

ACID-BASE BALANCE: BLOOD GASES

323.
A. Due to its high concentration in blood, the bicarbonate/carbonic acid pair is the most important buffer system in the blood. This buffer system is also effective in the lungs and in the kidneys in helping to regulate body pH. The other buffers that also function to help maintain body pH are the phosphate, protein, and hemoglobin buffer systems. The acetate buffer system is not used by the body to regulate pH.

324.
C. Pco_2 is an indicator of carbonic acid (H_2CO_3). The Pco_2 millimeters of mercury value (mm Hg) multiplied by the constant 0.03 equals the millimoles per liter (mmol/L) concentration of H_2CO_3 ($Pco_2 \times 0.03 = H_2CO_3$). Pco_2 can be measured using a pH/blood gas analyzer.

325.
A. Total CO_2 or carbon dioxide content is a measure of the concentration of bicarbonate, carbonate, carbamino compounds, carbonic acid, and dissolved carbon dioxide gas (Pco_2) in the plasma. Bicarbonate makes up approximately 95% of the total CO_2 content, but most laboratories are not equipped to directly measure bicarbonate. Therefore total CO_2 is generally quantified. The bicarbonate concentration may be estimated by subtracting the H_2CO_3 concentration (measured in terms of Pco_2 and converted to H_2CO_3) from the total CO_2 concentration.

326.
B. The most important buffer pair in the plasma is bicarbonate with carbonic acid. Use of the Henderson-Hasselbalch equation

$$pH = pK' + \log \frac{[salt]}{[acid]}$$

shows that the pH changes with the ratio of salt to acid, that is, bicarbonate to carbonic acid because pK' is a constant. For this buffer pair, apparent pK' = 6.1. When the ratio of the concentrations of bicarbonate to carbonic acid is 20:1 (log of 20 = 1.3), the pH is 7.4, that is:

$$pH = 6.1 + \log 20$$
$$7.4 = 6.1 + 1.3$$

The carbonic acid designation represents both the undissociated carbonic acid and the physically dissolved carbon dioxide found in the blood. Since the concentration of the undissociated carbonic acid is negligible compared to the concentration of physically dissolved carbon dioxide, the expression for carbonic acid concentration is usually written ($Pco_2 \times 0.03$).

327.
D. The acid-base equilibrium of the blood is expressed by the Henderson-Hasselbalch equation:

$$pH = pK' + \log \frac{cHCO_3^-}{[Pco_2 \times 0.03]}$$

In this buffer pair, pK' = 6.1. Normally, the ratio of the concentration of bicarbonate ions ($cHCO_3^-$) to the concentration of carbonic acid expressed as ($Pco_2 \times 0.03$) in the plasma is 20:1. The bicarbonate component of the equation is considered to be the "metabolic" component, controlled by the kidneys. The carbonic acid component is considered the "respiratory" component, controlled by the lungs. An excess of bicarbonate without a change in Pco_2 will increase the ratio of bicarbonate to carbonic acid. Therefore the pH will increase, that is, the plasma becomes more alkaline.

328.
C. The normal ratio of bicarbonate ions to dissolved carbon dioxide is 20:1 and pH = 6.1 + log 20/1. An excess of dissolved CO_2 (e.g., increase in Pco_2) will increase the denominator in the equation or decrease the ratio of bicarbonate ions to dissolved CO_2. The pH will decrease, that is, the plasma becomes more acid. The amount of dissolved CO_2 (Pco_2) in the blood is related to respiration. Hence, this condition is termed respiratory acidosis.

329.
B. It is possible to use arterial, venous, or capillary blood for blood gas analysis. The specimen of

choice for determining pulmonary dysfunction in adults is arterial blood. Analysis of arterial blood is the best indicator of pulmonary function, the capacity of the lungs to exchange carbon dioxide for oxygen. Po_2 and Pco_2 measurements from capillary blood are usually confined to infant sampling, and they are dependent on the patient preparation and sampling site. Venous blood should not be used for blood gas studies involving pulmonary problems because venous blood gas values also reflect metabolic processes. Furthermore, the reference range for Po_2 in venous blood varies drastically from arterial blood. Urine cannot be used to determine the acid/base status of a patient.

330.

B. Heparin is the best anticoagulant to use in drawing blood for blood gas analyses because it does not affect the value of the blood pH. This is also critical to Po_2 measurements because alterations in blood pH will cause concomitant changes in Po_2 values. Several heparin salts are available for use as anticoagulants. Sodium heparinate, 1000 U/mL, is commonly used. Ammonium heparinate may be substituted for the sodium salt when it is necessary to perform additional testing, such as electrolyte analysis, on the blood gas sample.

331.

A. When a blood specimen is drawn for gas analysis, it is important to avoid exposure of the specimen to air because of the differences in the partial pressures of carbon dioxide and oxygen in air and in blood. The Pco_2 in blood is much greater than the Pco_2 in air. Hence on exposure of blood to air, the total CO_2 and the Pco_2 both decrease, causing an increase in pH. Similarly, the Po_2 of air is much greater than that of blood, thus, the blood Po_2 increases on exposure to air.

332.

C. Glycolysis and other oxidative metabolic processes will continue in vitro by red blood cells when a whole blood specimen is left standing at room temperature. Oxygen is consumed during these processes, resulting in a decrease in Po_2 levels. A decrease of 3–12 mm Hg/hr at 37 °C has been observed for blood specimens exhibiting normal Po_2 ranges. This rate of decrease is accelerated with elevated Po_2 levels. Additionally, carbon dioxide is produced as a result of continued metabolism. An increase in Pco_2 levels of approxi-

mately 5 mm Hg/hr at 37 °C has been demonstrated. The increased production of carbonic acid and lactic acid during glycolysis contributes to the decrease in blood pH.

333.

D. The solubility coefficient of CO_2 gas (dissolved CO_2) in normal blood plasma at 37 °C is 0.03 mmol/L/mm Hg. The concentration of dissolved CO_2 found in plasma is calculated by multiplying the Pco_2 blood level by the solubility coefficient (0.03). The predominant components of total CO_2 are bicarbonate (95%) and carbonic acid (5%). The bicarbonate ion concentration in millimoles per liter can be calculated by subtracting the product of (0.03 mmol/L/mm Hg $\times$ Pco_2 mm Hg), which represents carbonic acid, from the total CO_2 concentration (millimoles per liter).

334.

C. pH, Pco_2 and Po_2 are measured directly from the specimen by utilizing electrodes. The pH and Pco_2 electrodes are potentiometric where the voltage produced across a semipermeable membrane to hydrogen ions or CO_2 gas is proportional to the "activity" of those ions in the patient's sample. Activity is measured in voltage whose value can be presented in terms of concentration. Po_2 is measured similarly, but using an amperometric electrode. For Po_2 a small charge is put on a cathode, and electrons are drawn off the cathode in proportion to the oxygen present. The O_2 becomes part of the circuit. The amount of electrons drawn is proportional to the amount of oxygen present. Bicarbonate and other parameters, such as base excess, are calculated by the instrument using pH and Pco_2 values and the Henderson/Hasselbalch equation.

335.

C. The red cell membrane is permeable to both bicarbonate and chloride ions. Chloride ions participate in buffering the blood by diffusing out of or into the red blood cells to compensate for the ionic change that occurs when bicarbonate enters or leaves the red blood cell. This is called the chloride shift.

336.

B. In the diabetic patient, diabetic ketoacidosis is one of the complications that may require emergency therapy. Blood glucose levels are usually in the range of 500–700 mg/dL but may be higher. The result is severe glycosuria that produces an osmotic diuresis leading to loss of water and depletion of body electrolytes. Lipolysis is accelerated as a result of insulin deficiency. The free fatty acids produced are metabolized to acetyl-coenzyme A units, which are converted in the liver to ketone bodies. Hydrogen ions are produced with ketone bodies (other than acetone), contributing to a decrease in blood pH. Ketoacids are also excreted in the urine, causing a decrease in urinary pH.

337.

D. One of the primary reasons for metabolic alkalosis, especially in infants, is vomiting. Hydrogen ions are lost in the vomit, and the body reacts to replace them in the stomach. Consequently, hydrogen is lost from the plasma. This loss of hydrogen is due to a metabolic as opposed to a respiratory reason. Salicylate poisoning, uncontrolled diabetes mellitus and renal failure all lead to metabolic acidosis either through an overproduction of ketone bodies, such as acetoacetic acid and beta-hydroxybutyric acid, or because of a reduced excretion of acid by the kidneys.

338.

D. Laboratory results from arterial blood gas studies in partially compensated respiratory alkalosis are as follows: pH slightly increased, Pco_2 decreased, HCO_3^- decreased, and total CO_2 decreased. Respiratory alkalosis is a disturbance in acid-base balance that is caused by hyperventilation associated with such conditions as fever, hysteria, and hypoxia. Respiratory alkalosis is characterized by a primary deficiency in physically dissolved CO_2 (decreased Pco_2). This decrease in the level of Pco_2 is due to hyperventilation, causing the accelerated loss of CO_2 by the lungs. This loss of CO_2 alters the normal 20:1 ratio of $cHCO_3^-/Pco_2$, causing an increase in the blood pH level. In respiratory alkalosis, since the initial defect is in the lungs, the kidneys respond as the major compensatory system. Ammonia production in the kidneys is decreased, Na^+–H^+ exchange is decreased with the retention of H^+, and bicarbonate reabsorption is decreased. By decreasing the bicarbonate reabsorption into the blood stream, the kidneys attempt to reestablish the 20:1 ratio and normal blood pH. In a partially compensated state, as the blood bicarbonate level decreases, the blood pH

begins to return toward normal but continues to be slightly alkaline. In a fully compensated state the blood pH is normal.

339.

C. Respiratory acidosis is a disturbance in acid-base balance that is caused by the retention of CO_2 by the lungs. This imbalance is associated with such conditions as bronchopneumonia, pulmonary emphysema, pulmonary fibrosis, and cardiac insufficiency. Respiratory acidosis is characterized by a primary excess in physically dissolved CO_2, which is quantified by measuring the blood Pco_2 level. The primary problem leading to an increase in the Pco_2 level is hypoventilation. This retention of CO_2 alters the normal 20:1 ratio of $cHCO_3^-/Pco_2$, causing a decrease in blood pH level. In respiratory acidosis, since the initial defect is associated with the lungs, the kidneys respond as the major compensatory system. The production of ammonia, the exchange of Na^+ for H^+ with the excretion of H^+, and the reabsorption of bicarbonate are all increased in the kidneys to compensate for the malfunction of the lungs. In cases where the defect is not within the respiratory center, the excess of Pco_2 in the blood can actually have a stimulatory effect on the center, causing an increase in the respiration rate. Thus compensation can also occur through CO_2 elimination by the lungs.

340.

A. There is a wide variety of conditions that will cause a shift of the dissociation curve of oxyhemoglobin to the left or to the right. A shift to the left will mean an increase in the affinity of hemoglobin for oxygen. Because of this increased affinity, there is also less oxygen delivered to the tissue for a given percent saturation of hemoglobin. When the curve is shifted to the right, there is a decrease in the affinity of hemoglobin for oxygen. Hence there is increased oxygen delivered to tissues for a given hemoglobin oxygen saturation. Oxyhemoglobin is a stronger acid than deoxyhemoglobin. Both exist in equilibrium in the blood. Increased hydrogen ion concentration shifts the equilibrium toward the deoxygenated form. This shift results in increased oxygen delivery to the tissue. The higher the concentration of 2,3-diphosphoglycerate in the cell, the greater is the displacement of oxygen, thus facilitating the release of oxygen at the tissue level. Increased Pco_2 and increased temperature will also have this same effect.

341.

A. Carbonic anhydrase (CA) is an enzyme found in red blood cells that catalyzes the reversible hydration of CO_2 to bicarbonate and a proton:

$$H_2O + CO_2 \overset{CA}{\rightleftarrows} HHCO_3$$

The proton, in turn, is buffered by the histidine portion of the hemoglobin molecule that activates the release of oxygen. It is at this point that oxyhemoglobin is converted to deoxyhemoglobin. In the alveoli of the lungs, CA catalyzes the conversion of H_2CO_3 to CO_2 and H_2O. The CO_2 is then exhaled. Carbonic anhydrase is an intracellular enzyme of erythrocytes and renal tubular cells, and it is not found normally in any significant concentration in the plasma. It is not associated with the oxygen dissociation curve.

342.

B. Base excess is a measure of the nonrespiratory buffers of the blood. They are hemoglobin, serum protein, phosphate, and bicarbonate. Therefore base excess reflects an abnormality in the buffer base concentration. Bicarbonate has the greatest influence on base excess, which is an indicator of metabolic function. The normal range for base excess is ±2.5 mmol/L. A quick estimation of base excess is to subtract the average "normal" reference bicarbonate level set by the laboratory from the measured bicarbonate level (e.g., if laboratory reference bicarbonate = 25 and patient's bicarbonate = 30, then Base Excess = (30 − 25) = +5; if patient's bicarbonate = 20, then Base Excess = (20 − 25) = −5. As demonstrated, a positive base excess is associated with metabolic alkalosis, and a negative base excess is associated with metabolic acidosis.

343.

C. The acid-base equilibrium of the blood is expressed by the Henderson-Hasselbalch equation:

$$pH = pK' + \log \frac{[HCO_3^-]}{[Pco_2 \times 0.03]}$$

For the stated problem, convert Pco_2 in mm Hg to dissolved CO_2, multiplying by the solubility coefficient of CO_2 gas: 44 mm Hg × 0.03 mmol/L/mm Hg = 1.32 mmol/L. Next, determine the bicarbonate concentration by finding the difference between the total CO_2 and dissolved CO_2 concentrations: 29 mmol/L − 1.32 mmol/L =

27.68 mmol/L. pK′ for the bicarbonate buffer system is 6.1. Therefore:

$$pH = 6.1 + \log \frac{[27.68]}{[1.32]}$$
$$pH = 6.1 + \log 20.97$$
$$pH = 6.1 + \log 20.1$$
$$pH = 6.1 + 1.32$$
$$pH = 7.42$$

344–347.

In evaluating acid-base balance, the pH, Pco_2, and total CO_2 of an arterial blood specimen are measured. The reference values of arterial whole blood at 37 °C for adults are:

$$pH = 7.35–7.45$$
$$Pco_2 = 35–45 \text{ mm Hg}$$
$$HCO_3^- = 22–26 \text{ mmol/L}$$
$$TCO_2 = 23–27 \text{ mmol/L}$$
$$Po_2 = 80–110 \text{ mm Hg}$$

Acid-base disturbances can be characterized into four basic disorders: metabolic alkalosis, metabolic acidosis, respiratory alkalosis, and respiratory acidosis.

$$pH = pK' + \log \frac{[HCO_3^-]}{[H_2CO_3]}$$

or

$$pH = pK' + \log \frac{[HCO_3^-]}{[Pco_2 \times 0.03]}$$

Normally the average ratio of bicarbonate to the concentration of carbonic acid is 20:1 resulting in a blood pH of 7.4. The HCO_3^- is represented in the measurement of total CO_2 value because 95% of the total CO_2 is HCO_3^-. The concentration of carbonic acid is calculated by multiplying the Pco_2 value by 0.03 (the solubility coefficient of CO_2 gas). The bicarbonate (base) represents the renal component of the acid-base balance. It is related to metabolic function. The dissolved carbon dioxide, measured as Pco_2, represents the respiration component, being related to respiratory function. Thus respiratory acidosis is characterized by an increase in blood Pco_2, whereas respiratory alkalosis is characterized by a decrease of blood Pco_2. Metabolic acidosis is characterized by a decrease in the blood bicarbonate levels, whereas metabolic alkalosis is related to an increase in blood bicarbonate levels. In acid-base disorders the compensatory changes occur in the component that is not the original cause of the imbalance if compensation can occur. Thus in an acid-base imbalance of respiratory origin, the kidneys exert the major corrective action. In an acid-base imbalance of metabolic origin, the lungs exert the major corrective action. Sometimes, a "mixed" or "double" problem of acidosis and alkalosis may exist due to more than one pathological process (e.g., a diabetic with asthma where both the respiratory and metabolic components indicate acidosis). If neither the respiratory nor the metabolic components indicate the condition of the patient (e.g., acidosis or alkalosis), then, most likely, there is something wrong with one or more of the blood gas results. In approaching acid-base problems, one should first key on the pH to determine the general condition (acidosis or alkalosis), then ask what is causing it—a change in bicarbonate or P_{CO_2} to determine if the problem is metabolic or respiratory, and finally look at the remaining component to see if there is compensation bringing the pH closer to 7.4. If there is no movement in the remaining component from the reference value, then there is no compensation or uncompensation.

344.

A. In this case the pH is increased indicating alkalosis. HCO_3^- is increased, which means it is a metabolic problem. The P_{CO_2} is also increased which indicates that the lungs are trying to compensate by retaining P_{CO_2} thus bringing the pH closer to 7.4.

345.

B. Here the pH is decreased indicating acidosis. The P_{CO_2} is increased, which indicates the problem is respiratory in nature. The HCO_3^- is unchanged from the reference range, which indicates that there is no compensation, thus the patient has uncompensated respiratory acidosis.

346.

C. The pH clearly indicates acidosis. Both the metabolic (decreased HCO_3^-) and respiratory (increased P_{CO_2}) components, however, indicate acidosis. There is no compensation seen in the results. Thus the patient has a double or mixed problem of acidosis.

347.

D. Here the pH and case information indicate alkalosis, but both the metabolic (decreased HCO_3^-) and respiratory (increased P_{CO_2}) components indicate acidosis. Most likely there is a problem/error in one or more of the measurements.

ENZYMES

348.

C. The majority of serum enzymes that are of interest clinically are of intracellular origin. These enzymes function intracellularly with only small amounts found in serum as a result of normal cellular turnover. Increased serum levels are due to tissue damage and necrosis where the cells disintegrate and leak their contents into the blood. Thus, elevated serum levels of intracellular enzymes are used diagnostically to assess tissue damage.

349.

B. Enzymes are proteins that act as catalysts. It is not practical to measure enzyme concentrations in a body fluid specimen but rather to assay enzymes according to their activity in catalyzing an appropriate reaction, that is, the conversion of substrate to product. An enzyme acts by combining with a specific substrate to form an enzyme-substrate complex, which then breaks down into product plus free enzyme, which is reused. A general form of the reaction is

$$[E] + [S] \rightleftarrows [ES] \rightarrow [P] + [E]$$

where $[E]$ = concentration of enzyme, $[S]$ = concentration of substrate, $[ES]$ = concentration of enzyme-substrate complex, and $[P]$ = concentration of product of the reaction. Since the rate of such a reaction is used as a measure of enzyme activity, it is important to consider the effect of substrate concentration on the rate of the reaction. The kinetics of the reaction are initially of the first order (i.e., the rate varies with the concentration of substrate as well as the concentration of enzyme) until there is sufficient substrate present to combine with all enzyme. The reaction rate then becomes zero order (i.e., the rate is independent of concentration of substrate and directly proportional to concentration of enzyme as measured by reaction rate) when substrate is present in excess. Hence it is desirable to use conditions that provide zero order kinetics when assaying enzyme activity.

350.

B. Michaelis and Menten proposed a basis for the theory of enzyme-substrate complexes and rate reactions. By measuring the velocity of the reaction at varying substrate concentrations, it is possible to determine the Michaelis constant (K_m) for any specific enzymatic reaction. K_m represents the specific concentration of substrate that is required for a particular reaction to proceed at a velocity that is equal to half of its maximum velocity. The K_m value tells something about the affinity of an enzyme for its substrate. When $[S] = K_m$, the velocity of the reaction is expressed as $V = \frac{1}{2} V_{max}$. In the graph shown with this question, the K_m of the reaction is represented by b. Since substrate must be present in excess to obtain zero order kinetics, the substrate concentration necessary would have to be at least 10 times the K_m, which is represented by d. Usually substrate concentrations 20–100 times the K_m are used to be sure that substrate is present in excess. Thus it is critical that the K_m value be determined experimentally.

351.

A. Factors that affect enzyme assays include temperature, pH, substrate concentration, and time of incubation. For each clinically important enzyme, the optimum temperature and pH for its specific reaction are known. When lower than optimum temperature or pH is employed, the measured enzyme activity will be lower than the expected activity value. As temperature increases, the rate of the reaction increases. Generally, a twofold increase in reaction rates will be observed with a 10 °C rise in temperature. However, once the optimum temperature is exceeded, the reaction rate falls off as enzyme denaturation occurs at temperatures ranging from 40 to 70 °C.

352.

D. An international unit (U) is defined as the enzyme activity that catalyzes the conversion of 1 μmol of substrate in 1 min under standard conditions. For determination of enzyme activity when a rate method is employed, the following equation is used:

$$\frac{\Delta A/min \times \text{total assay volume (mL)} \times 10^6 \text{ μmol/mol}}{\text{Absorptivity coefficient} \times \text{light path (cm)} \times \text{specimen volume (mL)}} = U/L$$

$$\frac{0.077 \times 3.02 \text{ mL} \times 10^6 \text{ μmol/mol}}{6.22 \times 10^3 \text{ L/mol·cm} \times 1 \text{ cm} \times 0.02 \text{ mL}} = 1869 \text{ U/L}$$

It is important to remember that the total assay volume includes the volume of reagent, diluent,

and sample used in the particular assay and that the total assay volume and specimen volume should be expressed in the same units.

353.

B. Enzymes are protein in nature. Like all proteins, they may be denatured with a loss of activity as a result of several factors (e.g., heat, extreme pH, mechanical agitation, strong acids, and organic solvents). Enzymes act as catalysts for the many chemical reactions of the body. Enzymes increase the rate of a specific chemical reaction by lowering the activation energy needed for the reaction to proceed. They do not change the equilibrium constant of the reaction; but rather, enzymes affect the rate at which equilibrium occurs between reactants and products.

354.

C. Serum alkaline phosphatase is elevated in several disorders, including hepatobiliary and bone diseases. For an accurate assay of most serum enzymes, the presence of hemolyzed red blood cells must be avoided because many enzymes are present in red cells. Serum aspartate transaminase (formerly known as glutamate-oxaloacetate transaminase, GOT) and lactate dehydrogenase are both enzymes that are elevated in acute myocardial infarction and liver disease.

355.

D. There are six major classes of enzymes. The International Commission of Enzymes of the International Union of Biochemistry has categorized all enzymes into one of these classes: oxidoreductases, transferases, hydrolases, lyases, isomerases, and ligases. Transferases are enzymes that catalyze the transfer of groups, such as amino and phosphate groups between compounds. Transferases frequently need coenzymes, such as pyridoxal-5'-phosphate (P-5'-P), for the amino transfer reactions. Aspartate and alanine aminotransferases, creatine kinase, and gamma-glutamyltransferase are typical examples.

356.

B. Hydrolases are enzymes that split molecules with the addition of water—for example, amylase, lipase, alkaline phosphatase, acid phosphatase, 5'-nucleotidase, and trypsin. They do not usually require coenzymes but often need activators. Aldolase and carbonic anhydrase are examples of the class of enzymes known as the lyases. Lyases are enzymes that split molecules between carbon-to-carbon bonds without the addition of water. The resulting products usually contain carbon double bonds.

357.

C. The oxidoreductases are enzymes that catalyze the addition or removal of hydrogen from compounds. These enzymes need a coenzyme, such as nicotinamide adenine dinucleotide (NAD) or its phosphorylated derivative NADP, as a hydrogen acceptor or donor in order to function. Lactate dehydrogenase and glucose-6-phosphate dehydrogenase are examples of oxidoreductases. Isomerases are those enzymes that catalyze intramolecular conversions such as the oxidation of a functional group by an adjacent group within the same molecule. Glucose phosphate isomerase is an example of this class of enzymes. Ligases are those enzymes that catalyze the union of two molecules accompanied by the breakdown of a phosphate bond in adenosine triphosphate (ATP) or a similar triphosphate. An example is glutamine synthetase.

358.

B. Aspartate and alanine aminotransferases catalyze the transfer of amino groups between amino acids and α-oxoacids. A prosthetic group, pyridoxal-5′-phosphate (P-5′-P), is required for the transfer of the amino group. In the aspartate aminotransferase (AST) reaction, AST catalyzes the transfer of an amino group from L-aspartate to α-oxoglutarate, with the amino group transfer mediated by P-5′-P, which is bound to the apoenzyme. The products formed are oxaloacetate and L-glutamate. By coupling this reaction with a malate dehydrogenase reaction, the decrease in absorbance of NADH as it is oxidized to NAD^+ can be followed at 340 nm. The change in absorbance will be proportional to the AST activity present in the serum specimen.

359.

D. Alanine aminotransferase (ALT), formerly known as glutamate pyruvate transaminase (GPT), and aspartate aminotransferase (AST), formerly known as glutamate oxaloacetate transaminase (GOT), are categorized as transferase enzymes. These older designations are still seen on reagent packaging. Through the transfer of amino groups, they catalyze the interconversion of amino acids and keto acids. ALT catalyzes the interconversion

of alanine and oxoglutarate to pyruvate and glutamate. The reaction is reversible. In viral hepatitis, both ALT and AST are elevated. In acute myocardial infarction, AST is elevated and ALT is normal or slightly increased.

$$\text{L-Alanine} + \alpha\text{-oxoglutarate} \underset{}{\overset{\text{ALT, P-5′-P}}{\rightleftarrows}} \text{pyruvate} + \text{L-glutamate}$$

360.

A. Lactate dehydrogenase (LD) is an intracellular glycolytic enzyme that exhibits increased serum concentrations with various types of tissue destruction. Since LD has five isoenzyme forms, it is possible to narrow down the site of tissue cell destruction to several areas by performing an electrophoretic separation of a serum specimen. An increase in the LD-5 and LD-4 fractions is suggestive of acute hepatic disease. It should be noted that LD-5 and LD-4 are not only the primary isoenzyme forms of liver tissue but also the primary isoenzyme forms of skeletal muscle. Electrophoretic separation of LD isoenzymes is not frequently performed, since the technique has been replaced by chemical methods that can be automated.

361.

A. Lactate dehydrogenase (LD, also abbreviated LDH) is found in all body tissues and is especially abundant in red and white blood cells. Hence hemolyzed serum will give falsely elevated results for LD. The enzyme catalyzes the conversion of lactate to pyruvate at pH 8.8–9.8 and pyruvate to lactate at pH 7.4–7.8, mediated by nicotinamide adenine dinucleotide (NAD). Serum specimens for LD isoenzyme determinations can be stored at room temperature for 2 or 3 days without appreciable loss of activity. Room temperature storage is necessary because LD-4 and LD-5 are labile in the cold. This is in contrast to most enzymes, which are more stable refrigerated or frozen.

362.

B. Lactate dehydrogenase (LD) exists in five isomeric forms called isoenzymes. The isoenzymes can be separated by electrophoresis. The fastest moving component is LD-1. LD-1 migrates the closest to the anode and, along with LD-2, is associated with heart muscle. The slowest component is LD-5; it is associated with the liver and skeletal muscle. In untreated pernicious anemia both the LD-1 and LD-2 levels are greater than normal.

When the myocardium is damaged, as in an acute myocardial infarction (AMI), the contents of the damaged myocardial cells spill out into the serum. Hence, the electrophoretic pattern for LD isoenzymes shows an elevation in LD-1 and LD-2 levels after an AMI.

363.

C. Enzymes catalyze specific reactions or closely related groups of reactions. Lactate dehydrogenase (LD), with nicotinamide adenine dinucleotide (NAD$^+$) as a hydrogen acceptor, catalyzes the oxidation of L-lactate to pyruvate and the reduction of NAD$^+$ to NADH. Since NAD$^+$ does not absorb light at 340 nm but NADH does, the production of NADH can be monitored as an increase in absorbance at 340 nm and related to the LD activity present in the specimen. Since this reaction is reversible, either the forward or reverse reaction can be used in the laboratory to quantify LD activity. Although the reaction equilibrium favors the formation of lactate from pyruvate, this reaction is less commonly used. It should be noted that the reference ranges for the two reactions are considerably different. Elevation of serum LD is associated with acute myocardial infarction, liver disease, pernicious anemia, malignant disease, and pulmonary embolism. It is also seen in some cases of renal disease, especially where tubular necrosis or pyelonephritis exists.

364.

B. In acute myocardial infarction (AMI), the initial increase in serum myoglobin levels occurs in 1 to 3 hours following onset of symptoms. Serial measurements need to be made since a single value is not diagnostic. When doubling of the initial value occurs within 1 to 2 hours, this is suggestive of AMI. In AMI, the myoglobin level will peak within 5 to 12 hours, with serum levels returning to normal within 18 to 30 hours. Since myoglobin is found in other tissues and is not cardiac specific, it is usually used in conjunction with troponin and CK-MB to assess the occurrence of AMI.

365.

C. Increased serum creatine kinase (CK), formerly called creatine phosphokinase (CPK), values are caused primarily by lesions of cardiac muscle, skeletal muscle, or brain tissue. CK increases in the early stages of Duchenne-type progressive muscular dystrophy. Assays of total CK and CK isoenzymes are commonly used in the diagnosis of myocardial infarction. Hypothyroidism causes a moderate increase in CK values. Elevation of this enzyme also occurs after vigorous muscular activity, in cases of cerebrovascular accidents (stroke), and after repeated intramuscular injections. In addition to quantifying total CK activity, isoenzymes may be determined by using electrophoretic, immunologic, or ion-exchange chromatography methods. Three isoenzymes have been identified: CK-1 or BB, primarily found in brain and nerve tissues with some in thyroid, kidney, and intestine; CK-2 or MB, primarily found in heart muscle; CK-3 or MM, primarily found in skeletal muscle but present in all body tissues. CK is not elevated in bone disease.

366.

C. Creatine kinase (CK) is found mainly in skeletal muscle, cardiac muscle, and brain tissue. It catalyzes the reversible reaction:

$$\text{creatine} + \text{adenosine triphosphate (ATP)} \underset{\text{pH 6.7}}{\overset{\text{pH 9.0}}{\rightleftarrows}}$$

$$\text{phosphocreatine} + \text{adenosine} \\ \text{diphosphate (ADP)}$$

Mg^{++} is required as an activator. The direction in which the reaction takes place, and hence the equilibrium point, depends on the pH. Measurement of CK activity is valuable in the early diagnosis of acute myocardial infarction. Its level rises 4 to 6 hours after infarction, reaches its peak at 18 to 30 hours, and returns to normal by the third day. In addition to quantifying total CK activity, electrophoresis may be performed to ascertain the presence of an MB band, which represents the heart tissue isoenzyme. Electrophoretically, the MB band moves to an intermediary position between the BB and the MM bands. The BB band travels fastest toward the anode and the MM band travels slowest, remaining in the gamma-globulin region. Electrophoretic separation of CK-MB has been widely replaced by immunologic and ion-exchange chromatography methods, which can be performed on automated instruments.

367.

B. The function of amylase to catalyze the hydrolysis of starch to dextrins, maltose, and glucose has been used as the basis for several methods over the years. The more commonly used methods today employ small oligosaccharides and 4-nitrophenyl-glycoside as substrates. In general, these methods can be automated, using an oxygen electrode system and UV or visible wavelength spectrophotometry to determine amylase activity.

368.

D. Gamma-glutamyltransferase (GGT) catalyzes the transfer of gamma-glutamyl groups from peptides to an appropriate acceptor. GGT is found in almost all cells. The highest amount of GGT is found in the kidney and slightly less in the liver and pancreas. Diagnostically, the assay of GGT is widely used to investigate hepatic disease. Increased values are seen in a variety of liver disorders and in conditions that are characterized by secondary liver involvement, including acute pancreatitis, pancreatic carcinoma, infectious mononucleosis, alcoholism, and cardiac insufficiency. Normal GGT levels are seen in bone disorders, in growing children, and during pregnancy.

369.

C. The main sources of alkaline phosphatase are liver, bone, intestine, and placenta. Elevated alkaline phosphatase is associated with liver disease and with both obstructive jaundice and intrahepatic jaundice. In most cases the alkaline phosphatase value in obstructive jaundice is higher than in intrahepatic jaundice. Increased values are also found in bone diseases such as Paget's disease; in pregnant women, especially in the third trimester of a normal pregnancy; and in normal growing children. In the presence of the latter conditions, when liver disease is also suspect, a gamma-glutamyltransferase (GGT) assay may be performed to aid in a differential diagnosis. GGT levels are normal in these conditions but elevated in liver disease.

370.

B. Alanine aminotransferase, aspartate aminotransferase, alkaline phosphatase, gamma-glutamyltransferase, and lactate dehydrogenase are enzymes for which the serum activities may be assayed to assess liver function. At the cellular level, alkaline phosphatase functions in the membrane border, gamma-glutamyltransferase functions in the cell membrane, and alanine aminotransferase functions both in the cytoplasm and mitochondria. With tissue damage and necrosis, the cells disintegrate and leak their contents into the blood. Since these enzymes are cellular enzymes, any increase in their activity levels in serum is indicative of tissue destruction. It is important to remember that these enzyme levels must be used in conjunction with other clinical data because enzymes generally are not organ specific, being found in several tissues.

371.

B. Amylase and lipase are the two most important enzymes in evaluating pancreatic function. The values of amylase and lipase activity are significantly elevated in acute pancreatitis and obstruction of the pancreatic duct. In most cases of acute pancreatitis, the lipase activity stays elevated longer than amylase activity.

372.

B. The quantification of serum prostate-specific antigen (PSA) has virtually replaced measurement of serum acid phosphatase for assessing carcinoma of the prostate. PSA measurement in conjunction with the digital rectal examination is recommended for prostate cancer screening. In addition, PSA can be used to stage and monitor therapy of prostatic cancer.

373.

B. Cholinesterase is a serum enzyme synthesized by the liver. It is also known as pseudo-cholinesterase to distinguish it from "true" cholinesterase (acetylcholinesterase) of erythrocytes. Although a number of disease states are associated with abnormal levels of this enzyme, cholinesterase levels are especially important in detecting organic insecticide poisoning of workers in the chemical industry and agriculture. Decreased cholinesterase levels and atypical enzyme forms are associated with prolonged apnea after succinylcholine administration during surgery. Propionylthiocholine is a commonly used substrate for measuring serum cholinesterase activity.

374.

C. For many years, the diagnosis of an acute myocardial infarction (AMI) was facilitated by assaying serum levels of aspartate aminotransferase (AST), lactate dehydrogenase (LD), creatine kinase (CK), and LD and CK isoenzymes. Today the clinical usefulness of AST and LD have been replaced primarily by troponin and to a lesser degree by myoglobin, while total creatine kinase (CK) and CK isoenzymes continue to play a role. While myoglobin will increase above the upper reference interval in 1–3 hours following AMI, it is not tissue specific for cardiac muscle and its application has found limited usefulness. Myoglobin will also be increased following skeletal muscle trauma. Troponin I and troponin T have proven to be useful markers, since each has a cardiac-specific isoform, cTnI and cTnT. cTnI appears to be more specific for cardiac muscle, since it has not been identified in regenerating or diseased skeletal muscle, while cTnT is made in small amounts by skeletal muscle. Total CK is elevated in AMI and takes 4–6 hours to rise above the upper reference interval. It is the increased level of CK-2 (CK-MB) that is more helpful in diagnosing AMI, but caution needs to be exercised here also since skeletal muscle injury can cause a similar increase.

375.

D. Osteitis deformans, also known as Paget's disease, is a chronic disorder of bone. This disorder is characterized by a significant increase in the serum alkaline phosphatase level. Gamma-glutamyltransferase will be normal in bone disease, since this enzyme is not found in bone tissue. However, in hepatobiliary disease both enzymes would characteristically be elevated.

376.

C. Obstruction of the biliary tree is also referred to as intrahepatic cholestasis. This disorder is characterized by significant elevations in the serum levels of alkaline phosphatase and gamma-glutamyltransferase. The serum levels of alanine and aspartate aminotransferases and lactate dehydrogenase are only slightly elevated. Early in the disease, the serum bilirubin level may be normal or only slightly elevated. In alcoholic cirrhosis, viral hepatitis, and infectious mononucleosis, only a slight to moderate elevation of alkaline phosphatase would be seen.

377.

A. Acute hepatitis is characterized by markedly elevated levels of serum alanine aminotransferase and aspartate aminotransferase, which may range from 10- to 100-fold greater than the reference values. Although alkaline phosphatase and gammaglutamyltransferase are increased, their elevations

are less notable than the aminotransferases. Alkaline phosphatase may range up to two times the reference range while gamma-glutamyltransferase may go as high as five times the reference range in acute hepatitis. Due to leakage of conjugated bilirubin from the hepatocytes, the urine bilirubin will be positive. With less conjugated bilirubin reaching the intestines, fecal urobilinogen will be less than normal.

378.

A. To aid in the diagnosis of skeletal muscle disease, measurement of creatine kinase (CK) would be most useful. CK yields the most reliable information when skeletal muscle disease is suspected. Other enzymes that are also useful to measure are aspartate aminotransferase and lactate dehydrogenase. Both of these enzymes will be moderately elevated, while creatine kinase is significantly increased.

379.

C. When an acute myocardial infarction occurs, creatine kinase (CK) is the first enzyme to become elevated in the blood, rising within 4 to 6 hours following chest pain. Aspartate aminotransferase (AST) exhibits a rise in the serum level within 6 to 8 hours. Lactate dehydrogenase (LD) shows an increase in 8 to 12 hours following infarction. Measurement of these three enzymes to assess acute myocardial infarction has been replaced by troponin, myoglobin, and CK-MB. However, awareness of the CK, AST, and LD patterns as well as other biochemical tests are useful in assessing organ complications that may arise during the period of acute myocardial infarction.

380.

C. Quantification of serum total creatine kinase, CK-2 (CK-MB) isoenzyme, and cardiac troponin I (cTnI) or cardiac troponin T (cTnT) is very useful in determining an acute myocardial infarction (AMI). Determining the presence and activity level of CK-2 (CK-MB) is valuable, since CK-2 levels can increase following an infarct, ranging from 6 to 30% of the total CK. Serial assessment of serum specimens is recommended with the initial specimen obtained at presentation, followed by blood collection at 3–6 hours, 6–9 hours, and 12–24 hours from the initial time. Since alkaline phosphatase isoenzymes are associated with liver, bone, intestinal, and placental tissues, its analysis would not contribute any significant information to determining the occurrence of an AMI.

381.

D. Reye's syndrome is associated with viral infections, exogenous toxins, and salicylate use. The disorder generally manifests itself in children from 2 to 13 years of age. The laboratory findings that support a diagnosis of Reye's syndrome include: increased levels of serum aspartate and alanine transaminases (greater than 3 times the reference range), increased plasma ammonia level (can exceed 100 μg/dL), and prolonged prothrombin time (3 sec or more than the control). In Reye's syndrome the serum bilirubin level is generally within the reference range.

382.

C. Lipase activity can be determined using a dilute olive oil emulsion as the substrate. The fatty micellar complexes absorb light as well as scatter light. Lipase catalyzes the hydrolysis of these triglyceride complexes, forming fatty acid and glycerol products. With the degradation of the micellar complexes, clearing of the reagent mixture occurs, causing changes in turbidity and light scatter. The rate at which the turbidity decreases can be monitored spectrophotometrically at 400 nm or the decrease in light scatter can be measured using a nephelometer. The rate of these changes can be equated to the lipase activity present in the serum specimen.

383.

D. Cystic fibrosis is inherited as an autosomal recessive trait. It is a systemic disease that affects the exocrine glands, causing gastrointestinal malabsorption, pancreatic insufficiency, and pulmonary disease. Cystic fibrosis is characterized by increased concentrations of chloride and sodium in sweat. With pancreatic insufficiency, the amount of lipase, amylase, trypsin, and bicarbonate secreted into the duodenum is decreased. Since the three enzymes contribute to digestion of fats, starches, and proteins, respectively, children with this disorder suffer from malabsorption.

ENDOCRINOLOGY

384.

C. The hypothalamus produces releasing factors or hormones that effect the release and synthesis of anterior pituitary hormones. The releasing hormones could have a stimulatory effect, as in the case of luteinizing hormone-releasing hormone (LH-RH) or an inhibitory effect as in the case of prolactin-inhibiting factor (PIF). The posterior lobe of the pituitary acts only as a storage area for vasopressin and oxytocin, which are manufactured in the hypothalamus. The posterior lobe of the pituitary gland does not effect any feedback control on the anterior lobe. The intermediate lobe secretes beta-melaninophore-stimulating hormone, which acts on the skin. It also does not effect any control over the anterior lobe. The adrenal medulla secretes catecholamines, which are not involved in any feedback mechanism to the pituitary gland.

385.

B. Adrenocorticotropic hormone (ACTH) stimulates the adrenal cortex to secrete cortisol and to a certain extent aldosterone. However, aldosterone is also regulated by sodium and potassium levels and more importantly by the renin-angiotensin system. Cortisol alone has an inhibitory effect or a negative feedback relationship to ACTH secretion by the pituitary. A low level of cortisol stimulates the hypothalamus to secrete corticotropin-releasing hormone (CRH), which in turn stimulates release of ACTH from the pituitary gland and causes the adrenal cortex to secrete more cortisol. Elevated levels of cortisol reverse this process. ACTH secretion is not inhibited by estrogen or progesterone levels.

386.

A. The corticosteroids, produced by the adrenal cortex, may be classified as glucocorticoids or mineralocorticoids. Cortisol is the primary glucocorticoid, and aldosterone is the primary mineralocorticoid. Aldosterone functions as a regulator of salt and water metabolism. Aldosterone promotes water retention and sodium resorption with potassium loss in the distal convoluted tubules of the kidney.

387.

B. Renin is a proteolytic enzyme secreted by the juxtaglomerular cells of the kidneys. In the blood, renin acts on renin substrate (angiotensinogen) to produce angiotensin I. An angiotensin-converting enzyme secreted by endothelial cells then converts angiotensin I to angiotensin II. It is the latter that is responsible for the vasoconstrictive action of renin release. Angiotensin III is a product of aminopeptidase on angiotensin II, and the action of angiotensin II and III is directed at modulating aldosterone secretion. Plasma renin activity, determined by radioimmunoassay, is assessed by quantifying the amount of angiotensin I produced by the action of renin on angiotensinogen using an initial kinetic assay.

388.

A. A low-salt diet, upright position, and diuretics cause a decrease in effective plasma volume. This decrease stimulates the renin-angiotensinogen system, which increases aldosterone secretion. Aldosterone promotes sodium retention and potassium loss.

389.

B. The hypothalamus, which secretes CRH, is sensitive not only to cortisol levels and stress but also to sleep-wake patterns. Thus plasma ACTH and cortisol levels exhibit diurnal variation or circadian rhythm. Cortisol secretion peaks at the time of awakening between 6 A.M. and 8 A.M. and then declines to the lowest level between early evening and midnight. After midnight the level again begins to increase. Specimens should be taken at 8 A.M. and 8 P.M. The evening cortisol level should be at least 50% lower than the morning result. In 90% of patients with Cushing's syndrome there is no diurnal variation. However, absence of the normal drop in the evening cortisol level is not specific for Cushing's syndrome. Other conditions, such as ectopic ACTH syndrome, blindness, hypothalamic tumors, obesity, acute alcoholism, and various drugs, alter normal circadian rhythm in cortisol secretion. To confirm Cushing's syndrome a dexamethasone suppression test may be performed.

390.

D. For differentiation of primary and secondary adrenal dysfunction, stimulation or suppression tests that depend on the feedback mechanism between cortisol and ACTH are performed. In the ACTH stimulation test, a patient with a low baseline serum cortisol level is given ACTH. The level of cortisol will increase slightly if the problem lies with the anterior pituitary gland, thus secondary adrenal insufficiency. This increase will be less than normal and may be somewhat delayed due to atrophy of the adrenal cortex as a result of the primary pituitary dysfunction. If the serum cortisol level does not change from baseline, the dysfunction is with the adrenal cortex, thus primary adrenal insufficiency.

391.

C. Only very small quantities, normally less than 2%, of the total adrenal secretion of cortisol appears in the urine as free cortisol. The majority of cortisol is either metabolized in various tissues or conjugated in the liver and excreted. It is only the serum unconjugated cortisol not bound to corticotropin binding globulin (CBG) or the conjugated cortisol that can be cleared by glomerular filtration in the kidney. Therefore, the measurement of free cortisol in the urine is a sensitive reflection of the amount of unbound cortisol in the serum. It is not a reflection of the amount of conjugated cortisol or the serum total cortisol but, rather, only the increased cortisol production that is not accompanied by an increase in serum levels of CBG.

392.

C. The probable diagnosis is Cushing's syndrome caused by adrenocortical carcinoma. In adrenocortical carcinoma, the urinary free cortisol and the serum cortisol levels would be elevated and the plasma ACTH level would be decreased. The carcinoma produces excess cortisol that, because of the feedback loop, turns off pituitary production of ACTH. Neither the low-dose dexamethasone suppression test nor the high-dose test are able to suppress cortisol production. Since dexamethasone is a cortisol analogue, it would normally suppress ACTH and cortisol levels in a healthy individual. All this data supports primary adrenal dysfunction caused by an adrenal carcinoma. If the elevated cortisol level was due to a pituitary adenoma or ectopic ACTH lung cancer, the ACTH level would also be increased. Addison's disease is caused by hypofunction of the adrenal cortex.

393.

B. The adrenogenital syndrome, congenital adrenal hyperplasia, is due to a deficiency in specific enzymes needed for the synthesis of cortisol and aldosterone. Because cortisol production is blocked, the pituitary increases its secretion of adrenocorticotropic hormone (ACTH), causing adrenal hyperplasia and hypersecretion of cortisol precursors. There are eight recognized types of inherited enzyme defects in cortisol biosynthesis. The most common type of defect is the lack of 21-hydroxylase, occurring in 95% of the cases. Conversion of 17α-hydroxyprogesterone to 11-deoxycortisol is impaired, causing accumulation of 17α-hydroxyprogesterone, which is metabolized to pregnanetriol. An increased plasma 17α-hydroxyprogesterone level is diagnostic and can be determined by radioimmunoassay. Determinations of serum testosterone and urinary pregnanetriol elevations are also diagnostic of this disorder. Virilization takes place in this syndrome because cortisol precursors are shunted to produce weak androgens [e.g., dehydroepiandrosterone (DHEA) and androstenedione]. These androgens are converted peripherally to testosterone in large-enough amounts to create this condition. The second most common defect is 11β-hydroxylase deficiency with an accumulation of 11-deoxycortisol. 3β-Hydroxysteroid dehydrogenase-isomerase deficiency and C-17,20-lyase/17α-hydroxylase deficiency are examples of other enzyme defects seen in this disorder. A testicular or adrenal tumor may cause symptoms similar to this syndrome; however, these tumors would be acquired in contrast to congenital disorders.

394.

D. Testosterone is the most potent of the body's androgens. One of the major functions of the testes is to produce testosterone. It is metabolized to the 17-ketosteroids, etiocholanolone and androsterone, but testosterone is not itself a 17-ketosteroid. The 17-ketosteroids, dehydroepiandrosterone (DHEA), androsterone, and androstenedione, all have androgenic properties but are much weaker than testosterone.

395.

B. The pituitary gland produces protein hormones such as adrenocorticotropic hormone, thyroid-stimulating hormone, follicle-stimulating hormone, growth hormone, and prolactin. Steroid hormones include C_{21} corticosteroids and progestins, C_{19} androgens, and C_{18} estrogens. The corticosteroids are secreted only by the adrenal glands, but the other steroids are secreted by the ovaries, testes, adrenal glands, and placenta to a varying extent, depending on the individual's sex.

396.

C. 17β-Estradiol (E_2) is the most potent estrogen. 17β-Estradiol is considered to be the true ovarian hormone because it is secreted almost entirely by the ovaries. In contrast, estrone (E_1) is produced from circulating C_{19} neutral steroids (e.g., androstenedione) and is also synthesized from 17β-estradiol. Estriol (E_3) is derived almost exclusively from 17β-estradiol and has little clinical significance except in pregnancy. The measurement of 17β-estradiol is used to evaluate ovarian function.

397.

C. In pregnant women the level of chorionic gonadotropin (CG) is highest during the first trimester, then it stabilizes to a lower level during the rest of the pregnancy. In the first trimester the level of pregnanediol is slightly higher than that found in nonpregnant women during the luteal phase of the menstrual cycle. As pregnancy progresses, the placenta secretes more progesterone, which peaks midway into the third trimester and then levels off. It should be noted that pregnanediol is a biologically inactive metabolite of progesterone that is sometimes measured in urine. After the second month of pregnancy, estriol levels steadily increase as the placenta takes over estrogen production.

398.

C. The triple test for Down's syndrome includes quantification of α-fetoprotein (AFP), unconjugated estriol (uE_3), and chorionic gonadotropin (CG) in the maternal serum. These measurements should be done between 16 and 18 weeks gestation, and they are useful in detecting neural tube defects and Down's syndrome. In Down's syndrome, the AFP and uE_3 levels are low, while the CG level is elevated. These test results are related to gestational age and expressed as a multiple of the median (MoM), meaning the maternal serum result is divided by the median result of the corresponding gestational population.

399.

A. Progesterone production can be monitored by measuring plasma progesterone or urinary pregnanediol, the major metabolite of progesterone. In the follicular stage of the menstrual cycle, only a small amount of progesterone is secreted. In the luteal stage, or the time from ovulation to menstruation, progesterone levels rapidly increase. Hence serial assays of plasma progesterone or urinary pregnanediol can be used to identify the time of ovulation. If pregnancy does not occur, progesterone quickly decreases approximately 24 hours before menstruation. If there is no ovulation, then there is no corpus luteum formation and no cyclic rise in pregnanediol levels.

400.

D. Luteinizing hormone (LH) is secreted only by the anterior pituitary. A protein hormone, chorionic gonadotropin (CG) appears soon after conception and is thus used for early detection of pregnancy. Human placental lactogen (HPL), also a protein hormone, is produced only by the placenta and is measurable between the seventh and ninth weeks. HPL steadily increases throughout pregnancy and peaks near term. Analysis of HPL for placental dysfunction has been successful; however, it is not widely used for this purpose. During pregnancy the placenta is the main source of estrogen and progesterone. Both hormones are needed for the maintenance of pregnancy.

401.

D. The formation of estriol during pregnancy involves mainly the fetoplacental unit. Dehydroepiandrosterone sulfate (DHEA-S) and its 16α-hydroxy-DHEA-S derivative are formed mainly by the fetal adrenal glands and to a lesser degree by the liver. The fetus possesses 16α-hydroxylase activity, which is needed to convert dehydroepiandrosterone sulfate (DHEA-S) to 16α-hydroxy-DHEA-S. The 16α-hydroxy-DHEA-S compound is metabolized by the placenta to estriol. The placenta lacks certain enzymes needed for the conversion of simple precursors such as acetate, cholesterol, and progesterone to estrogens. Thus, the placenta must rely on immediate precursors produced in the fetus. In the case of estriol, the placenta utilizes the 16α-hydroxy-DHEA-S precursor made in the adrenal glands of the fetus. The latter compound crosses into the placenta, which takes over with the necessary enzymes to complete the synthesis of estriol. This estriol produced in the placenta is rapidly reflected in the maternal plasma and far exceeds maternal synthesis of estriol. Thus measurement of

estriol in the maternal blood or urine is a sensitive indicator of the integrity of the fetoplacental unit. A defect in either the fetus or the placenta will be reflected by a decrease in estriol production.

402.

D. The concentration of estriol in maternal plasma or in a 24-hour sample of maternal urine is often used as an indicator of fetal distress or placental failure. A single value of either serum or urine estriol has relatively little value unless it can be related accurately to the gestational week. When sequential estriol determinations are made during pregnancy, a pattern of stable or steadily falling values may indicate a problem pregnancy. For serum or urine estriols, any individual value that is 30–50% less than the previous value or the average of the previous 3 days' values is significant.

403.

D. Acetate, cholesterol, progesterone, and the male sex hormones testosterone and androstenedione all serve as precursors for the synthesis of estrogens. The major pathway for conversion of testosterone to estradiol is in the ovaries. The major pathway for conversion of androstenedione to estrone is outside the ovaries.

404.

C. During the menstrual cycle, follicle-stimulating hormone (FSH) levels decrease in the later part of the follicular stage. Luteinizing hormone (LH) gradually increases during the follicular stage. At midcycle, both FSH and LH levels spike. Following this spike, in the luteal stage or second half of the menstrual cycle, FSH and LH levels gradually decrease. In postmenopausal women the ovaries stop secreting estrogens. In response the gonadotropins, FSH and LH, rise to their highest levels. The reason is the feedback system between estrogen secretion by the gonads and the secretion of releasing factors by the hypothalamus; a decreased estrogen level causes increased secretion of FSH-releasing factor and LH-releasing factor.

405.

C. Ectopic hormones are hormonal substances produced by benign and malignant tumors derived from tissues that do not normally secrete those hormones. Examples of ectopic hormone production would be ACTH production by oat cell carcinoma of the lung and growth hormone production by bronchogenic carcinomas of the lung. Cortisol and growth hormone are normally secreted by the adrenal gland and anterior pituitary gland, respectively. Ectopic hormones are not in all cases chemically identical to the native hormone but may be similar enough to cross-react in immunoassay methods for the native hormone.

406.

A. At the cellular level, the site of action of the peptide and catecholamine hormones is different from that of the steroid and thyroid hormones. The peptide and catecholamine hormones bring about their effects by combining with receptors on or in the cell membranes of the target cells. In some cases, this binding to the membrane results in activation of adenylate cyclase, which sets in motion the so-called second-messenger mechanism of hormone action. On the other hand, steroid and thyroid hormones act predominantly by diffusing through the target cell membranes and combining with cytoplasmic or nucleic receptors to form a complex that then brings about the hormone's action.

407.

C. The adrenal medulla produces 80% epinephrine and 20% norepinephrine (noradrenalin). Metanephrine is a metabolite of epinephrine. Dopamine, a catecholamine, is a precursor of norepinephrine. Norepinephrine is converted to epinephrine by an enzyme, N-methyltransferase, which is present almost exclusively in the adrenal medulla. A tumor of the chromaffin tissue, called a pheochromocytoma, secretes excessive amounts of epinephrine. Ninety percent of pheochromocytomas are in the adrenal medulla. The increased levels of epinephrine from the pheochromocytoma cause hypertension. Although hypertension caused by a pheochromocytoma is rare, a correct diagnosis is very important because pheochromocytoma is one of the few causes of hypertension that is curable by surgery.

408.

A. The majority of pheochromocytomas (rare tumors) occur in the adrenal medulla, causing increased secretion of the catecholamines. As a screening test for this disorder, quantification of urinary metanephrine, the methylated product of epinephrine, is suggested since false negatives seldom occur. Follow-up testing should include measurement of urinary vanillylmandelic acid

(VMA), since VMA is the primary metabolite of epinephrine and norepinephrine.

409.

B. Antidiuretic hormone (ADH), also known as vasopressin, is a peptide hormone secreted by the posterior pituitary gland under the influence of three major stimuli: decreased serum osmolality, increased blood volume, or psychogenic factors. ADH increases the renal reabsorption of water by increasing the permeability of the collecting ducts, with the result that body water is retained and urine osmolality increases. Diabetes insipidus is the syndrome that results from decreased secretion of ADH from any cause. Serum levels of ADH can be measured, but usually the measurement of serum and urine osmolality is sufficient to indicate the severity of the disease.

410.

A. C-peptide is formed in the pancreatic beta cells during the proteolytic conversion of proinsulin to insulin. Approximately equimolar quantities of C-peptide and insulin are secreted into the blood, but the serum ratio is 5 to 15:1 because the liver removes insulin rapidly while C-peptide is not removed. Therefore, radioimmunoassay for C-peptide is useful in evaluating pancreatic beta cell function. In several clinical situations the measurement of C-peptide is warranted. These include: insulinoma, a hypoglycemic condition, where C-peptide is elevated; identification of surreptitious injection of insulin, since C-peptide is absent from commercially available insulin; and follow-up assessment after total pancreatectomy, since C-peptide would be undetectable. Since measurable amounts of C-peptide are not present in diabetic ketoacidosis, this information is of little use in managing the disorder.

411.

C. Serotonin (5-hydroxytryptamine or 5-HT) is synthesized from tryptophan in a variety of tissues, with the majority found in the argentaffin (enterochromaffin) cells of the intestine. Abdominal carcinoid is a metastasizing tumor of those cells and is associated with excessive production of serotonin. Serotonin in the blood is found almost exclusively in the platelets and is rapidly oxidized in the lungs to 5-hydroxyindoleacetic acid (5-HIAA), its major urinary metabolite. Urinary levels of 5-HIAA may also be increased by eating foods such as bananas and avocados, which are rich in serotonin, by the use of certain drugs such as the phenothiazines, and by carcinoid tumors.

412.

D. Somatostatin is also known as growth hormone-inhibiting hormone (GHIH). Somatostatin is a 14-amino-acid peptide that is secreted by the hypothalamus and is an inhibitor of growth hormone (somatotropin) secretion by the pituitary. It is also secreted by a variety of other organs and is a powerful inhibitor of insulin and glucagon secretion by the pancreas. Somatostatin can be measured by radioimmunoassay methods, but its concentration in the peripheral circulation is extremely low, making it likely that its action is mostly at or near the site of secretion.

413.

B. Growth hormone (somatotropin) is a polypeptide secreted by the anterior pituitary. It is essential to the growth process of cartilage, bone, and a variety of soft tissues. It also plays an important role in lipid, carbohydrate, and protein metabolism of adults. During the growth phase of humans, hyposecretion of somatotropin results in dwarfism, whereas hypersecretion, conversely, causes pituitary gigantism. After the growth phase, hypersecretion of somatotropin causes acromegaly. Diagnosis of hypersecretion or hyposecretion of growth hormone usually requires the use of suppression or provocative tests of growth hormone release. Growth hormone levels may be quantified using immunoradiometric, chemiluminescence, and radioimmunoassay methods.

414.

C. Somatomedins, insulin-like growth factors I and II, is the designation given to a family of small peptides whose formation in the liver is under the control of growth hormone. The somatomedins exhibit similar activity as insulin and are active in stimulating many aspects of cell growth, particularly that of cartilage. Blood levels of somatomedin have been determined by radioimmunoassay methods, and acromegalic adults have been shown to have significantly elevated levels in comparison with normal adults.

415.

A. Calcitonin is a calcium-lowering hormone secreted by the parafollicular or C cells of the thyroid. Cal-

citonin acts as an antagonist to parathyroid hormone (PTH) action on the bone and kidneys. Medullary carcinoma of the thyroid is a neoplasm of the parafollicular cells that usually results in elevated serum levels of calcitonin. If the fasting calcitonin level is within the normal reference interval in a patient with suspected medullary carcinoma, a provocative calcium infusion test is often useful in improving the sensitivity of the test.

416.

A. Thyroglobulin is a glycoprotein in which the thyroid hormones are stored in the thyroid gland. When tyrosine residues of the thyroglobulin are iodinated, MIT and DIT are formed. These iodotyrosine residues are not hormones. T_3 and T_4 are the hormones produced by the thyroid, being formed by the coupling of either MIT or DIT. T_4 is the predominant form of the thyroid hormones secreted into the circulation, having a concentration in the plasma significantly greater than T_3. However, in terms of physiological activity, T_3 must be considered because it is four to five times more potent than T_4. Thus the overall contribution of T_3 to the total physiological effect of the thyroid hormones on the body is significant.

417.

B. The thyroid gland is composed of two lobes connected by a structure called the isthmus. The lobes consist of many follicles. The follicle, in the shape of a sphere, is lined with a single layer of epithelial cells. The epithelial cells produce T_3 and T_4, which are stored in the thyroglobulin molecule. Within the lumen of the follicle is a colloid. Thyroglobulin, secreted by the epithelial cells, makes up 90% of the colloid. As the epithelial cells synthesize the thyroid hormones, the hormones are stored in the thyroglobulin molecule. Thyroglobulin is then secreted into the colloid of the follicular lumen. When the thyroid hormones are needed, they are absorbed by the epithelial cells from their storage site, and through proteolysis the hormones are released from fragments of the thyroglobulin molecule. T_3 and T_4 are then secreted by the cells into the blood.

418.

A. A small amount of reverse T_3 (rT_3) is made in the thyroid gland, but the majority is made from peripheral deiodination of T_4. rT_3 varies from T_3 in that rT_3 contains one iodine atom in the tyrosyl ring and two iodines in the phenolic ring, while T_3 has two iodines in the tyrosyl ring and one iodine in the phenolic ring. rT_3 does not have any physiological action as it is metabolically inactive. However, increased levels of rT_3 are associated with nonthyroidal illness (NTI) that also manifests with decreased levels of total T_3.

419.

C. Thyroid-stimulating immunoglobulins (TSI) are IgG autoantibodies that bind to the thyroid-stimulating hormone (TSH) receptor sites on thyroid cell membranes, thus preventing TSH from binding. The TSI autoantibodies interact with the receptors similarly to TSH, thus stimulating the thyroid to secrete thyroid hormones. Since TSI does not respond to the negative feedback system as does TSH, hyperthyroidism is the end result. The majority of patients with Graves' hyperthyroid disease exhibit high titers of TSI. Currently, the suggested term for autoantibodies that bind to TSH receptor sites is thyrotropin-receptor antibodies (TRAbs).

420.

C. Graves' disease is a name given to a diffusely hyperactive thyroid that produces thyrotoxicosis. Thyrotoxicosis results from elevated levels of thyroid hormone; therefore, laboratory results for free thyroxine (FT_4) and free triiodothyronine (FT_3) would be increased, thyroid hormone binding ratio (THBR) increased, and thyroid-stimulating hormone (TSH) decreased. In hyperthyroidism, the THBR is increased because thyroxine-binding globulin (TBG) is saturated with endogenous T_4; thus more labeled T_3 is taken up by the resin. TSH levels are decreased because of the negative-feedback control of the thyroid hormones on the anterior pituitary.

421.

C. Hypothyroidism is a systemic disorder in which the thyroid gland does not secrete sufficient thyroid hormone. Myxedema is commonly used synonymously for hypothyroidism. Hypothyroidism can result from various diseases. If the disease affects the thyroid itself, it is referred to as primary hypothyroidism. If there is TSH deficiency of the pituitary gland, it is termed secondary hypothyroidism. Tertiary hypothyroidism is caused by hypothalamic failure that results in a decreased secretion of thyrotropin-releasing hormone. Thyroid failure in the newborn is termed "cretinism."

The free T_4 level and the thyroid hormone binding ratio (THBR) are decreased because of inadequate secretion of hormones. Since the thyroid hormones are low in concentration, the feedback mechanism to the anterior pituitary gland is triggered to increase production of TSH.

422.

B. To distinguish between a hypothalamic disorder and a disorder of the pituitary gland, thyroid-releasing hormone (TRH) is administered. In the case of a hypothalamic disorder (tertiary hypothyroidism), the TRH administered will cause an increased excretion of pituitary hormone, TSH. However, if the disorder originates in the pituitary gland (secondary hypothyroidism), the administration of TRH will have no effect on the pituitary gland and thus no increased excretion of TSH. Since the values of TSH were low before and remained low after administration of TRH, the disorder is secondary hypothyroidism. Primary hypothyroidism is caused by failure of the thyroid gland itself and is not evaluated by use of the TRH stimulation test. Iodine deficiency would cause high levels of TSH. Administration of TRH is not used to evaluate this disorder.

423.

B. Antibodies to thyroglobulin and thyroid cell microsomes are produced in several thyroid diseases. Very high antibody titers for antithyroglobulin antibodies and the detection of antimicrosomal antibodies are highly suggestive of Hashimoto's thyroiditis (type of hypothyroidism). These antibodies are also frequently detected in primary myxedema and Graves' disease by means of hemagglutination methods. It should be noted that antithyroid antibodies do occur in other thyroid diseases, but their prevalence is less. These antibodies have also been detected in 5–10% of the normal population.

424.

C. Almost all the triiodothyronine (T_3) and thyroxine (T_4) hormones are reversibly bound to the serum proteins, thyroxine-binding globulin (TBG), thyroxine-binding prealbumin (TBPA), and albumin. Most T_3 is bound to TBG, whereas 70% of T_4 is bound to TBG, 20% to TBPA, and 10% to albumin. T_3 has a lower affinity for TBG and TBPA than T_4. Thyroglobulin is manufactured and stored in the thyroid follicle and is not released into the circulation.

425.

C. Due to increased protein synthesis, the binding capacity of thyroxine-binding globulin (TBG) is increased in situations such as pregnancy and administration of oral contraceptives. The increased total thyroxine (Total T_4) levels in these situations do not reflect the functional state of the thyroid gland. It is important when interpreting total T_4 levels to take into consideration situations such as these. Free T_4 is not affected by variations in thyroxine-binding proteins and better reflects the metabolic state that is euthyroid. However, use of the thyroid hormone binding ratio (THBR), which measures the unoccupied binding sites of TBG, in conjunction with the free and total T_4 levels permits a better interpretation of thyroid function. By this process it can be seen where the primary change occurs, whether in the level of T_4 or in TBG-binding capacity.

426.

B. In cases of peptic ulcer, treatment may include surgery that severs the vagus nerve. This severing is known as vagotomy, which, if complete, prevents the secretion of gastrin and HCl by the stomach. The Hollander insulin test is performed to assess the completeness of the vagotomy. If the vagotomy is complete, the hypoglycemia caused by the administration of insulin will not exert its normal stimulatory effect on gastric HCl and pepsinogen secretion.

427.

C. Gastrin is the designation given to a family of protein hormones produced by the mucosal cells of the gastric antrum. Once secreted, gastrin is carried in the blood to the fundic cells, causing release of hydrochloric acid. Serum gastrin levels are markedly elevated in the Zollinger-Ellison syndrome, a neoplastic proliferation of the non-beta cells of the pancreatic islets. Gastrin levels may also be elevated in pernicious anemia, duodenal ulcer disease, and gastric ulcer disease.

428.

D. Enzyme-multiplied immunoassay technique (EMIT) is an example of a homogeneous immunoassay technique. A homogeneous assay is one in which separation of the bound and free fraction is unnecessary. The antigen is labeled with an enzyme and competes with the unknown antigen for binding sites on the antibody. The enzyme-labeled antigen that remains in the free fraction is enzymatically active. Therefore the free, labeled antigen can be determined by its action on a substrate in the presence of bound labeled fraction. The other techniques mentioned in the question, RIA, ELISA, and IRMA, are termed heterogeneous immunoassays because they require the physical separation of the bound from the free fraction prior to actual measurement.

429.

D. A number of radioactive and nonradioactive immunoassay methods have been developed for the quantification of hormones. The overall principle involved is the same. That is, the substance to be measured reacts with a specific macromolecule of limited binding capacity; frequently this binder is an antibody. All these assays are similarly dependent on the closeness with which the unknown species and the standard react with the binder. These assays differ only in the specific reagents used. RIA uses radioactive labeled and unlabeled antigen. The ELISA system depends on enzyme-labeled antigen. CPB is a general term for any system that uses serum protein or tissue receptors for binding agents. In IRMA the antibody is radioactively labeled, unlike RIA, in which the antigen is labeled. Nonradioactive methods, based on antigen-antibody reactions, include such assays as fluorescence polarization immunoassay (FPI), enzyme-multiplied immunoassay technique (EMIT), and chemiluminescence assays. While hormones may be quantified using high-performance liquid chromatography (HPLC), its principle is based on differential partitioning of compounds and not on antigen-antibody reactions as the immunoassays.

430.

A. In radioimmunoassay a competition exists between radioactively labeled antigen and unlabeled antigen (serum sample) for binding sites on the antibody. The less unlabeled antigen present in the assay mixture, the greater will be the binding of labeled antigen to antibody. It follows that when low levels of unlabeled antigen are present, the number of counts per minute recorded by a scintillation counter of the bound fraction will be greater because of the increased number of antibody sites occupied by labeled antigen. The number of counts per minute in the free fraction would correspondingly be low, since the majority of labeled antigen would be in the antibody-bound form.

TOXICOLOGY AND THERAPEUTIC DRUG MONITORING

431.
D. The term *carboxyhemoglobin saturation* refers to the fraction of circulating hemoglobin combined with carbon monoxide. Nonsmokers generally have carboxyhemoglobin saturations ranging from 0.5 to 1.5%. Fatal carbon monoxide poisoning is usually associated with carboxyhemoglobin saturations of more than 60%, and acute symptoms begin to appear at saturations of 20%. Cigarette smokers exhibit levels of 8–9% carboxyhemoglobin but, occasionally, saturations of greater than 16% have been reported in heavy smokers.

432.
D. Gas-liquid chromatography (GLC) is one of the few methods that can quantify ethanol reliably in the presence of isopropanol (2-propanol) or other alcohols. Examples of the analytical problems associated with quantifying alcohols are as follows: isopropanol significantly cross-reacts (6%) in the widely used alcohol dehydrogenase (ADH) method for ethanol; other alcohols will cross-react with dichromate methods for ethanol; and other alcohols will cross-react with the permanganate-chromotropic acid method, which is sometimes used for the identification of methanol. Since GLC is not generally available in stat laboratories, for patients with suspected exposure to alcohols other than ethanol, a variety of other laboratory and clinical findings are often used.

433.
A. A significant fraction of absorbed isopropanol is metabolized to acetone and rapidly excreted in the urine. Because of isopropanol's relatively low molecular weight, exposure to this compound will in most cases significantly increase the patient's serum osmolality. Of course, other alcohols will have a similar effect. Urine osmolality exhibits a wide variability throughout the day and therefore would be of little use in determining isopropanol exposure. Serum sodium would be only secondarily affected by isopropanol exposure.

434.
D. Reinsch's test is applied to urine and is based on the ability of copper to reduce most metal ions to their metallic states in the presence of acid. Cyanide is not a metal and therefore will not be reduced. Increased urinary levels of arsenic, bismuth, antimony, and mercury will coat the copper with dull black, shiny black, blue-black, and silver-gray deposits, respectively. The test is intended as a rapid screening method only, and results should be confirmed by more sensitive and specific methods.

435.
B. Heroin (diacetylmorphine), an abused drug, is a derivative of morphine. The morphine used in its synthesis is generally obtained from opium. Although heroin itself is not pharmacologically active, it does have a rapid onset of action. It is converted quickly to 6-acetylmorphine and then hydrolyzed to morphine, both of which are pharmacologically active. So heroin abuse can be detected by measuring its metabolite morphine in the blood or urine.

436.
B. Morphine, codeine, and heroin are collectively referred to as opiates. Codeine is found in many prescription medicines and is rapidly metabolized after absorption into morphine and norcodeine. Because blood concentrations of most opiates are low even in overdose, screening is usually done on the urine. Immunoassay or colorimetric methods can be used for screening purposes, but chromatography is generally required for quantification of specific compounds. Gas chromatography/mass spectroscopy (GC/MS) is useful for the quantification of morphine and codeine.

437.
B. THC (Δ^9-tetrahydrocannabinol) is the principal active component of marijuana. Homogeneous enzyme immunoassay methods test for the presence of THC metabolites, especially 11-nor-Δ^9-THC-9-carboxylic acid, which is the primary urinary metabolite. Metabolites appear in urine within hours of smoking and continue to be detectable for 3 to 10 days following exposure.

438.

B. Cocaine is an abused drug and not available for therapeutic use. After absorption, cocaine in the blood is rapidly converted into ecgonine and benzoylecgonine. Because of the kidney's concentrating effect, examination of the urine for the metabolites is a sensitive method of determining exposure to cocaine.

439.

C. After absorption, lead is distributed into an active pool in the blood and soft tissue and a storage pool in bone, teeth, and hair. In blood, the majority is found in erythrocytes, with only minor quantities in plasma or serum. Lead is mainly excreted by the kidney; hence urine or whole blood would be appropriate specimens for determining lead exposure. Provision for lead-free sample containers is a major requirement. Lead analysis can be done accurately by flameless atomic absorption or anodic stripping voltammetry.

440.

B. Lead interferes in heme biosynthesis at several stages, the last of these being the incorporation of iron into the tetrapyrrole ring. This alteration in biosynthesis results in the formation and accumulation of zinc protoporphyrin (ZPP), with zinc replacing the iron in the tetrapyrrole ring. Free erythrocyte protoporphyrin is the extraction product of the zinc metabolite and is a sensitive screening method for determining lead exposure above 25 μg/dL. The test is not as specific as accurate determination of lead content, however, because iron deficiency anemia and erythropoietic protoporphyria give false-positive results. Caution must be exercised in monitoring children under 6 years of age, since the Centers for Disease Control and Prevention have defined the acceptable blood level for lead to be less than 10 μg/dL in young children. At this level, ZPP and erythrocyte protoporphyrin assays are not sufficiently sensitive.

441.

D. After absorption, mercury rapidly accumulates in many organs and in the central nervous system, with only minor quantities found in the blood. The excretion of mercury by the kidney generally forms the basis for measurement of exposure. The preferred specimen in screening for exposure to methanol or acetaminophen is serum. Whole blood is required for determining carbon monoxide exposure, since practically all the inhaled carbon monoxide is found in erythrocytes bound to hemoglobin. The percent carboxyhemoglobin saturation of whole blood can be determined by differential spectrophotometry.

442.

C. The term *half-life* refers to the time required for a 50% decrease in serum drug concentration after absorption and distribution are complete. The more complete descriptive term is drug elimination half-life. It requires 5–7 half-life periods for drug concentration to reach steady state. At steady state the drug concentration is in equilibrium with the dose administered rate and the elimination rate. Knowledge of a drug's half-life is important both for planning therapy and for monitoring drug concentration. In disease states, particularly involving the kidney and liver, half-life may be significantly altered and lead to accumulations of the drug or its metabolites in the blood.

443.

C. The Trinder reaction or modification is used almost routinely in the determination of salicylate and is based on the colorimetric reaction with ferric ions. The availability of rapid quantification in cases of salicylate overdose has been particularly useful because of the necessity of determining the drug's elimination half-life. Most clinically used thin-layer chromatographic (TLC) methods are insensitive to the presence of salicylate. Because the colorimetric reaction used for determining the presence of phenothiazines with ferric perchloricnitric (FPN) reagent is dependent on ferric ions also, false-positive reactions in the ferric ion methods for salicylate may be expected.

444.

D. Hepatotoxicity is common in acetaminophen overdose. It is particularly important to be able to determine the acetaminophen serum level rapidly so that the elimination half-life of the drug can be estimated. Hepatic necrosis is more common when the half-life exceeds 4 hours and is very likely when it exceeds 12 hours. The concentration of acetaminophen can be measured by high-performance liquid chromatography (HPLC), colorimetric, EMIT, and fluorescence polarization methods.

445.

A. The barbiturates are classified pharmacologically according to their duration of action. Phenobarbital is long acting, amobarbital and butabarbital are intermediate acting, and pentobarbital and secobarbital are short acting. In general, the long-acting barbiturates have higher therapeutic and toxic levels than the shorter-acting barbiturates. In cases of overdose, it is important to be able to identify the type of barbiturate in the blood for correct therapy. Measurement of specific barbiturates usually requires chromatography or immunoassay.

446.

B. Tobramycin and gentamicin are examples of aminoglycoside antibiotics. Their use has been associated with both nephrotoxicity and ototoxicity. Drug concentration monitoring of patients taking the aminoglycosides requires an analytic system with good precision and accuracy over a wide range since both peak and trough levels are usually monitored. The trough level is used mainly as a measure of nephrotoxicity, whereas the peak level is useful in determining whether adequate therapy is being given to eliminate the causative organism.

447.

C. Although digoxin, nortriptyline, and quinidine have various effects on cardiac arrhythmias, they do not have metabolites with similar activity. Procainamide is an antiarrhythmic drug and has at least one metabolite with the same activity, namely, *N*-acetylprocainamide (NAPA). Because of differences in half-life, NAPA may accumulate in the blood and produce toxic effects even with therapeutic levels of procainamide.

448.

A. Drugs in the free state are able to elicit a pharmacologic response. It is the free drug that is able to cross cell membranes and to bind at receptor sites. In the protein-bound state, drugs are unable to enter tissues and interact at receptor sites.

449.

B. Acute glomerulonephritis is characterized by hematuria and albuminuria. The hypoalbuminemia results in less protein-bound drug and an increase in free drug. Thus more free drug is available in the circulation to enter the tissues. Such a situation may result in severe side effects and even toxic effects. Therefore, to properly regulate drug dosages, it is advisable to measure free drug levels in blood, rather than total drug levels, whenever possible.

450.

B. The term *free drug* refers to the fraction of drug in the plasma not bound to protein. For the determination of free drug concentrations, urine would not be the proper specimen because the rate of drug excretion depends mainly on conjugation or metabolism and not on protein binding. In preparation of a protein-free filtrate of plasma, the drugs bound to protein would also enter the filtrate because they are dissociated when the protein is denatured. Saliva is a form of plasma ultrafiltrate and with some restrictions as to sampling and type of drug analyzed can be used for free-drug monitoring. Methods for equilibrium dialysis and for preparation of ultrafiltrates of plasma are now available and can provide excellent samples for free-drug analyses of some compounds.

451.

C. Tacrolimus, formerly known as FK-506, is an antibiotic that functions as an immunosuppressant in organ transplantation, especially in liver transplants. By inhibiting interleukin production it blocks lymphocyte proliferation. Adverse reactions to the drug include nephrotoxicity, nausea, vomiting, and headaches. Other immunosuppressant drugs include cyclosporine, mycophenolic acid, and sirolimus. Methotrexate is an antineoplastic drug, amiodarone is an antiarrhythmic drug, and paroxetine is an antidepressant drug.

452.

B. Theophylline, a xanthine with bronchodilator activity, is widely used in the treatment of asthma. Because of its availability and potential toxicity, it can also be subject to accidental overdose. Chromatographic methods are effective in separating theophylline from caffeine and theobromine, which are two commonly occurring and potentially interfering xanthines. However, most clinical thin-layer chromatographic (TLC) methods are relatively insensitive to the xanthines, and suspected theophylline overdose should be confirmed by high-performance liquid chromatographic (HPLC) or immunoassay methods.

453.

D. Following absorption, primidone is metabolized primarily to phenobarbital and secondarily to phenylethylmalonamide (PEMA). Both metabolites have anticonvulsant activity, and both have a longer half-life than primidone. Generally, only serum phenobarbital and primidone concentrations are monitored. Determination of phenobarbital is particularly important when another anticonvulsant phenytoin is also administered because the metabolic rate of primidone conversion to phenobarbital may be increased, with a resulting accumulation of phenobarbital in the blood.

454.

A. Amitriptyline, doxepin, and imipramine and their active metabolites nortriptyline, nordoxepin, and desipramine, respectively, are tricyclic compounds particularly useful in the treatment of endogenous depression. These compounds are lipid soluble and therefore highly protein bound in the plasma. Although toxic concentrations of these drugs often lead to cardiac arrhythmias, low concentrations have been found to have antiarrhythmic activity. Because of these varying biological effects at differing serum concentrations, there is a need both for monitoring in cases of therapy and screening for toxic effects in cases of overdose.

455.

B. Lithium is used in the treatment of manic depression. Because of the small difference between therapeutic and toxic levels in the serum, accurate measurements of lithium concentrations are essential. It is also important to standardize the sample drawing time in relation to the previous dose. In the flame photometric method, sodium and potassium ions have strong emission bands which may contribute to the lithium signal. For this reason, concentrations of potentially interfering metal ions approximating the serum levels are used in the standards.

456.

C. The collection of blood samples for therapeutic drug monitoring requires both the selection of the proper time for sampling and the recording of that time on the report. It is essential that the drug level be related in time to the time of the previous and/or the next drug administration. Collection of blood samples is generally avoided during the drug's absorption and distribution phases. When peak levels of the drug are required, the blood sample must be drawn at a specified time after drug administration. Trough levels are most reliably determined by collecting the blood sample before the next drug administration.

457.

C. Persons involved in therapeutic drug monitoring should consider not only the properties of the various drugs but also the populations to which they are administered. The neonate is particularly susceptible to drug toxicity because of renal and hepatic immaturity, which leads to an increased drug half-life in comparison with that seen in adults. The neonatal pattern of drug elimination is reversed rapidly several weeks after birth, and children generally metabolize drugs more rapidly than adults. With the onset of puberty, the rate of drug metabolism generally slows and approaches the adult rate of drug use.

458.

C. Within the systemic circulation a drug will either remain free or will bind to protein. Generally, acidic drugs bind to albumin, and basic drugs bind to such globulins as alpha$_1$-acid glycoprotein. Occasionally a particular drug may bind to both types of protein.

459.

D. Chlorpromazine (thorazine®) and thioridazine are examples of phenothiazines and are used in the treatment of psychoses. Although the drugs themselves have a relatively short half-life, metabolites may be found in the urine for many weeks after cessation of therapy. Screening for phenothiazines is often done by specific chromatographic techniques or by the less specific ferric perchloric-nitric (FPN) colorimetric reagent. Quantification is done by HPLC and fluorescence polarization immunoassay (FPIA).

460.

A. Phenytoin is the recommended name for the anticonvulsant diphenylhydantoin. Because of its wide use and toxicity at high concentrations, phenytoin is often the subject of overdose. Thin-layer chromatography or spectrophotometry is used for screening. Quantification usually requires gas- or high-performance liquid chromatography or immunoassay, e.g., EMIT, RIA, FPIA.

461.

D. Diazepam (Valium®) is an example of a benzodiazepine. This group of drugs is used for the treatment of anxiety. Oxazepam is an active metabolite of diazepam and is also available as a prescribed drug (Serax®). Detection of oxazepam glucuronide in the urine is used as a screening method for diazepam. Quantification of the benzodiazepines may be achieved using HPLC.

462.

D. The major active metabolite of procainamide is *N*-acetylprocainamide (NAPA). Procainamide is an antiarrhythmic drug that is used to treat such disorders as premature ventricular contractions, ventricular tachycardia, and atrial fibrillation. Since procainamide and its metabolite NAPA exhibit similar and cumulative effects, it is necessary that both be quantified to assess therapy. Methods for their analysis include GC, HPLC, FPIA, and EMIT.

463.

A. Theophylline is a bronchodilator that is used to treat asthma. The therapeutic range is 10–20 μg/mL, and it must be monitored to avoid toxicity. Use of theophylline has been replaced where possible with β-adrenergic agonists which are available in the inhaled form.

464.

D. The enzyme-multiplied immunoassay technique (EMIT) employs a homogeneous enzyme immunoassay method. This means that physical separation of the free labeled antigen from the antibody-bound labeled antigen is not necessary for measurement. This is possible because only the free labeled antigen remains active. In the EMIT system the antigen is labeled with an enzyme (e.g., glucose-6-phosphate dehydrogenase). This is in contrast to radioimmunoassay (RIA), which employs a radioactive label (e.g., ^{125}I). Determination of the drug concentration in the serum sample is made when the free enzyme-labeled drug reacts with substrate and coenzyme, resulting in an absorbance change that is measured spectrophotometrically. The drug in the serum sample is the unlabeled antigen in the assay, and it competes with the labeled drug for the binding sites on the antibody.

465.

B. The components needed in the enzyme-multiplied immunoassay technique (EMIT) include the free unlabeled drug (unlabeled antigen) in the serum specimen, antibody specific to the drug being quantified, enzyme-labeled drug (labeled antigen), and substrate and coenzyme specific for the enzyme. In this method the enzyme is coupled to the drug, producing an enzyme-labeled drug also referred to as an enzyme-labeled antigen. This enzyme-labeled complex competes with free unlabeled drug in the serum sample for the binding sites on the antibody. EMIT therapeutic drug monitoring assays are available for a variety of drugs that are included in the categories of antimicrobial, antiepileptic, antiasthmatic, cardioactive, and antineoplastic drugs. The EMIT system is not limited only to drug assays but is also available for hormone testing.

466.

C. In the EMIT assay, antibody specific to the drug being quantified is added to the serum sample that contains the drug. Substrate and coenzyme specific for the enzyme label being used are added. Finally, the enzyme-labeled drug (free labeled antigen) is added to the mixture. The drug in the serum sample and the enzyme-labeled drug compete for the binding sites on the antibody. The binding of the enzyme-labeled drug to the antibody causes a steric alteration that results in decreased enzyme activity. This steric change prevents the substrate from reacting at the active site of the enzyme, leaving only the free enzyme-labeled drug able to react with the substrate and coenzyme. The resulting enzyme activity, measured at 340 nm, is directly proportional to the concentration of the drug in the serum sample. The greater the amount of enzyme activity measured, the greater is the concentration of free enzyme-labeled drug, and therefore the greater is the concentration of drug in the serum sample.

467.

C. Since the conception of radioimmunoassay (RIA), in the early 1960s, the method has been applied to a wide variety of substances that are present in the blood in very small concentrations. Categories of ligands for which RIA methods have been developed include drugs, hormones, vitamins, and enzymes. Electrolytes are commonly quantified using ion-selective electrodes. Some drugs that are assayed by RIA include digoxin, digitoxin, gentamicin, amikacin, kanamycin, sisomicin, tobramycin, phenobarbital, phenytoin, and theophylline. RIA methods are available for the vitamins B$_{12}$ and folic acid. Creatine kinase–MB isoenzyme and prostatic acid phosphatase, a tumor marker, are enzymes for which RIA methods are available. The list of hormones that are assayed by RIA is extensive. Some of these hormones are thyroxine, triiodothyronine, thyroid-stimulating hormone, follicle-stimulating hormone, luteinizing hormone, estradiol, estriol, beta-chorionic gonadotropin, cortisol, prolactin, aldosterone, insulin, gastrin, testosterone, and prostaglandins. Many of the RIA methods are being replaced by automated, nonradioactive immunoassays where enzyme labels and fluorogenic labels are used.

VITAMINS

468.

A. High-performance liquid chromatography (HPLC) is a commonly used technique for the measurement of vitamins. Measurement by HPLC tends to be rapid, sensitive, and specific. Other techniques employed include spectrophotometric, fluorometric, and microbiological assays.

469.

B. Ascorbic acid is commonly known as vitamin C. Since humans are unable to synthesize ascorbic acid, it is necessary that it be taken in through the diet. If ascorbic acid is not ingested in a sufficient amount, a deficiency develops that leads to the disease known as scurvy. Scurvy is characterized by bleeding gums, loose teeth, and poor wound healing.

470.

B. The term *lipid* encompasses a large group of compounds, including the sterols, fatty acids, triglycerides, phosphatides, bile pigments, waxes, and fat-soluble vitamins. Vitamins A, D, E, and K are classified as fat-soluble vitamins. Thiamine (B$_1$), riboflavin (B$_2$), pyridoxine (B$_6$), cyanocobalamin (B$_{12}$), niacin, pantothenic acid, lipoic acid, folic acid, inositol, and ascorbic acid (C) are classified as water-soluble vitamins and as such are not lipid compounds.

471.

C. The definitive test for the diagnosis of steatorrhea (fat malabsorption) is the fecal fat determination that usually is done with a 72-hour collection. Carotenoids are a group of fat-soluble compounds that are precursors of vitamin A (retinol). The carotenoids are not synthesized in humans, and their absorption depends on intestinal fat absorption. Therefore, the serum carotene level is sometimes used as a simple screening test for steatorrhea. In addition to steatorrhea, other conditions such as poor diet, liver disease, and high fever can result in below-normal carotene levels. Folic acid and vitamins C and B$_{12}$ are water soluble and would not be useful for determining fat absorption.

472.

C. Vitamin B$_{12}$ (cyanocobalamin) is a cobalt-containing vitamin that is necessary for normal erythropoiesis. Intrinsic factor is a gastric protein that specifically binds vitamin B$_{12}$ and carries it to the ileum for absorption. The transcobalamins are a group of plasma proteins, some of which bind vitamin B$_{12}$ and some of which bind both vitamin B$_{12}$ and cobalamin analogs. The cobalophilins (R proteins) are those transcobalamins that can also bind the cobalamin analogs.

473.

A. Vitamin B$_{12}$ is a water-soluble vitamin. It is absorbed in the gastrointestinal tract by way of a substance called intrinsic factor. Deficiency of vitamin B$_{12}$ produces a megaloblastic anemia. Anemia caused by a deficiency of vitamin B$_{12}$ because of a lack of intrinsic factor (IF) is called pernicious anemia. The Schilling test (with and without IF) is used to diagnose pernicious anemia. It is helpful in distinguishing pernicious anemia from other malabsorption syndromes. A positive Schilling test indicates low absorption of B$_{12}$ without IF and normal absorption with IF. However, in diseases of the small bowel, low absorption occurs with and without IF.

474.

A. The designation vitamin D applies to a family of essential fat-soluble sterols that includes vitamin D$_3$ or cholecalciferol. This compound can either be absorbed directly or synthesized in the skin from 7-dehydrocholesterol with the help of ultraviolet irradiation. For physiological functioning, vitamin D_3 must be metabolized first by the liver to 25-hydroxyvitamin D_3 and then by the kidney to the final hormonal product, 1,25-dihydroxyvitamin D_3 (calcitriol). The kidney also synthesizes 24,25-dihydroxyvitamin D_3 by an alternate pathway. This compound does not have the hormonal activity of calcitriol, but because of its similar structure and relatively high concentration in the serum, it has complicated the determination of serum calcitriol.

475.

D. Adequate amounts of vitamin K are required for the synthesis of prothrombin by the liver. Since prothrombin is an essential component of the clotting system, a deficiency of vitamin K leads to a deficiency of prothrombin, which results in a delayed clot formation. Several closely related compounds having vitamin K properties include phylloquinones, which are synthesized in plants, and menaquinones, which are synthesized by bacteria. Since the intestinal flora may not be developed sufficiently in the newborn, vitamin K (menaquinone) deficiency can occur. This leads to increased clotting time, which may result in hemorrhagic disease in infancy.

476.

B. Riboflavin (vitamin B_2) is a constituent of two redox coenzymes, flavin mononucleotide (FMN) and flavin-adenine dinucleotide (FAD). These coenzymes, in combination with appropriate proteins, form the flavoprotein enzymes, which participate in tissue respiration as components of the electron-transport system. The property that enables them to participate in electron-transport is their ability to exist in the half-reduced form (FADH) and in the fully reduced form ($FADH_2$).

477.

A. A deficiency in thiamin (vitamin B_1) is associated with beriberi and Wernicke-Korsakoff syndrome. In general, thiamin deficiency affects the nervous and cardiovascular systems. Thiamin deficiency is sometimes seen in chronic alcoholics and in the elderly.

REFERENCES

Bishop, M. L., Duben-Engelkirk, J. L., and Fody, E. P. (Eds.) (2000). *Clinical Chemistry Principles, Procedures, Correlations,* 4th ed. Philadelphia: Lippincott Williams & Wilkins.

Burtis, C. A., and Ashwood, E. R. (Eds.) (2001). *Tietz Fundamentals of Clinical Chemistry,* 5th ed. Philadelphia: W. B. Saunders.

Haven, M. C., Tetrault, G. A., and Schenken, J. R. (Eds.) (1995). *Laboratory Instrumentation,* 4th ed. New York: Van Nostrand Reinhold.

Henry, J. B. (Ed.) (2001). *Clinical Diagnosis and Management by Laboratory Methods,* 20th ed. Philadelphia: W. B. Saunders.

Kaplan, L. A., and Pesce, A. J. (1996). *Clinical Chemistry Theory, Analysis, and Correlation*, 3rd ed. St. Louis: Mosby-Year Book.

Westgard, J. O., Quam, E., and Barry, T. (Eds.) (1998). *Basic QC Practices*. Madison, WI: WesTgard® Quality Corporation.

2 Hematology

contents

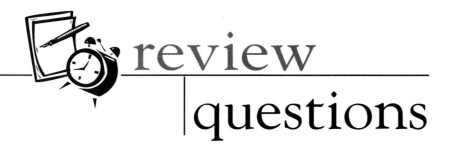

review questions

INSTRUCTIONS Each of the questions or incomplete statements that follow comprises four suggested responses. Select the *best* answer or completion statement in each case.

HEMATOPOIESIS

1. What is the first type of cell produced by the developing embryo?
   A. Erythrocyte
   B. Granulocyte
   C. Lymphocyte
   D. Thrombocyte

2. What percentage of bone cavities in the adult is filled by fatty tissue?
   A. 10%
   B. 25%
   C. 50%
   D. 75%

3. Which of the following blood cells is *not* produced in the bone marrow of normal adults?
   A. Neutrophil
   B. Monocyte
   C. Lymphocyte
   D. Thrombocyte

4. In an adult, what are the two best areas for obtaining active bone marrow by aspiration?
   A. Vertebra, tibia
   B. Sternum, tibia
   C. Posterior iliac crest, tibia
   D. Posterior iliac crest, sternum

5. What is the normal ratio of myeloid to erythroid precursors in bone marrow (M:E ratio)?
   A. 1:1
   B. 1:2
   C. 1:5
   D. 4:1

6. In myelopoiesis, which is the first developmental stage to present with primary granules?
   A. Myeloblast
   B. Promyelocyte
   C. Myelocyte
   D. Metamyelocyte

7. In the third month of gestation, what is the primary site of hematopoiesis?
   A. Liver
   B. Marrow of long bones
   C. Spleen
   D. Yolk sac

8. The mechanism that relays information about oxygen levels to the erythropoietin-producing tissue is thought to be located in the
   A. Brain
   B. Kidney
   C. Liver
   D. Spleen

9. Premature release of erythrocytes in the circulation due to increased erythropoietin stimulation results in
   A. Anisochromia
   B. Poikilocytosis
   C. Stress reticulocytes
   D. Smaller than normal reticulocytes

10. Which is the correct definition for "half-life" when applied to red blood cells?
    A. Mean erythrocyte life span
    B. Time at which 50% of a given number of erythrocytes have been destroyed
    C. Time at which half the amount of injected ^{59}Fe appears in the bone marrow
    D. Time at which half the amount of injected ^{59}Fe appears in circulating red cells

11. In what area of the bone marrow does hematopoiesis take place?
    A. Cords
    B. Endosteum
    C. Endothelium
    D. Sinuses

12. Which of the following substances will produce cohort labeling of red blood cells?
    A. ^{51}Cr
    B. ^{59}Fe
    C. Evans blue dye
    D. Ashby agglutination technique

13. Which of the following cells produces one of its own growth hormones?
    A. Basophil
    B. Erythrocyte
    C. Lymphocyte
    D. Neutrophil

14. What is the approximate total blood volume in an adult?
    A. 1 L
    B. 2 L
    C. 6 L
    D. 12 L

15. To which of the following cell lines is the CFU-S multipotential stem cell *not* a precursor?
    A. Erythrocytes
    B. Monocytes
    C. Megakaryocytes
    D. Lymphocytes

16. Of the following cells, which is never found in the peripheral circulation in its mature form?
    A. Myeloblast
    B. Promyelocyte
    C. Promonocyte
    D. Megakaryocyte

17. Stem cells comprise what proportion of nucleated bone marrow cells?
    A. 1 of 10
    B. 1 of 100
    C. 1 of 1000
    D. 1 of 10,000

18. As most blood cells mature, which of the following is characteristic?
    A. Cell diameter increases
    B. Nucleus to cytoplasm ratio (N:C) decreases
    C. Nuclear chromatin becomes less condensed
    D. Basophilia of the cytoplasm increases

19. Which of the following describes erythropoietin?
    A. Renal hormone that regulates marrow red cell production
    B. Marrow hormone secreted by developing erythroblasts
    C. Produced primarily by the liver
    D. Absent in anephric individuals

20. Liver biopsy in a patient with hepatomegaly revealed red and white blood cell precursor cells identical to those found in the bone marrow. Of the following conditions, the one where this type of scenario would most likely be found is
    A. Viral or fungal infection
    B. Acquired immune deficiency syndrome (AIDS)
    C. Lymphoproliferative disease
    D. Severe hemolytic anemia

ERYTHROCYTES

21. What is the average life span of a normal red blood cell?
    A. 1 day
    B. 10 days
    C. 60 days
    D. 120 days

22. The Na^+-K^+ pump is an important mechanism in keeping the red blood cell intact. Its function is to maintain a high level of
    A. Intracellular Na^+
    B. Intracellular K^+
    C. Serum Na^+
    D. Serum K^+

23. Which of the following are components of the hemoglobin A molecule?
    A. One heme molecule, four globin chains
    B. Two heme molecules, two globin chains
    C. Four heme molecules, two globin chains
    D. Four heme molecules, four globin chains

24. Which of the following describes the process known as *culling*?
    A. Release of red cells from the bone marrow
    B. Binding of hemoglobin by transport proteins
    C. Incorporation of iron into the hemoglobin molecule

D. Removal of abnormal red cells by the spleen

25. What does methemoglobin contain?
    A. Ferric form of iron
    B. Ferrous form of iron
    C. Sulfur attached to the heme iron
    D. Carbon monoxide molecule attached to the heme iron

26. Hemoglobin electrophoresis, carried out on cellulose acetate (alkaline pH) on the blood of a stillborn infant, revealed a single band that migrated farther towards the anode than did the Hb A control. What is the most likely composition of the stillborn infant's hemoglobin?
    A. Four beta-globin chains
    B. Four gamma-globin chains
    C. Two alpha-globin and two beta-globin chains
    D. Two alpha-globin and two gamma-globin chains

27. A *senescent* red blood cell is one that has
    A. Been hemolyzed
    B. Lived its life span
    C. Become deformed
    D. Become a reticulocyte

28. What cellular characteristic of red blood cells is described by the term *poikilocytosis*?
    A. Size
    B. Shape
    C. Presence of nuclear material
    D. Concentration of hemoglobin

29. Howell-Jolly bodies are composed of
    A. DNA
    B. Iron
    C. Mitochondria
    D. Endoplasmic reticulum

30. When schistocytes are reported on a peripheral blood smear, what would one expect to see?
   A. Red cell fragments
   B. Red cells with blunt projections
   C. Red cells with sharp projections
   D. Red cells with intracellular rod-shaped crystals

31. Which of the following red cell inclusions is characteristically found in lead poisoning?
   A. Basophilic stippling
   B. Heinz bodies
   C. Howell-Jolly bodies
   D. Pappenheimer bodies

32. Rouleaux of red blood cells when seen in the monolayer of a differential smear is charactcristic of
   A. Megaloblastic anemia
   B. Myelofibrosis
   C. Myelogenous leukemia
   D. Myeloma

33. Which of the following would most likely be associated with the inclusion body seen in Color Plate 1?
   A. Myelofibrosis
   B. After transfusion
   C. Post splenectomy
   D. Iron deficiency anemia

34. Which of the following is characteristically seen in abetalipoproteinemia?
   A. Acanthocytes
   B. Codocytes
   C. Echinocytes
   D. Stomatocytes

35. What term describes a mature red blood cell that contains nonhemoglobin iron granules?
   A. Acanthocyte
   B. Drepanocyte
   C. Echinocyte
   D. Siderocyte

36. Which of the following is associated with a "shift to the left" in the oxygen dissociation curve?
   A. Decreased pH
   B. Decreased oxygen affinity
   C. Decreased oxygen delivery
   D. Presence of 2,3-bisphosphoglycerate

37. In regard to hemoglobin E Saskatoon $\alpha_2\beta_2^{\ 22\,\text{Glu}\,\rightarrow\,\text{Lys}}$ (an abnormal hemoglobin), all the following statements are correct *except*
   A. There are two normal alpha chains.
   B. Glutamic acid replaces lysine on position 22 of the beta chains.
   C. Electrophoretic mobility is similar to that of other E hemoglobins.
   D. Glutamic acid is normally found at position 22 of the beta chain.

38. An increase in which of the following factors will result in an immediate increase of oxygen delivery to the tissues?
   A. pH
   B. Altitude
   C. 2,3-bisphosphoglycerate levels
   D. Erythropoietin levels

39. A patient with an MCV of 107 fL, hyper-segmented neutrophils, and markedly decreased intrinsic factor, would most likely have which of the following red cell inclusions?
   A. Siderotic granules
   B. Heinz bodies
   C. Basophilic stippling
   D. Howell-Jolly bodies

40. Which of the following inclusions is *not* seen on Wright's stained smears?
   A. Basophilic stippling
   B. Döhle bodies

C. Heinz bodies

D. Toxic granulation

41. Which of the following conditions is *not* usually associated with the presence of schistocytes on the peripheral blood smear?
    A. Disseminated intravascular coagulation (DIC)
    B. Prosthetic heart valves
    C. Severe burns
    D. Lead poisoning

42. Which technique is commonly used to separate red cell membrane proteins?
    A. Polyacrylamide gel electrophoresis (PAGE)
    B. Radial immunodiffusion (RID)
    C. Immunoelectrophoresis (IEP)
    D. High-performance liquid chromatography (HPLC)

43. A patient has slight splenomegaly with mild anemia. Which of the following abnormalities would you *not* expect to have been instrumental in creating this condition?
    A. Heinz bodies
    B. Hypochromia
    C. Target cells
    D. Howell-Jolly bodies

44. What is the most mature red blood cell seen in Color Plate 2?
    A. Basophilic normoblast
    B. Polychromatophilic normoblast
    C. Orthochromic normoblast
    D. Pronormoblast

45. Lecithin-cholesterol acyltransferase (LCAT) is an enzyme associated with
    A. Red cell glycolysis
    B. Maintaining hemoglobin reduction
    C. Erythrocyte membrane synthesis
    D. Generation of 2,3-bisphosphoglycerate

46. Which of the following pathways is a source of 2,3-bisphosphoglycerate?
    A. Krebs (citric acid) cycle
    B. Hexose monophosphate (pentose phosphate) pathway
    C. Phosphogluconate pathway
    D. Rapoport-Luebering shunt

47. Which of the following red blood cell precursors is the last stage to undergo mitosis?
    A. Pronormoblast
    B. Basophilic normoblast
    C. Polychromatophilic normoblast
    D. Orthochromic normoblast

48. Hemoglobin F is composed of two alpha-globin chains and two
    A. Beta-globin chains
    B. Delta-globin chains
    C. Epsilon-globin chains
    D. Gamma-globin chains

49. A 69-year-old male patient is brought to the Emergency Room with pallor, lethargy, and mild tachycardia. His CBC and differential smear reveal a hemoglobin of 7.5 g/dL, a hematocrit of 30% (0.3 L/L), an MCV of 112 fL, large platelets, and hypersegmented neutrophils. A decrease in which of the following may have created this condition?
    A. Intrinsic factor
    B. Cyanocobalamin
    C. Transcobalamin
    D. Pepsin

50. A tech performs a reticulocyte count and observes 63 reticulocytes among 1000 erythrocytes on a smear. What is the reported count?
    A. 0.63%, which is a decreased value
    B. 6.3%, which is within the reference range
    C. 6.3%, which is an increased value
    D. 63%, which is an increased value

51. Red blood cells with a mean corpuscular volume (MCV) of 105 fL should correlate with a peripheral blood smear appearance of
    A. Polychromasia
    B. Poikilocytosis
    C. Hypochromia
    D. Macrocytosis

52. Where does conjugation of bilirubin occur?
    A. Kidney
    B. Spleen
    C. Liver
    D. Bone marrow

53. Which protein is primarily responsible for transport of hemoglobin dimers resulting from intravascular hemolysis?
    A. Hemopexin
    B. Albumin
    C. Hemosiderin
    D. Haptoglobin

54. During periods of increased erythropoiesis, which of the following may be seen in increased numbers on the peripheral smear?
    A. Stomatocytes
    B. Red cell fragments
    C. Target cells
    D. Shift cells

55. Where do the early and late stages of heme synthesis occur?
    A. On ribosomes
    B. In mitochondria
    C. In cytoplasm
    D. In nucleoli

56. Spectrin is a protein that occupies a major role in
    A. Red blood cell membrane structure
    B. Protoporphyrin synthesis
    C. Hemoglobin reduction
    D. Hemoglobin degradation and transport

57. What is the function of reduced glutathione (GSH) in the red blood cell?
    A. Generates ATP
    B. Maintains anion balance during the "chloride shift"
    C. Inactivates intracellular oxidants that accumulate
    D. Prevents oxygen uptake by hemoglobin

58. In what way are myoglobin and hemoglobin similar to each other?
    A. Identical oxygen dissociation curves
    B. Heme molecules and polypeptide chains in their structure
    C. Interchangeable oxygen transport functions
    D. Identical molecular weights

59. Which of the following describes ceruloplasmin, an iron-associated protein?
    A. A beta-globulin synthesized by the liver
    B. A storage protein found in mucosal cells of the intestine
    C. An enzyme responsible for iron mobilization
    D. Responsible for iron recovery during hemoglobin degradation

60. Where is hemoglobin F found?
    A. Only in fetal cells
    B. Only in patients with hemoglobinopathies
    C. In a small percentage of erythrocytes in adults
    D. In small amounts in all adult red cells

ERYTHROCYTE DISORDERS

61. Impaired DNA metabolism is characteristic of
    A. Hemoglobin C disease
    B. Iron deficiency anemia
    C. Sideroblastic anemia
    D. Folic acid deficiency

62. Which of the following is associated with glucose-6-phosphate dehydrogenase (G6PD) deficiency?
    A. Microcytic red cells
    B. Precipitation of hemoglobin
    C. Faulty heme synthesis
    D. Hemoglobins with low oxygen affinities

63. Which of the following is a red blood cell membrane defect that results in increased complement deposition?
    A. Pyruvate kinase deficiency
    B. Paroxysmal nocturnal hemoglobinuria
    C. Hereditary elliptocytosis
    D. Stomatocytosis

64. Color Plate 3 shows the peripheral blood of a 16-year-old female with a sporadic history of dizzy spells, fainting, and jaundice. This patient also had a history of sporadic abdominal pain related to gallstones. Upon physical examination, she exhibited mild splenomegaly. Direct antiglobulin tests were negative, hematocrit was 0.32 L/L (32%), hemoglobin was 112 g/L (11.2 g/dL), and red cell indices were normal. Based on history and peripheral blood morphology, which of the following statements is most likely *true*?
    A. Hemoglobin S will be revealed by electrophoresis.
    B. Tests to confirm iron deficiency should be ordered.
    C. An intrinsic hereditary defect of red cells should be suspected.
    D. The anemia is secondary to spleen and gallbladder disorders.

65. A 15-month-old male was seen in the Emergency Room with a femur fracture. History revealed that the break had occurred from a fall down the stairs. The child had been seen three times previously in the Emergency Room for otitis media and pneumonia.

Upon physical examination, the physician noted hepatosplenomegaly, extreme pallor, and a slight arrhythmia. A complete blood count revealed the following:

WBC	10.2×10^9/L (10.2×10^3/μL)
RBC	3.05×10^{12}/L (3.05×10^6/μL)
Hemoglobin	61 g/L (6.1 g/dL)
Hematocrit	0.17 L/L (17%)
MCV	55.7 fL
MCH	20 pg
MCHC	359 g/L (35.9 g/dL)
RDW	21%

The differential revealed morphology as seen in Color Plate 4. Hemoglobin electrophoresis was ordered and results are as follows:

HgbF	97%
HgbA$_2$	3%
HgbA	0%

Which condition is most likely causing the hematologic abnormalities?
    A. Bart's hydrops fetalis
    B. Cooley's anemia
    C. Hereditary abetalipoproteinemia
    D. Sickle cell trait

66. A 25-year-old male graduate student was seen in the campus clinic complaining of abdominal pain for 3 days. A complete blood count revealed the following:

WBC	7.0×10^9/L (7.0×10^3/μL)
RBC	2.90×10^{12}/L (2.90×10^6/μL)
Hemoglobin	85 g/L (8.5 g/dL)
Hematocrit	0.25 L/L (25%)
MCV	86.2 fL
MCH	29.3 pg
MCHC	340 g/L (34.0 g/dL)
RDW	21%

The peripheral smear revealed the red blood cell morphology seen in Color Plate 5. Of what condition is this suggestive?

A. Hemoglobin H disease
B. Hemoglobin S-S disease
C. Hemoglobin S-C disease
D. Hereditary persistence of Hemoglobin F

67. In children, pica is most commonly associated with which of the following conditions?

A. Hemochromatosis
B. Lead poisoning
C. Iron deficiency anemia
D. Pernicious anemia

68. The acid serum lysis (Ham) test is used to screen patients for which disorder?

A. Glucose-6-phosphate dehydrogenase deficiency
B. Paroxysmal nocturnal hemoglobinuria
C. Pyruvate kinase deficiency
D. Paroxysmal cold hemoglobinuria

69. Which of the following statements about sickle cell anemia is *false*?

A. Asplenism may result from repeated sickling crises.
B. Heterozygous persons may be partly protected from infection by falciparum malaria.
C. Hemoglobin S is more soluble in dithionite than is normal hemoglobin.
D. Microhematocrits (centrifuge-based) may be falsely elevated when cells are sickled.

70. The red blood cells seen in Color Plate 6 were noted in a patient with renal insufficiency. What are these cells known as?

A. Acanthocytes
B. Blister cells
C. Burr cells
D. Target cells

71. Which of the following disorders is most often associated with ringed sideroblasts in the bone marrow?

A. Hemolytic anemias
B. Folate deficiencies
C. Dyserythropoiesis
D. Disturbances of heme synthesis

72. Which of the following conditions is *not* usually associated with marked reticulocytosis?

A. Drug-induced autoimmune hemolytic anemia
B. Sickle cell anemia
C. Thalassemia
D. Pernicious anemia

73. Hereditary stomatocytosis is manifested physiologically by changes in

A. Hemoglobin oxygen affinity
B. Membrane cation permeability
C. Efficiency of hemoglobin reduction
D. Glycolytic ATP production

74. In addition to an increase in red blood cells, which of the following is characteristic of polycythemia vera?

A. Decreased platelets, decreased granulocytes
B. Normal platelets, decreased granulocytes
C. Increased platelets, normal granulocytes
D. Increased platelets, increased granulocytes

75. Which of the following describes erythropoietin production in polycythemia vera?

A. Normal
B. Greatly increased
C. Mildly decreased
D. Greatly decreased

76. What values would you expect to obtain on hemoglobin and hematocrit determinations

done immediately after a major hemorrhage, if the patient had normal hemoglobin and hematocrit values prior to the hemorrhage?
A. Both normal
B. Both decreased
C. Hemoglobin decreased, hematocrit normal
D. Hemoglobin normal, hematocrit decreased

77. Which of the following is characteristic of aplastic anemia?
A. Microcytic, hypochromic
B. Microcytic, normochromic
C. Normocytic, hypochromic
D. Normocytic, normochromic

78. When viewing Color Plate 7, the red blood cell with the elongated projection is known as a(n) _____ and may be seen in _____.
A. Acanthocyte, liver disease
B. Codocyte, mechanical cell damage
C. Drepanocyte, myelofibrosis
D. Dacrocyte, myelofibrosis

79. A patient with normocytic, normochromic anemia secondary to small cell carcinoma may be exhibiting an anemia characterized as
A. Hemolytic
B. Megaloblastic
C. Myelophthisic
D. Sideroblastic

80. Idiopathic aplastic anemia is best defined as a form of anemia that
A. Has no identifiable cause
B. Is caused by a physician's treatment
C. Is caused by ionizing radiation
D. Is found in children with Down's syndrome

81. Which of the following is a true red blood cell aplasia?
A. Bernard-Soulier
B. Fanconi
C. Diamond-Blackfan
D. Chédiak-Higashi

82. Causes of absolute secondary erythrocytosis include all the following *except*
A. Pulmonary disease
B. High-altitude adjustment
C. Dehydration
D. Defective oxygen transport

83. In the fluorescent spot test for pyruvate kinase (PK) deficiency, if PK is present, it will
A. Catalyze the reaction of phosphoenol-pyruvate (PEP) to phenol alcohol
B. Catalyze the reaction of phosphoenol-pyruvate (PEP) to pyruvate
C. React with pyruvate and NAD to produce fluorescent NADH
D. Utilize lactate to produce pyruvate from phosphoenolpyruvate (PEP)

84. A Schilling test gave the following results: 1% excretion of radioactive vitamin B_{12} in the urine without intrinsic factor (IF); 7% excretion of radioactive vitamin B_{12} in the urine when vitamin was given along with IF. What do these results suggest?
A. Malabsorption
B. Steatorrhea
C. *Diphyllobothrium latum* infestation
D. Primary pernicious anemia

85. Tropical sprue has the peripheral blood picture of
A. Malaria
B. Thalassemia
C. Iron deficiency
D. Megaloblastic anemia

86. The peripheral smear on a newborn demonstrated cells as seen in Color Plates 2 and 8. This infant's complete blood count revealed a hemoglobin of 115 g/L (11.5 g/dL) and hematocrit of 0.34 L/L (34%). The mother was D negative and had exhibited no atypical antibodies in the antibody screen test. The cells demonstrated in the peripheral smear are possibly indicative of
    A. Post-partum fetal-maternal hemorrhage
    B. Erythroblastosis fetalis
    C. Hemoglobinopathy
    D. Extramedullary erythropoiesis

87. Serum ferritin is a good indicator of the amount of
    A. Cytochrome iron
    B. Storage iron
    C. Hemoglobin iron
    D. Transferrin saturation

88. In what form is the majority of storage iron found?
    A. Apoferritin
    B. Transferrin
    C. Hemosiderin
    D. Hemachromatin

89. What is an excess of storage iron called?
    A. Hemochromatosis
    B. Sideroblastosis
    C. Raynaud's disease
    D. Goodpasture's syndrome

90. The majority of iron found in an adult is a constituent of
    A. Ferritin
    B. Myoglobin
    C. Hemoglobin
    D. Hemosiderin

91. What is the most common cause of iron deficiency?

A. Bleeding
B. Gastrectomy
C. Inadequate diet
D. Intestinal malabsorption

92. In a patient with hypochromic, microcytic anemia, it is necessary to distinguish between iron deficiency and
    A. Anemia of chronic infection
    B. Hereditary spherocytosis
    C. Heterozygous thalassemia
    D. Pernicious anemia

93. In the anemia of chronic disease, what are the characteristic serum iron and transferrin levels?
    A. Serum iron decreased, transferrin decreased
    B. Serum iron decreased, transferrin increased
    C. Serum iron normal, transferrin normal
    D. Serum iron increased, transferrin increased

94. The most important effect of lead poisoning is on the
    A. Liver
    B. Kidney
    C. Neurologic system
    D. Erythrocyte development

95. What cellular appearance best characterizes the peripheral smear seen in Color Plate 9?
    A. Anisocytosis
    B. Poikilocytosis
    C. Anisocytosis and poikilocytosis
    D. Normocytic

96. What is the most likely genetic defect in the hemoglobin of cells seen in Color Plate 10?
    A. $\alpha_2^A \beta^{6\ Lys \rightarrow Val}$
    B. $\alpha_2^A \beta^{6\ Glu \rightarrow Val}$
    C. $\alpha_2^{6\ Glu \rightarrow Val} \beta_2^A$
    D. $\alpha_2^{6\ Glu \rightarrow Lys} \beta_2^A$

97. On what is the classification of sickle cell trait versus sickle cell disease based?
    A. Severity of the clinical symptoms
    B. Number of irreversibly sickled cells (ISCs)
    C. Proportion of sickle hemoglobin present in any one cell
    D. Presence of heterozygous or homozygous hemoglobin S

98. Which of the following is the most appropriate treatment for sickle cell anemia?
    A. Urea
    B. Supportive therapy
    C. Hyperbaric oxygen
    D. Iron

99. Which of the following values can be used to indicate the presence of a hemolytic anemia?
    A. Hemoglobin
    B. Hematocrit
    C. Erythrocyte count
    D. Reticulocyte count

100. In which of the following would an increase in hemoglobin A_2 be found?
    A. Homozygous alpha thalassemia
    B. Heterozygous alpha thalassemia
    C. Heterozygous beta thalassemia
    D. Heterozygous delta-beta thalassemia

101. What is the mechanism of the hemolytic process in glucose-6-phosphate dehydrogenase deficiency?
    A. Culling
    B. Osmotic pressure changes
    C. Complement attachment
    D. Oxidative denaturation

102. How is hereditary spherocytosis treated?
    A. Removal of the spleen
    B. Removal of the liver
    C. Intramuscular vitamin B_{12} injections
    D. Therapeutic phlebotomy

103. The following results were obtained on an autohemolysis test:

	Control Hemolysis	Patient Hemolysis
Whole blood plus no additive	0.4%	10.0%
Whole blood plus glucose	0.4%	0.5%
Whole blood plus adenosine triphosphate	0.4%	0.5%

The patient's results are consistent with
    A. Glucose-6-phosphate dehydrogenase deficiency
    B. Hereditary spherocytosis
    C. Pyruvate kinase deficiency
    D. Paroxysmal nocturnal hemoglobinuria

104. Of the following hemolytic anemias, which one is acquired?
    A. Glucose-6-phosphate dehydrogenase deficiency
    B. Abetalipoproteinemia
    C. Pyruvate kinase deficiency
    D. Paroxysmal nocturnal hemoglobinuria

105. Which of the following antibodies is associated with paroxysmal cold hemoglobinuria?
    A. Anti-e
    B. Anti-I
    C. Ham
    D. Donath-Landsteiner

106. What does measuring the total iron binding capacity (TIBC) represent?
    A. Amount of free iron in serum
    B. Circulating protein-bound iron
    C. Amount of iron that transferrin can bind
    D. Indirect measurement of iron stores

107. A technologist examined a Wright's stained peripheral smear and saw what appeared to be small, irregular, dark-staining granules in the mature erythrocytes. A second smear was stained with Prussian blue and a positive result was obtained. Based on this information, what should these granules be called?
    A. Cabot rings
    B. Heinz bodies
    C. Reticulum
    D. Siderotic granules

108. Spherocytes are characteristic of all the following *except*
    A. Rh disease of the newborn
    B. ABO disease of the newborn
    C. March hemoglobinuria
    D. Autoimmune hemolytic anemia

109. Which of the following statements about hereditary spherocytosis is *true*?
    A. Abnormally shaped cells are produced in the bone marrow.
    B. Cell mechanical fragility is decreased.
    C. Splenectomy can relieve the rate of red cell destruction.
    D. Red cell osmotic fragility is decreased.

110. Which of the following statements about hereditary elliptocytosis (HE) is *true*?
    A. Characteristic oval shape is found in reticulocytes and mature erythrocytes.
    B. About 50% of affected individuals display hemolytic anemia.
    C. Cellular defect involves the lipid composition of the membrane.
    D. HE cells are abnormally permeable to Na^+.

111. Which of the following statements about hemoglobin mobility during electrophoresis is correct when the procedure is performed at a pH of 8.4?
    A. Hemoglobin S moves faster than hemoglobin A
    B. Hemoglobin A moves faster than hemoglobin C
    C. Hemoglobin C moves faster than hemoglobin A
    D. Hemoglobin C moves faster than hemoglobin F

112. Which of the following statements about hemoglobin C disease is *false*?
    A. Valine is substituted for glutamic acid at position 6 of the beta chain.
    B. Target cells (codocytes) are frequently seen on peripheral smears.
    C. Osmotic fragility of red cells is decreased.
    D. The disorder is less severe than sickle cell disease.

113. Which of the following is associated with sickle cells?
    A. Increased osmotic fragility
    B. Decreased mechanical fragility
    C. Increased deformability
    D. Promote spleen destruction

114. Which of the following findings would *not* be expected in a patient with hemolytic anemia?
    A. Increased unconjugated bilirubin
    B. Microcytosis and hypochromia of peripheral red cells
    C. Decreased haptoglobin concentration
    D. Peripheral smear polychromasia

115. Which of the following statements about intrinsic hemolytic anemia is *false*?
    A. The patient's red cells have a shortened survival time in the patient.
    B. The defects are usually acquired rather than inherited.
    C. Not all the patient's red cells may display the defect.
    D. Hemolysis may be either intravascular or extravascular.

116. Which of the following statements about iron absorption is *true*?
   A. Absorption occurs in the ileum.
   B. The mucosal cell always absorbs the correct amount of iron to meet needs.
   C. Absorption increases when erythropoietic activity increases.
   D. Alkaline pH favors absorption.

117. A cellulose acetate electrophoresis revealed a large band of hemoglobin in the hemoglobin S position. This band quantified as 95%. The peripheral smear revealed 70% target cells and the solubility test was negative. Based on this information, what is the hemoglobin?
   A. Hemoglobin Bart's
   B. Hemoglobin C
   C. Hemoglobin D
   D. Hemoglobin S

118. With what disorder is a decrease in the plasma level of hemopexin associated?
   A. Severe intravascular hemolysis
   B. Onset of myelofibrosis
   C. Polycythemia vera
   D. Increased iron stores

119. The Miller disk is used for
   A. Red blood cell counts on a hemocytometer
   B. Reticulocyte counts
   C. Eosinophil counts
   D. Platelet counts using phase microscopy

120. Acquired reversible sideroblastic anemias are associated with all the following *except*
   A. Thalassemia major
   B. Chloramphenicol use
   C. Isoniazid treatment
   D. Acute alcohol ingestion

121. Which of the following statements about the relative anemia of pregnancy is *false*?

   A. It is due to a relative reduction in number of erythrocytes.
   B. It is normochromic and normocytic.
   C. It does not produce an oxygen deficit for the fetus.
   D. It can coexist with iron deficiency anemia.

122. The anemia found in hypothyroidism is
   A. Hypochromic, microcytic
   B. Caused by lack of cellular oxygen demand
   C. Caused by lack of iron absorption
   D. Due to increased red cell destruction

123. Which of the following statements about aplastic anemia is *false*?
   A. Stem cell disorder
   B. Lymphocytes decreased
   C. Bleeding associated with decreased platelet production
   D. Peripheral red blood cell counts reduced

124. Polycythemia is characterized by all the following *except*
   A. Hyperviscosity of the blood
   B. Increased plasma volume
   C. Tendency for thrombosis
   D. Increased red cell mass

125. An increase in erythropoietin is *not* a normal compensating mechanism in which of the following conditions?
   A. Renal tumors
   B. Heavy smokers
   C. Cardiovascular disease
   D. Pulmonary disease

126. Which of the following diseases results from decreased globin chain synthesis?
   A. Thalassemia
   B. Pernicious anemia
   C. Hereditary spherocytosis
   D. Heinz body anemia

127. Which of the following characterizes iron deficiency anemia?
    A. Decreased serum iron, decreased transferrin saturation, normal ferritin
    B. Decreased serum transferrin, decreased transferrin saturation, decreased ferritin
    C. Increased serum transferrin, decreased transferrin saturation, decreased ferritin
    D. Increased serum transferrin, increased transferrin saturation, decreased serum iron

128. Fetal hemoglobin differs from adult hemoglobin in that hemoglobin F
    A. Has a lower oxygen affinity
    B. Resists elution from red cells with acid solutions
    C. Is no longer synthesized after birth in a normal individual
    D. Has four identical globin chains

129. The hemolysis associated with infection by malaria organisms is due to the
    A. Release of merozoites from erythrocytes
    B. Invasion of erythrocytes by merozoites
    C. Host's immunologic response to infected erythrocytes
    D. Toxins produced by the malarial organism

130. A tech received a blood sample that contained EDTA as the anticoagulant. The total volume was only 1.5 mL. A smear was prepared and stained with Wright's stain. When examined microscopically, the majority of cells appeared to have many evenly distributed, uniform-size blunt spicules on the surface. How should this cellular appearance be interpreted?
    A. An anemic condition requiring further testing
    B. Acanthocytes caused by using incorrect technique during slide preparation
    C. Artifacts caused by a dirty spreader slide
    D. Crenated cells caused by incorrect blood:anticoagulant ratio

131. A failure to generate sufficient ATP is characteristic of red blood cells with
    A. Pyruvate kinase deficiency
    B. Glucose-6-phosphate dehydrogenase deficiency
    C. Hereditary spherocytosis
    D. Methemoglobin reductase deficiency

132. Which of the following anemias is characterized by microcytic, hypochromic red blood cells?
    A. Pernicious anemia
    B. Autoimmune hemolytic anemia
    C. Beta thalassemia
    D. Aplastic anemia

133. With which of the following are acanthocytes (spur cells) associated?
    A. Severe burns
    B. Abetalipoproteinemia
    C. Hemoglobinopathies
    D. Microangiopathic destruction

134. Basophilic stippling of red blood cells represents
    A. Precipitated hemoglobin
    B. Aggregated ribosomes
    C. Nuclear fragments
    D. Excess iron deposits

135. Thinning of bones and deformation of facial bone structure seen in beta thalassemia is a
    A. Consequence of disturbances in calcium metabolism
    B. Result of hyperplastic marrow activity
    C. Secondary disorder due to immunologic response
    D. Result of increased fibroclast activity

136. Dacrocytes are associated with
   A. Marrow replacement disorders
   B. Thermal injury (severe burns)
   C. Intrinsic membrane abnormalities
   D. Fragmentation by intravascular fibrin deposits

137. Which of the following represents an anemia that would present with a high red cell distribution width (RDW)?
   A. Hemolytic anemia with compensation
   B. Anemia accompanying myelofibrosis
   C. Pernicious anemia
   D. Anemia of chronic blood loss

138. Splenomegaly would be a common finding in all the following disorders *except*
   A. Thalassemia
   B. Hereditary spherocytosis
   C. Polycythemia vera
   D. Folic acid deficiency

LEUKOCYTES

139. Functionally, white blood cells are divided into
   A. Granulocytes, nongranulocytes
   B. Polymorphonuclears, mononuclears
   C. Phagocytes, immunocytes
   D. Granulocytes, lymphocytes

140. Normally, what is the largest white blood cell found in the peripheral blood?
   A. Eosinophil
   B. Neutrophil
   C. Lymphocyte
   D. Monocyte

141. Typically, what is the amount of time a granulocyte spends in the circulation before migrating into the tissues?
   A. Less than 1 day
   B. About 3 days
   C. Up to 5 days

   D. More than 10 days

142. What percentage of neutrophils in the peripheral blood constitutes the circulating pool?
   A. 100%
   B. 80%
   C. 50%
   D. 30%

143. What is the major phagocytic cell involved in the initial defense against pathogens such as bacteria?
   A. Neutrophil
   B. Eosinophil
   C. Basophil
   D. Monocyte

144. What is the growth factor that is primarily responsible for regulating granulocyte and monocyte production?
   A. Erythropoietin (EPO)
   B. Colony stimulating factor (GM-CSF)
   C. Interleukin (IL)
   D. Thrombopoietin (TPO)

145. What does the granulocyte mitotic pool in the bone marrow contain?
   A. Myeloblasts and promyelocytes
   B. Band and segmented forms
   C. The majority of marrow granulocytes
   D. Myelocytes and metamyelocytes

146. A "shift to the left," when used to describe a cell population, refers to
   A. Increased cells in the blood due to redistribution of marginating and circulating blood pools
   B. An increase in immature blood cells following release of bone marrow pools
   C. A cell production "hiatus" or gap
   D. A higher percentage of lymphocytes than neutrophils

147. Which of the following is characteristic of agranulocytosis?
    A. Neutrophils without granules
    B. Decreased numbers of granulocytes, red cells, and platelets
    C. Immature granulocytes in the peripheral blood
    D. Decreased numbers of granulocytes

148. T lymphocytes are characterized by all the following *except*
    A. Secrete cytokines
    B. Synthesize antibody
    C. Comprise majority of cells in blood lymphocyte pool
    D. Regulate immune response

149. An adult has a total white blood cell count of 4.0×10^9/L (4.0×10^3/μL). The differential count is as follows: polymorphonuclear neutrophils (PMNs) 25%, lymphocytes 65%, bands 5%, and monocytes 5%. The normal absolute value range for lymphocytes is 1.0–4.0 $\times 10^9$/L. Which of the following statements is true?
    A. The percentage of lymphocytes is normal
    B. There is an absolute lymphocytosis
    C. There is a relative lymphocytosis
    D. There is both an absolute and a relative lymphocytosis

150. Which of the following statements is correct?
    A. Hypersegmented neutrophils have greater than six nuclear lobes.
    B. Auer rods are composed of fused primary granules.
    C. Toxic granules are prominent secondary granules.
    D. Döhle bodies are agranular patches of DNA.

151. All the following factors are associated with variations in the total white blood cell count *except*
    A. Age
    B. Exercise
    C. Emotional stress
    D. Sex

152. With which of the following is an absolute neutrophil count of 1.0×10^9/L associated?
    A. Shortness of breath
    B. Bleeding tendencies
    C. Risk of infection
    D. No clinical symptoms

153. Which of the following statements about basophils is *false*?
    A. Morphologically, basophils resemble tissue mast cells
    B. Membrane receptors bind IgG, initiating anaphylactic reactions
    C. Basophilic granules contain heparin and histamine
    D. Granules are water soluble

154. What is the most mature cell that can undergo mitosis?
    A. Myeloblast
    B. Promyelocyte
    C. Myelocyte
    D. Metamyelocyte

155. Production of primary granules ceases and production of secondary granules commences with what cell stage?
    A. Myeloblast
    B. Promyelocyte
    C. Myelocyte
    D. Metamyelocyte

156. Which of the following statements about eosinophils is *false*?

A. They contain a type of peroxidase that is distinct from that of neutrophils.

B. Eosinophilic granules contain lysozyme.

C. Eosinophils are a first line defense against parasites.

D. Major basic protein is a component of eosinophil granules.

157. Which of the following is characteristic of primary granules?

A. Coated with a phospholipid membrane

B. Called azurophilic or specific granules

C. Contain myeloperoxidase and lactoferrin

D. Present in promyelocyte stage only

158. Which of the following are indicators of a neutrophilic response to tissue damage or inflammatory stimuli?

A. Toxic granules and Döhle bodies in the neutrophils

B. Vacuoles and Barr bodies in the neutrophils

C. Hypersegmented neutrophils and Auer bodies

D. Pyknotic neutrophils and Russell bodies

159. What is the term for cell movement through blood vessels to a tissue site?

A. Diapedesis

B. Opsonization

C. Margination

D. Chemotaxis

160. Vasodilation and bronchoconstriction would be associated with which blood cell?

A. Eosinophils

B. Monocytes

C. Neutrophils

D. Basophils

161. On what basis can B and T lymphocytes be distinguished?

A. Differences in cytoplasmic basophilia as seen on Wright's-stained smears

B. Monoclonal antibody reactions to surface and cytoplasmic antigens

C. Cytoplasmic granularity and overall cell size

D. Morphology consistent with "reactive"-type lymphocytes

162. Cells that produce immunoglobulins in response to antigenic stimulation are designated

A. Sézary cells

B. Plasma cells

C. Virocytes

D. Thymocytes

163. Which of the following statements about neutrophils is *false*?

A. Suppress allergic reactions caused by basophils

B. Have surface receptors for IgG and complement components

C. Contain alkaline phosphatase and muramidase

D. Act in nonspecific phagocytosis and are destined to die

164. Which of the following characteristics would be *least* likely to distinguish large lymphocytes from monocytes?

A. Indentation of the cytoplasmic margin by adjacent red blood cells

B. Presence of large azurophilic granules

C. Absence of fine granules in the cytoplasm

D. Chromatin pattern in the nucleus

165. Which of the following is characteristic of metamyelocytes?

A. Appearance of specific granules

B. Indentation of nucleus

C. Absence of nucleoli

D. Color of cytoplasm

166. Lymphocyte concentrations in the peripheral blood are greatest during what age interval?
    A. Young child (1 to 4 years)
    B. Older child (4 to 15 years)
    C. Young adult (16 to 40 years)
    D. Older adult (40 to 70 years)

167. Normal lymphoid stem cells would be expected to demonstrate which of the following markers?
    A. SIgM, a surface membrane immunoglobulin
    B. CIg, a cytoplasmic immunoglobulin
    C. TdT, a cytoplasmic enzyme
    D. CALLA, a surface antigen

168. Which of the following statements about macrophages is *incorrect*?
    A. They are mature tissue forms of blood monocytes.
    B. Macrophages serve as antigen presenting cells to the immune system.
    C. Quantity of lysosomes and acid hydrolases decrease during maturation.
    D. They help remove dead cells and debris (necrophagocytosis).

169. Antigen independent lymphopoiesis occurs in primary lymphoid tissue located in the
    A. Liver and kidney
    B. Spleen and lymph nodes
    C. Peyer's patches and spleen
    D. Thymus and bone marrow

170. Which of the following is *not* produced by neutrophils during the respiratory burst?
    A. Hydroxyl radicals (OH^-)
    B. Hydrogen peroxide (H_2O_2)
    C. Superoxide anion (O_2^-)
    D. Myeloperoxidase

LEUKOCYTE DISORDERS

171. In patients with infectious mononucleosis, which blood cells are infected by the causative agent?
    A. Monocytes
    B. T lymphocytes
    C. B lymphocytes
    D. Histiocytes

172. Which of the following statements about hairy cell leukemia is *true*?
    A. It is an acute disease, primarily affecting young adults.
    B. Splenomegaly is an unusual finding.
    C. Hairy cells contain tartrate resistant acid phosphatase (TRAP).
    D. Hairy cells are abnormal T lymphocytes.

173. The lymphoid cells seen in FAB type L3 are morphologically similar to those of
    A. Burkitt's lymphoma
    B. Hodgkin's lymphoma
    C. Mycosis fungoides
    D. Chronic lymphocytic leukemia (CLL)

174. The presence of both immature neutrophils and nucleated erythrocytes in the peripheral blood is most accurately called a
    A. Neutrophilic left shift
    B. Regenerative left shift
    C. Neutrophilic leukemoid reaction
    D. Leukoerythroblastic reaction

175. In which anomaly is a failure of granulocytes to divide beyond the band or two-lobed stage observed?
    A. Pelger-Huët
    B. May-Hegglin
    C. Alder-Reilly
    D. Chédiak-Higashi

176. Eosinophils are increased in all the following *except*
    A. Cushing's disease
    B. Allergic disorders

C. Skin disorders

D. Parasitic infection

177. Which of the following represents the principal defect in chronic granulomatous disease?

A. Chemotactic migration

B. Phagocytosis

C. Lysosomal formation and function

D. Oxidative respiratory burst

178. In which of the following disorders is the nitroblue tetrazolium test (NBT) considered diagnostic?

A. Pelger-Huët anomaly

B. Alder-Reilly anomaly

C. May-Hegglin anomaly

D. Chronic granulomatous disease (CGD)

179. A patient with normal hemoglobin and WBC values, a persistently elevated platelet count ($> 1000 \times 10^9$/L), increased marrow mega-karyocytes, and a history of frequent bleeding and clotting episodes most likely has

A. Polycythemia vera (PV)

B. Myelofibrosis with myeloid metaplasia

C. Essential thrombocythemia (ET)

D. Chronic myelocytic leukemia (CML)

180. An adult patient with massive splenomegaly has mild anemia, a slightly elevated WBC count, and an LAP score of 170. The blood smear shows teardrop erythrocytes and leukoerythroblastosis. In addition, the bone marrow aspirate was a "dry tap." These findings are most consistent with

A. Chronic myelocytic leukemia

B. Primary myelofibrosis

C. Primary polycythemia

D. Primary thrombocythemia

181. The blood cells shown in Color Plate 11 are frequently caused by all the following infections *except*

A. Epstein-Barr virus (EBV)

B. *Bordetella pertussis* (whooping cough)

C. Cytomegalovirus (CMV)

D. *Toxoplasma gondii* (toxoplasmosis)

182. The most common type of chronic lymphocytic leukemia (CLL) in the United States involves the

A. B cell

B. Null cell

C. T cell

D. Plasma cell

183. Which of the following is increased in Waldenström's macroglobulinemia?

A. IgA

B. IgE

C. IgG

D. IgM

184. A leukemoid reaction is an increase in peripheral blood cells associated with

A. A preleukemic state

B. An extreme infectious response

C. The presence of leukemia

D. A fibrotic bone marrow

185. A significant finding in systemic lupus erythematosus (SLE) is an LE cell that is

A. A phagocyte with crystalline inclusion bodies

B. Aggregated cells coated with antibody

C. A phagocyte with ingested red cells

D. A phagocyte with an ingested nuclear mass

186. In which of the following is progression to acute leukemia *least* likely?

A. Chronic myelocytic leukemia

B. Refractory anemia with excess blasts (RAEB)

C. Refractory anemia with excess blasts in transformation (RAEB-t)

D. Chronic lymphocytic leukemia

187. A Gaucher's cell is best described as a macrophage with
   A. "Wrinkled" cytoplasm due to an accumulation of glucocerebroside
   B. "Foamy" cytoplasm filled with unmetabolized sphingomyelin
   C. Pronounced vacuolization and deposits of cholesterol
   D. Abundant cytoplasm containing storage iron and cellular remnants

188. Which of the following suggests a diagnosis of Hodgkin's disease rather than other lymphoproliferative disorders?
   A. An absolute lymphocytosis with mature appearing lymphocytes
   B. Predominance of immature B cells with irregular nuclear clefts
   C. Circulating T cells with a convoluted, cerebriform nucleus
   D. Presence of giant Reed-Sternberg cells binucleated with prominent nucleoli

189. The blood findings shown in Color Plate 12 of a patient with leukemia are most suggestive of therapy with
   A. Corticosteroids (e.g., prednisone)
   B. A folate antagonist (e.g., methotrexate)
   C. Growth factor (e.g., GM-CSF)
   D. Chloramphenicol

190. The FAB type of acute myelogenous leukemia most often associated with disseminated intravascular coagulation is
   A. M2
   B. M3
   C. M4
   D. M5

191. Which of the following is *not* commonly found in acute nonlymphocytic leukemias (ANLLs)?
   A. Neutropenia
   B. Thrombocytopenia
   C. Hepatosplenomegaly
   D. Lymphadenopathy

192. The peripheral blood shown in Color Plate 13 is from a 69-year-old female. Her WBC count was 83×10^9 cells/L ($83 \times 10^3/\mu L$) and her platelet count was normal. Based on the smear morphology and this information, what is the most likely diagnosis?
   A. Acute lymphoblastic leukemia
   B. Chronic lymphocytic leukemia
   C. Waldenström's disease
   D. Viral infection

193. The patient whose bone marrow is shown in Color Plate 14 most likely has a(n)
   A. Acute leukemia
   B. Chronic leukemia
   C. Dysmyelopoietic disorder
   D. Aplastic anemia

194. Multiple myeloma is characterized by the presence in urine of large amounts of
   A. IgM antibodies
   B. IgG heavy chains
   C. IgG light chains
   D. Beta microglobulins

195. Which of the following is *not* usually classified as a myeloproliferative disorder?
   A. Polycythemia vera
   B. Essential thrombocythemia
   C. Multiple myeloma
   D. Chronic myelocytic leukemia

196. The Philadelphia chromosome is a reciprocal translocation of material between chromosomes
   A. 8 and 14
   B. 8 and 21
   C. 9 and 22
   D. 15 and 17

197. The Philadelphia chromosome is present in approximately 90% of patients with
    A. Acute lymphocytic leukemia
    B. Chronic lymphocytic leukemia
    C. Acute monocytic leukemia
    D. Chronic myelocytic leukemia

198. Which of the following would be *least* helpful in distinguishing chronic myelocytic leukemia (CML) from a leukemoid reaction?
    A. Presence of marked leukocytosis with increased neutrophilic bands, metamyelocytes, and myelocytes
    B. Leukocyte alkaline phosphatase (LAP) score
    C. Presence of splenomegaly
    D. Presence of neutrophils with Döhle bodies and toxic granulation

199. The cytoplasmic inclusion present in the cell shown in Color Plate 15
    A. Excludes a diagnosis of acute myelogenous leukemia
    B. Stains positive with leukocyte alkaline phosphatase (LAP)
    C. Stains positive with myeloperoxidase (MPO)
    D. Identifies the cell as a malignant lymphoblast

200. Which of the following is a typical finding in chronic leukemias at onset?
    A. Symptoms of infection and bleeding
    B. Severe thrombocytopenia
    C. Severe anemia
    D. Elevated leukocyte count

201. In what condition would a leukocyte alkaline phosphatase (LAP) score of 10 most likely be found?
    A. Bacterial septicemia
    B. Late pregnancy
    C. Polycythemia vera
    D. Chronic myelocytic leukemia

202. All the following are associated with neutrophilia *except*
    A. Staphylococcal pneumonia
    B. Crushing injury
    C. Infectious hepatitis
    D. Neoplasms (tumors)

203. An absolute monocytosis may be seen in all the following *except*
    A. Tuberculosis
    B. Recovery stage of acute bacterial infection
    C. Collagen disorders
    D. Infectious mononucleosis

204. Coarse PAS positivity is found most often in the leukemic cells of
    A. Acute myelocytic leukemia, M2
    B. Acute lymphocytic leukemia, L1
    C. Acute myelomonocytic leukemia, M4
    D. Acute monocytic leukemia, M5

205. Diagnostic criteria for classifying the myelodysplastic syndromes include all the following *except*
    A. Unexplained anemia refractory to treatment
    B. Hypogranular and hyposegmented neutrophils
    C. Abnormal platelet size and granulation
    D. Hypercellular bone marrow with greater than 30 percent blasts

206. Naphthol AS-D chloroacetate esterase (specific) is usually positive in _____ cells and alpha-naphthyl acetate esterase (nonspecific) is useful for identifying blast cells of _____ lineage.
    A. Granulocytic, monocytic
    B. Monocytic, granulocytic
    C. Granulocytic, lymphocytic
    D. Monocytic, megakaryocytic

207. The familial disorder featuring pseudo-Döhle bodies, thrombocytopenia, and large platelets is called
    A. May-Hegglin anomaly
    B. Chédiak-Higashi syndrome
    C. Pelger-Huët anomaly
    D. Alder-Reilly anomaly

208. Alder-Reilly anomaly is an abnormality of
    A. Lysosomal fusion
    B. Nuclear maturation
    C. Oxidative metabolism
    D. Mucopolysaccharide metabolism

209. What is the initial laboratory technique for the diagnosis of monoclonal gammopathies?
    A. Immunologic markers of marrow biopsy cells
    B. Cytochemical staining of marrow and peripheral blood cells
    C. Serum and urine protein electrophoresis
    D. Cytogenetic analysis of marrow cells

210. Which of the following statements about Hodgkin's disease is *false*?
    A. Bimodal incidence with respect to age of patient
    B. Staging determines extent of disease and treatment course
    C. Stage IV has best prognosis
    D. Males have higher incidence than females

211. The blast cells shown in Color Plate 16 are CD14 and CD33 positive, Sudan black B positive, specific esterase positive, and non-specific esterase positive. Which FAB classification of acute leukemia is *most consistent* with the immunophenotyping and cytochemical staining results?
    A. L1
    B. M2
    C. M4
    D. M5

212. Which type of leukemia is associated with the best prognosis for a cure?
    A. Chronic lymphocytic leukemia in elderly
    B. Acute lymphocytic leukemia in children
    C. Acute myelocytic leukemia in children
    D. Chronic myelocytic leukemia in young adults

213. What is the key diagnostic test for Hodgkin's lymphoma?
    A. Bone marrow biopsy
    B. Lymph node biopsy
    C. Spinal tap
    D. Skin biopsy

214. A hypercellular bone marrow and myeloid:erythroid (M:E) ratio of 8:1 is most characteristic of
    A. Chronic myelocytic leukemia
    B. Primary polycythemia
    C. Beta thalassemia major
    D. Aplastic anemia

215. A 60-year-old patient presents with extreme fatigue. Her blood and bone marrow findings are as follows: severe anemia with a dual RBC population, 3 % marrow blasts, and numerous ringed sideroblasts. This information is most consistent with
    A. Refractory anemia (RA)
    B. Refractory anemia with ringed sideroblasts (RARS)
    C. Refractory anemia with excess blasts (RAEB)
    D. Refractory anemia with excess blasts in transformation (RAEB-t)

216. Which of the following is *not* a mechanism by which neutropenia may be produced?
    A. Marrow injury
    B. Marrow replacement
    C. Recent strenuous exercise
    D. Drug suppression

217. Usual findings in polycythemia vera include all the following *except*
    A. Pancytosis
    B. Increased red cell mass
    C. Increased erythropoietin (EPO) level
    D. Increased blood viscosity

218. In what disorder is significant basophilia most commonly seen?
    A. Hairy cell leukemia
    B. Multiple myeloma
    C. Acute lymphocytic leukemia
    D. Chronic myelogenous leukemia

219. Di Guglielmo's syndrome or FAB acute leukemia type M6 is characterized by increased
    A. Promyelocytes and lysozyme activity
    B. Marrow megakaryocytes and thrombocytosis
    C. Marrow erythroblasts and multinucleated red cells
    D. Marrow monoblasts and monocytes

220. The blood findings present in Color Plate 17 are most often associated with
    A. Plasma cell dyscrasias
    B. Lipid storage diseases
    C. Sézary syndrome
    D. Mycosis fungoides

221. Myeloid metaplasia refers to
    A. Displacement of normal marrow cells by abnormal elements
    B. Hematopoietic failure
    C. Extramedullary hematopoiesis
    D. Tumors (neoplasms) of the bone marrow

222. Which of the following statements about non–Hodgkin's lymphoma is *true*?
    A. Lymphadenopathy most common presenting symptom
    B. Initially systemic disease rather than localized tumor

C. Often associated with multiple bone lesions
D. Proliferation of malignant cells primarily involving bone marrow

METHODOLOGY

223. Which combination of reagents is used in measuring hemoglobin?
    A. Hydrochloric acid and *p*-dimethyl-aminobenzaldehyde (Ehrlich's reagent)
    B. Potassium ferricyanide and potassium cyanide (Drabkin's reagent)
    C. Sodium bisulfite and sodium metabisulfite
    D. Sodium citrate and hydrogen peroxide

224. What is the fastest-moving hemoglobin on an alkaline electrophoresis at pH 8.4?
    A. A
    B. F
    C. H
    D. S

225. A patient with suspected sickle cell trait has negative solubility test results, but hemoglobin electrophoresis at pH 8.4 shows an apparent A-S pattern. What is the most likely explanation?
    A. Patient has hemoglobin AS, and the solubility test is incorrect.
    B. Patient has hemoglobin AA, and the electrophoresis is incorrect.
    C. Patient has hemoglobin AD or AG, and both procedures are correct.
    D. Tests need to be repeated; impossible to determine which procedure is correct.

226. All the following are true of the solubility test for Hemoglobin S *except*
    A. Hemoglobin S polymerizes when deoxygenated.
    B. Testing performed on a 2-day-old infant can result in a false negative result.
    C. Sickle cell trait can be differentiated from sickle cell anemia with this test.
    D. The test is positive in Hemoglobin C_{Harlem}.

227. All the following will cause a falsely low ESR *except*
   A. ESR tube is slanted
   B. EDTA tube is clotted
   C. EDTA tube is one-third full
   D. EDTA specimen is 24 hours old

228. A platelet count of 96×10^9/L (96,000/μL) is obtained on an automated instrument from an EDTA blood sample. Smear evaluation reveals the presence of platelet clumps. The specimen is redrawn using sodium citrate as the anticoagulant, and a count of 300×10^9/L (300,000/μL) is obtained. What is the correct platelet count to report?
   A. 270×10^9/L
   B. 300×10^9/L
   C. 330×10^9/L
   D. 360×10^9/L

229. To best preserve cellular morphology, differential smears from an EDTA specimen should be made no later than
   _____ hour(s) after collection.
   A. 1
   B. 3
   C. 12
   D. 24

230. The blood smear made on a patient with polycythemia vera is too short. What should one do to correct this problem?
   A. Decrease the angle of the spreader slide
   B. Increase the angle of the spreader slide
   C. Put the angle of the spreader slide to 25 degrees
   D. Use a smaller drop of blood

231. Wright's stain is a mixture of
   A. Crystal violet and safranin
   B. Brilliant green and neutral red
   C. New methylene blue and carbolfuchsin
   D. Polychrome methylene blue and eosin

232. What is the reason for red blood cells to be bright red when stained with Wright's stain?
   A. Bright red is the correct color for red blood cells
   B. The stain is too alkaline
   C. The buffer is too acidic
   D. The smear was not washed long enough

233. In a reticulocyte count, 1000 red blood cells were counted, and 60 of them were reticulocytes. What is the reticulocyte count expressed in percent?
   A. 0.06
   B. 0.6
   C. 6.0
   D. 60.0

234. Using the percent reticulocyte from Question 233 and an RBC count of 3.00×10^{12}/L $(3.00 \times 10^6$/μL), what is the calculated absolute reticulocyte count?
   A. 1.8×10^9/L
   B. 18×10^9/L
   C. 180×10^9/L
   D. 1800×10^9/L

235. The Sudan black B stain shown in Color Plate 18 is a stain for
   A. Glycogen
   B. Lipids
   C. Myeloperoxidase
   D. Acid phosphatase

236. The following numbers were obtained in evaluating leukocyte alkaline phosphatase (LAP) activity in neutrophils. What is the score?

0	1	2	3	4
32	24	21	15	8

   A. 100
   B. 143
   C. 175
   D. 241

237. Perl's Prussian blue is a stain used to detect
    A. DNA
    B. RNA
    C. Iron
    D. Glycogen

238. Which of the following red cell inclusions stains with *both* Perl's Prussian blue and Wright's stain?
    A. Howell-Jolly bodies
    B. Basophilic stippling
    C. Pappenheimer bodies
    D. Heinz bodies

239. What is the depth of the space between the counting platform and the coverslip on a hemacytometer?
    A. 0.01 mm
    B. 0.10 mm
    C. 1.00 mm
    D. 0.1 cm

240. When both sides of a hemacytometer are counted, a total of 308 cells are seen. The dilution used is 1:20, and the total area counted is 8 mm². What is the WBC count?
    A. 3850/mm³
    B. 7700/mm³
    C. 15,400/mm³
    D. 38,500/mm³

241. Which set of results indicates that an error in measurement has occurred?

	RBC × 10¹²/L	Hgb g/dL	Hct %
A.	3.00	9.0	26.5
B.	3.10	11.0	27.0
C.	3.25	9.8	29.5
D.	3.50	10.7	31.5

242. A *falsely* high MCHC of 365 g/L (36.5 g/dL) on an automated instrument could be caused by all the following *except*

A. Hereditary spherocytosis
B. Hyperlipidemia
C. Presence of a cold agglutinin
D. Instrument sampling or mixing error

243. What is the basis for the Coulter principle of electronic particle counting?
    A. Angle of laser beam scatter by the particles
    B. Amplification of an electrical current by the particles
    C. Impedance of an electrical current by the particles
    D. Change in optical density of the solution containing the particles

244. A clinically significant difference between two electronic cell counts is indicated when the standard deviation is greater than
    A. ±1.0
    B. ±1.5
    C. ±2.0
    D. ±3.0

245. Right-angle scatter in a laser-based cell counting system is used to measure
    A. Cell size
    B. Cytoplasmic granularity
    C. Cell number
    D. Immunologic (antigenic) identification

246. A white blood cell count is done on an automated impedance cell counter from a patient with β-thalassemia major, as seen in Color Plate 19. What is the WBC result?
    A. Falsely increased because of numerous nucleated red blood cells (nRBCs)
    B. Falsely increased because of red cell fragments
    C. Falsely decreased because of nRBCs
    D. An accurate quantification of the WBC concentration (no error due to this disorder)

247. The hemoglobin A$_2$ quantification using anion exchange chromatography will be valid in
    A. Hemoglobin C disease
    B. Hemoglobin E trait
    C. Hemoglobin O trait
    D. β-thalassemia minor

Questions 248–250 refer to the osmotic fragility graph.

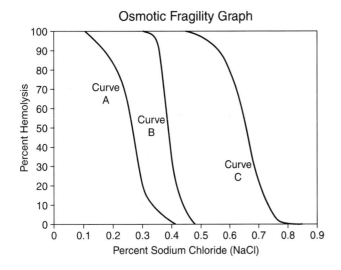

248. Using the osmotic fragility graph shown, which of the following is correct?
    A. Curve A is normal
    B. Curve C is normal
    C. Curve A shows increased osmotic fragility
    D. Curve C shows increased osmotic fragility

249. What type of cell would generate curve C?
    A. Codocyte
    B. Dacrocyte
    C. Drepanocyte
    D. Spherocyte

250. What is a common cause for the presence of the type of cells that will produce curve A?
    A. Aging
    B. Globin chain disorders

C. Enzyme deficiency
D. Leaking membrane

251. To establish a standard curve for reading hemoglobin concentration
    A. A commercial control material is used
    B. A wavelength of 640 nm is employed
    C. Certified standards are used
    D. A patient blood sample of known hemoglobin concentration is used

252. Which of the following does *not* represent a source of error when measuring hemoglobin by the cyanmethemoglobin method?
    A. Excessive anticoagulant
    B. High white blood cell count
    C. Lipemic plasma
    D. Scratched or dirty hemoglobin measuring cell

253. Which of the following statements about microhematocrits is *false*?
    A. Centrifuging for too long causes falsely low results.
    B. The buffy coat is excluded from the hematocrit reading.
    C. Hemolysis causes falsely low results.
    D. Units for hematocrit are L/L (SI) or percent (conventional units).

254. The erythrocyte sedimentation rate (ESR) is influenced by the phenomenon seen in Color Plate 17. All the following factors contribute to this phenomenon and thus affect the ESR *except*
    A. Size of the red blood cells
    B. Shape of the red blood cells
    C. Hemoglobin content of the red blood cells
    D. Composition of the plasma

255. An EDTA blood sample run on an automated impedance cell counter has generated a warning flag at the upper region of the platelet histogram shown. The presence of all the following could cause this warning flag *except*

A. Nucleated RBCs

B. Microcytic RBCs

C. EDTA-dependent platelet agglutinins

D. Giant platelets

Platelet Histogram

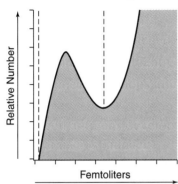

256. To evaluate normal platelet numbers in an appropriate area of a blood smear, approximately how many platelets should be observed per oil immersion field?

A. 1–4

B. 4–10

C. 8–20

D. 20–50

257. Which of the following statements about reticulocyte counts is *false*?

A. Staining can occur for more than 5 minutes.

B. A supravital stain is used.

C. RBC inclusions can result in falsely elevated counts.

D. Polychrome methylene blue stain is used.

258. When are automated cell counters required to have a calibration check performed?

A. At least every three months

B. After replacement of any major part

C. After performing monthly maintenance

D. When the control values are greater than 2 standard deviations from the mean

259. A blood sample was run through an automated cell counter and the following results were ob-

tained: RBC 3.52×10^{12}/L (3.52×10^6/µL), Hgb 120 g/L (12.0 g/dL), Hct 0.32 L/L (32.0%), MCH 34.1 pg, MCHC 375 g/L (37.5 g/dL). An aliquot of the specimen is centrifuged, determined to be lipemic, and the hemoglobin is corrected using the plasma blank procedure. The "hemoglobin" obtained on plasma is 2.0 g/dL. Using this data, what is the correct hemoglobin to report in g/dL?

A. 11.4

B. 11.0

C. 10.6

D. 10.2

260. Which of the following procedures could be performed on a hemolyzed blood sample?

A. Hemoglobin

B. Hemoglobin and platelet count

C. RBC count and hematocrit

D. No results are reportable

261. For which of the following procedures would heparin be a recommended anticoagulant?

A. Platelet count

B. Coagulation tests

C. Smear-based red cell morphology

D. Osmotic fragility

262. In the platelet count procedure utilizing phase microscopy

A. Platelets appear dark against a light background.

B. The entire ruled counting surface of the hemacytometer is used.

C. Ammonium oxalate will lyse the WBCs.

D. Platelets should be counted immediately after addition to the hemacytometer.

263. What is the quality control term used to describe the reproducibility of a test?

A. Accuracy

B. Precision

C. Standard deviation

D. Specificity

CASE HISTORIES

Use the following information to answer questions 264–268.

The peripheral blood shown in Color Plate 19 is from an 8-month-old Sicilian boy with the following results on a hematology impedance analyzer: WBC 31.0×10^9/L $(31.0 \times 10^3$/μL); RBC 2.50×10^{12}/L $(2.50 \times 10^6$/μL); hemoglobin 45 g/L (4.5 g/dL); hematocrit 0.16 L/L (16%); platelet count 340×10^9/L (340,000/μL); reticulocyte count 8.0%; differential smear normal, except for 110 nucleated red blood cells/100 WBCs; serum iron elevated; serum iron binding capacity (TIBC) decreased; serum ferritin elevated.

264. What is the corrected white blood cell count?
   A. 4.6×10^9/L
   B. 12.5×10^9/L
   C. 14.8×10^9/L
   D. 18.4×10^9/L

265. What would be the appearance of the child's red blood cells on a peripheral smear?
   A. Hypochromic, microcytic
   B. Hypochromic, normocytic
   C. Normochromic, normocytic
   D. Normochromic, microcytic

266. The CBC, serum iron, TIBC, and ferritin levels are most characteristic of
   A. β-Thalassemia minor
   B. Iron deficiency anemia
   C. α-Thalassemia minor
   D. β-Thalassemia major

267. What form(s) of hemoglobin will be detected on this child using hemoglobin electrophoresis?
   A. A
   B. A and F
   C. A, increased A_2, F
   D. F

268. Why is it difficult to diagnose this disorder in a newborn?

A. The liver is immature.
B. The beta chains are not fully developed.
C. It is similar to ABO erythroblastosis.
D. There are normally many erythrocyte precursors in the peripheral blood.

Use the following information to answer questions 269–271.

Sally, an 80-year-old woman with rheumatoid arthritis, lives alone. She gets around with great difficulty. In addition to the pain of the arthritis, she has increasing complaints of being tired. Her blood values are as follows: WBC 5.2×10^9/L $(5.2 \times 10^3$/μL); RBC 3.49×10^{12}/L $(3.49 \times 10^6$/μL); hemoglobin 97 g/L (9.7 g/dL); hematocrit 0.29 L/L (29%); MCV 83 fL; MCHC 339 g/L (33.9 g/dL); serum iron and total iron binding capacity (TIBC) both decreased, serum ferritin slightly elevated.

269. If the serum iron is 22 μg/dL and the TIBC is 150 μg/dL, what is the percent transferrin?
   A. 7%
   B. 10%
   C. 15%
   D. 38%

270. The results of the CBC and iron studies in this case are most characteristic of
   A. β-Thalassemia minor
   B. Iron deficiency
   C. Sideroblastic anemia
   D. Anemia of chronic disorders

271. In addition to rheumatoid arthritis, all the following are associated with the anemia described above *except*
   A. Chronic gastrointestinal blood loss
   B. Hodgkin's disease
   C. Congestive heart failure
   D. Systemic lupus erythematosus

Use the following information to answer questions 272–274.

The peripheral blood shown in Color Plate 12 is from Amy, a 21-year-old vegetarian college student who has been living primarily on tea and toast for the past 9 months because she finds dining hall food distasteful. She complains of being tired, and the following results are obtained when a complete blood cell count is done: WBC 2.5×10^9/L (2.5×10^3/μL); RBC 2.10×10^{12}/L (2.10×10^6/μL); hemoglobin 85 g/L (8.5g/dL); hematocrit 0.24 L/L (24%); platelet count 110×10^9/L (110,000/μL); MCV 114 fL; MCHC 350 g/L (35.0 g/dL); reticulocyte count 0.8%; and differential count 64% polymorphonuclear neutrophils (PMNs) and 36% lymphocytes.

272. What test(s) should be done *first* to determine a diagnosis in this patient?
A. Vitamin B_{12} and folate levels
B. Iron studies
C. Bone marrow examination
D. Osmotic fragility

273. In the absence of neurological symptoms, the anemia in this patient is most likely caused by a lack of
A. An enzyme
B. Iron
C. Folic acid
D. Intrinsic factor

274. In addition to the findings seen in Color Plate 12, other abnormalities seen in this general classification of anemia include all the following *except*
A. Target cells
B. Teardrop cells
C. Howell-Jolly bodies
D. Giant platelets

Use the following information to answer questions 275–277.

Linda, a 45-year-old Scandinavian woman with white hair, appears older than her stated age. She complains to her physician of weakness, a tingling sensation in her lower extremities, and shortness of breath. Her laboratory values are as follows: WBC 3.4×10^9/L (3.4×10^3/μL); RBC 1.90×10^{12}/L (1.90×10^6/μL); hemoglobin level 86 g/L (8.6 g/dL); hematocrit 0.25 L/L (25%); MCV 132 fL; MCHC 344 g/L (34.4 g/dL); and platelet count 100×10^9/L (100,000/μL). Cabot rings are noted on the peripheral smear.

275. All the following disorders are possible causes of the patient's anemia *except*
A. Liver disease
B. Vitamin B_{12} deficiency
C. Folic acid deficiency
D. Malabsorption syndromes

276. What would a Schilling test performed on this patient most likely show?
A. Part I abnormal, Part II abnormal
B. Part I abnormal, Part II normal
C. Part I normal, Part II normal
D. Part I normal, Part II would not be done

277. Which of the following statements about megaloblastic anemia is *true*?
A. Pharmaceutical doses of folate reverse the neurologic symptoms of PA.
B. Intramuscular vitamin B_{12} will reverse the neurologic symptoms of PA.
C. Oral doses of vitamin B_{12} will cure PA.
D. Vitamin B_{12} is absorbed in the duodenum.

Use the following information to answer questions 278–280.

James, a 32-year-old black man, had been healthy until he began taking primaquine for prevention of malaria. He went to his physician because he felt faint and his urine was black.

278. What is the most likely cause of this hemolytic episode?
A. G6PD deficiency
B. Hereditary spherocytosis
C. Sickle cell disease
D. Pyruvate kinase deficiency

279. What is the defect associated with the disorder described in this case?

   A. Amino acid substitution

   B. Intrinsic red blood cell membrane defect

   C. Enzyme deficiency in the hexose monophosphate shunt

   D. Enzyme deficiency in the Embden-Meyerhof pathway

280. When exposed to oxidants, what do patients with this disorder form?

   A. Döhle bodies

   B. Heinz bodies

   C. Howell-Jolly bodies

   D. Pappenheimer bodies

Use the following information to answer questions 281–283.

Stephanie, a 6-month-old child who has been breast-fed since birth, was brought to the laboratory for a routine hematologic examination. The following results were obtained on a complete blood cell count: WBC 9.5 × 10^9/L (9.5 × 10^3/μL); RBC 2.70 × 10^{12}/L (2.70 × 10^6/μL); hemoglobin 67 g/L (6.7 g/dL); hematocrit 0.25 L/L (25%); MCV 73.5 fL; MCHC 268 g/L (26.8 g/dL); RDW 19%. Abnormal RBC morphology present included pencil forms and target cells. The reticulocyte count was 0.2%.

---

281. What is the most probable cause of anemia in this 6-month-old child?

   A. Folate deficiency

   B. Hereditary spherocytosis

   C. Iron deficiency

   D. Erythroblastosis fetalis

282. When iron requirements exceed iron absorption, what event will occur first?

   A. Increased total iron binding capacity

   B. Decreased serum iron

   C. Decreased hemoglobin

   D. Decreased ferritin

283. What is the absolute reticulocyte count for this child?

   A. 0.05 × 10^9/L

   B. 0.5 × 10^9/L

   C. 5 × 10^9/L

   D. 50 × 10^9/L

Use the following information to answer questions 284–288.

The peripheral blood shown in Color Plate 20 and the bone marrow shown in Color Plate 14 are from Kathryn, a 5-year-old girl, who has a fever and sore throat. On examination, bruising, petechiae, and pallor are noted. Her laboratory values are as follows: WBC 110 × 10^9/L (110 × 10^3/μL); RBC 1.70 × 10^{12}/L (1.70 × 10^6/μL); hemoglobin 55 g/L (5.5 g/dL); hematocrit 0.16 L/L (16%); and differential count 92% blasts, 7% lymphocytes.

---

284. Which of the following would you expect to most accurately reflect the child's platelet count?

   A. 10 × 10^9/L

   B. 100 × 10^9/L

   C. 200 × 10^9/L

   D. 400 × 10^9/L

285. What type of leukemia is this child most likely to have?

   A. Acute lymphocytic leukemia

   B. Acute myelogenous leukemia

   C. Chronic lymphocytic leukemia

   D. Chronic myelogenous leukemia

286. Which of the following cytochemical stains would most likely be positive in the blast cells of this patient?

   A. Myeloperoxidase

   B. Leukocyte alkaline phosphatase

   C. Periodic acid-Schiff

   D. Nonspecific esterase

287. Terminal deoxyribonucleotidyl transferase (TdT) is found in 90% of the cases of

A. Acute lymphocytic leukemia

B. Chronic lymphocytic leukemia

C. Acute myelogenous leukemia

D. Chronic myelogenous leukemia

288. The presence of CD2, CD5, CD7 and the absence of CD10 (CALLA) are associated with

A. B-cell acute lymphocytic leukemia

B. T-cell acute lymphocytic leukemia

C. Acute myelomonocytic leukemia (FAB M4)

D. Acute monocytic leukemia (FAB M5)

Use the following information to answer questions 289–292.

The Sudan black B stain in Color Plate 18 and the peripheral blood smear in Color Plate 16 are from Richard, an 82-year-old man. He complained of malaise and nosebleeds. The physician noted the patient was febrile and had petechiae. CBC results were as follows: WBC 20.0×10^9/L $(20.0 \times 10^3/\mu L)$; RBC 2.58×10^{12}/L $(2.58 \times 10^6/\mu L)$; hemoglobin 77 g/L (7.7g/dL); hematocrit 0.24 L/L (24 %); platelet count 32×10^9/L (32,000/μL); and differential count 95% blasts, 5% monocytes. A bone marrow examination revealed 80% cellularity and 97% blasts. Special stains showed the blasts were Sudan black B and myeloperoxidase positive, specific esterase positive. The nonspecific esterase stain was positive with blasts demonstrating inhibition by the addition of sodium fluoride. PAS stain was negative.

---

289. What is the most likely diagnosis for this patient?

A. Acute myelogenous leukemia (FAB M1)

B. Acute myelomonocytic leukemia (FAB M4)

C. Acute monocytic leukemia (FAB M5)

D. Myelodysplastic syndrome

290. In addition to the special stain results, what test would be the most useful in diagnosing the above disorder?

A. Muramidase

B. Calcium

C. Uric acid

D. Lactate dehydrogenase (LD)

291. For the diagnosis of acute leukemia, the percentage of bone marrow blasts must be greater than

A. 5

B. 10

C. 30

D. 50

292. All the following underlying conditions are known to predispose a patient to acute leukemia *except*

A. Viral infection

B. Bacterial infection

C. Chronic bone marrow dysfunction

D. Congenital chromosome abnormalities

Use the following information to answer questions 293–296.

Matthew, a 72-year-old man, is seen in the emergency room complaining of fatigue and recent weight loss. Laboratory tests were performed and showed the following: WBC 2.6×10^9/L $(2.6 \times 10^3/\mu L)$; RBC 2.79×10^{12}/L $(2.79 \times 10^6/\mu L)$; hemoglobin 92 g/L (9.2 g/dL); hematocrit 0.27 L/L (27%); RDW 21.5%; platelet count 42×10^9/L (42,000/μL); and differential count 42% segmented neutrophils, 45% band neutrophils, 3% lymphocytes, 3% metamyelocytes, 4% myelocytes, 3% blast, and 4 nRBC/100 WBC. Morphologic changes noted on the differential smear include poor granulation and hyposegmentation of the neutrophils, giant platelets that display poor granulation, oval-macrocytes, basophilic stippling, Cabot rings, Pappenheimer bodies, and Howell-Jolly bodies. Three micromegakaryocytes are seen per 100 WBCs. Serum B_{12} and folate levels are normal.

---

293. What is the most likely diagnosis for this patient?

A. Myelodysplastic syndrome

B. Degenerative left shift

C. Pernicious anemia

D. Chronic myelogenous leukemia

294. What is the expected appearance of the bone marrow in this disorder?
    A. Hypocellular; blasts greater than 30%
    B. Hypocellular; blasts less than or equal to 30%
    C. Hypercellular; blasts greater than 30%
    D. Hypercellular; blasts less than or equal to 30%

295. If the bone marrow in this patient had 15% blasts, what would the FAB classification for this myelodysplastic syndrome most likely be?
    A. Chronic myelomonocytic leukemia (CMML)
    B. Chronic myelogenous leukemia (CML)
    C. Refractory anemia with ringed sideroblasts (RARS)
    D. Refractory anemia with excess blasts (RAEB)

296. All the following are true of myelodysplastic syndromes *except*
    A. MDS is "preleukemic" and frequently terminates in acute leukemia.
    B. Treatment for MDS is only supportive and not a cure.
    C. Median survival for all types of MDS is 5 years.
    D. Best survival rates are in patients with the lowest blast percent.

Use the following information to answer questions 297–300.

Craig, a 55-year-old white man, reported to the hematology laboratory for routine blood work as part of a yearly physical. He had been feeling tired for the last few months. His complete blood counts were: WBC 45.0 × 10^9/L (45.0 × 10^3/μL); RBC 4.10 × 10^{12}/L (4.10 × 10^6/μL); hemoglobin 123 g/L (12.3 g/dL); hematocrit 0.37 L/L (37.0%); platelet count 400 × 10^9/L (400,000/μL); differential count showed polymorphonuclear neutrophils 50%, bands 8%, metamyelocytes 5%, myelocytes 7%, lymphocytes 28%, and monocytes 2%.

297. Which of the following pairs of blood disorders should be considered and differentiated with this particular blood picture?
    A. Neutrophilic leukemoid reaction and chronic myelogenous leukemia
    B. Chronic myelogenous leukemia and chronic lymphocytic leukemia
    C. Chronic myelogenous leukemia and acute myelogenous leukemia
    D. Acute myelogenous leukemia and neutrophilic leukemoid reaction

298. Which stain should be used to differentiate a neutrophilic leukemoid reaction from chronic myelogenous leukemia?
    A. Sudan black B
    B. Periodic acid-Schiff reagent (PAS)
    C. Nitroblue tetrazolium (NBT)
    D. Leukocyte alkaline phosphatase (LAP)

299. Which of the following is a myeloproliferative disorder characterized by the presence of the Philadelphia chromosome?
    A. Polycythemia vera
    B. Essential thrombocythemia
    C. Chronic myelogenous leukemia
    D. Myelofibrosis with myeloid metaplasia

300. How does the presence of the Philadelphia chromosome in this malignant disorder affect the prognosis?
    A. It is not prognostic.
    B. The prognosis is better when the chromosome is present.
    C. The prognosis is better when the chromosome is not present.
    D. Progression to acute lymphocytic leukemia will occur if the chromosome is present.

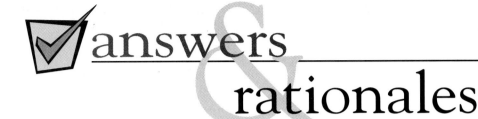

answers & rationales

HEMATOPOIESIS

1.

A. The need for oxygen delivery to developing tissues results in the production of erythrocytes prior to other blood cells. Erythropoiesis commences in the yolk sac as early as the fourteenth day of embryonic development. Myelopoietic and lymphopoietic activities begin when the liver and spleen become sites of production at six to nine weeks of gestation.

2.

C. In the infant, there is an increased demand for blood formation because of the rate of growth. All bone marrow cavities will produce cells. As the growth rate slows, there is less need for active marrow. Fatty infiltration of marrow becomes noticeable at about 4 years of age. It comprises 50% of the total marrow space in the adult.

3.

C. Lymphocytes are produced in the peripheral lymphatic tissue such as the lymph nodes in the adult. Precursor cells of the lymphocytic cell line are found in the bone marrow, but it is in the secondary lymphatic organs that reproduction takes place. Granulocytes (i.e., neutrophils, basophils, and eosinophils), as well as monocytes and thrombocytes, are formed in the bone marrow.

4.

D. Unlike the infant, in which all bone marrow is capable of forming blood cells, the active marrow in an adult is confined to the flat bones of the skeleton such as the sternum and posterior iliac crest. Although the spinous processes of the vertebrae contain active marrow, these sites are not often used for aspiration in adults because of the danger of damage to the spinal cord. Although sternal puncture also may present a possibility of serious damage to underlying structures, this site is often used because of its easy accessibility.

5.

D. Myeloid precursors outnumber erythroid precursors by about 3 or 4 to 1 in the bone marrow. Although there are many more red blood cells in the peripheral blood than granulocytes, red blood cells have a much longer life span. Granulocytes, therefore, require a more continual production than erythrocytes.

6.

B. The promyelocyte is the first cell to present with primary granules. The cell that can first be recognized as granulocytic is the myeloblast. This cell has no granules. The appearance of the primary granules after 3 to 5 mitotic divisions of the myeloblast signifies the promyelocyte stage.

7.

A. The liver of the fetus assumes primary responsibility for hematopoiesis about the second month of gestation. From the third to sixth months, the spleen is also involved, but the primary site remains the liver. At around the seventh gestational month, the bone marrow becomes the primary hematopoietic site. By birth, the liver and spleen have ceased hematopoiesis.

8.

B. Erythropoietin production is currently thought to be controlled by the amount of oxygen present in the kidney. Either the glomeruli or the juxtaglomerular cells are thought to be actual sensor sites. Although the liver and spleen can be sites of extramedullary cell production, they are not considered essential to the feedback mechanism in erythropoietin production.

9.

C. When the bone marrow is stressed, younger reticulocytes are released. These cells are larger than normal. The premature cells are called "stress" or "shift" reticulocytes. The stress reticulocyte contains more filamentous reticulum than a mature reticulocyte.

10.

B. A given number of tagged cells are injected into an individual. ^{51}Cr is the most commonly used radioisotope. The time during which half (50%) of the radioactively labeled cells are lost from the circulation is called the half-life. This measurement is valuable in the diagnosis of hemolytic anemias.

11.

A. Bone marrow consists of vessels, nerves, hematopoietic cells at various levels of maturation, and reticuloendothelial cells encased in a membrane lining called the endosteum. The vascular system empties into a system of sinuses (venous sinusoids). A layer of endothelium lines these sinusoids. The blood cell formation occurs in the hematopoietic cords located outside of the sinusoids.

12.

B. Cohort labeling involves the marking of a group of cells that are all the same age. This is accomplished by using a radioactive material that will be incorporated into the developing cell. ^{59}Fe serves this function in erythrocytes. ^{51}Cr and the Ashby agglutination technique produce random labels, whereas Evans blue dye is a label for plasma.

13.

C. T Lymphocytes are able to secrete their own growth factor. Other blood cells require the addition of a specific growth hormone produced by other cells. For example, the hormonal influence for red blood cells is erythropoietin, which is produced by the renal cells.

14.

C. The total blood volume includes both formed (cellular) elements and fluid elements (plasma). The total of both is about 12 pints or 6 L. Cells account for about 45% or 2.7 L, and plasma accounts for 55% or 3.3 L.

15.

D. Lymphocytes emerge as a distinct cell line from the pluripotential stem cell (PSC) at the same time that the multipotential stem cell or Colony Forming Unit-Spleen (CFU-S) arises. The CFU-S differentiates into erythrocytic, megakaryocytic, eosinophilic, and granulocytic-monocytic committed stem cells. Lymphoid stem cells migrate to secondary lymphoid tissues to differentiate into specialized types of lymphocytes.

16.

D. The mature megakaryocyte is the largest hematopoietic cell in the bone marrow. Its size prevents the cell from passing through the venous sinuses into the peripheral circulation. In some myeloproliferative diseases, such as acute megakaryocytic leukemia, micromegakaryoblasts may be found. On very rare occasions, these cells may be seen in peripheral circulation.

17.

C. About 1 in 1000 nucleated marrow cells are believed to be stem cells of one type or another. Since these cells are morphologically similar to small lymphocytes, evidence for their prevalence is derived from cell culture studies. Immunologic techniques are available to identify and distinguish various types of stem cells.

18.

B. The nucleus to cytoplasm ratio decreases as blood cells mature. Blood cells generally become smaller, the nuclear chromatin condenses, nucleoli become less prominent, and cytoplasm loses its deep blue basophilia when stained with Wright's stain. Exceptions include megakaryocytes (they grow larger as cytoplasm accumulates) and plasma cells (increased RNA and protein synthesis produces a deep basophilia).

19.

A. Erythropoietin is a hormone that increases red blood cell production in the bone marrow by its action on erythrocyte precursors. It has been isolated and has been found to be a glycoprotein with a molecular weight of about 39,000. Although primarily produced by the kidney, there seems to be a site of extrarenal production, possibly the liver, because nephrectomized animals will still show about 10–15% of the normal level.

20.

D. Cell production outside of the marrow space takes place when the bone marrow is unable to meet its production demands. This may occur in severe hemolytic anemia. Splenic cell production may also occur in myelofibrosis, where it is probably an extension of the disease process.

ERYTHROCYTES

21.

D. Red blood cells survive in a normal individual about 4 months, or 120 days. The entire life span of the normal red cell is spent inside the vascular tree, making it easier to determine the rate of production and destruction. Most erythrocyte destruction occurs in the reticuloendothelial system.

22.

B. The erythrocyte has a semipermeable membrane that allows water and some anions, such as chloride (Cl^-) and bicarbonate (HCO_3^-), to enter the cell rapidly. Sodium ions (Na^+) enter the cell and potassium ions (K^+) leave the cell slowly but continuously. In order to maintain a high intracellular K^+ concentration and remove excess Na^+, ATP-dependent cationic pumps expel Na^+ and take in K^+.

23.

D. Hemoglobin is a conjugated protein composed of globin chains and ferroheme molecules. Two types of globin chains are produced by polyribosomes (in adult hemoglobin, or hemoglobin A, alpha and beta), each of which attach to a ferroheme. First, a subunit consisting of an alpha-globin chain with its associated heme is assembled. Then two subunits associate to form the final molecule, which consists of two alpha-globin chains and two beta-globin chains, each with their associated heme,

making a total of four polypeptide chains and four ferrohemes.

24.

D. Culling is the process of removal of red blood cells from the circulation by the spleen. The spleen removes senescent (aged) and abnormal red blood cells from the circulation. The spleen recognizes subtle abnormalities in the cell. It then sequesters and removes the cells.

25.

A. Hemoglobin in which the ferrous iron molecule (Fe^{2+}) has been oxidized to the ferric state (Fe^{3+}) is known as methemoglobin. Carboxyhemoglobin is hemoglobin with a CO attached to the iron molecule. The action of hydrogen sulfide on heme produces sulfhemoglobin. Abnormalities in the globin chains are known as hemoglobinopathies.

26.

B. In infants with homozygous alpha-thalassemia-1, no alpha-globin chains are produced. Consequently the infants have nearly 100% hemoglobin Bart's, which consists of four gamma-globin chains. This hemoglobin migrates farther towards the anode than Hb A. Since Hb Bart's has a very high oxygen affinity, it is useless for delivery of oxygen to the tissues making its presence incompatible with life.

27.

B. A senescent red blood cell is one that has lived its life span. Repeated passes through the spleen deplete the cells of glucose and decrease their surface area. The red cells are then removed from the circulation by the reticuloendothelial system. Specifically, the spleen recognizes subtle abnormalities in these cells, sequesters and destroys them.

28.

B. Variation in the shape of erythrocytes is commonly referred to as poikilocytosis. Anisocytosis is the term used when differences in the sizes of red cells are described. Color in red cells is designated as normochromic (normal) or hypochromic (indicating a decrease from the normal).

29.

A. In red blood cells in which nuclear maturation and division are incomplete, such as those found in megaloblastic anemia, remnants of nuclear material may remain after the nucleus has been extruded. These are called Howell-Jolly bodies. They may also be found in individuals without a spleen who lack the normal pitting function that rids red cells of inclusions. Pitting is a process where splenic macrophages remove inclusions while leaving the rest of the cell intact.

30.

A. Schistocytes, or schizocytes, are fragments of red cells. Their presence indicates some form of mechanical damage. They should be distinguished from acanthocytes (sharp projections) and echinocytes (blunt projections).

31.

A. The presence of lead causes an inhibition of several of the enzymes important in the manufacture of heme. Among these is pyrimidine 5′-nucleotidase, which is normally responsible for degradation of ribosomal ribonucleic acid (RNA). The lack of this enzyme apparently allows remnants of aggregated, incompletely degraded RNA to remain in the cell cytoplasm. It is this material that appears on Wright's stain as punctate basophilic stippling.

32.

D. The presence of rouleaux is a characteristic finding in myeloma because of the increased concentration of immunoglobulins in the blood plasma. The immunoglobulins are produced by the plasma cells that make up the tumors. Teardrop-shaped cells tend to be characteristic of myelofibrosis.

33.

C. In viewing Color Plate 1, the inclusion in the red blood cell is a nuclear remnant known as a Howell-Jolly body. The spleen generally removes cells containing Howell-Jolly bodies. Post splenectomy, the cells remain in the circulation. These inclusions may also be seen in hemolytic anemias such as sickle cell, megaloblastic anemia, and conditions with splenic atrophy.

34.

A. Acanthocytes are red cells with sharp pointed projections and are characteristic of abetalipoproteinemia. Discocytes are normal cells. Echinocytes are crenated, but the projections are rounded. Codocytes are target cells, and stomatocytes have a slit-like central pallor.

35.

D. Siderocytes are adult cells that contain nonhemoglobin iron. Reticulocytes may commonly contain small amounts of iron. Siderocytes may be found in abnormalities where there is an iron utilization problem (such as thalassemia or sideroblastic anemia). Echinocytes are burred cells, acanthocytes have sharp points, and drepanocytes are sickle cells.

36.

C. A "shift to the left" in the oxygen dissociation curve means that a higher percentage of the hemoglobin will retain more of its oxygen at a given pressure. Thus affinity will be greater and oxygen delivery will be reduced. This will lead to a compensatory increase in red cells in an attempt to increase the amount of oxygen available to the tissues. A higher or more alkaline pH is associated with decreased oxygen dissociation.

37.

B. Hemoglobin nomenclature indicates a number of things. Saskatoon is the geographical area in which the hemoglobin was first found. The letter E indicates an electrophoretic mobility similar to other previously named E hemoglobins. The symbol α_2 or α_2^A indicates the presence of normal adult, or A, alpha chains. The designation $\beta_2^{\;22\;Glu\;\rightarrow\;Lys}$ indicates that lysine residues have replaced glutamic acid on position 22 of the beta chains.

38.

C. Increased 2,3-BPG (formerly, 2,3-DPG) levels decrease the affinity of hemoglobin for oxygen. Increased pH (alkalinity) enhances oxygen affinity and thus inhibits delivery to the tissues. Less oxygen is available at higher altitudes, affecting blood saturation and delivery to tissues. An increase in erythropoietin will affect red cell production, but does not have an immediate or direct impact on oxygen delivery.

39.

D. Megaloblastic anemias are associated with nuclear maturation abnormalities. Howell-Jolly bodies are nuclear remnants frequently seen in these anemias. Cabot rings may also occur, but these are very rare. Heinz bodies represent precipitated hemoglobin, basophilic stippling is associated with toxic injury, and siderotic granules occur with defective iron utilization. Reticulofilamentous precipitates indicate the presence of reticulocytes, usually decreased or normal in megaloblastic anemias.

40.

C. Heinz bodies do not stain distinctively with Wright's stain. They can be visualized on wet preps with phase microscopy or by using vital stains, such as crystal violet. They consist of denatured hemoglobin and appear in Wright's stain as "normal" hemoglobin. Döhle bodies and toxic granulation are seen in white blood cells; these and the other inclusions are visible with Wright's stain.

41.

D. Lead poisoning interferes with heme synthesis but does not result in red blood cell fragmentation. Increased intravascular deposits of fibrin in disseminated intravascular coagulation (DIC) cut red cells into pieces. The presence of artificial surfaces, such as heart valves, can cause mechanical damage. Thermal injury also results in schistocyte formation.

42.

A. The red blood cell membrane is dissolved with a detergent, sodium dodecyl sulfate (SDS). The membrane proteins are separated by polyacrylamide gel electrophoresis (PAGE) and then stained with either Coomassie blue or with periodic acid-Schiff (PAS). The major protein bands are numbered (eight stain with Coomassie blue and four stain with PAS), the basis for a provisional nomenclature.

43.

B. Red cell nuclei and inclusions such as Heinz bodies and Howell-Jolly bodies are normally removed by the pitting action of splenic macrophages. Target cells contain abnormal amounts of cholesterol or increased surface area and are also destroyed by the spleen. Hypochromia denotes a decrease in hemoglobin content, and the spleen does not affect these cells.

44.

C. The orthochromic normoblast or metarubricyte is the most mature stage seen in Color Plate 2. It is also the last stage of the red blood cell to contain a nucleus. The less mature cell is the polychromatophilic normoblast. The reticulocyte is the first nonnucleated stage.

45.

C. Lecithin-cholesterol acyltransferase (LCAT) is an enzyme associated with erythrocyte membrane synthesis. It catalyzes the formation of esters from cholesterol. Because red cell membrane cholesterol is in rapid equilibrium with plasma cholesterol, activity of this enzyme helps determine membrane lipid composition. Deficiencies of LCAT result in target cells with increased cholesterol content.

46.

D. The Rapoport-Luebering shunt of the Embden-Meyerhof pathway bypasses the formation of 3-phosphoglycerate directly from 1,3-bisphosphoglycerate. Instead, bisphosphoglycerate mutase catalyzes the formation of 2,3-BPG. The production of 2,3-BPG results in the loss of ATP formation. This is one of only two such steps during anaerobic glycolysis.

47.

C. The polychromatophilic normoblast (rubricyte) is the last red cell stage capable of mitosis. Each pronormoblast produces two basophilic normoblasts and each of these cells also produces two mitotic divisions. Polychromatophilic normoblasts divide twice, the last resulting in orthochromic normoblasts with highly condensed nuclei. The latter are incapable of further division.

48.

D. Fetal hemoglobin (Hb F) consists of two alpha and two gamma globin chains. Adult hemoglobin (Hb A) is made up of alpha and beta globin chains, and hemoglobin A_2 contains delta chains. Epsilon chains are found in embryonic hemoglobins (Gower 1 and 2).

49.

A. Intrinsic factor is a 45,000-dalton glycoprotein secreted by the gastric mucosa. It combines with dietary vitamin B_{12} to effect absorption in the small intestine. Inadequate secretion of intrinsic factor results in pernicious anemia.

50.

C. An observation of 63 reticulocytes of 1000 total erythrocytes results in a reported count of 6.3%.

Reference ranges are commonly given as 0.5–1.5% or 0.5–2.0%. Values higher than 2.0% indicate increased erythroid production, most often in response to hypoxia associated with hemolytic or hemorrhagic anemias.

51.

D. Erythrocytes with large volumes (MCV > 100 fL) should appear as macrocytes on a peripheral blood smear. In this case, the macrocytosis is slight and may not be apparent, particularly if considerable size variation (anisocytosis) is also present. Hypochromia and polychromasia refer to staining of the red cell due to hemoglobin content and RNA content, respectively. Poikilocytosis refers to variation in cell shape.

52.

C. Bilirubin is formed by the extravascular degradation of hemoglobin in the reticuloendothelial system, primarily in the spleen. Unconjugated bilirubin (indirect) is transported by the plasma to the liver, where it is converted to a glucuronide (conjugated or direct bilirubin). This posthepatic bilirubin is excreted via the gallbladder and intestines.

53.

D. Haptoglobin forms a 1:1 complex with alpha-beta dimers of hemoglobin. The large size of this complex prevents filtration of the hemoglobin through the kidneys, where it can cause renal damage. Haptoglobin can be depleted in the plasma during major hemolytic events, such as malarial attacks, transfusion reactions, and other causes of severe intravascular red cell destruction.

54.

D. Shift cells are large diffusely basophilic cells seen on a peripheral smear during intense erythrocyte production. The diffuse basophilic nature of these cells is the result of RNA remaining in the young cell. These cells may not be identified as reticulocytes based on the Wright's stained smear.

55.

B. Heme synthesis begins in the mitochondria with the formation of aminolevulinic acid. Formation of the pyrrole ring structure occurs in the cytoplasm, resulting in the synthesis of coproporphyrinogen III. The final stages of porphyrin synthesis occur again in the mitochondria, culminating in the formation of heme.

56.

A. Spectrin comprises about 25% of all red cell membrane protein, forming a cytoskeleton with other proteins, such as actin, protein 4.1, and ankyrin. Spectrin consists of two alpha and two beta chains (pairs of alpha-beta dimers). Stability of the cytoskeleton complex requires phosphorylation by protein kinase, an ATP-dependent process.

57.

C. Reduced glutathione (GSH) counteracts oxidants that accumulate in the red cell. These occur as a result of normal metabolic activities and increase during infections and as a result of treatment by some drugs. In the absence of GSH or as a result of enzyme deficiencies in the hexose monophosphate pathway, oxidant accumulation can lead to oxidation and precipitation of hemoglobin.

58.

B. The structures of hemoglobin and myoglobin are similar in that they are made of polypeptide globin chains and heme molecules. A hemoglobin molecule contains four of each while myoglobin is constructed with one globin chain and one heme. Myoglobin functions differently with regard to oxygen dissociation and cannot be used interchangeably with hemoglobin.

59.

C. Ceruloplasmin is an alpha$_2$-glycoprotein found in the serum. It contains copper and weighs 120,000–160,000 daltons. Ceruloplasmin oxidizes iron after release from mucosal cells.

60.

C. Hemoglobin F production decreases after birth, composing less than 1% of total hemoglobin in adults. Only a small percentage of the circulating erythrocytes (< 8%) in adults contain hemoglobin F. In certain conditions, such as thalassemia and some hemoglobinopathies, restriction of normal beta chain production can be compensated by increased production of gamma chains and formation of hemoglobin F.

ERYTHROCYTE DISORDERS

61.

D. Deficiencies of folic acid (folate) and vitamin B$_{12}$ result in abnormal DNA synthesis and a resultant delay in nuclear maturation. These anemias are also categorized as megaloblastic because the red cell precursors are large. The other anemias are characterized by defects of heme (sideroblastic anemia and iron deficiency anemia) or globin synthesis (hemoglobin C disease).

62.

B. G6PD deficiency compromises the ability of the glutathione reduction pathway to prevent the oxidation of hemoglobin. Oxidative stress may occur from infections, certain drugs, or during the immediate postnatal period. The oxidized hemoglobin precipitates in the form of Heinz bodies.

63.

B. Paroxysmal nocturnal hemoglobinuria (PNH) is an intrinsic defect of red cells that have a high affinity for complement, leading to intravascular hemolysis. Membrane defects, not affecting complement deposition, are present in hereditary elliptocytosis and stomatocytosis, while pyruvate kinase deficiency involves the glycolytic pathway. Sideroblastic anemias result from defects in heme synthesis.

64.

C. The peripheral blood as seen in Color Plate 3 shows numerous elliptocytes (ovalocytes). If they were artifacts due to smear preparation, they would be oriented in the same direction. Hereditary elliptocytosis is associated with a hemolytic anemia in only about 10% of the cases, but the presence of an enlarged spleen is further evidence of ongoing extravascular destruction. Gallstones are a common complication in patients with clinical manifestations of this inherited disorder.

65.

B. Cooley's anemia or β-Thalassemia major would be the appropriate diagnosis in this case. This condition is caused by the inheritance of two β-thalassemia alleles. This results in production of virtually no hemoglobin A or A_2 because no beta globin chains are produced. The primary hemoglobin produced is hemoglobin F. The anemia results from the lack of normal hemoglobin production. Nucleated red blood cells and target cells, as seen in Color Plate 4, are common. Basophilic stippling may also be seen. These children are plagued with anemia and recurrent infections.

66.

C. As seen in Color Plate 5, the presence of S-C crystals on the peripheral blood smear provides a positive diagnosis of hemoglobin S-C disease. These crystals are often distinguished by one or more blunt projections that protrude from the cell membrane. Numerous target cells are additional clues when crystals are rare or absent. The diagnosis should always be confirmed by hemoglobin electrophoresis.

67.

B. Pica may be associated with iron deficiency (usually a cause rather than an effect) in adults. In children, pica is most commonly associated with lead poisoning, resulting from the ingestion of lead-based paint from walls, on toys, or from other objects. Pica describes a number of bizarre eating practices (ice, clay, and chalk) that have been documented for particular cultures.

68.

B. The acid serum lysis test is used to diagnose paroxysmal nocturnal hemoglobinuria (PNH). Red blood cells in these patients are abnormally sensitive to complement deposition. Lysis is most likely at night when blood pH decreases slightly. In the Ham test, patient erythrocytes are incubated with serum at pH 6.5–7.0, and red cell lysis is compared to normal controls. Other red cells, such as spherocytes and those sensitized by antibodies, may also lyse. The test can be repeated with heat-inactivated serum to remove complement.

69.

C. The hemoglobin solubility test, using dithionite, can distinguish between hemoglobins with reduced solubility (such as hemoglobin S) and normal hemoglobin variants, such as Hb C_{Harlem}. Some hemoglobins that result in Heinz body formation, may also give positive solubility test results. Positive results should be confirmed by electrophoresis.

70.

C. The cells demonstrated in Color Plate 6 are burr cells. Acanthocytes resemble burr cells but have fewer, more irregular and more blunt projections than burr cells. A blister cell is one that appears to have a vacuole-like area. Most likely caused by mechanical damage. A fibrin strand will cause this type of damage. Target cells or codocytes have a central area of hemoglobin surrounded by a colorless ring that gives them a bell or "Mexican hat" shape.

71.

D. Ringed sideroblasts result from the accumulation of nonferritin iron deposits in mitochondria surrounding the erythroblast nucleus. The deposits are secondary to a defect in heme synthesis or in iron metabolism within the erythroblast. The defect may be either hereditary or acquired, involving one of several steps in the heme pathway.

72.

D. Reticulocytosis is indicative of increased red blood cell production and release by the marrow, a normal response in conditions involving red cell destruction or loss. Usually, the reticulocyte count is not elevated in a patient with megaloblastic anemia, such as pernicious anemia. If the relative count is elevated (> 2.0%), it usually reflects the decrease in mature red blood cells; the absolute count will usually be normal or decreased, indicating the hypoproliferative nature of this disorder.

73.

B. The major defect in hereditary stomatocytosis is altered permeability of the red cell membrane to Na^+ and K^+ ions. A net gain of sodium within the cell leads to increased water entry and the appearance of a swollen cell with a slit-like area of pallor. The disorder is probably heterogeneous in that a number of specific membrane constituent defects have been postulated.

74.

D. Polycythemia vera (PV) belongs to the group of disorders commonly characterized as "myeloproliferative." In these disorders, there appears to be a defect in the multipotential stem cell. Although the major increase in PV is in red blood cells, there are also increases in granulocytes and platelets, particularly in the early stages of the disease.

75.

D. The increased production of cells in PV is not due to the activity of erythropoietin. The production of erythropoietin is almost completely suppressed in this disorder. The stem cell is reacting to some as-yet-unknown stimulus.

76.

A. Since red blood cells and plasma are lost together, the hemoglobin and hematocrit will not reflect the severity of an acute hemorrhage until the lost blood volume begins to be replaced by the formation of plasma. The restoration of a normal blood volume is usually complete by 72 hours. It is then that the hemoglobin and hematocrit will reach their lowest point, and they will begin to rise only with the release of newly formed cells.

77.

D. The multipotential stem cell defect in aplastic anemia results in a cell that is normocytic and normochromic, or occasionally slightly macrocytic. There is no hypochromia because of the lack of interference with hemoglobin synthesis by the developing erythrocyte. The occasional slight macrocytosis that occurs may result from an accelerated marrow transit time.

78.

D. The red blood cell with the elongated projection, seen in Color Plate 7, is a dacrocyte or tear drop cell. Dacrocytes are most often seen in myelofibrosis or disorders of marrow replacement. Drepanocytes or sickle cells are observed during sickling crisis of sickle cell anemia. Codocytes or target cells may be seen in conditions where the membrane structure is abnormal as well as in hemoglobin C-C and S-C disorders. Acanthocytes are cells with a few irregularly shaped thornlike projections and are seen in conditions such as alcoholic cirrhosis as well as a rare inherited condition known as abetalipoproteinemia.

79.

C. Myelophthisic anemia is an anemia of bone marrow failure seen in patients with carcinoma who are experiencing bone marrow replacement with abnormal cells. The anemia is a hypoproliferative anemia. There is no hemolysis involved and the cells are normocytic, normochromic.

80.

A. Any idiopathic disorder is one for which there is no apparent cause. Ionizing radiation is a well-known cause of aplasia. Iatrogenic disorders are those that result from treatments for a different disorder; for example, aplasia will result from chloramphenicol treatment for bacterial disease.

81.

C. Diamond-Blackfan is a congenital disorder that depresses only red blood cell production. Fanconi's is a congenital disorder of the hematologic stem cell that results in aplasia of all cell lines. Bernard-Soulier is a disorder with giant platelets, and Chédiak-Higashi is a qualitative disorder of granulocytes.

82.

C. Dehydration is a cause of relative erythrocytosis. High altitude adjustment, pulmonary disease, and defective oxygen transport are all causes of absolute secondary erythrocytosis. Absolute primary erythrocytosis is known as polycythemia vera.

83.

B. Pyruvate kinase (PK) catalyzes the reaction of phosphoenolpyruvate (PEP) to pyruvate while converting ADP to ATP. The pyruvate then reacts with a fluorescent NADH to produce lactate and a non-fluorescent NAD. This second reaction requires the presence of lactate dehydrogenase (LD). A normal reaction is characterized by the loss of fluorescence.

84.

D. Primary pernicious anemia is a disorder in which the lack of intrinsic factor (IF) prevents the absorption of vitamin B_{12} from the intestine. The Schilling test involves administration of radioactive B_{12} by mouth and the measurement of excreted radioactive B_{12} in a 24-hour urine collection. When this is abnormal (below 7%), a second dose of radioactive B_{12} is given along with external IF, and the radioactivity in a 24-hour urine collection is again assayed. A defect in absorption caused by the lack of IF will be corrected when IF is present; defects caused by other types of malabsorption syndromes or competitive inhibition (fish tapeworm, bacterial overgrowth) will not be corrected.

85.

D. Tropical sprue is a malabsorption syndrome of unknown origin. The peripheral blood has a characteristic megaloblastic appearance. This is due, first, to a lack of folate, followed by a lack of vitamin B_{12}.

86.

B. The nucleated red blood cells seen in Color Plate 2 and the polychromatophilic cells of Color Plate 8 are indicative of possible erythroblastosis fetalis. The neonate has experienced some hemolysis of the red blood cells. The bone marrow is compensating by releasing nucleated red cells and reticulocytes, represented by the polychromatophilic cells. The incompatibility may be an IgG form of an ABO antibody. Hemoglobinopathies, unless not compatible with life, are not often diagnosed at birth but rather as the fetal hemoglobin begins to convert to adult hemoglobin.

87.

B. Serum ferritin is considered to be a good indicator of storage iron in most individuals. Its measurement is not useful in some cases of familial hemochromatosis where normal levels may be found even in the presence of high amounts of serum iron. The transferrin saturation level, or serum iron divided by the amount of iron capable of being absorbed by transferrin, will also be high in these instances. A lack of hemoglobin iron will be reflected by the amount of color in the red cell (hypochromia).

88.

C. When iron is removed from the heme of destroyed red blood cells, it is combined with a protein shell, apoferritin. The combination of the iron micelle and apoferritin is called ferritin. Ferritin is further consolidated into larger aggregates that are visible by light microscopy and are called hemosiderin. Most storage iron is found as hemosiderin.

89.

A. Exposure to increased quantities of iron, causing macrophage overload and expansion of storage sites, is called hemochromatosis. It is commonly associated with disorders in which there is an increased need for transfusion, such as thalassemia major. There is also a familiar form in which there is increased iron absorption.

90.

C. Of the 3000–4000 mg of iron present in a normal adult, around 2500 mg is contained in the hemoglobin circulating in erythrocytes. Most of the remainder, 500–1500 mg, is found in storage iron such as hemosiderin or ferritin. A much smaller amount of iron is contained in muscle myoglobin and enzymes.

91.
A. The majority of body iron is found in the hemoglobin of circulating erythrocytes. This means that any form of bleeding will lead to excessive iron loss. Iron balance is normally very tightly controlled through absorption rather than excretion.

92.
C. Both iron deficiency anemia and thalassemia are hypochromic, microcytic anemias. In iron deficiency a lack of heme synthesis is the cause, whereas thalassemia is the result of the lack of globin chain production. The anemia of chronic infection is characterized by normochromic, normocytic cells. The cells in pernicious anemia are macrocytic, whereas those in spherocytosis are microcytic but well filled with hemoglobin.

93.
A. Serum iron is low in both iron deficiency anemia and the anemia of chronic disorders. Transferrin concentration is low in the anemia of chronic disorders, whereas it is high in iron deficiency. Morphologically the red blood cells are very similar in iron deficiency and thalassemia, but the serum iron level is high with a normal transferrin level in thalassemia.

94.
C. Although the punctate basophilic stippling found in lead poisoning in erythrocytes is widely used as a diagnostic tool, the anemia present is usually not severe. The presence of lead inhibits the formation of heme, with a consequent increase in erythrocyte protoporphyrin and urinary coproporphyrin III. The most significant effect of these compounds is the production of a neurological deficit.

95.
A. In Color Plate 9, the red blood cells represented display anisocytosis. Anisocytosis is a variation in cell size. Poikilocytosis represents a variation in cell shape. While there may be small variations in shape, the majority of cells are discoid in shape. Normocytic cells would be uniform size and shape while conforming to the disc shape cell, approximately 7 μm in diameter.

96.
B. The cells visualized in Color Plate 10 are sickle cells. The substitution of a valine for the glutamic acid normally found in the sixth position of the beta-polypeptide chain in hemoglobin A causes the cells to undergo the characteristic shape change that gave the sickle cell its name. A substitution on both genes (or the homozygous state) results in sickle cell disease, whereas a single gene mutation causes the sickle cell trait, a much milder disorder. The molecular formula $\alpha_2^A \beta^{6\,Lys \to Val}$ is designated hemoglobin C.

97.
D. The number of irreversibly sickled cells (ISCs) and the proportion of S hemoglobin within the cells contribute collectively to the severity of sickle cell disorders. The classification of "trait" vs. "disease" is not based on the severity of symptoms. It is the differentiation of the presence of the single (AS-heterozygous) or double (SS-homozygous) S gene that determines whether the condition is classified as the trait (AS) or the disease (SS).

98.
B. Hyperbaric oxygen will reverse the sickling process, but it will also suppress erythropoietin, which stimulates the bone marrow to produce adequate replacement erythrocytes. Urea prevents sickling and has had experimental trials, but since it has had severe adverse side effects, it is not now used. Treatment at this time is still supportive and symptomatic.

99.
D. Reticulocytosis is characteristic of hemolytic anemias because of the continued increased need for replacement cells. The hemoglobin, hematocrit, and erythrocyte count are usually low. These decreased values are found primarily in anemias of production but anemias of destruction may demonstrate similar results.

100.
C. Individuals with heterozygous beta thalassemia will have approximately twice as much hemoglobin A_2 as genetically normal persons. This results from decreased production of beta globin chains and increased delta chain production. Alpha thalassemia results in a decrease or absence in

production of alpha globin chains. Delta-beta thalassemia would affect the levels of production of both delta and beta globin chains and would most likely decrease the level of hemoglobin A_2 production.

101.

D. Oxidative denaturation is the primary mechanism of the hemolytic process. When glucose-6-phosphate dehydrogenase (G6PD) is deficient, the red blood cells cannot generate sufficient reduced glutathione (GSH) to detoxify hydrogen peroxide. The hemoglobin molecule is oxidized to methemoglobin and denatures forming Heinz bodies. These Heinz bodies induce the rigidity of the cell and hemolysis occurs as the cells try to pass through the microcirculation.

102.

A. The membrane defect present in hereditary spherocytosis is accentuated by the passage of the red blood cell through the spleen. The spleen has a low glucose concentration that prevents the red cell from generating sufficient adenosine triphosphate (ATP) to maintain the elasticity of the membrane and the Na^+-K^+ pump. Eventually, the red cell will be trapped and destroyed. Removal of the spleen causes the red cell to survive normally.

103.

B. Spherocytes deplete their energy supply quickly in the absence of a source of glucose. This is due to a membrane defect that allows leakage. Because they can no longer manufacture ATP, the cells take on water and lyse. The addition of either glucose or ATP will correct this lysis.

104.

D. All the disorders listed are intrinsic forms of hemolytic anemia. Paroxysmal nocturnal hemoglobinuria (PNH) is the major exception to the rule that every form of this type of anemia is genetic. Although PNH may appear at any age, it is an acquired disorder.

105.

D. Paroxysmal cold hemoglobinuria (PCH) is caused by an antibody that reacts in the cold, named the Donath-Landsteiner (DL) antibody. It is usually of the anti-P specificity. Anti-I is frequently the cause of cold autoimmune hemolytic anemia, while anti-e causes warm autoimmune conditions.

106.

C. Total iron binding capacity (TIBC) represents the amount of iron that the circulating transferrin could bind if it were saturated. In this test, the transferrin is measured indirectly by adding ferric (Fe^{3+}) iron to the serum, allowing it to bind to the unsaturated sites on transferrin. Unbound iron is then removed and the sample analyzed for the remaining iron that is bound to transferrin.

107.

D. Siderotic granules are composed of iron. The reaction of the granules with Prussian blue is positive, indicating the presence of iron. Cabot rings are believed to be remnants of microtubules or fragments of nuclear membrane. Reticulocytes and Heinz bodies are seen only when stained with supravital stain.

108.

A. Spherocytes are produced as a result of some form of membrane injury to the cell. In autoimmune hemolytic anemia (AIHA), this injury is antibody mediated; in March hemoglobinuria it is physical damage. The presence of microspherocytes is one way to differentiate ABO hemolytic disease of the newborn from other forms of this disorder.

109.

C. The structural abnormality seen in spherocytosis is due to a loss of membrane surface, not abnormal production. The round cell shape causes increased osmotic fragility. Clinically the symptoms may vary from severe to essentially none. Splenectomy allows the cells to maintain a normal life span, since it is in the slow passage through the spleen that the cellular destruction takes place.

110.

D. In hereditary elliptocytosis (HE) the red blood cells show increased Na^+ permeability due to any of several membrane defects linked to this autosomal dominant disorder. These include deficiencies in protein band 4.1, spectrin, and ankyrin, but not lipid constituents. The characteristic oval or elliptical shape is seen only in mature red blood cells.

111.

B. In order of movement rate from the origin at pH 8.4, hemoglobin A moves fastest (farther) than any of the hemoglobins listed. From fastest to slowest, the order is: Hb A, Hb F, Hb S, and Hb C. Rate of movement depends on the number and charge of amino acids that are influenced by the electrical field.

112.

A. Hemoglobin C disease results from a homozygous substitution of lysine for glutamic acid at the beta-6 position. Valine substitution results in sickle cell disease. Target cells and decreased osmotic fragility are characteristic of hemoglobin C disease.

113.

D. Sickle cells are mechanically brittle but show increased resistance to osmotic change (decreased fragility) because of their shape. They adhere more readily to vascular endothelium than normal cells and they are less deformable. They are easily trapped in the small vessels of the spleen, leading to obstructive ischemia and eventual destruction of splenic tissue.

114.

B. Hemolytic anemias are usually normochromic, normocytic. Increased reticulocytes and polychromasia indicate a measured erythroid hyperplasia in response to the hypoxia. Increased unconjugated bilirubin results from hemoglobin degradation, and decreased haptoglobin results from its use as an intravascular transport protein for hemoglobin.

115.

B. Most intrinsic hemolytic anemias have a genetic basis, but many cells within the circulating population may appear normal. Both intravascular and extravascular hemolysis may be present, depending on the disorder, but most defective cells are removed by splenic macrophages. Because the cells have an intrinsic or intracorpuscular deficiency, the cells will have a shortened survival time whether they are in the patient or in a recipient.

116.

C. One of the reasons for increased iron absorption is the presence of a high level of erythropoiesis. Although the mucosal cell does act as a barrier in normal circumstances, this function is not absolute, and controls break down in the presence of large amounts of iron, causing an excess to be absorbed. Iron absorption depends on an acid pH, which is present in the jejunum for absorption.

117.

C. Hemoglobin D migrates in the same location as hemoglobin S, normal hemoglobin A_2, and hemoglobin F on cellulose acetate at alkaline pH. The negative solubility test rules out the presence of hemoglobin S. Target cells are seen in large numbers in homozygous hemoglobin D disease. The quantification of 95% differentiates homozygous from heterozygous states where less than 50% hemoglobin D would be seen.

118.

A. Hemopexin is a plasma globulin protein that carries free heme. It is decreased most often in severe intravascular hemolysis. The degree of hemopexin decrease is proportional to the concentration of free heme in the plasma and severity of hemolysis.

119.

B. Reticulocyte counts are done using the Miller disc. The disc is a calibrated disc placed in the ocular of the microscope. The field of view contains 2 squares, one inside of the other. The smaller, inside square is one-ninth the size of the outer square. The erythrocytes are counted in small square B and the reticulocytes in large square A. This is done in 20 fields. The reticulocyte count is then computed using a formula.

120.

A. Thalassemia major is a hereditary disorder that produces a quantitative reduction of beta chains. Production of adult hemoglobin is impaired. Acute alcohol ingestion, Isoniazid treatment, and Chloramphenicol use all may cause an acquired, reversible sideroblastic anemia. Discontinuing the offensive agent may reverse the effects.

121.

A. Although iron deficiency may be the most common cause of anemia in pregnancy, there is a mild form that develops in the third trimester in pregnant women with adequate iron levels. Although both erythrocytes and plasma increase during pregnancy, plasma increases in a higher proportion, causing a relative anemia. This increased blood volume actually increases oxygen delivery to both the mother and the fetus.

122.

B. Anemia of hypothyroidism is normocytic, normochromic. This anemia results from a lowered metabolism and decreased oxygen demand by the tissues. The erythropoietin levels also drop below normal resulting in a decrease in red blood cell production accordingly. Androgen deficiency found in male gonadal disorders also results in a decrease in erythropoietin production but is unrelated to hypothyroidism.

123.

B. Aplastic anemia is a disorder that affects the multipotential stem cell in the bone marrow, which leads to a decrease in erythrocytes, leukocytes, and platelets. Although lymphocyte numbers are frequently normal, infection is a serious problem because of the lack of granulocytes. The reduced number of platelets is responsible for the bleeding often seen. Bone marrow cellularity is reduced with the replacement of active marrow by fatty tissue.

124.

B. Polycythemia is characterized by an increase in blood viscosity and the total blood volume (hypervolemia). These effects are caused by an increase in the red cell mass. The resultant sluggish blood flow may lead to thrombosis and tissue hypoxia. Relative or "stress" polycythemia is characterized by a decrease in plasma volume.

125.

A. A need for the increased oxygen-carrying capacity provided by additional red blood cells is found in conditions such as pulmonary disease, where normal oxygenation is inhibited. A decrease in the ability of the cardiovascular system to appropriately circulate cells is another reason for increased erythrocytes. Individuals with a high level of methemoglobin, such as heavy smokers or persons with genetic disorders, cannot effectively unload oxygen. This results in a need for increasing the number of red blood cells to compensate. Renal tumors are associated with excess production of erythropoietin, leading to an inappropriate polycythemia.

126.

A. Alpha thalassemia results from a reduced rate of alpha-globin chain synthesis, and beta thalassemia results from a reduced rate of beta-globin chain synthesis. Pernicious anemia is caused by lack of vitamin B_{12}, while hereditary spherocytosis is a membrane protein abnormality. Heinz body anemias result from hemoglobin precipitation associated with unstable hemoglobin configurations or with enzyme deficiencies.

127.

C. Low serum iron and iron stores (represented by serum ferritin) characterize iron deficiency that is severe enough to result in anemia. The production of transferrin, the iron transport protein, increases as iron stores decrease. Transferrin saturation, an expression of the relative content of serum iron to serum transferrin, decreases dramatically.

128.

B. Hemoglobin F can be distinguished from Hb A in red blood cells by the acid elution technique of Kleihauer and Betke. Only hemoglobin F remains in red blood cells after exposure to a citric acid-phosphate buffer solution at pH 3.3. Hb F has a higher oxygen affinity than Hb A and it migrates more slowly on alkaline electrophoresis. A small percentage continues to be produced in normal persons after birth and in patients who are unable to synthesize delta and beta globin chains. No clinical manifestations are seen in patients with hereditary persistence of fetal hemoglobin (HPFH).

129.

A. The hemolytic crisis of malaria results from the rupture of erythrocytes containing merozoites. This event becomes synchronized to produce the fever and chill cycles that are characteristic of this infection. In severe infections, particularly those caused by *Plasmodium falciparum*, the massive intravascular hemolysis results in significant hemoglobinuria.

130.

D. The incorrect ratio of blood to anticoagulant caused the cells to shrink. This gave them the crenated appearance. This is an artifact as opposed to significant clinical finding. Acanthocytes are cells with fewer, less evenly spaced spicules.

131.

A. Pyruvate kinase (PK) is an enzyme of the Embden-Meyerhof pathway (anaerobic glycolysis). A deficiency of PK results in decreased ATP generation and a loss of normal membrane function. PK-deficient cells have a shortened survival time, but clinical manifestations vary widely.

132.

C. Beta thalassemia results from decreased beta globin synthesis and results in small red blood cells with decreased hemoglobin content. Iron deficiency also results in microcytic, hypochromic red cell morphology. Macrocytic cells are seen in pernicious anemia, and cells in the other listed conditions are usually normocytic.

133.

B. Acanthocytes are seen in abetalipoproteinemia and some liver disorders. They are distinguished from echinocytes in that the latter have short, sharp, regular projections (as in crenated red blood cells). Acanthocytes have large, irregular, and rounded projections that result from membranes with altered lipid content.

134.

B. Basophilic stippling is seen on Wright's-stain smears as bluish-black granules. The inclusions represent aggregations of ribosomes (RNA), often in association with metal poisoning and other disorders of hemoglobin synthesis. Precipitated hemoglobin forms Heinz bodies (not visible with Wright's stain), nuclear fragments are called Howell-Jolly bodies, and iron granules are Pappenheimer bodies.

135.

B. The demand for red blood cell replacement in severe thalassemia during early child development results in hyperproliferative marrow. Expansion of the marrow causes the bones to be thin and narrow. This may result in pathologic fractures. Facial bones have the Mongoloid appearance with prominence of the forehead, cheekbones, and upper jaw.

136.

A. Dacrocytes or teardrop red blood cells may result from conditions affecting marrow architecture, such as myelofibrosis. They may also result from removal of inclusions such as Heinz bodies by the spleen. Schistocytes or fragments are common in patients with severe burns and intravascular pathology.

137.

A. Increased red cell distribution width (RDW) is present when there is a heterogeneous cell population with cells of varying sizes. Hemolytic anemias will compensate by releasing cells that are immature and hence larger in size. Macrocytic anemias, such as pernicious anemia, usually represent a single population of large cells, while anemia of chronic blood loss and the anemia that accompanies myelofibrosis represent normocytic, normochromic anemias. Normocytic, normochromic anemias are those with a single cell population but a decreased number of overall cells.

138.

D. Splenomegaly is a common finding in hemolytic anemias because the spleen is the major source of extravascular destruction of red blood cells. Patients with hemoglobinopathies, such as sickle cell anemia, severe C disease, and thalassemias, also exhibit enlarged spleens for the same reason. Splenomegaly caused by extramedullary hematopoiesis is seen in about 75% of patients with polycythemia vera. Splenomegaly does occasionally occur in megaloblastic and iron deficiency anemias (incidence is less than 10%), but this finding would not be characteristic.

LEUKOCYTES

139.

C. The major function of leukocytes is defense, either by phagocytosis or by immune mechanisms. The phagocytic cells are the granulocytes and monocytes. The immune response is mediated by lymphocytes; however, monocytes play a role in immunity as antigen presenting cells. Leukocytes may be classified according to granularity as granulocytes and nongranulocytes or divided based on nuclear segmentation as polymorphonuclears (PMNs) and mononuclears.

140.

D. Monocytes have a diameter of about 20 μm, making them the largest cells in the peripheral blood under normal conditions. Eosinophils and neutrophils have diameters of about 12 μm. The small lymphocyte is 9 μm in diameter, similar to the red blood cell, which has a diameter of 6–8 μm. Large lymphocytes range in size from 11 to 16 μm in diameter.

141.

A. After granulocytes are released from the bone marrow, they remain in the circulation one day or less. Their major function takes place in the tissues. They migrate through the vessel walls to reach areas of inflammation very soon after release. The lifespan of the granulocyte is short; however, eosinophils and basophils appear to survive longer in the tissues than neutrophils.

142.

C. Approximately 50% of the neutrophils in the peripheral blood are found in the circulating pool. This is the pool measured when a total WBC count is done. Another 50% are found on the walls of the vessels (marginal pool). These pools are in constant exchange. Emotional or physical stress will cause a shift of cells from the marginal to the circulating pool, causing a transient rise in the total WBC count.

143.

A. Although some phagocytic activity has been attributed to the eosinophil, it is the segmented neutrophil and monocyte that have the greatest phagocytic activity. The neutrophil is the most important because of numbers and its ability to respond quickly. Monocytes arrive at the site of injury after the neutrophil to "clean up."

144.

B. The growth factor mainly responsible for regulating the production of granulocytes and monocytes is granulocyte-monocyte colony stimulating factor (GM-CSF), which acts on the committed stem cell CFU-GM. G-CSF and M-CSF also play roles in stimulating granulocyte and monocyte production, respectively. Erythropoietin (EPO) is the growth factor mainly responsible for stimulating erythrocyte production, and thrombopoietin (TPO) is responsible for regulating platelet production. Interleukins, particularly IL-3, influence multiple cell lines, including granulocytes and monocytes.

145.

A. The granulocyte mitotic pool contains the cells capable of division, which are the myeloblasts, promyelocytes, and myelocytes. The post-mitotic pool, or reserve, is the largest bone marrow pool and contains metamyelocytes, band and segmented forms. This pool is available for prompt release into the blood if needed (i.e., infection) and its early release is the cause of a "left shift."

146.

B. A "shift to the left" means an increase in immature neutrophilic cells in the blood caused by bone marrow release of cells in response to infection or tissue damage. A redistribution of the blood pools due to emotional or physical stimuli is characterized by an increased WBC count without a left shift. A cell "hiatus" refers to a population of cells in which there is a gap in the normal maturation sequence and is most often seen in acute leukemia in which there are many blasts and a few mature cells but no intermediate stages.

147.

D. Agranulocytosis refers to an absence of granulocytes in both the peripheral blood and bone marrow. A deficiency of granulocytes is found in cases of aplastic anemia, in which deficiencies in red cells and platelets also occur. The early release of cells from the bone marrow will result in immature cells in the blood but is not referred to as agranulocytosis. Neutrophils that exhibit little or no granulation may be called hypogranular or agranular.

148.

B. Antibodies are synthesized by plasma cells, which are end stage B lymphocytes that have transformed to plasma cells following stimulation by antigen. An end-product of T cell activation is the production of cytokines (lymphokines) such as interleukins and growth factors. T cells are surveillance cells that normally comprise the majority (~80%) of lymphocytes in the blood. T cells regulate the immune response by helping (T-helper cells) or suppressing (T-suppressor cells) the synthesis of antibody by plasma cells.

149.

C. Absolute values for cell types are obtained by multiplying the percentage of the type by the total number of cells. In this case, $4000/mm^3 \times 0.65 = 2600/mm^3$, or $2.6 \times 10^9/L$. Although estimates vary, the normal absolute count for lymphocytes is from 1.0 to $4.0 \times 10^9/L$. The normal percentage of lymphocytes is from 20 to 44%. There is a relative lymphocytosis (increase in percentage), but the absolute lymphocyte value is normal.

150.

B. Auer rods are seen in the cytoplasm of malignant cells, most often myeloblasts, and are composed of fused primary (nonspecific, azurophilic) granules. Hypersegmented neutrophils have greater than five lobes and are associated with B_{12} or folate deficiency. Toxic granules are primary granules with altered staining characteristics that stain in late stage neutrophils due to toxicity. Döhle bodies are agranular patches of RNA present in neutrophil cytoplasm and associated with toxic states.

151.

D. White blood cell count reference ranges for males and females are equivalent. WBC counts do change with age, being higher in newborns and children than in adults. Any change from basal conditions, such as exercise or emotional stress, will cause a transient leukocytosis due to a redistribution of blood pools.

152.

C. Neutropenia is associated with risk of infection. The degree of neutropenia correlates with the infection risk from high susceptibility ($< 1.0 \times 10^9$/L) to great risk ($< 0.5 \times 10^9$/L). Infection increases with degree and duration of the neutropenia. Shortness of breath and bleeding tendencies are clinical symptoms of anemia and thrombocytopenia, respectively.

153.

B. Basophils and tissue mast cells have receptors for IgE, which triggers degranulation when appropriate antigens are present and is responsible for severe hypersensitivity reactions (anaphylaxis). Basophils possess water-soluble granules that contain, among other substances, heparin and histamine (a vasodilator and smooth muscle contractor). Basophils have a segmented nucleus and the granules, while often scanty, overlie the nucleus. The mast cell has a single round nucleus and contains many more granules than the basophil.

154.

C. The last stage in the granulocytic series that divides is the myelocyte. Cells prior to and including this stage constitute the bone marrow mitotic pool. Nuclear chromatin progressively clumps and nucleoli are no longer present in the nondividing metamyelocyte stage that follows the myelocyte.

155.

C. Primary or nonspecific granule production begins and ends during the promyelocyte stage. The granules are distributed between daughter cells as mitotic divisions occur. Secondary or specific granule production begins with the myelocyte stage and continues during succeeding cell stages with the synthesis of products specific to the function of the particular granulocyte (neutrophil, eosinophil, or basophil).

156.

B. Eosinophils lack lysozyme, which is present in neutrophils and monocytes, and contain a distinctive peroxidase that differs biochemically from the myeloperoxidase of neutrophils and monocytes. Major basic protein is a component of the granules and is very important to the eosinophil's ability to control parasites. In addition, eosinophils play a role in modifying the allergic reactions caused by degranulation of basophils and mast cells.

157.

A. Primary granules, which appear in the promyelocyte stage, may be called azurophilic or nonspecific granules. Specific or secondary granules (neutrophilic, eosinophilic, basophilic) appear in the myelocyte stage. Primary granules contain hydrolytic enzymes (e.g., myeloperoxidase, lysozyme, acid phosphatase) and are coated with a phospholipid membrane. Lactoferrin is a component of neutrophil granules. Primary granules are often visible in the myelocyte stage but in later stage cells the primary granules, although present, are no longer visible by light microscopy under normal conditions.

158.

A. The presence of toxic granules, Döhle bodies, and/or vacuoles in the cytoplasm of neutrophils (segmented, band, metamyelocyte, and myelocyte stages) are indicative of a neutrophilic response to inflammation. The changes observed in the "toxic" neutrophil may occur in patients with severe burns, some malignancies, exposure to toxic drugs and chemicals, and acute infection (most often bacterial). A Barr body is a "drumstick"-shaped body of nuclear material found in the neutrophils of females that represent the inactive X chromosome and are of no significance. Auer bodies are seen in malignant myeloid cells. Hypersegmented neutrophils are associated with megaloblastic anemias but may be seen in long-term chronic infections. Pyknotic cells and vacuoles may be seen in overwhelming sepsis or old blood. Russell bodies are globular inclusions found in plasma cells that are composed of immunoglobulin.

159.

A. Diapedesis is the movement of cells (usually referring to neutrophils) from the blood stream into the tissues. Chemotaxis is the movement of cells directed by molecular stimuli. Margination is the attachment of neutrophils to the endothelial lining of the blood vessels. Opsonization is the coating of the organism by IgG or complement for recognition (by neutrophils).

160.

D. Basophil granules contain histamine, a potent vasodilator and smooth muscle contractor, which is responsible for the systemic effects seen in certain hypersensitivity reactions. Degranulation occurs when basophils or mast cells are coated with an IgE type of antibody that recognizes a specific allergen, such as bee venom or certain plant pollens. The resulting anaphylactic shock can be life threatening.

161.

B. Monoclonal antibodies (CD surface markers) to specific surface and cytoplasmic antigens can distinguish lymphocyte subpopulations and identify the development stage. Morphologic criteria such as size and granularity cannot be used to identify lymphocyte types. Both B lymphocytes and T lymphocytes can be "reactive" when responding to antigenic stimulation.

162.

B. Plasma cells are the most mature and specialized stage of the B lymphocyte, producing immunoglobulins (antibodies) in response to a specific antigen. Sézary cells are malignant T cells present in the blood of patients with Sézary syndrome, which is the leukemic phase of mycosis fungoides. Virocytes are reactive lymphocytes and thymocytes are immature T cells.

163.

A. A function of the eosinophil is to modify the severe allergic reactions caused by degranulation of the basophil. Neutrophils have receptors for the

opsonins IgG and complement and are the most important cell in the initial defense against acute bacterial infection. Neutrophils are nonspecific phagocytes, ingesting bacteria, fungi, dead cells, etc., and contain hydrolytic enzymes including muramidase (lysozyme) and alkaline phosphatase. Neutrophils die in the performance of their function and are removed by macrophages.

164.

B. Both monocytes and large lymphocytes can contain large azurophilic granules. Lymphocytes lack the fine granules that give monocytes a typical "ground glass" appearance. Indentation by adjacent red cells and a clumpy nuclear chromatin are characteristics of lymphocytes whereas monocytes have a linear chromatin pattern with folds and lobulations.

165.

B. Indentation of the nucleus (kidney shape) is the feature that characterizes the metamyelocyte stage. Specific granules begin forming in the myelocyte and persist through later stages. Cytoplasmic color is not a reliable feature as it is variable and may not differ significantly from the myelocyte or band stage. Nucleoli are absent in metamyelocytes and may not be visible in myelocytes.

166.

A. Young children have the highest peripheral lymphocyte concentrations, ranging from 4.0 to 10.5×10^9 cells/L at age 1 year and declining to 2.0–8.0×10^9 cells/L by 4 years of age. Lymphocyte counts decrease with age, due to a decrease in lymphocyte stimulation and processing of antigens, ranging from 1.0 to 4.0×10^9 cells/L in adults. In addition to the difference in lymphocyte number in children, the normal morphology of children's lymphocytes differs from that of adults. Patient age should be considered when deciding between normal and abnormal lymphocytes.

167.

C. Only TdT, the enzyme marker for terminal deoxynucleotidyl transferase, is present in the earliest lymphoid stem cells of the bone marrow. CALLA (CD10), SIgM, and CIg are present on B cells at later stages of development. TdT can be used to differentiate the leukemic cells of acute lymphocytic leukemia from acute myelogenous leukemia.

168.

C. Acid hydrolases and the number of lysosomes increase as the blood monocyte matures into the tissue macrophage. Macrophages have receptors for IgG and complement and serve as secondary phagocytes, ingesting debris and dead cells (usually neutrophils) at inflammation sites. Macrophages act in the immune response as antigen presenting cells by ingesting and exposing antigens for recognition by lymphocytes.

169.

D. Antigen independent lymphopoiesis occurs in primary lymphoid tissue located in the thymus and bone marrow. The formation of immunocompetent T and B cells from the lymphoid stem cell is influenced by environment (thymus) and interleukins. Antigen dependent lymphopoiesis occurs in secondary lymphoid tissue (spleen, lymph nodes, Peyer's patches) and begins with antigenic stimulation of immunocompetent T and B cells.

170.

D. Myeloperoxidase is an enzyme present in the primary granules, regardless of the phagocytic activity of the cell. The products produced during the respiratory burst, many of them short-lived, are generated in response to chemotactic activation and ingestion of microbes. Generation of oxygen metabolites is necessary for microbial killing.

LEUKOCYTE DISORDERS

171.

C. The Epstein-Barr virus (EBV) attaches to receptors on B lymphocytes and the virus is incorporated into the cell. The infection generates an intense immune response of T cells directed against infected B cells. It is the activated T lymphocytes that comprise the majority of reactive lymphocytes seen in the blood of patients with infectious mononucleosis. Other B cells produce nonspecific polyclonal (heterophile) antibody in response to the EBV infection.

172.

C. The malignant cells of hairy cell leukemia (HCL) stain positive with acid phosphatase in the presence of tartaric acid, i.e., hairy cells contain tartrate resistant acid phosphatase (TRAP). Normal cells stain acid phosphatase positive but staining is inhibited by the addition of tartrate. HCL is a chronic disorder, mainly confined to the elderly. Unlike many other lymphoproliferative disorders, the spleen shows marked enlargement, whereas lymph nodes show minimal changes. Hairy cells are considered to be malignant B cells.

173.

A. The lymphoid cells of acute lymphocytic leukemia FAB type L3 are morphologically identical to the cells of Burkitt's lymphoma. In both disorders, the malignant B cells are large and uniform in size, have moderately abundant basophilic cytoplasm, and prominent cytoplasmic vacuoles. The cells of chronic lymphocytic leukemia (CLL) are identical to the cells of small lymphocytic lymphoma (SLL). Mycosis fungoides and Sézary syndrome are different stages of a T cell lymphoma in which the skin is the early site of involvement.

174.

D. A leukoerythroblastic blood picture, which refers to the presence of both immature neutrophils and nucleated red cells, is most commonly associated with conditions involving bone marrow infiltration by malignant cells (leukemia, lymphoma) or replacement by fibrotic tissue. A neutrophilic left shift is defined as the presence of increased numbers of immature neutrophils in the blood without nucleated red cells. A regenerative left shift and a neutrophilic leukemoid reaction are characterized by varying degrees of leukocytosis and a neutrophilic left shift found in response to infection. In contrast, a degenerative left shift refers to leukopenia and a left shift that may occur if marrow pools are depleted in overwhelming infection.

175.

A. "True" Pelger-Huët anomaly is a benign autosomal dominant trait characterized by hyposegmentation of the granulocytes, coarse nuclear chromatin, and normal cytoplasmic granulation. The cells have no functional defect. It is of practical importance to recognize this anomaly so that it is not confused with a shift to the left due to infection. Acquired or "pseudo" Pelger-Huët is commonly associated with myeloproliferative disorders, myelodysplastic syndromes, or drug therapy. The cytoplasm of pelgeroid cells is frequently hypogranular.

176.

A. Eosinophils are decreased in Cushing's disease, in which the adrenal glands secrete large amounts of adrenocorticosteroids. Eosinophils are increased in allergic disorders, various skin diseases, and certain types of parasitic infections (especially those due to intestinal and tissue-dwelling worms). Eosinophilia is also seen in chronic myelocytic leukemia.

177.

D. Chronic granulomatous disease (CGD) is a hereditary disorder in which neutrophils are incapable of killing most ingested microbes. The disease is usually fatal because of defective generation of oxidative metabolism products, such as superoxide anions and hydrogen peroxide, which are essential for killing. Chemotaxis, lysosomes, phagocytosis, and neutrophil morphology are normal. Several variants of CGD have been described, with specific enzyme defects and different modes of inheritance. The more common type of CGD has a sex-linked inheritance pattern.

178.

D. Abnormal oxygen metabolism of neutrophils can be detected by nitroblue tetrazolium (NBT) dye reduction. Individuals with chronic granulomatous disease (CGD) lack the respiratory burst and fail to reduce the nitroblue tetrazolium dye, while normal activated phagocytes are able to reduce the NBT dye. The anomalies listed have normal NBT activity.

179.

C. Primary or essential thrombocythemia (ET) is a chronic myeloproliferative disorder in which the main cell type affected is the platelet. An extremely high number of platelets are produced; however, abnormal platelet function leads to both bleeding and clotting problems. The bone marrow shows megakaryocytic hyperplasia. Hemoglobin values and platelet counts are increased in polycythemia vera; CML is characterized by a high WBC count. Malignant thrombocythemia must be differentiated from a reactive thrombocytosis seen in patients with infection or following surgery. In reactive causes the platelet count is rarely over 1 million $\times 10^9$/L, platelet function is normal, and thrombocytosis is transient.

180.

B. The bone marrow is progressively replaced by fibrous tissue in myelofibrosis, a chronic myeloproliferative disorder. Attempts to aspirate bone marrow usually result in a "dry tap." A biopsy stain demonstrates increased fibrosis. The presence of teardrop-shaped red blood cells is an important feature of myelofibrosis. In addition, abnormal platelets, a leukoerythroblastic blood picture, and myeloid metaplasia in the spleen and liver are often associated with this disease. A high LAP score (reference range 13–160) and increased RBC mass are found in polycythemia vera; the LAP score is low in chronic myelocytic leukemia.

181.

B. A striking lymphocytosis may be seen in children with pertussis but normal lymphocytes, rather than reactive lymphocytes, are present. A relative and/or absolute lymphocytosis with reactive lymphocytes in various stages of activation (see Color Plate 11) is characteristic of infection caused by Epstein-Barr virus (EBV), cytomegalovirus, and toxoplasmosis. A positive heterophile antibody test can help distinguish infectious mononucleosis caused by EBV from conditions with a similar blood picture.

182.

A. B cell chronic lymphocytic leukemia (CLL) is by far the most common type found in the United States. T cell CLL is a rare and more aggressive disease. Immune dysfunction such as hypogammaglobulinemia or development of immune hemolytic anemia is associated with the malignant B cells of CLL.

183.

D. Waldenström's macroglobulinemia is caused by a proliferation of transitional B lymphocytes, called plasmacytoid lymphs, that secrete high amounts of monoclonal IgM. Because IgM is a macroglobulin, blood hyperviscosity is the cause of many of the symptoms found in this disease. Plasmapheresis reduces the IgM protein concentration.

184.

B. A leukemoid reaction is one that mimics the type of blood picture seen in leukemia. It is associated with extremely elevated leukocyte counts (often > 50 $\times 10^9$ cells/L) and is usually found in severe infection. The most common type of leukemoid reaction is neutrophilic but lymphocytic leukemoid reactions also occur. The leukocyte alkaline phosphatase stain can be used to distinguish neutrophilic leukemoid reactions due to bacterial infection from chronic myelogenous leukemia.

185.

D. An LE cell is described as a phagocyte that has ingested a homogeneous mass of nuclear material. The antinuclear antibody present in patients with systemic lupus erythematosus (SLE) depolymerizes nuclear material that stimulates phagocytosis by a neutrophil or a monocyte. Spontaneous formation of the LE cell phenomenon may occur *in vivo*.

186.

D. Progression to acute leukemia is a very unlikely event for patients with chronic lymphocytic leukemia. Patients with chronic myelocytic leukemia typically progress to "blast crisis," most often of myeloid type. Refractory anemia with excess blasts (RAEB) and refractory anemia with excess blasts in transformation (RAEB-t) are the most likely types of myelodysplastic syndrome to develop acute myelogenous leukemia.

187.

A. Gaucher's disease is a lipid storage disorder in which there is an accumulation of glucocerebroside in the macrophages due to a genetic lack of glucocerebrosidase, an enzyme required for normal lipid metabolism. Gaucher's cells are found in the liver, spleen, and bone marrow. Niemann-Pick disease is caused by a deficiency of sphingomyelinase in which "foamy" macrophages (Niemann-Pick cells) are filled with sphingomyelin. Normal macrophages may contain iron and other cellular debris.

188.

D. The presence of Reed-Sternberg cells in a lymph node biopsy is the diagnostic feature of Hodgkin's disease (HD). The Reed-Sternberg giant cell is usually binucleated and each lobe has a prominent eosinophilic nucleoli. Its origin is controversial. An absolute lymphocytosis with a predominance of mature appearing lymphocytes is characteristic of chronic lymphocytic leukemia. Circulating T cells with a convoluted nucleus (Sézary cells) are seen in Sézary syndrome, the leukemic phase of

mycosis fungoides. A predominance of immature B cells with nuclear clefts is most descriptive of cells seen in some types of peripherilized non–Hodgkin's lymphoma.

189.

B. A drug-induced megaloblastic anemia with macrocytic ovalocytes and hypersegmented neutrophils, as seen in Color Plate 12, is a common finding in patients receiving antifolate drugs such as methotrexate or hydroxyurea. Growth factors, which stimulate granulocyte and monocyte production, are used to rescue patients after high-dose chemotherapy. Chloramphenicol is an antibiotic with a known association for marrow suppression.

190.

B. The abnormal cells found in acute promyelocytic leukemia, FAB type M3, contain large numbers of azurophilic granules. These granules contain procoagulants that on release hyperactivate coagulation resulting in disseminated intravascular coagulation. Although other acute leukemias may initiate DIC, M3 is the one most often associated with coagulopathies.

191.

D. Although a hallmark of acute lymphocytic leukemia (ALL), lymphadenopathy is not associated with acute nonlymphocytic leukemia (ANLL). Hepatomegaly and splenomegaly are associated with both ALL and ANLL, as well as the presence of anemia, neutropenia, and thrombocytopenia. Common presenting symptoms are fatigue, infection, or bleeding. If untreated, both ALL and ANLL have a rapidly fatal course.

192.

B. Refer to Color Plate 13. Chronic lymphocytic leukemia (CLL) is characterized by an absolute lymphocytosis and a predominance of small, mature lymphocytes in the peripheral blood. Elevated leukocyte counts are usual and fragile; smudged lymphocytes may be present. CLL is most often seen in elderly patients, whereas acute lymphocytic leukemia (ALL) typically occurs in children and is characterized by immature lymphoid cells. Plasmacytoid lymphocytes may be found in the blood of individuals with Waldenström's disease. Viral infections are associated with a lymphocytosis and the presence of reactive lymphocytes that are heterogeneous in morphology. Reactive lymphocytes exhibit a variety of forms with regard to size and cytoplasmic staining intensity as compared to the homogeneous cell populations present in malignant disorders such as CLL and ALL.

193.

A. The "packed" bone marrow with predominantly immature blast cells and few normal precursor cells, as seen in Color Plate 14, is most indicative of a patient with acute leukemia. Although chronic leukemias often have a hypercellular marrow, the malignant cells are more mature or differentiated. Dysmyelopoietic syndromes are associated with a hypercellular bone marrow but the blast percent is not greater than 30%. Aplastic anemia is characterized by a hypocellular bone marrow with few cells.

194.

C. The excretion of large amounts of monoclonal IgG or other immunoglobulin light chains produces a characteristic M spike on serum and urine protein electrophoresis. In some cases, only the light chains are produced in excess. Since the light chains are easily cleared by the kidneys, they may appear only in the urine (Bence-Jones proteinuria).

195.

C. Multiple myeloma is a malignant lymphoproliferative disorder characterized by a clonal proliferation of plasma cells. Myeloproliferative disorders are characterized by a proliferation of bone marrow cells (granulocytic, monocytic, erythrocytic, megakaryocytic) with one cell type primarily affected. For example, the main cell type affected in polycythemia vera is the erythrocyte and the platelet is mainly affected in essential thrombocythemia. Transformation between the myeloproliferative disorders is frequent.

196.

C. The first chromosome abnormality associated with a malignancy was the Philadelphia chromosome which is a balanced translocation involving chromosomes 9 and 22. Approximately 90% of cases of chronic myelocytic leukemia have the t(9;22) in leukemic cells of the bone marrow and blood. Other translocations have diagnostic or prognostic significance with disorders as follows: t(8;21) with acute myelocytic leukemia, type M2, t(15;17) with acute promyelocytic leukemia, and t(8;14) with Burkitt's lymphoma.

197.

D. The Philadelphia chromosome (Ph) is an acquired translocation associated with about 90% of patients with chronic myelogenous leukemia (CML). The prognosis for CML patients with the Ph chromosome is better than for Ph chromosome negative patients. The most common chromosomal abnormalities are translocations that result from the movement of a DNA segment from one chromosome to another and are often associated with oncogene rearrangement.

198.

A. The blood picture of both chronic myelocytic leukemia (CML) and a neutrophilic leukemoid reaction is characterized by extremely high leukocyte counts with immature neutrophils. Splenomegaly is associated with CML rather than a leukemoid reaction. The presence of toxic granules and Döhle bodies would be typical of a leukemoid reaction caused by a severe bacterial infection. The LAP score is low in CML and high in a neutrophilic leukemoid reaction.

199.

C. In Color Plate 15, the malignant blast cell contains an Auer rod composed of fused primary granules which stains positive with myeloperoxidase and Sudan black B. Auer rods are not seen in lymphoblasts and their presence is diagnostic of acute nonlymphocytic leukemias such as acute myelocytic or acute myelomonocytic leukemia. Multiple auer rods may be seen in acute promyelocytic leukemia. Auer rods stain negatively with LAP, which detects the enzyme alkaline phosphatase in neutrophil granules.

200.

D. At presentation, patients with chronic leukemia (e.g., CLL or CML) consistently have elevated leukocyte counts, while individuals with acute leukemia may present with low, normal, or high leukocyte counts. The hallmark findings of anemia, thrombocytopenia, and neutropenia are often found in patients with acute leukemia at the time of diagnosis. Patients with chronic leukemia may have few symptoms at onset, with anemia and thrombocytopenia developing during progression of the disease.

201.

D. Leukocyte alkaline phosphatase (LAP) scores are usually low in patients with chronic myelocytic leukemia (CML). The LAP reflects alkaline phosphatase activity in neutrophils and the score is usually elevated in conditions where neutrophils are activated and/or increased in number, such as late pregnancy, bacterial infection, and polycythemia vera. The primary use of the LAP is to distinguish between the malignant cells of CML and a severe bacterial infection (leukemoid reaction). It may also be used to distinguish between CML and polycythemia vera (PV).

202.

C. Acute viral hepatitis is associated with lymphocytosis. The major causes of neutrophilia are bacterial infection, neoplastic tumors, and inflammatory responses to tissue injury. "Toxic" neutrophils may be present. Infection with organisms other than bacteria (fungi, some parasites, certain viruses) may also cause neutrophilia.

203.

D. Monocytes must be distinguished from reactive lymphocytes, which are the characteristic feature of infectious mononucleosis. Monocytosis occurring in the recovery stage of acute infections is considered a favorable sign. An increase in monocytes is associated with collagen disorders, tuberculosis, and malignant conditions such as myelodysplastic syndromes and monocytic leukemias.

204.

B. The periodic acid-Schiff (PAS) stain is used most often to detect intracellular glycogen deposits in the lymphoblasts of acute lymphocytic leukemia in which coarse clumps of PAS positive material may be observed. Myeloblasts and monoblasts usually show a faint staining reaction. The PAS can be used to distinguish the malignant erythroid precursors of erythroleukemia, which show strong PAS positivity, from normal erythrocytic cells that stain negative.

205.

D. Myelodysplastic syndromes (MDS) are characterized by a hypercellular bone marrow and up to 30% marrow blasts that distinguishes MDS from acute leukemia. The blood and bone marrow blast percentages differ and the risk of transformation to acute leukemia varies with the five FAB types of MDS. These disorders are characterized by one or more peripheral blood cytopenias along with features of abnormal growth (dyspoiesis) in the bone marrow. Abnormalities may be morphologic and/or functional. Criteria which help define the types of myelodysplastic syndrome include: megaloblastoid maturation of erythroid precursors, ringed sideroblasts, neutrophils with decreased granules and/or hyposegmentation, percent of monocytes, abnormal platelet morphology, circulating micromegakaryocytes, and degree of dyspoiesis.

206.

A. Naphthol AS-D chloroacetate esterase (specific) reacts strongly in granulocytic cells and alpha-naphthyl acetate esterase (nonspecific) stains positively in monocytic cells. The esterase stains are used to distinguish between types of acute myelogenous leukemia. The leukemic cells of FAB types M1 and M2 will stain positive with specific esterase and negative with nonspecific esterase. The leukemic cells of FAB type M5 will stain positive with nonspecific esterase and negative with specific esterase. The cells of FAB type M4 (AMML) will show positivity with both specific and nonspecific esterase.

207.

A. May-Hegglin anomaly is an autosomal dominant disorder in which large blue cytoplasmic structures that resemble Döhle bodies are found in the granulocytes and possibly the monocytes. Leukocytes are normal in function. Platelets are decreased in number and abnormally large. About one-third of patients have a prolonged bleeding time and mild to severe bleeding problem.

208.

D. Alder-Reilly anomaly is a hereditary autosomal recessive disorder caused by a deficiency of enzymes involved in the metabolism of mucopolysaccharides. Partially degraded mucopolysaccharides accumulate in various tissues, organs, and the leukocytes that are characterized by the presence of large azurophilic granules resembling toxic granulation. The inclusions do not affect leukocyte function and are referred to as Alder-Reilly bodies. The anomaly is often associated with facial and skeletal abnormalities, such as those seen in Hunter's syndrome and Hurler's syndrome. Lysosomal fusion with impaired degranulation is the defect in Chédiak-Higashi syndrome.

209.

C. Serum and urine protein electrophoresis detects the presence of an M spike, the first essential step in establishing the disorder as a monoclonal gammopathy such as multiple myeloma or Waldenström's disease. This can be followed by immunoelectrophoresis to determine the class of immunoglobulin or chain type. Immunologic markers, cytochemical stains, and cytogenetics are used in conjunction with cell morphology to diagnose malignant conditions.

210.

C. The prognosis is poor for patients with stage IV Hodgkin's disease in which there is widespread disease including bone marrow involvement. Stage I or II Hodgkin's disease has a very good prognosis for cure. The clinical course and treatment varies with the extent of disease and morphologic subtype (Rye classification). Hodgkin's disease has two peaks of occurrence: young adults (late twenties) and older adults (fifties). Men have about a 40% higher incidence of the disease than women.

211.

C. The acute leukemia indicated by these results is acute myelomonocytic leukemia, FAB type M4, which has both granulocytic and monocytic features. Note the monocytic characteristics of the blast cells in Color Plate 16. CD14 is a monocytic marker and CD33 is a marker for primitive myeloid cells. The SBB shows positive staining in both granulocytic and monocytic cells, the specific esterase stains positive in granulocytic cells, and the nonspecific esterase is positive in monocytic cells.

212.

B. Acute lymphoblastic leukemia (ALL) of children has the best prognosis. Other favorable factors include FAB type L1, children between ages 3 and 7, mild to moderate increases in the peripheral white count prior to treatment, and common ALL (CALLA) type. Leukemia in adults is less favorable; remissions are shorter and more difficult to induce.

213.

B. The test that would be the most beneficial for the diagnosis of Hodgkin's lymphoma is a lymph node biopsy. Lymphadenopathy is the major clinical presentation of Hodgkin's disease and early stages do not have bone marrow involvement. A skin biopsy would be indicated for diagnosis of mycosis fungoides, a T cell lymphoma of the skin. A bone marrow exam and spinal tap are important to the diagnosis of acute leukemias.

214.

A. A hypercellular bone marrow and high M:E ratio is most characteristic of the excessive granulocyte production that occurs in chronic myelocytic leukemia. Polycythemia vera typically has a hypercellular marrow with panhyperplasia and a normal or low M:E ratio. Beta thalassemia major is a severe hemolytic anemia in which RBC hyperplasia of the marrow is pronounced and a low M:E ratio is usual. Aplastic anemia is associated with a hypocellular marrow with a reduction of all cell lines and normal M:E ratio.

215.

B. Refractory anemia with ringed sideroblasts (RARS) is a myelodysplastic syndrome (MDS) that may also be referred to as primary or idiopathic sideroblastic anemia. The main findings that characterize this type of MDS include anemia with a heterogeneous population of red cells, a hypercellular bone marrow with < 5% blasts, and the presence of >15% ringed sideroblasts in the marrow (demonstrated with Prussian blue stain). RA and RARS are the least likely MDS types to progress to acute nonlymphocytic leukemia.

216.

C. Recent strenuous exercise or other physical and emotional stimuli cause a transient increase in the leukocyte count. This is due to a redistribution of the blood pools. Marrow injury to stem cells or marrow replacement by malignant cells causes neutropenia of varying degrees. Chemotherapeutic drugs suppress bone marrow production of neutrophils. Neutropenia may also be caused by immune mechanisms or viral infection.

217.

C. Primary polycythemia (vera) is a malignant myeloproliferative disorder characterized by autonomous marrow production of erythrocytes in the presence of low erythropoietin levels. Usual findings include increased RBC mass with elevated hemoglobin values and variable degrees of leukocytosis and thrombocytosis (pancytosis). Splenomegaly, a high LAP score, and problems caused by blood viscosity are typical.

218.

D. Basophilia (and eosinophilia) is a typical finding in patients with chronic myelocytic leukemia (CML). A progressive increase in basophil number suggests transformation of the disease to a more accelerated phase. Myeloproliferative disorders such as CML, polycythemia vera, or AML are often associated with peripheral basophilia, which is not a feature of lymphoproliferative disorders such as ALL.

219.

C. More than 50% of the marrow cells are erythroid in acute erythroleukemia, type M6. Giant erythroid precursors, bizarre and multinucleated red cells, and increased myeloblasts are found in the marrow and may appear in the blood. Patients with erythroleukemia typically evolve to acute leukemia indistinguishable from FAB types M1, M2, or M4.

220.

A. Plasma cell dyscrasias are clonal diseases involving malignant B cells in which overproduction of immunoglobulin is a hallmark and the presence of red cell rouleaux is a characteristic finding on the blood smear (refer to Color Plate 17). Excessive amounts of a monoclonal immunoglobulin result in the deposition of proteins on circulating red cells that causes red cell "coining." The erythrocyte sedimentation rate is extremely elevated in these disorders due to spontaneous rouleaux formation.

221.

C. The production of hematopoietic cells in sites outside of the bone marrow can be referred to as myeloid metaplasia or extramedullary hematopoiesis. Hematopoiesis, with the exception of lymphopoiesis, is normally confined to the bone marrow during postnatal life. Production of erythroid, myeloid, and megakaryocytic elements can be established in the liver and spleen, similar to that which occurs during embryonic development.

Myeloid metaplasia is frequently associated with myelofibrosis, a condition in which the marrow is gradually replaced by fibrotic tissue.

222.

A. Prominent lymphadenopathy is the most consistent finding in non–Hodgkin's lymphoma at presentation but lymphoma may arise in the spleen, liver, or GI tract. Lymphomas begin as localized tumors involving lymphoid tissue that spread to the bone marrow and blood. Leukemias are initially systemic disorders primarily involving the bone marrow and blood at onset. Bone lesions are associated with multiple myeloma. Several classification systems for the non–Hodgkin's lymphoma exist, which use morphologic criteria, immunologic markers, and correlations between histologic type and clinical course of the disease to classify this group of heterogeneous disorders.

METHODOLOGY

223.

B. The standard assay for hemoglobin utilizes potassium ferricyanide. This solution, formerly called Drabkin's reagent, is now called cyanmethemoglobin (HiCN) reagent. The ferricyanide oxidizes hemoglobin iron from ferrous to ferric, and the potassium cyanide stabilizes the pigment as cyanmethemoglobin for spectrophotometric measurement.

224.

C. Hemoglobin H is composed of four beta-globin chains. Since the beta chain of hemoglobin is comprised of 146 amino acids in comparison with 141 amino acids in alpha chains, there is a greater net negative charge. This causes hemoglobin H to move farthest from the point of origin towards the anode (+) in an alkaline electrical field.

225.

C. Hemoglobins S, D, and G all migrate to the same location on the hemoglobin electrophoresis gel at an alkaline pH. However, since hemoglobins D and G are nonsickling hemoglobins, tests based on sickle formation under decreased oxygen tension will have negative results. These hemoglobins can be further differentiated by their movement on agar gel at an acid pH, where hemoglobins D and G will migrate with hemoglobin A, not with hemoglobin S.

226.

C. When the sample is deoxygenated, reduced hemoglobin S polymerizes, resulting in a cloudy solution. A false negative can be obtained if the quantity of hemoglobin S is below the sensitivity of the method, which can be seen in newborns and anemic patients. Although this procedure is a screening test for hemoglobin S detection, it is positive in the presence of any sickling hemoglobin, such as hemoglobin C_{Harlem}.

227.

A. A slanted tube increases the ESR. Fibrinogen concentration is proportional to the rate of rouleaux formation. A clotted sample, which lacks fibrinogen, causes a falsely decreased ESR. The EDTA tube for ESR must be at least half-full, and the test must be set up within 4 hours of draw; failure to follow these guidelines results in poikilocytosis that will inhibit rouleaux formation.

228.

C. Some patients develop EDTA-dependent platelet agglutinins caused by an IgM or IgG platelet-specific antibody. To correct for this, the sample can be redrawn in sodium citrate and rerun. The dilution factor of blood to anticoagulant in sodium citrate is 9:1. To compensate for this dilution factor, the platelet count obtained must be multiplied by 1.1. (300×10^9/L $\times$ 1.1 = 330×10^9/L)

229.

B. Blood smears should be made within 3 hours of collection from blood anticoagulated with ethylenediaminetetraacetic acid (EDTA). Although some of the blood cells may still be normal in blood kept longer, others (especially granulocytes) may deteriorate. Vacuolation of neutrophils can appear as an artifact in blood kept past this time. The age of the blood may also affect the visual quality when the slide is stained.

230.

A. The angle normally used for the spreader slide when a smear is made is 25 degrees. Increasing the angle will produce a shorter, thicker smear. Decreasing the angle will produce a longer, thinner smear.

231.

D. One type of Romanowsky stain is the Wright's stain. It is the most popular blood stain in the

United States. It is a polychrome stain consisting of methylene blue and eosin. This combination causes multiple colors to appear on staining. Brilliant green and neutral red are used in a supravital stain for Heinz bodies. Crystal violet and safranin are used in Gram's stain for bacteria.

232.

C. When red blood cells are stained correctly with Wright's stain, their color is pink to orange-red. They will appear bright red in the presence of an acid buffer. Staining elements such as white cells, which stain with a more basic pH, will not take up the stain adequately in this instance. Inadequate washing and an alkaline stain or buffer mixture results in a smear that is excessively blue.

233.

C. The formula for calculating a reticulocyte count in percent is

$$\frac{\text{Number of reticulocytes counted}}{\text{Total number of RBCs counted}} \times 100$$

In the case described in Question 233,

$$\% \text{Reticulocytes} = \frac{60}{1000} \times 100 = 6.0\%$$

Since the error in reticulocyte counts is high, it is desirable to count a larger number of cells or use a standardized counting method such as the Miller disc.

234.

C. The formula used to calculate the absolute reticulocyte count is

$$\frac{\text{Reticulocyte percent}}{100} \times \text{RBC} (10^{12}/\text{L}) \times 1000$$

Multiplication by 1000 is done to report the results in SI units of 10^9/L.

In this case, $\frac{6.0 \times 3.00}{100} \times 1000 = 180 \times 10^9$/L

235.

B. As visualized in Color Plate 18, Sudan black B is a histochemical stain for lipids, including steroids, phospholipids, and neutral fats. It is widely used as a tool to differentiate the blasts of acute lymphocytic leukemia (ALL) from those of acute non-lymphocytic leukemia (ANLL). Blasts in ALL are negative, whereas those in ANLL will show some degree of positivity.

236.

B. An LAP score is determined by first multiplying the number of cells found by the degree of positivity (i.e., 24 × 1 = 24). These numbers are then added to obtain a final score. In this instance, 0 + 24 + 42 + 45 + 32 = 143.

237.

C. When stained with a mixture of potassium ferricyanide and hydrochloric acid, nonheme iron stains bright blue. This is the most common stain used for storage iron. It can be used on bone marrow to identify sideroblasts, peripheral blood to identify the presence of siderocytes, or urine for hemosiderin testing, among other uses.

238.

C. Pappenheimer bodies are iron deposits associated with mitochondria, and they stain with both procedures, Perl's Prussian blue and Wright's stain. A cell that contains Pappenheimer bodies is called a siderocyte. Howell-Jolly bodies and basophilic stippling can be visualized with Wright's stain, whereas Heinz bodies require a supravital stain to be seen.

239.

B. Depth on a standard counting chamber is 0.10 mm. The formula to calculate volume is $V = A \times D,$ where V is volume, A is area, and D is depth. When the counting chamber is used, the area may change, depending on the number of ruled squares counted, but the depth remains constant.

240.

B. The standard formula for hemacytometer counts expressed in mm^3 is

$$\frac{\text{total number cells counted} \times \text{dilution factor}}{\text{area counted} \times \text{depth}}$$

In this instance

$$\frac{308 \times 20}{8 \text{ mm}^2 \times 0.10 \text{ mm}} = \frac{6160}{0.8 \text{ mm}^3} =$$

$$7700/\text{mm}^3 = 7.7 \times 10^9/\text{L}$$

241.

B. The Rule of Three states that RBC × 3 = Hgb and Hgb × 3 = Hct ±3 in error-free results. These rules apply only for normocytic, normochromic erythrocytes. One check to determine if an error has occurred is to determine the MCHC. An MCHC should be less than 360 g/L (36 g/dL) in error-free results. The MCHC is calculated by dividing hemoglobin by hematocrit, and multiplying by 100. In instance (B), the MCHC is 407 g/L (40.7 g/dL) and the rules of three are broken. All other answers follow the rules.

242.

A. The only *true* cause of a high MCHC is the presence of spherocytes, as may be seen in hereditary spherocytosis. Since the MCHC is a calculation using the hemoglobin and hematocrit, anything causing those parameters to be wrong will affect the MCHC. The occurrence of a falsely high MCHC is much more common than the presence of spherocytes, and specimen-troubleshooting procedures must be undertaken in order to obtain reportable results.

243.

C. The Coulter principle uses electrical impedance as a means of measuring cell count and size. Blood cells are nonconductors of electrical current; they create a resistance/impedance of current in a diluent solution that is conductive. When the suspension is forced through a small aperture, the current flow is interrupted by the presence of the cells. A pulse is generated. The number of pulses generated is proportional to the number of particles present, and the size of the pulse generated is proportional to the size of the cell.

244.

C. To show a significant difference, a second cell count needs to be greater than ±2 standard deviations (±2 s) from the first count. For example, if a WBC count is 12.0 × 10^9/L (12.0 × 10^3/μL) with 2 s of ±0.5, then a succeeding count must be greater than 12.5 × 10^9/L (12.5 × 10^3/μL) or less than 11.5 × 10^9/L (11.5 × 10^3/μL) to be considered significantly different. Using ±2 s, 95% confidence limits are achieved; 95% confidence limits predict a range that values should fall within 95% of the time.

245.

B. Right-angle scatter of a laser beam increases with granularity of the cytoplasm. Forward-scatter is used to enumerate cells and determine their relative size. The presence of specific antigens in the cytoplasm or on the cell surface is determined by immunofluorescence after reactions with appropriate antibodies.

246.

A. β-Thalassemia major is a disorder in which large numbers of nucleated red blood cells (nRBCs) are found (refer to Color Plate 19). Impedance instruments count nuclei as WBCs. An automated instrument cannot differentiate between the nucleus of a white blood cell and the nucleus of an nRBC, and both will be counted as WBCs. The presence of 5 or more nRBCs/100 WBCs can result in a falsely elevated white blood cell count, and a correction must be made as follows:

Corrected WBC count =

$$\text{Observed count} \times \frac{100}{100 + \#nRBCs/100 \text{ WBCs}}$$

247.

D. Hemoglobin A_2 values up to 3.5% are considered normal. Values between 3.5% and 8.0% are indicative of β-thalassemia minor. Hemoglobins C, E, and O have net electrical charges similar to hemoglobin A_2. They elute off with hemoglobin A_2 using anion exchange (column) chromatography, causing an invalid hemoglobin A_2 result. If the hemoglobin A_2 quantification using column chromatography yields a result greater than 8.0%, one of these interfering hemoglobins should be considered.

248.

D. In the test for osmotic fragility, red blood cells are added to decreasing concentrations of sodium chloride. Normal plasma salt concentration is 0.85%. Normal red blood cells shown in curve B will show beginning hemolysis at approximately 0.45% concentration, and complete hemolysis at a 0.30% concentration. Red cells that lyse at a higher concentration than normal show increased osmotic fragility and decreased resistance to lysis.

249.

D. The spherocyte cannot withstand reduced osmotic pressure because it has a decreased surface to volume ratio. It is unable to expand as much as normal discocytes, so even small amounts of fluid entering the spherocyte will cause lysis. Spherocytes are seen in hereditary spherocytosis, severe burns, and immune hemolytic anemias.

250.

B. Curve A indicates decreased osmotic fragility and increased resistance to lysis. This is a characteristic of target cells, also known as codocytes. This type of cell is seen in thalassemias and hemoglobinopathies, which are globin chain disorders. All the other disorders produce cells that have normal or increased osmotic fragility.

251.

C. Standards are commercially available to generate a hemoglobin concentration curve. The absorbance of each solution is read against a reagent blank at 540 nm on a spectrophotometer. Patient blood samples and commercial control materials can be used to assess precision and other quality control parameters.

252.

A. Anything that causes an increase in absorbance will cause a hemoglobin that is read spectrophotometrically to be falsely high. It is necessary to correct for this type of error, such as making a plasma blank in the case of lipemia or icterus. WBCs are present in the hemoglobin dilution and usually do not interfere. When the WBC count is extremely high, their presence will cause cloudiness, increasing the absorbance in the hemoglobin measuring cell and resulting in a falsely high hemoglobin concentration. Excessive anticoagulant does not affect hemoglobin readings.

253.

A. When a microhematocrit is spun at 10,000–15,000 g for 5 minutes, maximum packing is achieved. Spinning a longer time has no affect on the result. White cells and platelets form a buffy coat, distinct from the packed cell volume. Hemolysis damages the RBC membrane and allows for more packing. Results are expressed in liters per liter (L/L), although the older traditional term, percent, is still widely used.

254.

C. The erythrocyte sedimentation rate (ESR) measures the rate of fall of red cells through plasma. ESR increases when cells become stacked (rouleaux, as seen in Color Plate 17); this decreases when cells are not normal discocytes. Larger cells (macrocytes) and fewer cells (anemia) fall faster. Plasma containing increased proteins, such as fibrinogen and globulins, promote rouleaux formation and an elevated ESR. Hemoglobin content does not affect the ESR.

255.

A. Impedance counters measure RBCs and platelets using the same dilution. To differentiate the two, sizing thresholds are used. Particles between 2–20 fL are counted as platelets, and particles larger than 35 fL are counted as RBCs. Small RBCs, clumped and giant platelets fall in the overlap area between platelets and RBCs, generating a warning flag. Nucleated RBCs are larger than normal RBCs and are not mistaken for platelets.

256.

C. A platelet estimate is obtained by multiplying the average number of platelets per oil immersion field (in an erythrocyte monolayer) by 20,000. The reference range for a platelet count is $150–450 \times 10^9$/L. Approximately 8–20 platelets per oil immersion field will represent a normal platelet concentration of approximately $160–400 \times 10^9$/L. This method assumes the red blood cell count is normal. If it is not, alternate platelet estimate procedures may need to be performed.

257.

D. A living cell stain using new methylene blue is performed for reticulocyte counts. Reticulocytes should not be stained for less than 5 minutes, but elapsed times of greater than this are not critical. Howell-Jolly bodies, Pappenheimer bodies, crenated cells, and refractile artifacts can be mistaken for reticulocyte inclusions. Polychrome methylene blue is used in the Wright's stain for peripheral blood smear staining.

258.

B. All laboratories that are College of American Pathologists (CAP) certified are required to calibrate with commercially available calibrators at least once every 6 months. Calibration must be checked if any major part or lengthy tubing is replaced, or if optical alignment is adjusted. A calibration procedure can be verified using commercially available controls.

259.

C. The lipemic plasma interference level can be determined by performing a hemoglobin test on the plasma only. The amount of interference is equal to the plasma hemoglobin value multiplied by the decimal *plasma* fraction, also called the plasmacrit. The plasmacrit is 1 − Hct L/L. In this instance the plasmacrit is 1 − 0.32 L/L, or 0.68 L/L. The amount of interference is then subtracted from the original hemoglobin to determine the true hemoglobin value. In this instance

Original Hgb − (plasmacrit × plasma hemoglobin)
= Corrected Hgb

or

12.0 g/dL − (0.68 L/L × 2.0 g/dL) = 10.6 g/dL

Once this correction has been done, the MCH and MCHC are recalculated using the corrected hemoglobin.

$$MCH = \frac{10.6 \times 10}{3.52} = 30.1 \text{ pg}$$

$$MCHC = \frac{10.6 \times 100}{32.0} = 33.1 \text{ g/dL (331 g/L)}$$

260.

A. Hemoglobin is still valid on a hemolyzed specimen, since RBC lysis is the first step in the cyanmethemoglobin method. The red blood cell count depends on the presence of intact red blood cells. Red blood cell fragments caused by hemolysis may be as small as platelets and affect instruments that utilize sizing criteria to differentiate the two. Therefore, samples for these procedures should be recollected.

261.

D. Heparin is recommended for osmotic fragility and red cell enzyme studies, because it results in less lysis and membrane stress than other anticoagulants. Heparin induces platelet clumping and is unacceptable for the platelet count. Heparin is unacceptable for coagulation test procedures because it binds with antithrombin III to neutralize many enzymes, especially thrombin. This would cause very long coagulation test results. EDTA is recommended for most routine hematology procedures, especially for Wright's-stained smears. Sodium citrate or EDTA can be used for sedimentation rates.

262.

A. When counting platelets, only the central square (1 mm^2) is counted on each side of the hemacytometer. Platelets appear round or oval and may have dendrites. These characteristics can help distinguish them from debris, which is irregularly shaped and often refractile. White cells are not lysed; they may be counted, using a different ruled area of the hemacytometer. Platelets will be easier to count if allowed to settle for 10 minutes, because they will appear in the same plane of focus.

263.

B. Precision is the term used to describe the reproducibility of a method that gives closely similar results when one sample is run multiple times. An accurate method is one that gives results that are very close to the true value. Laboratories must have procedures that are both accurate and precise.

CASE HISTORIES

264.

C. WBC counts done by an impedance cell counter must be corrected when nucleated red blood cells (nRBCs) are present (see Color Plate 19), since such instruments do not distinguish between white and red nucleated cells. This correction is done according to the following formula:

Corrected WBC count =

$$\text{Observed count} \times \frac{100}{100 + \#nRBCs \text{ per } 100 \text{ WBCs}}$$

In this instance:

Corrected WBC count =

$$31.0 \times 10^9/\text{L} \times \frac{100}{100 + 110} = 14.8 \times 10^9/\text{L}$$

265.

A. The appearance of red cells on a differential smear may be predicted by calculating the red cell indices.

$$\text{MCV} = \frac{\text{Hct} \times 10}{\text{RBC}} = \frac{16\% \times 10}{2.50 \times 10^{12}/\text{L}} = 64.0 \text{ fL}$$

$$\text{MCH} = \frac{\text{Hgb} \times 10}{\text{RBC}} = \frac{4.5 \text{ g/dL} \times 10}{2.50 \times 10^{12}/\text{L}} = 18.0 \text{ pg}$$

$$\text{MCHC} = \frac{\text{Hgb} \times 100}{\text{Hct}} = \frac{4.5 \text{ g/dL} \times 100}{16\%}$$
$$= 28.1 \text{ g/dL} (281 \text{ g/L})$$

The mean corpuscular volume (MCV), mean corpuscular hemoglobin (MCH), and mean corpuscu-

lar hemoglobin concentration (MCHC) are all below the reference range. This indicates a cell that is small (microcytic) with a reduced hemoglobin concentration (hypochromic). These indices refer to averages and do not necessarily reflect the actual appearance of cells in which there is great diversity in size and shape.

266.

D. Children with β-thalassemia major, also known as Cooley's anemia, do not use iron effectively to make heme because of a genetic defect causing a decreased rate of production of structurally normal globin chains. In addition, they receive frequent transfusions due to severe anemia. The result is hemochromatosis with a high serum iron and storage iron. None of the other anemias listed are hemolytic, and thus would not explain the high number of nucleated RBCs.

267.

D. β-Thalassemia major is characterized by a lack of ability to produce beta-globin chains, resulting in a decrease or complete absence of hemoglobin A. Hemoglobin F, a compensatory hemoglobin that contains 2 alpha and 2 gamma globin chains, is frequently the only hemoglobin present. Hemoglobin A_2 is classically increased in heterozygous β-thalassemia, but it is variable in homozygous β-thalassemia.

268.

B. The predominant hemoglobin present at birth is hemoglobin F, which consists of two alpha and two gamma globin chains. It is not until about 6 months of age that beta chain production is at its peak. At this point, hemoglobin A (two alpha and two beta chains) replaces hemoglobin F as the predominant hemoglobin. A deficiency in the production of these chains will not be apparent until this beta-gamma switch has occurred.

269.

C. The formula for calculation of transferrin saturation is as follows:

Transferrin saturation %

$$= \frac{\text{Serum iron } (\mu g/dL) \times 100}{\text{TIBC } (\mu g/dL)}$$

In this case,

$$\text{Transferrin saturation } \% = \frac{22 \times 100}{150} = 15\%$$

Since the reference range for saturation is 20–45%, this is a low saturation.

270.

D. The anemia of chronic disorders is caused by a lack of release of storage iron from the macrophages. These patients have iron, but are unable to utilize it. Iron stores are usually normal or elevated. This condition is also thought to result in impaired response to erythropoietin by the bone marrow.

271.

A. The most common anemia among hospitalized patients is anemia of chronic disease. Patients with chronic infections, inflammatory disorders, and neoplastic disorders develop this type of anemia. The typical presentation is of a normocytic, normochromic anemia, but microcytic and hypochromic anemia can develop in long-standing cases. Chronic blood loss can cause iron deficiency, a microcytic, hypochromic anemia.

272.

A. Both megaloblastic anemias and nonmegaloblastic anemias are characterized by the presence of macrocytic, normochromic red cells. Vitamin B_{12} and folic acid are coenzymes necessary for DNA synthesis. Lack of either one causes megaloblastic anemia. Maturation asynchrony is evident in both the peripheral blood and bone marrow. The bone marrow examination is done after Vitamin B_{12} and folate levels because of its invasive nature. Vitamin B_{12} and folic acid levels are normal or increased in nonmegaloblastic anemias. Iron studies are useful in the diagnosis of microcytic, hypochromic anemias.

273.

C. The most common causes of megaloblastic anemia are pernicious anemia and folate deficiency. Pernicious anemia is caused by a lack of intrinsic factor production in the stomach, which is necessary for the absorption of vitamin B_{12}. Since there are large stores of vitamin B_{12} in the liver, it takes from 1 to 4 years for the deficiency to manifest itself. Pernicious anemia is noted for neurological complications and is seen more commonly among people of British and Scandinavian ancestry. Folate is a water-soluble vitamin for which there are few bodily stores. A diet poor in green vegetables and meat products can result in folate deficiency in 2–4 months.

274.

A. The general classification of anemia described here is megaloblastic anemia. The lack of vitamin B_{12} and folate affects DNA production. All dividing cells will show nuclear abnormalities, resulting in megaloblastic changes. In the neutrophil, as seen in Color Plate 12, this takes the form of hypersegmentation (six or more lobes). Enlarged, fragile cells are formed, many of which die in the bone marrow, never making it out into circulation. Macrocytic red blood cells are oval. Pancytopenia is the usual finding. The reticulocyte absolute value if calculated is $13 \times 10^9/\text{L}$, which is low. Inclusions are a common finding. One cause of a nonmegaloblastic macrocytic anemia, which has round cells such as target cells instead of oval cells, is liver disease.

275.

A. The red blood cells are macrocytic and normochromic. The patient is pancytopenic. Cabot rings, which are remnants of spindle fibers that form during mitosis, can be seen in disorders of DNA synthesis. They are not associated with nonmegaloblastic anemia such as liver disease. Further investigation of serum folate and vitamin B_{12} levels is warranted. Dietary history is important. Malabsorption syndromes decrease the absorption of many nutrients, including vitamin B_{12} and folate.

276.

B. Intrinsic factor, needed for vitamin B_{12} absorption, is secreted by the parietal cells. Individuals with pernicious anemia (PA) are incapable of absorbing vitamin B_{12} due to a lack of or antibodies to intrinsic factor. There may be anti–parietal cell autoantibodies present in PA. There is also an associated lack of gastric acidity in this disorder. Achlorhydria is not diagnostic for PA, since it may occur in other disorders (such as severe iron deficiency), but it is confirmatory evidence of the problem. The Schilling test is used to differentiate pernicious anemia from malabsorption syndromes. Part I includes having the patient ingest a tablet of radioactive ^{57}Co-labeled cobalamin. This part will be abnormal in both PA and malabsorption syndromes. Part II is performed in the same manner as Part I, with the addition of a tablet containing intrinsic factor. Patients with PA will have a normal Part II, whereas patients with malabsorption syndromes will still be abnormal. Part II is only performed on patients who initially have an abnormal Part I.

277.

B. Intrinsic factor is necessary for absorption of vitamin B_{12} from the ileum. Giving vitamin B_{12} orally will not increase absorption. Although pharmaceutical doses of folate will correct the megaloblastic changes of PA, they will not correct the neurological symptoms. For this reason, correct diagnosis is crucial.

278.

A. The adult red blood cell in glucose-6-phosphate dehydrogenase (G6PD) deficiency is susceptible to destruction by oxidizing drugs. This occurs because the mechanism for providing reduced glutathione, which keeps hemoglobin in the reduced state, is defective. Primaquine is one of the best-known drugs that may precipitate a hemolytic episode. Ingestion of fava beans can also elicit a hemolytic episode in some patients.

279.

C. G6PD deficiency, a sex-linked disorder, is the most common enzyme deficiency in the hexose monophosphate shunt. Most patients are asymptomatic and go through life being unaware of the deficiency unless oxidatively challenged. Pyruvate kinase, an enzyme in the Embden-Meyerhof pathway, is necessary to generate ATP. ATP is needed for red blood cell membrane maintenance. Patients with a pyruvate kinase deficiency have a chronic mild to moderate anemia.

280.

B. Reduced glutathione levels are not maintained due to a decrease in NADPH production. Methemoglobin (Fe^{3+}) accumulates and denatures in the form of Heinz bodies. Heinz bodies cause rigidity of the RBC membrane, resulting in red cell lysis.

281.

C. Iron deficiency causes a microcytic, hypochromic anemia that is prone to develop in milk-fed infants. The anemia occurs because of the lack of red blood cell production needed to maintain growth, due to the lack of iron available in a diet that consists primarily of milk. Hereditary spherocytosis results in RBCs that are normal to low normal in size, with an MCHC possibly greater than 360 g/L (36 g/dL). Folate deficiency causes a macrocytic, normochromic anemia. Erythroblastosis fetalis is a hemolytic disease of the newborn caused by red blood cell destruction by antibodies from the mother that would no longer exist in the circulation of a 6-month-old child.

282.

D. The development of iron deficiency occurs in three stages. They are the iron depletion stage, the iron deficient erythropoiesis stage, and the iron deficiency anemia stage. Iron stores are the first to disappear, so the serum ferritin level is the earliest indicator of iron deficiency anemia.

283.

C. In iron deficiency anemia, red blood cell production is restricted due to lack of iron, and the reticulocyte absolute value reflects this ineffective erythropoiesis. The formula used to calculate the absolute reticulocyte count is

Absolute reticulocytes $=$
$$\frac{\text{Reticulocytes \%}}{100} \times \text{RBC} (10^{12}/\text{L}) \times 1000$$

The 1000 in the calculation is to convert to SI units (10^9/L).

In this case,

$$\frac{0.2}{100} \times 2.70\,(10^{12}/\text{L}) \times 1000 = 5 \times 10^9/\text{L}$$

The normal absolute reticulocyte count is approximately $18\text{–}158 \times 10^9$/L.

284.

A. Petechiae and ecchymoses (bruises) are primary hemostasis bleeding symptoms seen in quantitative and qualitative platelet disorders. Although estimates vary, spontaneous bleeding does not usually occur until platelet numbers are less than 50×10^9/L. The malignant disorder represented by this case is noted for thrombocytopenia.

285.

A. A high percentage of blast cells are seen in both peripheral blood and bone marrow, as demonstrated in Color Plates 20 and 14, respectively. The leukemic "gap," or "hiatus," between normal and abormal cells indicates the presence of an acute leukemia. The triad of symptoms seen in acute leukemia is neutropenia, anemia, and thrombocytopenia. Both types of chronic leukemia will show the presence of more intermediate and adult cell forms. Acute lymphocytic leukemia is the leukemia most likely to be found in this age group.

286.

C. Periodic acid-Schiff stains glycogen in lymphoblasts. The myeloperoxidase stain is positive in myeloid cells. Monocytes show a positive reaction to the nonspecific esterase stain, which is inhibited by sodium fluoride. Leukocyte alkaline phosphatase is useful in the diagnosis of chronic granulocytic leukemia.

287.

A. Terminal deoxyribonucleotidyl transferase (TdT) is a nuclear enzyme (DNA polymerase) found in stem cells and precursor B- and T-lymphoid cells. High levels of TdT are found in 90% of ALL's. TdT has been found in up to 10% of cases of AML, but in lower levels than are present in ALL. This enzyme is not found in mature lymphocytes.

288.

B. There are now at least 130 recognized human leukocyte antigens, each of which has been given a CD (cluster designation) number. CD 2, 5, and 7 are seen on T-cells. CALLA, the common acute lymphoblastic leukemia antigen, is seen in early pre-B cells. Distinct CD markers have been identified for cells of both lymphoid and myeloid stem cell lineage.

289.

B. The bone marrow blast percent is high enough to indicate an acute leukemia. Sudan black B, myeloperoxidase, and specific esterase stains are positive in the presence of the myeloid cell line. The nonspecific esterase stain is positive with a number of different cell lines, including monocytes. When sodium fluoride is added to the incubation mixture, the staining reaction of monocytes is inhibited or absent.

290.

A. An increase in cell turnover causes hyperuricemia and elevated LD levels. Increased bone resorption frequently causes hypercalcemia. These three findings can be found in any acute leukemia. Murami-

dase (lysozyme) is a hydrolytic enzyme found in the monocytic cell line, and it is elevated in serum and urine of patients with acute leukemia with a monocytic component (FAB M4 and M5).

291.

C. When a diagnosis of AML or myelodysplastic syndrome is suspected, a bone marrow examination is performed. The French-American-British (FAB) approach to the diagnosis of acute leukemia requires the presence of greater than 30% blasts in the bone marrow. A normal bone marrow blast percent is 0–2%. Myelodysplastic syndromes have bone marrow blast percent ranges from 0 up to 30%.

292.

B. HTLV-I is implicated in T-cell leukemia and lymphoma in Japan. The Epstein-Barr virus is associated with Burkitt's lymphoma in Africa. Chronic bone marrow dysfunction can be caused by exposure to radiation, drugs, and chemicals such as benzene. Myelodysplastic syndromes and myeloproliferative disorders are "preleukemic" because they have a high incidence of terminating in acute leukemia. Paroxysmal nocturnal hemoglobinuria, aplastic anemia, multiple myeloma, and lymphoma are stem cell disorders that are particularly noted for transformation into acute leukemia. Genetic susceptibility is associated with Klinefelter's and Down's syndromes, both of which have chromosomal abnormalities. It is likely that more than one factor is responsible for the evolution of an acute leukemia.

293.

A. The myelodysplastic syndromes (MDS) are pluripotential stem cell disorders characterized by one or more peripheral blood cytopenias. Bone marrow examination is necessary for diagnosis. There are prominent maturation abnormalities of all three cell lines in the bone marrow. Megaloblastoid erythrocyte maturation is present that is not responsive to B_{12} or folic acid therapies. While many of the red blood cell inclusions noted in this case can be seen in a megaloblastic anemia such as pernicious anemia, this patient has a normal vitamin B_{12} and folate level. This patient has hyposegmentation of neutrophils, whereas megaloblastic anemias present with hypersegmentation of neutrophils. Of the disorders listed, the only one associated with dyshematopoiesis of all cell lines is myelodysplastic syndrome.

294.

D. In most cases of myelodysplastic syndrome (MDS), the bone marrow is hypercellular with erythroid hyperplasia. MDS is considered a disease of the elderly. Since normal cellularity decreases with age, interpretation of cellularity must take the age of the patient into account. FAB criteria for a diagnosis of MDS are related to bone marrow blast percent, which must be 30% or less.

295.

D. In RAEB at least two cell lines exhibit cytopenia, and all cell lines show evidence of dyshematopoiesis. Poor granulation and pseudo-Pelger-Huët anomaly is seen. There are less than 5% blasts in the peripheral blood, and 5–20% blasts in the bone marrow. Platelets exhibit poor granulation, giant forms, and the abnormal maturation stage of micromegakaryocytes. The five FAB classifications of MDS are RA, RARS, RAEB, CMML, and RAEB-t. CML is a myeloproliferative disorder, not a myelodysplastic syndrome.

296.

C. The myelodysplastic syndromes are refractory to treatment, and patients are supported using blood products dependant on their cytopenias. The median survival rate for all types of MDS is less than 2 years. RAEB and RAEB-t have the highest percentage of blasts, and the lowest survival rates. At this time, bone marrow transplant offers the only chance for a cure, and it is the treatment of choice in patients less than 50 years old. Studies have shown that the incidence of MDS is greater than the incidence of AML in the 50–70-year-old age group. Up to 40% of the MDSs, transform into acute leukemia.

297.

A. A neutrophilic leukemoid reaction represents a normal body response to a severe infection. It is a benign proliferation of WBCs. Toxic changes to the neutrophils such as toxic granulation, vacuoles, and Döhle bodies are present. Chronic myelogenous leukemia (CML) is a myeloproliferative disorder, a malignant proliferation of leukocytes not in response to infection. No toxic changes are present in CML. These two disorders both display a "left" shift, and can be confused with each other.

298.

D. Leukocyte alkaline phosphatase activity is increased in severe infections such as the neutrophilic leukemoid reaction, polycythemia vera, and during the last trimester of pregnancy. It is greatly reduced in chronic myelogenous leukemia, although it may increase during blast crisis of this disease. Periodic acid-Schiff and Sudan black B are used to differentiate ALL from AML. Nitroblue tetrazolium is used to detect oxidative deficiencies in chronic granulomatous disease, a functional WBC disorder.

299.

C. The Philadelphia chromosome is found in the precursor cells for erythrocytes, granulocytes, and platelets in about 90% of the cases of CML. It is not found in PV. It is an acquired chromosome abnormality that results from a reciprocal translocation between chromosomes 9 and 22 (t[9;22]). The chromosome abnormality can be detected even when the patient is in remission.

300.

B. Patients who have the Philadelphia chromosome have a less aggressive disease and better prognosis than those who do not. Some cases of CML terminate in an acute lymphocytic leukemia. However, this outcome cannot be predicted by the presence or absence of the Philadelphia chromosome.

REFERENCES

Beutler, E. (Ed.) (1995). *Williams Hematology,* 5th ed. New York: McGraw-Hill.

Brown, B. A. (1993). *Hematology Principles and Procedures,* 6th ed. Philadelphia: Lea & Febiger.

Carr, J. H., and Rodak, B. F. (1999). *Clinical Hematology Atlas.* Philadelphia: W. B. Saunders.

Harmening, D. M. (Ed.) (1997). *Clinical Hematology and Fundamentals of Hemostasis,* 3rd ed. Philadelphia: F. A. Davis.

McKenzie, S. B. (1996). *Textbook of Hematology,* 2nd ed. Philadelphia: Williams & Wilkins.

Stiene-Martin, E. A., Lotspeich-Steininger, C. A., and Koepke, J. A. (Eds.) (1998). *Clinical Hematology-Principles, Procedures, Correlations,* 2nd ed. Philadelphia: Lippincott.

Turgeon, M. L. (1993). *Clinical Hematology: Theory and Procedures,* 2nd ed. Boston: Little and Brown and Co.

3 Hemostasis

contents

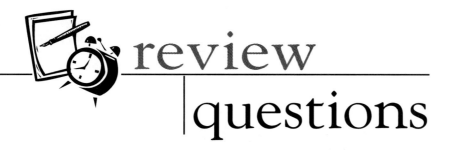

review questions

INSTRUCTIONS Each of the questions or incomplete statements that follow comprises four suggested responses. Select the *best* answer or completion statement in each case.

---

1. The hemorrhagic problems associated with scurvy are due to a deficiency of _____, which is a cofactor required for collagen synthesis.
   A. Vitamin C
   B. Prothrombin
   C. Vitamin K
   D. Protein C

2. Approximately how many platelets does an average megakaryocyte generate?
   A. 1
   B. 50
   C. 175
   D. 2000

3. Thrombocytopenia may be caused by all the following *except*
   A. Post-splenectomy
   B. Chemotherapy
   C. Decreased thrombopoietin
   D. Aplastic anemia

4. During the hemostatic process, platelets interacting with and binding to other platelets is referred to as
   A. Adhesion
   B. Aggregation
   C. Release
   D. Retraction

5. In platelet aggregation studies, certain aggregating agents induce a biphasic aggregation curve. To what is the second phase of aggregation directly related?
   A. Formation of fibrin
   B. Changes in platelet shape
   C. Release of endogenous ADP
   D. Release of platelet factor 3

6. The platelet aggregation pattern drawn below is characteristic of what aggregating agent?
   A. ADP
   B. Collagen
   C. Ristocetin
   D. Thrombin

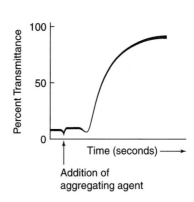

7. What is the operating principle of a platelet aggregometer?
   A. Aggregation on a foreign surface: Platelet aggregation is directly proportional to the difference in platelet counts performed before and after PRP is passed through a column of glass beads
   B. Change in optical density: As platelets aggregate, the optical density of the platelet-rich plasma decreases
   C. Electrical impedance: Platelet aggregates are counted as they pass through an aperture, temporarily interrupting the flow of current between two electrodes
   D. Pulse editing: editing electronically generated pulses can differentiate the number of free platelets versus platelet aggregates

8. Which of the following is a platelet aggregation agent that characteristically yields a biphasic pattern when used in optimal concentration?
   A. Arachidonic acid
   B. Collagen
   C. Epinephrine
   D. Ristocetin

9. Which therapeutic agent affects platelet function?
   A. Aspirin
   B. Coumadin®
   C. Heparin
   D. Streptokinase

10. A potent inhibitor of platelet aggregation released by endothelial cells is
    A. Epinephrine
    B. Prostacyclin
    C. Ristocetin
    D. Thromboxane A_2

11. What is the approximate normal mean platelet volume (MPV) expressed in femtoliters (fL)?

A. 5
B. 7
C. 10
D. 18

12. The platelet parameter PDW refers to the
    A. Average platelet volume
    B. Cell weight *vs.* density
    C. Capacity to adhere to foreign surfaces
    D. Variation in cell size

13. Which of the following describes normal histograms showing platelet size distribution?
    A. Bimodal, nonskewed
    B. Nonskewed, broad flat peak
    C. Right-skewed, single peak
    D. Single peak, Gaussian distribution

14. All the following are normal maturation stages of platelets *except*
    A. Megakaryoblast
    B. Promegakaryocyte
    C. Micromegakaryocyte
    D. Megakaryocyte

15. For the performance of manual platelet counts, what is the recommended type of microscopy?
    A. Electron
    B. Dark-field
    C. Light
    D. Phase

16. Twenty microliters of blood are diluted in 1.98 mL of diluent. This dilution is plated on both sides of a Neubauer-ruled counting chamber. A total of 356 cells is seen when both large center squares are counted. What is the platelet count expressed as the number of cells per liter?
    A. 100×10^9/L
    B. 178×10^9/L
    C. 356×10^9/L
    D. 712×10^9/L

17. What size threshold range does the electrical impedance method use to count particles as platelets?
    A. 0–10 fL
    B. 2–20 fL
    C. 15–40 fL
    D. 35–90 fL

18. In storage pool diseases, platelets are primarily deficient in
    A. ADP
    B. Platelet factor 3
    C. Thrombasthenin
    D. Thromboxane A_2

19. What is the specimen of choice for routine coagulation testing?
    A. Heparin
    B. 3.2% (0.109 M) sodium citrate
    C. 3.8% (0.129 M) sodium citrate
    D. Sodium oxalate

20. The ratio of anticoagulant to blood for coagulation procedures should be 1 to
    A. 4.5
    B. 7.0
    C. 9.0
    D. 10.0

21. The liver is the site of synthesis of all the following *except*
    A. Factor VIII
    B. Plasminogen
    C. Protein C
    D. von Willebrand's factor

22. When thrombin binds with thrombomodulin on the endothelial cell surface, thrombin can
    A. Activate Protein C
    B. Activate Factor V and Factor VIII
    C. Convert fibrinogen to fibrin
    D. Stimulate platelet aggregation

23. What is the coagulation factor that has a sex-linked recessive inheritance pattern?
    A. Factor V
    B. Factor IX
    C. Factor X
    D. von Willebrand's factor

24. Which of the following is associated with individuals having a Prekallikrein deficiency?
    A. Bleed into the joints
    B. Inherit it as an autosomal dominant disorder
    C. Can have thrombotic complications
    D. Have delayed bleeding at the incision site following surgery

25. A soybean extract is used in specimen collection tubes for fibrin degradation product (FDP) tests to prevent
    A. Activation of the coagulation system
    B. Activation of the fibrinolytic system
    C. Further fibrinogen degradation
    D. Precipitation of the fibrinolytic products

26. The thrombin time will be prolonged in the presence of all the following *except*
    A. Elevated fibrinogen degradation products
    B. Heparin
    C. Factor I deficiency
    D. Factor II deficiency

27. What would be the expected screening test results for a patient with a fibrin stabilizing factor deficiency?
    A. Prothrombin time prolonged
    B. Activated partial thromboplastin time prolonged
    C. Prothrombin time and activated partial thromboplastin time prolonged
    D. Prothrombin time and activated partial thromboplastin time normal

28. What is the role of vitamin K in relation to the vitamin K–dependent group of clotting factors?
    A. A precursor to the active factors
    B. Conversion of the circulating precursors to active forms
    C. Carboxylation of precursors to form functional factors
    D. Regulation of the activity of these factors

29. All the following are complexes that must form for blood coagulation to occur *except*
    A. VIIa, Tissue Factor, Ca^{++}
    B. IXa, VIII, Ca^{++}, PF3
    C. Xa, V, Ca^{++}, PF3
    D. XIIa, kallikrein, HMWK

30. What is von Willebrand's factor?
    A. Phospholipid required for several reactions in the coagulation sequence
    B. Plasma protein that binds platelets to exposed subendothelium
    C. Plasma protein with procoagulant activity in the intrinsic coagulation system
    D. Platelet membrane glycoprotein that attaches the cell to injured vessel walls

31. Fibrin strands are cross-linked and the fibrin clot stabilized by the activity of
    A. α_2-Antiplasmin
    B. Factor XIIIa
    C. Plasmin
    D. Thrombin

32. Activation of the fibrinolytic system is accomplished by all the following *except*
    A. XIIa
    B. XIa
    C. Kallikrein
    D. Tissue plasminogen activator

33. Which of the following enzymatically degrades the stabilized fibrin clot?
    A. Plasminogen
    B. Plasmin
    C. Prothrombin
    D. Thrombin

34. The activity of the lupus anticoagulant appears to be directed against
    A. Factor V
    B. Factor VIII
    C. Factor IX
    D. Phospholipid

35. Heparin works as an inhibitor to clotting by
    A. Chelating calcium ions
    B. Preventing activation of prothrombin
    C. Antagonizing vitamin K's role in factor synthesis
    D. Enhancing the inhibitory effects of antithrombin III

36. Approximately 80% of inhibition of the clotting system is attributed to
    A. Antithrombin III
    B. Protein C
    C. Protein S
    D. Tissue factor pathway inhibitor

37. Why is the activated partial thromboplastin time (APTT) *not* the procedure of choice for detecting a platelet factor 3 (PF3) deficiency?
    A. Platelet-rich plasma is used for this test
    B. The reagent contains a substitute for PF3
    C. PF3 is unstable in the reagent used for this test
    D. PF3 does not function in the system being tested

38. Measurement of the time required for fibrin formation when thrombin is added to plasma evaluates the
    A. Fibrinogen concentration
    B. Prothrombin concentration

C. Extrinsic clotting system

D. Intrinsic clotting system

39. A fibrinogen performed on the fibrometer using the standard 1:10 dilution with Owren's buffer does not read on the standard curve. A 1:5 dilution is performed, and it is 250 mg/dL when read off the curve. What is the concentration of fibrinogen to be reported in mg/dL?

A. 500 mg/dL

B. 250 mg/dL

C. 125 mg/dL

D. 50 mg/dL

40. All the following are true of the International Normalized Ratio (INR) *except*

A. INR is dependent on reagents and instrumentation used

B. INR is calculated using the PT ratio taken to the power of the ISI value

C. The World Health Organization recommends reporting the INR on patients on long-term oral anticoagulant therapy

D. The desired INR on a patient on coumadin® is between 2.0 and 2.5, but may be higher depending on the cause of the patient's hypercoagulable state

41. A prolonged APTT result is obtained on a patient diagnosed as having acute disseminated intravascular coagulation (DIC). The patient has not yet been treated for this syndrome. How can the prolonged APTT be explained?

A. In addition to DIC, the patient is deficient in a factor required for the intrinsic pathway

B. DIC is characterized by synthesis of less stable coagulation factors, which deteriorate rapidly in the circulation

C. Continuous activation of the coagulation system uses some factors more rapidly than the liver can synthesize them

D. The patient has been misdiagnosed, since a prolonged APTT indicates the problem is deficient, not excessive, coagulation

42. All the following test results are characteristic of disseminated intravascular coagulation (DIC) *except*

A. Decreased fibrinogen concentration

B. Negative test for degradation products

C. Decreased platelet count

D. Prolonged prothrombin time test

43. The principle of _____ methods depends on cleavage of synthetic substrates by an active serine protease.

A. Chromogenic

B. Photo-optical

C. Mechanical

D. Immunodiffusion

44. Cell counts are performed on a fingerstick specimen from a female patient. The results are

Hgb	142 g/L (14.2 g/dL)
Hct	0.43 L/L (43.0%)
Platelet count	178×10^9/L

In the erythrocyte monolayer of this patient's peripheral blood smear, an average of 10 platelets per field are seen under $1000\times$ magnification. Based on these data, what should you do?

A. Report the results, since the platelet count and platelet estimate correlate

B. Recollect a specimen for a repeat platelet count, since the platelet count and estimate do not correlate

C. Examine the periphery of the blood smear for clumping, since the platelet count and estimate do not correlate

D. Repeat the platelet count on the available specimen

45. Blood for an APTT was collected from a 5-year-old boy named Horace. During the venipuncture, Horace had to be restrained by several people and still managed to be a moving target. Even though the situation was traumatic for everyone present, the blood specimen was obtained. The APTT controls were in range. The result of the APTT on Horace was 18.0 seconds (reference range 22.0–38.0 seconds). Which of the following interpretations would apply to Horace's APTT result?
    A. APTT abnormal due to a factor deficiency
    B. APTT invalid due to contamination with tissue juices
    C. Tube was probably not full, resulting in a falsely short time
    D. Based on age of patient, result was within acceptable range

46. A 4-year-old child is seen in the emergency room with petechiae and a platelet count of 15×10^9/L. She has no previous history of bleeding problems. Three weeks earlier she had chicken pox. The physician advises the parents to keep the child off the playground to avoid injury, and the child will recover within several weeks to a month with no further treatment. What condition does this child most likely have?
    A. Essential thrombocythemia
    B. Idiopathic thrombocytopenic purpura
    C. Thrombotic thrombocytopenic purpura
    D. Wiskott-Aldrich syndrome

47. Laboratory results on a patient with a severe bleeding problem are as follows

Platelet count	193×10^9/L
Bleeding time	>15 min
Prothrombin time	12.0 sec (control 12.0 sec)
APTT	92.0 sec (control 32.0 sec)

Platelet aggregation	Normal response to ADP, collagen, epinephrine; no response with ristocetin

These results are consistent with
A. Christmas disease
B. Hemophilia A
C. Glanzmann's thrombasthenia
D. von Willebrand's disease

48. Laboratory results on a patient with a severe bleeding problem are as follows:

Platelet count	125×10^9/L
MPV	16.0 fL (reference range 7.4–10.4 fL)
Bleeding time	>15 min
Prothrombin time	12.0 sec (control 12.0 sec)
APTT	32.0 sec (control 32.0 sec)
Platelet aggregation	Normal response to ADP, collagen, epinephrine; no response with ristocetin

These results are consistent with
A. Bernard-Soulier syndrome
B. von Willebrand's disease
C. Glanzmann's thrombasthenia
D. Ehlers-Danlos syndrome

49. The following results are obtained on a patient with a severe bleeding problem

Platelet count	256×10^9/L
Bleeding time	>15 minutes
Clot retraction	Deficient
Platelet aggregation	Normal response to ristocetin; weak response to ADP, collagen, epinephrine

These results are characteristic of
A. von Willebrand's disease
B. Glanzmann's thrombasthenia

C. Storage pool diseases

D. Christmas disease

50. Laboratory tests requested on a patient scheduled for early morning surgery the following day include a platelet count and CBC. An automated platelet count performed on the specimen is 57×10^9/L ($57,000/\mu$L). In the monolayer area of the peripheral blood smear there are approximately 10–12 platelets per oil immersion field, many of which are encircling neutrophils. All CBC results fall within the reference ranges. Controls are in range. Based on this information, what is the best course of action?

A. Report all the results, since the instrument is functioning properly

B. Immediately alert the physician so that cancellation of surgery can be considered

C. Thoroughly mix specimen and repeat platelet count; if results remain the same, report all results and indicate platelet count has been checked

D. Have specimen recollected by fingerstick directly into diluting fluid for platelet count

51. Results on a patient presenting with sudden severe hemorrhagic problems are as follows:

Bleeding time	Normal
Prothrombin time	Normal
Activated partial thromboplastin time	Prolonged
APTT 1:1 mixing study	No correction

These clinical manifestations and laboratory results are consistent with

A. Coumadin® therapy

B. von Willebrand's disease

C. Hemophilia A

D. Presence of a circulating inhibitor

52. Jessica, a famous author, is visiting her cousin, whose neighbor has been found unconscious in the bedroom. Jessica, while snooping through the neighbor's bathroom, finds a box of rat poison in the back of a cabinet covered by a shower cap. The rat poison contains a coumarin derivative, and Jessica thinks this poison may have been given to the neighbor in an attempt on his life. Jessica explains her finding to the detective in charge and recommends that a laboratory test be performed on the individual's blood to determine whether coumarin could be responsible for the neighbor's unconscious state. What test will show coumarin's effect on the patient's blood?

A. Bleeding time

B. Platelet count

C. Prothrombin time

D. Thrombin time

53. The following results are obtained on a patient

WBC	24.7×10^9/L ($24.7 \times 10^3/\mu$L)
RBC	6.20×10^{12}/L ($6.20 \times 10^6/\mu$L)
Hgb	186 g/L (18.6 g/dL)
Hct	0.56 L/L (56.0 %)
Plt	79×10^9/L ($79,000/\mu$L)
PT	19.3 sec (control 12.0 sec)
APTT	81.2 sec (control 32.0 sec)

The WBC, RBC, Hgb, Hct, and Plt were performed on blood collected in an evacuated tube containing EDTA. The PT and APTT were performed on blood collected in an evacuated tube containing sodium citrate. The standard collection procedure was followed, and all tests were performed within the appropriate time limits. Based on this information, which of the following statements best explains the prolonged coagulation test results?

A. Coagulation reactions require platelet factor 3; availability of this component is insufficient when the platelet count is below 100×10^9/L (100,000/μL)

B. The ratio of anticoagulant to blood is critical; the volume of anticoagulant must be decreased when the HCT is greater than 55%

C. The PT and APTT evaluate the extrinsic and intrinsic pathways, respectively. Prolongation of both tests indicates a deficiency of a factor common to both systems

D. Coagulation reactions are inhibited by a product released by leukocytes; this inhibitory activity becomes significant when the leukocyte count is greater than 20×10^9/L (20×10^3/μL)

54. Forgetful Frank, a phlebotomist at Hospital X, collected a tube of blood for an APTT at 6:47 A.M. The blood was collected in a tube with sodium citrate. He forgot to deliver the tube of blood to the lab until around 4:30 P.M. During the intervening time the blood specimen was on Frank's blood collection tray while he continued to collect specimens. Which of the following best describes the expected results?

A. Sodium citrate is a preservative as well as an anticoagulant, so the test results should be accurate

B. Blood collected in sodium citrate will not give accurate results in coagulation tests, since some factors are unstable in this anticoagulant

C. Unreliable results are expected, since some factors deteriorate rapidly at room temperature

D. Exposure of the plasma to erythrocytes for several hours has probably inactivated the factors, so the specimen will yield inaccurate results

55. The following results are obtained on a 3-year-old boy with sudden severe hemorrhagic problems:

Bleeding time	Normal
Prothrombin time	Normal
Activated partial thromboplastin time	Prolonged
APTT 1:1 mixing study	Correction
Platelet aggregation	Normal with ristocetin, ADP, collagen, and epinephrine

These clinical manifestations and laboratory results are consistent with

A. Aspirin
B. von Willebrand's disease
C. Hemophilia A
D. Heparin

56. An APTT and PT are requested on a patient scheduled for emergency surgery. On an optical density clot detection system, normal and abnormal controls for both tests are within range, but the patient's results are extremely prolonged. The patient's tests have been performed in duplicate, but there is sufficient plasma, which is dark amber, to repeat the tests. What is the best course of action to follow?

A. Report the results immediately by phone, emphasizing that the tests were run in duplicate, and the controls are within range

B. Request a new specimen and repeat the procedures using freshly diluted controls

C. Repeat the procedures on an instrument that detects clot formation electromechanically

D. Inform the physician that accurate results are impossible

57. An APTT on a 46-year-old male patient admitted for minor surgery is markedly abnormal, whereas the PT is within the normal range. The patient has no clinical manifestations of a bleeding problem and has no personal or fam-

ily history of bleeding problems, even following dental extraction. Several family members have been treated for thrombotic episodes. The prolonged APTT is corrected with a 1:1 mixing study using normal plasma. Based on these laboratory results and the clinical history, what factor deficiency would be expected?

A. II

B. VIII

C. XII

D. XIII

58. A 25-year-old obstetrical patient at 35 weeks gestation is admitted through the emergency room. She has bleeding in the genitourinary tract, and there are visible petechiae and ecchymoses. The following laboratory results are obtained

Platelet count	Decreased
Prothrombin time	Prolonged
Activated partial thromboplastin time	Prolonged
Fibrinogen	Decreased
Thrombin time	Prolonged
D-Dimer	Positive
FDP	Positive
AT III	Decreased
RBC morphology	Schistocytes present

These laboratory results are consistent with

A. Primary fibrinolysis

B. DIC with secondary fibrinolysis

C. Factor II deficiency

D. Heparin therapy

59. A 57-year-old man with prostate cancer is admitted to the intensive care unit with severe bleeding problems. The following laboratory results are obtained

Platelet count	Normal
Prothrombin time	Prolonged
Activated partial thromboplastin time	Prolonged
Fibrinogen	Decreased
Thrombin time	Prolonged
D-Dimer	Negative
FDP	Positive
AT III	Normal
RBC morphology	Schistocytes absent

These laboratory results are consistent with

A. Primary fibrinolysis

B. DIC with secondary fibrinolysis

C. Factor II deficiency

D. Coumadin® therapy

60. Which of the following is a component of platelet alpha granules?

A. ADP

B. Calcium ions

C. Serotonin

D. von Willebrand's factor

61. What may be the cause of defective clot retraction?

A. Lack of the platelet receptor glycoprotein Ib

B. Lack of the platelet receptor IIb/IIIa for fibrinogen

C. Insufficient storage of ADP

D. Absence of von Willebrand's factor

62. Thrombocytosis is a characteristic of

A. Disseminated intravascular coagulation

B. Splenomegaly

C. Polycythemia vera

D. Idiopathic thrombocytopenic purpura

63. Endothelial cells lining vessel walls release products involved in all the following functions except

A. Inhibiting platelet aggregation

B. Activating the fibrinolytic system

C. Changing thrombin from a procoagulant to an anticoagulant

D. Cross-linking fibrin monomers

64. Abnormal platelet function is the suspected cause of the bleeding problem in a patient who has a normal platelet count. Which of the following laboratory procedures gives information with regard to platelet function and, therefore, could provide pertinent information as to the cause of the bleeding problem?
    A. Activated partial thromboplastin time
    B. Prothrombin time
    C. Thrombin time
    D. Bleeding time

65. Which coagulation factors are referred to as "vitamin K–dependent"?
    A. I, V, VIII, XIII
    B. II, V, IX, XII
    C. II, VII, IX, X
    D. XI, XII, Fletcher, Fitzgerald

66. Which pharmaceutical agent works as an inhibitor to the fibrinolytic system?
    A. Aspirin
    B. DDAVP
    C. EACA
    D. Streptokinase

67. Which factors are consumed in clotting and, therefore, absent in serum?
    A. I, V, VIII, XIII
    B. I, II, V, VIII, XIII
    C. II, VII, IX, X
    D. VIII, IX, XI, XII

68. A severe vitamin K deficiency will affect all the following *except*
    A. Fibrinogen
    B. Stable factor
    C. Christmas factor
    D. Protein C

69. All the following are associated with thrombosis *except*
    A. Factor V Leiden mutation
    B. Hypofibrinogenemia
    C. Lupus anticoagulant
    D. Prothrombin 20210 mutation

70. A patient with coronary artery disease is admitted to the hospital with venous thrombosis. What medication can be administered that will lyse the clot?
    A. Aspirin
    B. Coumadin®
    C. Heparin
    D. Tissue plasminogen activator

71. Reversal of a heparin overdose can be achieved by
    A. Vitamin K
    B. Protamine sulfate
    C. Antithrombin III
    D. Warfarin

72. Which of the following describes Protein C?
    A. Is a vitamin K–dependent plasma protein
    B. Activates factors V and VIII:C
    C. Is an inhibitor of fibrinolysis
    D. Is synthesized by endothelial cells

73. Fitzgerald factor is another name for
    A. Factor II
    B. Factor VIII
    C. Factor IX
    D. High-molecular-weight kininogen

74. The one-stage prothrombin time will detect deficiencies in the _____ pathway(s) when calcium and an extract of tissue such as brain are added to plasma.
    A. Extrinsic
    B. Extrinsic and common
    C. Intrinsic
    D. Intrinsic and common

75. D-Dimers are degradation products of
    A. Noncross-linked fibrin
    B. Cross-linked fibrin
    C. Fibrinogen
    D. Plasmin

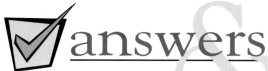

answers & rationales

1.

A. Vascular integrity is influenced by vitamin C intake. In the absence of vitamin C, collagen is not formed properly. Vitamin C deficiency is associated with capillary fragility and the primary hemostasis bleeding symptoms of petechiae and mucosal bleeding.

2.

D. Each megakaryocyte produces approximately 2000–4000 platelets. A single megakaryocyte can generate this large number of cells because platelets are nonnucleated fragments of their cytoplasm. The number of platelets generated by a megakaryocyte depends on its cell size, which is directly related to the number of endomitotic divisions before cytoplasmic fragmentation.

3.

A. Once platelets are released from the bone marrow, approximately two-thirds of them are in circulation and one-third of them are sequestered in the spleen. Once the spleen has been surgically removed, there is no storage site for platelets, and they all circulate. Splenomegaly is a cause of thrombocytopenia due to increased sequestration.

4.

B. Aggregation refers to attachment of platelets to other platelets. Adhesion refers to platelets interacting with damaged vessel walls; retraction describes one of the final steps in coagulation in which the fibrin-platelet plug retracts. Release is the process by which platelet granule contents are secreted.

5.

C. In platelet aggregation studies, the addition of the aggregating agent may induce an initial aggregation phase followed by a secondary wave. The initial phase is the result of the interaction of the agent with the platelet. The second phase is thought to depend on release of nonmetabolic ADP from platelet granules, which promotes additional aggregation.

6.

B. Collagen is the only aggregating agent that includes a single wave response preceded by a lag phase. During the lag phase collagen stimulates platelets to release their granule contents. ADP released from the platelets then initiates platelet aggregation.

7.

B. When an aggregating agent is added to platelet-rich plasma (PRP), which is an optically dense suspension, the platelets normally stick to each other, forming platelet aggregates. As additional platelets aggregate, the cell suspension becomes clearer with a few large clumps of cells. At maximum aggregation the specimen is relatively clear, allowing light transmission, which is only partially obstructed by a few platelet aggregates.

8.

C. Of the responses listed, epinephrine is the aggregating agent that typically gives a biphasic pattern. ADP and thrombin also give biphasic patterns when used in optimal concentrations. Arachidonic acid causes a rapid secondary wave of platelet aggregation. Collagen and ristocetin induce uniphasic aggregatory responses.

9.

A. Aspirin inhibits the enzyme cyclo-oxygenase in the prostaglandin pathway, preventing formation of thromboxane A$_2$. Thromboxane A$_2$ is needed for release of platelet granule contents in primary hemostasis. Without the release reaction, platelets will not aggregate. The platelets affected by aspirin are nonfunctional for the lifespan of the platelet. The other agents listed affect the coagulation factors in secondary hemostasis.

10.

B. Prostacyclin, also referred to as PGI$_2$, is the most potent inhibitor of platelet aggregation known. Injured endothelial cells release prostacyclin. Epinephrine and ristocetin induce platelet aggregation. Thromboxane A$_2$, generated by platelets via the prostaglandin pathway, also induces platelet aggregation.

11.

C. The average volume of normal platelets is approximately 10 fL. This platelet parameter is equivalent to the erythrocyte parameter, mean corpuscular volume (MCV). The term femtoliter has replaced cubic micron (micrometer) as the unit of expression for this parameter.

12.

D. PDW is an abbreviation for platelet distribution width. This parameter measures the uniformity of platelet size. It is the platelet equivalent of the red cell parameter RDW. It represents the coefficient of variation of the platelet population.

13.

C. A histogram showing platelet size distribution is made by plotting platelet size (x axis) *vs.* number (y axis). The resulting curve is usually a single, right-skewed peak. This reflects a larger number of platelets in the lower size range with a "tail" of larger cells to the right of the majority.

14.

C. Micromegakaryocytes, also known as dwarf megakaryocytes, are thought to be megakaryocytes that have lost their ability to undergo endomitosis. They can be seen in the peripheral blood of patients with myelodysplastic syndromes or myeloproliferative disorders. They may resemble lymphocytes, but cytoplasmic blebs can help to identify them as micromegakaryocytes.

15.

D. Phase microscopy is currently recommended for manual platelet counts. This allows satisfactory discrimination between platelets and debris, a major problem in manual counts. Light microscopy may also be used; however, differentiating between platelets and debris is more difficult than with phase microscopy.

16.

B. Twenty microliters of blood (0.02 mL) added to 1.98 mL of diluting fluid gives a dilution of 1:100; the dilution factor is 100. The standard formula for hemacytometer counts expressed in mm^3 is

$$\frac{\text{total number cells counted} \times \text{dilution factor}}{\text{area counted} \times \text{depth}}$$

The correct equation for this problem is:

$$\frac{356 \times 100}{2 \text{ mm}^2 \times 0.10 \text{ mm}} = 178{,}000 = 178 \times 10^3/\text{mm}^3$$

When expressed as the number of cells per liter, the platelet count is 178×10^9/L (178,000/μL).

17.

B. In the electrical impedance method for counting platelets, particles between 2 and 20 fL will be classified as platelets by the analyzer's computer. The normal average platelet volume is 10 fL. One dilution is used for counting and sizing of platelets and red blood cells. In the electrical impedance method, size thresholds differentiate the two.

18.

A. Platelets in storage pool disease are deficient in dense-granule associated ADP. These platelets lack the intrinsic ADP that is normally released when the platelets are stimulated. This accounts for a poor response to aggregation agents.

19.

B. NCCLS standards recommend 3.2% sodium citrate. 3.8% sodium citrate is a higher concentration than is needed to anticoagulate normal blood samples. Sodium oxalate, when recalcified in the test procedures, forms insoluble precipitates that can interfere with instruments that use optical density endpoint determinations. Heparin is unacceptable for coagulation testing.

20.

C. The optimum ratio of anticoagulant to blood should be one part anticoagulant to nine parts blood. A 1:9 ratio is sufficient for sodium citrate to prevent coagulation by binding all available calcium in the blood sample, but insufficient to make calcium a rate-limiting factor when the specimen is recalcified during the test. A tube that is not full causes falsely long clotting times.

21.

D. The liver produces most of the clotting factors as well as inhibitors to clotting. A patient with liver disease has impaired synthesis of these clotting factors and inhibitors. Endothelial cells and megakaryocytes produce von Willebrand's factor.

22.

A. Thrombomodulin, an endothelial cell receptor, has the ability to change the specificity of thrombin from a procoagulant to an anticoagulant. Once bound to thrombomodulin, thrombin has anticoagulant properties due to its activation of protein C. protein C, along with its cofactor protein S, can then exert negative feedback on the clotting system by inactivating factor V and factor VIII.

23.

B. Factor IX and Factor VIII are the only sex-linked recessive hemostatic defects. von Willebrand's factor deficiency and dysfibrinogenemia are inherited as autosomal dominant disorders. Factor V, factor X, and most of the other inherited hemostatic disorders have an autosomal recessive inheritance pattern.

24.

C. Prekallikrein (Fletcher factor) deficiency is inherited as an autosomal recessive disorder. There are usually no significant bleeding problems with this disorder. Prekallikrein is an activator of the fibrinolytic system. Prekallikrein deficient patients cannot lyse clots efficiently and are prone to thrombosis. Fibrinolytic and anticoagulant therapies are indicated in patients who develop thrombosis.

25.

C. When used in blood collection tubes for FDP procedures, soybean enzyme inhibitors allow the quantification of *in vivo* FDP by preventing additional fibrin/fibrinogen degradation after blood is drawn. Without the inhibitors fibrin/fibrinogen degradation continues, falsely elevating the FDP level. The FDP test is positive in the presence of *either* fibrin *or* fibrinogen degradation products.

26.

D. The thrombin time is a test that measures fibrinogen. Thrombin reagent is added to undiluted patient plasma, and the time it takes for fibrinogen conversion to fibrin is measured. Anything that interferes with the ability of thrombin to convert fibrinogen to fibrin will prolong the test. Heparin, and degradation products X and E inhibit thrombin. Factor II is not measured in the thrombin time, since the reagent used is thrombin (II_a).

27.

D. Thrombin converts fibrinogen to the fibrin monomer. Fibrin monomers spontaneously polymerize to form the fibrin polymer. This is the endpoint of clot-based PT and APTT tests. This fibrin polymer is unstable. Factor XIIIa, also known as fibrin stabilizing factor, produces double bonds to create a stable fibrin polymer after the endpoint of the PT and APTT has been reached. The 5M urea clot solubility test is performed when factor XIII deficiency is suspected.

28.

C. Vitamin K acts in a carboxylation step in which the precursors of factors II, VII, IX, and X are made functional. The carboxylated forms are capable of binding calcium. The uncarboxylated precursors lack calcium-binding sites. The activity of the activated forms of these factors depends on their ability to bind calcium.

29.

D. The intrinsic, extrinsic, and common pathways each have a complex that must form for blood coagulation to occur. The intrinsic complex of IXa, VIII, and Ca^{++} occurs on the platelet surface (PF3) and activates factor X. The extrinsic complex of VIIa, tissue factor, and Ca^{++} activates factor X as well as factor IX. Factor IX activation by the extrinsic complex provides a link between the intrinsic and extrinsic systems. The prothrombin-converting complex of Xa, V, Ca^{++}, and PF3 is responsible for converting prothrombin to thrombin.

30.

B. von Willebrand's factor (vWF) is a portion of the plasma protein known as the factor VIII/von Willebrand's factor complex. Its function is to bind to platelet membrane glycoprotein Ib and form a bridge between the platelet and exposed subendothelium in primary hemostasis. vWF is a carrier protein for factor VIII:C, but vWF does not have coagulant activity in secondary hemostasis as factor VIII:C does.

31.

B. Activated factor XIII is a transglutaminase that cross-links fibrin monomers between glutamine and lysine residues. Fibrin monomers that are not cross-linked lack the stability to maintain the hemostatic plug, as evidenced by the bleeding problems experienced by individuals deficient in factor XIII. Thrombin contributes to the formation of the fibrin clot, which is degraded by plasmin. Once the fibrin clot has been lysed and plasmin is free in circulation, α_2-antiplasmin quickly neutralizes plasmin.

32.

B. Once activated, three of the four contact factors activate both the intrinsic clotting system and provide intrinsic activation of the fibrinolytic system. The only contact factor that does not activate the fibrinolytic system is factor XI. Extrinsic activation of the fibrinolytic system is achieved by the release of tissue plasminogen activator by damaged endothelial cells.

33.

B. Plasmin, the active form of plasminogen, is the enzyme responsible for degrading fibrin into several different fragments. The D-Dimer test is abnormal when there is excessive fibrinolytic activity. Prothrombin is the inactive precursor of thrombin that cleaves fibrinogen to form fibrin, which is stabilized by the activity of factor XIII.

34.

D. An IgG or IgM immunoglobulin occasionally occurs in systemic lupus erythematosus that interferes with coagulation. This inhibitor is called the lupus anticoagulant, although it also occurs in other autoimmune disorders. Its activity appears to be directed against the phospholipid portion of the prothrombinase complex (Xa-V-phospholipid-calcium).

35.

D. Heparin forms a complex with antithrombin III to inhibit coagulation. The heparin-antithrombin III complex rapidly inhibits thrombin and other activated coagulation factors. Coagulation may be inhibited by coumarin and related compounds, which antagonize vitamin K activity. Several anticoagulants, such as sodium citrate and EDTA, prevent fibrin formation by combining with calcium ions, which serve as cofactors in several reactions.

36.

A. Antithrombin III is the most important naturally occurring inhibitor to clotting. It inhibits most of the serine proteases. The serine protease that antithrombin III does not inhibit, VIIa, is inhibited by tissue factor pathway inhibitor. The cofactors factor V and factor VIII are not serine proteases. Protein C and its cofactor, protein S, inhibit them. ATIII is called the heparin cofactor, because in its absence heparin is not an inhibitor to clotting.

37.

B. The reagent used in the APTT procedure is a phospholipid extract that substitutes for platelet factor 3 in coagulation reactions. Platelet-poor plasma is used, so thrombocytopenia does not affect the APTT test. Platelet factor 3 functions in the intrinsic and prothrombin-converting complexes that must form for blood coagulation to occur.

38.

A. Thrombin is the active enzyme that converts fibrinogen to fibrin. When thrombin is added to plasma, the rate of fibrin formation depends only on the concentration of fibrinogen. Fibrin formation is the last step in a sequence of reactions and does not evaluate prior steps such as those involved in the other responses.

39.

C. A 1:5 dilution is used when the time obtained on a patient sample is greater than the longest time used in preparation of the standard curve. A 1:5 dilution is twice as concentrated as the standard 1:10 dilution. The value read off the curve must be divided by 2 to take into account the alternate dilution factor used.

40.

A. The World Health Organization recommends using the INR to monitor patients on stabilized coumadin® therapy because it is *independent* of the reagent or instrument used. It is a means of standardizing the reporting of prothrombin times (PTs) worldwide. The INR is calculated by many instruments and laboratory information systems, but can be calculated manually.

$$INR = \left[\frac{Patient\ PT\ (in\ seconds)}{Control\ PT\ (in\ seconds)} \right]^{ISI}$$

Where:

INR is the International Normalized Ratio

ISI is the International Sensitivity Index of the thromboplastin source. This value is determined by the manufacturer of the thromboplastin reagent. The closer to 1.00 the ISI, the more sensitive the thromboplastin reagent is in detecting factor deficiencies.

Patient PT is the prothrombin time value for the patient.

Control PT is the mean prothrombin time value of the normal range.

41.

C. As coagulation occurs *in vivo,* some factors are consumed just as they are when blood is allowed to clot in a test tube *in vitro.* The factors consumed during coagulation are fibrinogen, prothrombin, and factors V, VIII, and XIII. Results of laboratory procedures relying on one or more of these factors will be affected. All these factors except factor XIII contribute to the reactions evaluated in the APTT procedure.

42.

B. During disseminated intravascular coagulation, platelets and factors are consumed in the coagulation process. Factors particularly affected are I, II, V, VIII, and XIII. Consumption of platelets and these factors will usually prolong the prothrombin time test and decrease the platelet count and fibrinogen concentration. The APTT test is also prolonged. The fibrinolytic system is activated by systemic intravascular coagulation; therefore, serum fibrin/fibrinogen degradation products are elevated. FDP and D-Dimer tests will both be positive.

43.

A. The proteolytic activity of antithrombin III after activation to a serine protease can be assayed via methods that employ synthetic substrates. The cleavage of the synthetic substrate by an active serine protease will yield a chromogenic compound. Chromogenic methods can also be used to assay other substances such as plasminogen, protein C, and heparin.

44.

A. The results should be reported. A platelet estimate is obtained by multiplying the average number of platelets per oil immersion field (in an erythrocyte monolayer) by 20,000. This number is based on a normal erythrocyte count, which must be considered when comparing the platelet count and estimate. The estimate in this example is 200×10^9/L. This agrees with the platelet count. All the other responses assume that the platelet count and estimate do not agree.

45.

B. A clean venipuncture is required for coagulation testing. Contamination with tissue juices, which contain tissue thromboplastin, causes a falsely short test result. In this case, the description of the traumatic venipuncture indicates that the result might be invalid due to exposure to tissue thromboplastin. A tube that is not full would cause a falsely long time.

46.

B. Acute idiopathic thrombocytopenic purpura is mainly seen in young children. A viral infection often precedes the onset of symptoms by several weeks. In 90% of patients with acute ITP, there is an increase in IgG immunoglobulin attached to the surface of the platelets. Spontaneous remission occurs in most patients within 2 to 6 weeks of the onset of the illness. A chronic form of ITP, believed to be a different disease, is seen in adults.

47.

D. The patient's platelet count is within the reference range, but the bleeding time is prolonged. This indicates a platelet function problem. The coagulation tests indicate a problem in the intrinsic clotting system (factors XII, XI, IX, VIII, Fitzgerald, and Fletcher). The one disorder in which both platelet function and the coagulant property of factor VIII are affected is von Willebrand's disease. A synonym for von Willebrand's factor is the ristocetin cofactor. In its absence, platelets will not aggregate with ristocetin. The platelet aggregation pattern confirms this diagnosis.

48.

A. Bernard-Soulier syndrome is a platelet adhesion defect that can be mistaken for von Willebrand's disease. Platelets in this syndrome lack the glycoprotein Ib receptor, which is necessary for von Willebrand's factor to attach to the platelet. Both disorders give identical platelet aggregation patterns. Differentiating characteristics are that Bernard-Soulier syndrome is noted for giant platelets and varying degrees of thrombocytopenia. Since von Willebrand's factor is present in Bernard-Soulier syndrome, the APTT is normal.

49.

B. Since the platelet count is within the reference range, the prolonged bleeding time is due to a qualitative platelet disorder. Poor clot retraction and platelet aggregation are characteristic of thrombasthenia. Clot retraction is normal in storage pool diseases and von Willebrand's disease, and platelets are normal in Christmas disease, which is caused by factor IX deficiency. Thrombasthenia can be further differentiated from von Willebrand's disease by platelet aggregation studies.

50.

D. The best course of action is to have the specimen recollected without anticoagulant. According to the description of the peripheral blood smear, platelets encircled the neutrophils, a phenomenon referred to as platelet satellitism. This "pseudothrombocytopenia" occurs when the blood of some individuals is anticoagulated with EDTA. Recollecting the specimen using sodium citrate sometimes corrects this problem. If sodium citrate is used, the platelet count must be multiplied by 1.1 to account for the dilution factor.

51.

D. A 1:1 mixing study using normal plasma contains all components necessary to correct a prolonged coagulation test result caused by a factor deficiency. Failure of normal plasma to correct the APTT result indicates the presence of a circulating inhibitor. Hemophilia A and von Willebrand's disease are both factor deficiencies that would result

in correction when a 1:1 mixing study is performed. Coumadin® causes a multiple acquired defect of the prothrombin group factors that would correct with a mixing study. von Willebrand's disease would give a prolonged bleeding time. Heparin and the lupus anticoagulant are examples of circulating inhibitors.

52.

C. Coumarin and related compounds are vitamin K antagonists. By interfering with the function of vitamin K in the synthesis of factors II, VII, IX, and X, coumarin derivatives prolong test results that depend on one or more of these factors. These factors are synthesized, but are not functional. Of the procedures listed, only the prothrombin time depends on the presence of these factors.

53.

B. The usual blood-to-anticoagulant ratio is 9:1. If a volume of blood contains more RBCs and less plasma, this ratio will be affected. There will be excess anticoagulant in the plasma. Excess sodium citrate, which acts as an anticoagulant by binding calcium ions, will bind the reagent calcium added back to the test plasma during the procedure, making this component rate limiting and falsely prolonging the results.

54.

C. Factor V deteriorates rapidly at room temperature, and factor VIII is also relatively labile. Blood for coagulation studies should be tested within 2 to 4 hours of draw, depending upon whether the specimen has been centrifuged. Sodium citrate is the appropriate anticoagulant for coagulation procedures.

55.

C. Hemophilia A is inherited as a sex-linked recessive disorder of factor VIII:C. Mothers are carriers who pass the disease on to male offspring. This disorder is strictly a secondary hemostasis defect, so tests for primary hemostasis such as the bleeding time and platelet aggregation studies are normal. Factor deficiencies correct when a 1:1 mixing study is performed; presence of heparin in the sample would result in no correction of the mixing study. Aspirin affects platelets in primary hemostasis.

56.

C. The dark amber color of icteric plasma may interfere with fibrin formation detection by instruments measuring a change in optical density. The change in optical density may be insufficient for detection. The most accurate results in this situation can be obtained by performing the procedure on an electromechanical fibrin detection instrument that does not rely on optical clot detection.

57.

C. An abnormal APTT that corrects with a 1:1 mixing study and a normal PT indicate a deficiency of one of the intrinsic system factors; extrinsic and common factors are not responsible for the prolonged APTT if the PT is normal. Of the responses listed, factors II and XIII can be eliminated because the former is common to both pathways and the latter does not contribute to fibrin formation, the end point of these reactions. Factor VIII deficiency causes bleeding into muscles and joints. Factor XII deficiency does not result in bleeding. Since factor XII is an activator of fibrinolysis, however, a deficiency of factor XII can result in thrombosis.

58.

B. DIC is a consumption coagulopathy in which factors are used up in systemic clotting faster than the liver can synthesize them. When the clotting system is activated, the fibrinolytic system is simultaneously activated. Degradation products form that will cause the FDP and D-Dimer tests for degradation products to be positive. Antithrombin III inhibits serine proteases, but it is quickly overwhelmed in the systemic clotting that occurs. Platelets are consumed in clotting, and red blood cells fragment as they encounter fibrin strands in circulation.

59.

A. Primary fibrinolysis is an unusual disorder in which the fibrinolytic system is activated, but not in response to clot formation. Plasmin degrades factors V, VIII, and fibrinogen. There is no fibrin clot to lyse, so there are no fibrin degradation products formed. The D-Dimer test is considered to be a specific marker of fibrinolysis because it is only positive in the presence of fibrin degradation products. The FDP test is positive in the presence of fibrin *or* fibrinogen degradation products. Tests that are abnormal in DIC due to the systemic clotting are normal in primary fibrinolysis.

60.

D. Alpha granules contain a number of substances including von Willebrand's factor, platelet factor 4, beta thromboglobulin, platelet-derived growth factor, fibrinogen, fibronectin, and factor V. The dense bodies contain nonmetabolic ADP, ATP, calcium, and serotonin. Granules compose part of the organelle zone of the platelet structure.

61.

B. Glanzmann's thrombasthenia is a disorder characterized by absent or defective platelet receptors for fibrinogen. Clot retraction in these patients is either absent or reduced. Neither insufficient ADP storage, absence of von Willebrand's factor, nor absence of the platelet receptor glycoprotein Ib affects clot retraction. Lack of glycoprotein Ib, the von Willebrand's factor receptor site, causes the platelet adhesion defect seen in Bernard-Soulier disease.

62.

C. Polycythemia vera, a hemopoietic stem cell disorder characterized by excessive production of erythrocytic, granulocytic, and megakaryocytic cells in the bone marrow, is usually accompanied by thrombocytosis. ITP, DIC, and splenomegaly are all characterized by a decreased platelet count. In ITP, platelet destruction is mediated by immune mechanisms. Platelets are consumed in DIC and sequestered in an individual with an enlarged spleen.

63.

D. Endothelial cells release prostacyclin, which is a potent inhibitor of platelet aggregation. They also release tissue plasminogen activators, which initiate the fibrinolytic system. When thrombin binds with thrombomodulin on the endothelial cell surface, the specificity of thrombin changes. Rather than converting fibrinogen to fibrin, thrombin complexed with thrombomodulin activates Protein C. Protein C along with Protein S inhibits clotting by "turning off" factors V and VIII. Factor XIII is responsible for cross-linking fibrin monomers, but it is not a component of endothelial cells.

64.

D. The bleeding time test is a primary hemostasis screening test for platelet and vascular function. Since a platelet factor 3 substitute is a component of the partial thromboplastin reagent, neither the number nor function of platelets is evaluated in the APTT. Both the partial thromboplastin time and the prothrombin time are secondary hemostasis screening tests and, therefore, do not evaluate platelet function. The thrombin time measures the availability of functional fibrinogen.

65.

C. The Prothrombin group factors II, VII, IX, and X are called vitamin K–dependent factors. Vitamin K is needed by the liver to synthesize functional circulating forms of these factors. The fibrinogen group of I, V, VIII, XIII and the contact group of XII, XI, Fletcher, and Fitzgerald factors are not vitamin K–dependent.

66.

C. Epsilon-aminocaproic acid (EACA) is useful in the treatment of primary fibrinolysis because it stops the activation of plasminogen to plasmin. Aspirin is a platelet inhibitor. DDAVP (desamino-D-arginine-vasopressin) is useful in treating von Willebrand's disease and occasionally in Hemophilia A. DDAVP induces release of stored von Willebrand's factor in endothelium. Streptokinase is an activator of the fibrinolytic system.

67.

B. Factors VIII, XIII, and fibrinogen are consumed during coagulation and are absent in serum. Little if any factor V is present in serum. Only very little prothrombin remains, but it quickly disappears from serum.

68.

A. Vitamin K is required for liver synthesis of functional clotting factors II, VII, IX, and X and for synthesis of the coagulation inhibitors protein C and S. A deficiency of vitamin K decreases the concentrations of these proteins and subsequently prolongs test results depending on one or more of them. Factor VII is also known as stable factor, and factor IX is also known as Christmas factor.

69.

B. The most common hereditary thrombotic disorder is factor V Leiden. An abnormal factor V molecule is synthesized that is resistant to the inhibitory affects of protein C. A synonym for factor V Leiden is Activated Protein C Resistance (APCR). While other causes of activated protein C resistance

exist, up to 90% of patients with APCR have the factor V Leiden mutation. The prothrombin 20210 mutation, in which an abnormal factor II molecule is synthesized, is the second most common hereditary thrombotic disorder. Presence of the lupus anticoagulant causes an acquired thrombotic disorder. While hereditary dysfibrinogenemia frequently causes thrombosis, hypofibrinogenemia causes bleeding tendencies.

70.

D. Tissue plasminogen activator, streptokinase, and urokinase are thrombolytic therapies that will exogenously activate the fibrinolytic system and lyse the clot. Coumadin® and heparin can be administered to prevent the formation of new clots. Aspirin will prevent platelet aggregation.

71.

B. A heparin overdose can result in hemorrhage. If bleeding becomes life-threatening, protamine sulfate can be given. Heparin will dissociate from anthithrombin III if protamine sulfate is administered, because heparin has a higher affinity for protamine sulfate. Vitamin K can be administered in the management of bleeding for patients who overdosed with warfarin, which is a synonym for coumadin®.

72.

A. Protein C, a glycoprotein produced in the liver, is a potent inhibitor of coagulation. The activation of protein C, by the thrombin/thrombomodulin complex, will cause the inactivation of factors V and VIII:C. Protein C is a vitamin K–dependent protein.

73.

D. Fitzgerald factor is also referred to as high-molecular-weight kininogen (HMWK). Deficiency of HMWK is inherited as an autosomal recessive trait. Patients who are HMWK deficient do not have bleeding complications, but are prone to thrombotic episodes since HMWK is an activator of the fibrinolytic system.

74.

B. The prothrombin time test measures the coagulant activity of the extrinsic and common pathway factors of I, II, V, VII, and X. The reagent used for the prothrombin time test contains calcium and tissue thromboplastin. Thromboplastin is an extract of tissue such as brain or placenta. The activated partial thromboplastin time test measures all coagulation factors present in the intrinsic and common pathways except factor XIII. Calcium, a phospholipid source, and an activating agent, such as kaolin, silica, or celite, are present in the reagents used for the activated partial thromboplastin time.

75.

B. The primary function of the fibrinolytic system is fibrin clot lysis, thus keeping the vascular system free of deposited fibrin and fibrin clots. Fibrinolysis occurs when plasminogen, a single-chain glycoprotein found in plasma, is converted into plasmin, which will act on fibrinogen and/or non-cross-linked fibrin, degrading them into smaller fragments (i.e., fibrinogen/fibrin degradation products). D-Dimers are degradation products caused by the action of plasmin on cross-linked fibrin.

REFERENCES

Beutler, E. (Ed.) (1995). *Williams Hematology,* 5th ed. New York: McGraw-Hill.

Bick, R. L. (1992). *Disorders of Thrombosis & Hemostasis: Clinical and Laboratory Practice.* Chicago: ASCP Press.

Harmening, D. M. (Ed.) (1997). *Clinical Hematology and Fundamentals of Hemostasis,* 3rd ed. Philadelphia: F. A. Davis.

McKenzie, S. B. (1996). *Textbook of Hematology,* 2nd ed. Philadelphia: Williams & Wilkins.

Stiene-Martin, E. A., Lotspeich-Steininger, C. A., and Koepke, J. A. (Eds.) (1998). *Clinical Hematology-Principles, Procedures, Correlations,* 2nd ed. Philadelphia: Lippincott.

4

Immunology

contents

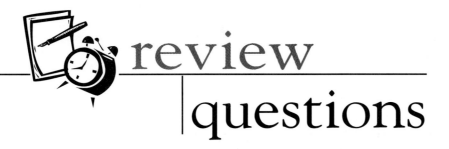

INSTRUCTIONS Each of the questions or incomplete statements that follow comprises four suggested responses. Select the *best* answer or completion statement in each case.

1. Color Plate 21 depicts a monomeric immunoglobulin molecule. The portion of the molecule indicated by the dotted red circle and the red arrow is called the
   A. Fab fragment
   B. Fc fragment
   C. Heavy chain
   D. Hinge region

2. A hapten is
   A. A carrier molecule for an antigen that is not antigenic alone
   B. A determinant capable of stimulating an immune response only when bound to a carrier
   C. An immunoglobulin functional only in the presence of complement
   D. Half of an immunoglobulin molecule

3. Which of the following characteristics is not true for B cells?
   A. Become memory cells
   B. Contain surface immunoglobulins
   C. Differentiate into plasma cells
   D. Secrete the C5 component of complement

4. A lymphokine is
   A. A soluble mediator produced by granulocytes and affecting lymphocytes
   B. A soluble mediator produced by lymphocytes
   C. A soluble mediator produced by plasma cells
   D. An antibody that reacts with lymphocytes

5. Monocytes and macrophages play a major role in the mononuclear phagocytic system. For an antibody-coated antigen to be phagocytosed, what part of the antibody molecule fits into a receptor on the phagocytic cell?
   A. Fab region
   B. Fc region
   C. Hinge region
   D. Variable region

6. The DQ antigens in the HLA system
   A. Are detected by antibody activity
   B. Are detected by mixed lymphocyte culture or the polymerase chain reaction (PCR)
   C. Are inherited as recessive traits
   D. Are not important in transplantation

7. The HLA complex is located primarily on
   A. Chromosome 3
   B. Chromosome 6
   C. Chromosome 9
   D. Chromosome 17

8. HLA antigens are found on
   A. All nucleated cells
   B. Red blood cells only
   C. Solid tissue only
   D. White blood cells only

9. Which of the following is more likely to be diagnostic of recent acute infection?
   A. A total antibody titer of 2 followed by a titer of 16
   B. A total antibody titer of 80
   C. A total antibody titer of 80 followed by a titer of 40
   D. An antibody titer of 80 that is IgG

10. A young woman shows increased susceptibility to pyogenic infections. Upon assay, she shows a low level of C3. Which of the following statements is probably not true?
    A. She has an autoimmune disease with continual antigen-antibody activity causing consumption of C3
    B. She has decreased production of C3
    C. She has DiGeorge syndrome
    D. She may produce an inactive form of C3

11. What is the predominant type of antibody found in the serum of neonates born after full-term gestation?
    A. Infant IgA
    B. Infant IgD
    C. Infant IgG
    D. Maternal IgG

12. What type of cell predominates in the germinal centers of lymph nodes?
    A. B cells
    B. Macrophages
    C. Natural killer cells
    D. T cells

13. The major class of immunoglobulin found in adult human serum is

   A. IgA
   B. IgE
   C. IgG
   D. IgM

14. Which class of immunoglobulin possesses delta heavy chains?
    A. IgA
    B. IgD
    C. IgE
    D. IgG

15. Which class of immunoglobulin possesses 10 antigenic binding sites?
    A. IgA
    B. IgD
    C. IgG
    D. IgM

16. Color Plate 22 represents a dimeric IgA molecule. The structure printed in red and indicated by the red arrow is called the
    A. Heavy chain
    B. Hinge region
    C. J-piece
    D. Light chain

17. Which class of immunoglobulin binds to basophils and mast cells to mediate immediate hypersensitivity reactions?
    A. IgA
    B. IgD
    C. IgE
    D. IgG

18. Which class of immunoglobulin has four subclasses?
    A. IgA
    B. IgE
    C. IgG
    D. IgM

19. When performing the enzyme multiplied immunoassay technique (EMIT), how is the ligand in the patient's serum detected?
    A. Agglutinates by binding to antibody-coated latex beads
    B. Binds to enzyme-labeled antibody
    C. Competes with enzyme-labeled antigen for binding to a specific antibody
    D. Forms antibody-antigen complex and precipitates

20. Adjuvants are added to vaccines to
    A. Decrease toxicity
    B. Increase absorption
    C. Increase specificity
    D. Increase the immune response

21. An example of immune injury due to the deposition of antigen-antibody complexes is
    A. Acute glomerulonephritis
    B. Bee-sting allergy
    C. Contact dermatitis
    D. Penicillin allergy

22. The serologically detectable antibody produced in rheumatoid arthritis (RA) is of the class
    A. IgA
    B. IgE
    C. IgG
    D. IgM

23. In bone marrow transplantation, immuno-competent cells in the donor marrow may recognize antigens in the recipient and respond to those antigens. This phenomenon is an example of
    A. Acute rejection
    B. Chronic rejection
    C. Graft-vs.-host-disease (GVHD)
    D. Hyperacute rejection

24. The method used to determine MHC Class I compatibility between a donor and a recipient involves
    A. Fluorescent-labeled antigen
    B. Mixed lymphocyte cultures
    C. Sensitized RBCs
    D. Specific typing antibodies

25. Arthus reactions are initiated by
    A. IgE antibody
    B. IgG antibody
    C. IgM antibody
    D. T cell activity

26. In individuals allergic to bee venom, hyposensitization protocols may be initiated. These are designed to promote the formation of
    A. IgA
    B. IgE
    C. IgG
    D. IgM

27. After exposure to antigen, the first antibodies that can be detected belong to the class
    A. IgA
    B. IgG
    C. IgE
    D. IgM

28. Corneal tissue may be transplanted successfully from one patient to another because
    A. Anticorneal antibodies are easily suppressed
    B. Corneal antigens do not activate T cells
    C. The cornea is nonantigenic
    D. The cornea occupies a privileged site not usually seen by the immune system

29. A kidney transplantation from one identical twin to another is an example of
    A. A xenograft
    B. An allograft
    C. An autograft
    D. An isograft

30. In Bruton's disease, measurement of serum immunoglobulins would show
    A. Elevated levels of IgE
    B. Elevated levels of IgG
    C. Normal levels of IgG and IgM but reduced levels of IgA
    D. The absence of all immunoglobulins

31. Antigenically identical tumors produced in different animals are most commonly produced by
    A. Bacteria
    B. Chemicals
    C. Radiation
    D. Viruses

32. The lymphokine able to cause proliferation and differentiation of B cells is
    A. Interleukin 2
    B. Interleukin 4
    C. Interleukin 5
    D. Interleukin 9

33. Which cell is the principle source of interleukin 2?
    A. B cell
    B. Monocyte
    C. Plasma cell
    D. T cell

34. Diagnostic reagents useful for detecting antigen by the coagglutination reaction may be prepared by binding antibody to killed staphylococcal cells via the Fc receptor of staphylococcal protein A. The class of antibody bound by this protein is
    A. IgA
    B. IgD
    C. IgG
    D. IgM

35. A major advantage of passive immunization as opposed to active immunization is that
    A. Antibody is available more quickly
    B. Antibody persists for the life of the recipient
    C. IgM is the predominant antibody class provided
    D. Oral administration can be used

36. The strength with which a multivalent antibody binds a multivalent antigen is termed the
    A. Affinity
    B. Avidity
    C. Reactivity
    D. Valence

37. How does the secondary immune response differ from the primary immune response?
    A. IgG is the predominant antibody class produced in the secondary immune response
    B. The antibody levels produced are higher in the secondary immune response
    C. The lag phase (the time between exposure to antigen and production of antibody) is shorter in the secondary immune response
    D. All the above

38. After activation of the complement system, leukocytes and macrophages are attracted to the site of complement activation by
    A. C1
    B. C5a
    C. C8
    D. IgM

39. The type of immunity that follows the injection of an antigen is termed
    A. Active
    B. Adaptive
    C. Innate
    D. Passive

40. The type of immunity that follows the injection of antibodies synthesized by another individual or animal is termed
    A. Active
    B. Adaptive

C. Innate

D. Passive

41. Male sterility may be caused by an autoantibody against sperm cells. The body can make these antibodies because
    A. The testes constitute an immunologically privileged site
    B. The sperm cell has alloantigens
    C. The sperm cell develops altered antigens
    D. Sperm cell antigens develop after self-tolerance is induced

42. The agglutination pattern shown in Color Plate 23 was observed while performing an antibody titration. This agglutination pattern is an example of
    A. A prezone reaction
    B. A prozone reaction
    C. An inactive antigen
    D. Incomplete complement inactivation

43. The antibody most frequently present in systemic lupus erythematosus (SLE) is directed against
    A. Myelin
    B. Nuclear antigen
    C. Surface antigens of bone marrow stem cells
    D. Surface antigens of renal cells

44. The rapid plasma reagin (RPR) for syphilis does not need to be read microscopically because the antigen is
    A. Cardiolipin
    B. Complexed to charcoal
    C. Complexed to latex
    D. Inactivated bacterial cells

45. The Venereal Disease Research Laboratory (VDRL) test for syphilis is classified as a(n)
    A. Agglutination reaction
    B. Flocculation reaction

C. Hemagglutination reaction

D. Precipitation reaction

46. One of the causes of a false-positive VDRL test is
    A. Brucellosis
    B. Rocky Mountain spotted fever
    C. Systemic lupus erythematosus (SLE)
    D. *Treponema pallidum* infection

47. Which of the following ions is necessary in complement fixation tests?
    A. Fe^{3+}
    B. Mg^{2+}
    C. Mn^{2+}
    D. Zn^{2+}

48. A cause of false-positive results in the rapid plasma reagin (RPR) test for syphilis is
    A. Gastroenteritis
    B. Gonococcal urethritis
    C. Infectious mononucleosis
    D. Streptococcal pharyngitis

49. IgM antibodies are known to react well in complement fixation (CF) tests. Because of this, CF tests for antibodies should
    A. Be positive early in the course of the disease
    B. Be useful in identifying antibodies responsible for a delayed hypersensitivity reaction
    C. Be useful in identifying antibodies responsible for anaphylactic reactions
    D. Detect transplacental antibodies

50. Which of the following serologic tests is commonly performed by an immunofluorescence method?
    A. Antinuclear antibody (ANA)
    B. Antistreptolysin O (ASO)
    C. Heterophile antibody
    D. Venereal Disease Research Laboratory (VDRL) test for syphilis

51. Which of the following will invalidate a test for antistreptolysin O (ASO)?
    A. A reference serum titer within one dilution of the stated value
    B. Fifty percent lysis in the complement control tube
    C. Fifty percent lysis of the red cells in the hemolysin control
    D. No hemolysis in the red cell control

52. In the enzyme-linked immunosorbent assay (ELISA) system, the visible reaction is due to a reaction between
    A. Enzyme and substrate
    B. Fluorescent dye and bacteria
    C. Group-specific red cells and antibody
    D. Latex particles and antibody

53. The commonly used specific diagnostic test for infection by the hepatitis C virus (HCV) is
    A. An elevated alanine aminotransferase (ALT) level
    B. Negative tests for antibodies to hepatitis A and hepatitis B in the presence of jaundice
    C. The presence of anti-delta antibody
    D. The presence of anti-HCV antibody

54. For a substance to be immunogenic it must be
    A. A linear molecule
    B. A lipid
    C. Less than 5,000 molecular weight
    D. Recognized as nonself

55. There is no bursa of Fabricius in humans. Which of the following is considered the site of B-cell differentiation in adult humans?
    A. Bone marrow
    B. Liver
    C. Spleen
    D. Thymus

56. Which of the following statements about immunoglobulin light chains is true?
    A. Each immunoglobulin monomer has either one kappa or one lambda chain
    B. There are two types, kappa and lambda
    C. They consist of constant regions only
    D. They form part of the Fc fragment

57. Which of the following statements applies to the Fc fragment of an immunoglobulin molecule?
    A. It consists of the entire heavy chain
    B. It contains the antigen binding sites of the molecule
    C. It contains the variable region of the heavy chain
    D. It is produced by the action of papain on a complete immunoglobulin molecule

58. Monoclonal antibodies are produced by
    A. Cultured T cells
    B. Human plasma cells
    C. Hybridomas
    D. Mouse plasma cells

59. Which of the following statements about monoclonal antibodies of the same clone is true?
    A. They are highly specific
    B. They are produced by a malignant cell
    C. They have the same idiotype
    D. All the above

60. Skin testing is a useful diagnostic tool in a number of disorders such as tuberculosis. Which of the following statements about skin testing is true?
    A. A positive test depends on preformed antibody
    B. Sensitivity to a particular antigen may be transferred from one individual to another by sensitized lymphocytes

C. The intensity of the response correlates directly with the clinical activity of the disease

D. The maximum response will occur immediately

61. Large granular lymphocyte (LGL) is synonymous with
   A. Cytotoxic T cell
   B. Helper T cell
   C. Natural killer cell
   D. Suppressor T cell

62. Which of the following have been identified as B cell surface markers?
   A. C3 receptor
   B. Immunoglobulin
   C. MHC class II antigens
   D. All the above

63. Which of the following is not a characteristic of T cells?
   A. Able to bind antigen
   B. Antibody synthesis
   C. Possess CD1 antigen
   D. Protection against intracellular parasites

64. The mechanism responsible for pathology in autoimmune diseases is
   A. Circulating immune complexes
   B. Lack of intracellular killing after neutrophil phagocytosis of bacteria
   C. Non-specifically activated T cells
   D. The inability to activate B cells

65. Which complement protein is present in the greatest concentration in human serum?
   A. C1
   B. C2
   C. C3
   D. C4

66. Which class of antibody, referred to as incomplete antibody, is able to agglutinate RBCs after antihuman globulin is added?

A. IgA
B. IgE
C. IgG
D. IgM

67. An Ouchterlony gel diffusion plate is depicted in Color Plate 24. The center well contains antibody and the peripheral wells contain antigens labeled 1 through 4. What is the relationship between the antigen in well 2 and the antigen in well 3?
   A. 2 is part of 3
   B. 3 is part of 2
   C. They are identical
   D. They are unrelated

68. An Ouchterlony gel diffusion plate is depicted in Color Plate 24. The center well contains antibody and the peripheral wells contain antigens labeled 1 through 4. What is the relationship between the antigen in well 2 and the antigen in well 4?
   A. Cannot be determined
   B. They are identical
   C. They are unrelated
   D. They react incompletely with the antibody

69. Which of the following complement proteins is not part of the membrane attack complex?
   A. C4
   B. C5
   C. C7
   D. C9

70. Which of the following is characteristic of contact hypersensitivity reactions?
   A. Caused by preformed IgE antibody
   B. Characterized by infiltration of neutrophils into the area of reaction
   C. The primary symptoms often occur in the respiratory tract
   D. Usually due to a hapten

71. Which of the following statements about the test for C-reactive protein (CRP) is true?
    A. It correlates with neutrophil phagocytic function
    B. It is an indicator of ongoing inflammation
    C. It is diagnostic for rheumatic fever
    D. It measures patient antibody

72. In the classic pathway of complement activation
    A. C1q is activated by the presence of a single Fab region
    B. C3 is activated by binding C-reactive protein
    C. C3 is split into C3a and C3b
    D. The sequence of activation is C1, C2, C3, C4

73. The alternate pathway for complement activation
    A. Bypasses steps C1-C4
    B. Can be activated by bacterial capsule polysaccharides
    C. Can be activated by properdin
    D. All the above

74. A cut on a person's finger becomes contaminated with the bacterium *Staphylococcus aureus*. The first defense by the immune system consists of a response by
    A. B cells
    B. Monocytes
    C. Neutrophils
    D. T cells

75. A patient is suspected of having hereditary angioedema. Which of the following conditions would be found in this patient if this is the correct diagnosis?
    A. An increase in C1INH
    B. An increase in C1qrs
    C. An increase in C4
    D. An increase in complement activity

76. A 3-year-old male child presents with a history of recurring bacterial pneumonia. A test for T-cell function gives a normal result, lymphocyte counts are normal, and a CH50 test is normal. You would expect the child to have
    A. An abnormal thymus
    B. Defective C1q
    C. Lack of functional B cells
    D. Repeated fungal infections

77. In the enzyme-linked immunosorbent assay (ELISA) test
    A. A radioactive label is required
    B. Antigen-antibody interaction is indicated by a color change
    C. The enzyme system is always attached to patient antibody
    D. The method is useful only for detecting antibody as opposed to antigen

78. A serum test for HbsAg gives a positive result. This result indicates that the person from whom the serum was taken
    A. Had a hepatitis B infection in the past but overcame the infection
    B. Has either the active or chronic form of hepatitis B infection
    C. Is not infectious for the hepatitis B virus
    D. Was immunized recently against the hepatitis B virus

79. What is the indicator system used in the complement fixation test?
    A. Enzyme labeled antihuman globulin
    B. Fluorescent labeled antihuman globulin
    C. Guinea pig complement
    D. Sensitized sheep red blood cells

80. The idiotype of an immunoglobulin antibody
    A. Defines the heavy chain
    B. Defines the light chain
    C. Is constant for all immunoglobulins of an individual
    D. Is the variation within the variable region

81. The lymphokine most important for increased natural killer cell activity and decreased viral replication in cells is
   A. Interferon gamma
   B. Interleukin 3
   C. Interleukin 4
   D. Interleukin 5

82. The type of immunity following the transfer of lymphocytes from an immune host to a nonimmune host is
   A. Active
   B. Adaptive
   C. Innate
   D. Passive

83. Autoimmune disease is thought to arise when self-reactive T or B lymphocytes
   A. Are anergized
   B. Are deleted
   C. Are sufficiently activated to cause a prolonged, substantial inflammatory response
   D. Remain indifferent (unactivated)

84. Rheumatic heart disease sometimes occurs after Group A streptococcal infections. In this condition, an autoimmune response attacks the tissue of the heart valves. This phenomenon is an example of
   A. Epitope spreading
   B. Molecular mimicry
   C. Polyclonal B-cell activation
   D. Preferential activation of Th1 cells

85. "Superantigens" found in toxins produced by some strains of *Staphylococcus aureus* and Group A streptococcus are examples of
   A. Epitope spreading
   B. Molecular mimicry
   C. Polyclonal T-cell activation
   D. Preferential activation of Th1 cells

86. Typically, with no antirejection treatment, the fate of an allograft from an ABO-compatible individual is
   A. Acceptance
   B. Acute rejection
   C. Chronic rejection
   D. Hyperacute rejection

87. A living donor is being sought for a child who requires a kidney transplant. The best odds of finding an MHC-compatible donor occur between the child and
   A. A sibling (brother or sister)
   B. An unrelated individual
   C. The child's father
   D. The child's mother

88. Cells that can act as APCs for exogenous antigens include
   A. All nucleated cells
   B. B lymphocytes, macrophages/ monocytes, and dendritic cells
   C. Only B lymphocytes
   D. T lymphocytes

89. The T cell receptor (TCR) recognizes antigen
   A. As a peptide complexed to an MHC class II molecule on the surface of an APC
   B. As an intact molecule on the surface of a bacterium, fungus, or parasite
   C. As free-floating, degraded antigen fragments in body fluids
   D. When the antigen is complexed with its specific antibody

90. Activated $CD4^+$ T_H cells produce and respond to interleukin-2 (IL-2). This process is an example of
   A. Autocrine stimulation
   B. Clonal selection
   C. Paracrine stimulation
   D. T-cell activation

91. B lymphocytes and T lymphocytes are derived from
    A. Hematopoietic stem cells
    B. Macrophages or monocytes
    C. Mucosa-associated lymphoid tissue (MALT)
    D. The fetal liver

92. Contact dermatitis is mediated by
    A. B lymphocytes
    B. Macrophages
    C. Polymorphonuclear cells
    D. T lymphocytes

93. In the radioallergosorbent test (RAST) for the quantitation of IgE, what does a high count per minute (cpm) suggest?
    A. Allergen was improperly adsorbed to solid phase
    B. High concentration of IgE in patient's serum
    C. High levels of IgG nonspecifically binding to solid phase
    D. Pipetting error

94. A 5-year-old boy suffering from fever, inflamed cervical lymph nodes, multiple skin abscesses, and granulomas was admitted to the hospital. Pertinent lab results included

    WBC: 15,000/μL

    Differential: 72% PMN

         20% lymphocytes

         5% monocytes

         2% eosinophils

         1% basophils

    Total immunoglobulins: elevated

    CH_{50}: normal

    Serum protein electrophoresis: normal

    Skin test against *Candida* antigens: positive

    Nitroblue tetrazolium (NBT): negative

    T cell conA stimulation: normal

Which of the following describes his immune deficiency?
    A. Anergy
    B. B cell deficiency
    C. Defective neutrophil function
    D. T cell deficiency

95. An 18-year-old female presented with fever, sore throat, lethargy, and tender cervical lymphadenopathy. Relevant findings included splenomegaly and lymphocytosis with many large atypical lymphocytes. Heterophile antibody tests were negative. Further laboratory results were

	IgG titer	IgM titer
Cytomegalovirus (CMV)	20	0
Epstein-Barr virus (EBV) VCA	0	80
Toxoplasma	0	0

What conclusion can be made concerning the diagnosis?
    A. Acute CMV infection
    B. Acute EBV infection
    C. Acute toxoplasmosis
    D. Autoimmune disease

96. A male infant had been well until about 5 months of age, at which time he was diagnosed as having otitis media and bronchitis caused by *Haemophilus influenzae*. Over the next several months he presented with streptococcal pneumonia and giardiasis. At 10 months of age a serum protein electrophoresis showed a virtual lack of gamma globulins. Quantitative serum levels were as follows: 75 mg/dL IgG and undetectable levels of IgM, IgA, and IgE. There were a normal number of T cells and they exhibited normal mitogen stimulation.

What disease does this child most likely suffer from?

A. Combined immunodeficiency

B. DiGeorge's syndrome

C. Iatrogenic immunodeficiency

D. X-linked agammaglobulinemia

97. An antibody titration is depicted in Color Plate 25. In this titration, a 0.2 mL aliquot of a patient's serum sample was added to 0.8 mL of saline, and this mixture was labeled tube #1. A 0.5 mL sample was removed from tube #1 and placed into another tube, labeled tube #2, and 0.5 mL of saline was added. This procedure was repeated thru tube #10. The dilutions were assayed for antibody to an infectious agent. How should the antibody titer be reported?

A. 1:512

B. 512

C. 1:640

D. 640

98. Typically, with no antirejection treatment, the fate of an autograft is

A. Acceptance

B. Acute rejection

C. Chronic rejection

D. Hyperacute rejection

99. An example of a minor histocompatibility antigen is

A. The ABO blood group "AB"

B. The H-Y antigen

C. The MHC Class I antigen HLA-B27

D. None of the above

100. When an antigen and an antibody react, bonds are formed between the two molecules. These bonds may be

A. Covalent bonds

B. Hydrogen bonds

C. Ionic bonds

D. All the above

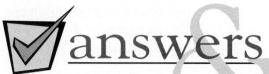

answers & rationales

1.

A. The basic structure of all immunoglobulins is two light chains joined to two heavy chains by disulfide bridges. The amino terminals of both the heavy and light chains, together, constitute the Fab fragment (antigen binding fragment). The carboxyl terminals of the heavy chains constitute the Fc fragment. The hinge region is the area at the center of the "Y," near the carboxyl terminals of the light chains.

2.

B. Haptens are substances that are not immunogenic by themselves. These molecules are not large or complex enough to stimulate the immune system. When bound to a carrier, they are capable of stimulating a specific immune response.

3.

D. The ability to convert to plasma cells and memory cells following clonal proliferation is characteristic of B cells. In addition, B cells carry surface immunoglobulins that react to a specific antigen. The liver is the source of complement components.

4.

B. Lymphokines are soluble mediators of cellular immunity reactions. They are produced most often by T lymphocytes. Antibodies are produced by plasma cells.

5.

B. The Fc region of an IgG molecule fits into an Fc receptor (FcR) on macrophages and monocytes. The Fc receptor binds to specific amino acid residues in the Fc region of the immunoglobulin. The variable region of immunoglobulin binds to the antigen.

6.

B. Unlike the A, B, and C antigens in the HLA system that can be identified serologically, the DP, DQ, and DR antigens must be determined by mixed lymphocyte culture or the polymerase chain reaction (PCR). Like the other HLA antigens, they are inherited codominantly. The HLA-DP, DQ, and DR antigens are important for transplant immunology.

7.

B. The HLA system is part of a larger region known as the major histocompatibility complex; it is located on chromosome 6. The region is located on the short arm of the chromosome. Chromosome 15 contains one HLA gene, B2M. The murine major histocompatibility genes are located on chromosome 17 of the mouse.

8.

D. Human leukocyte antigens (HLA) are a group of antigens originally described on human white cells. It is now known that they are found on all nucleated cells of the body, including solid tissue cells. HLA antigens are not found on red blood cells.

9.

A. The most significant indicator of acute recent or current infection is the presence of a rising antibody titer. A fourfold or greater rise in titer, from 2 to 16, is significant. Even relatively high antibody titers that are IgG may indicate past infection. IgM is produced first following bacterial infections.

10.
A. C3 may be decreased owing to a genetic defect that caused deficient production. Because complement is usually measured immunologically by radial immunodiffusion, the activity of the molecule is not determined. In certain autoimmune disorders such as systemic lupus erythematosus, continual complement activation leads to low levels; however, susceptibility to pyogenic infections is not a feature of autoimmune diseases. DiGeorge syndrome is a deficiency in T cells.

11.
D. Antibody production is antigen induced. Because the fetus develops in a sequestered site, it makes very little immunoglobulin. Maternal IgG is able to cross the placenta and is the primary antibody found in infant's circulation.

12.
A. The germinal centers of lymph nodes are where B cells undergo transformation after antigen stimulation. T cells are located primarily in the paracortex, while the medullary cord is the location of plasma cells. B cells located within the germinal centers are called follicular center cells.

13.
C. Immunoglobulin G is the predominant class of immunoglobulin found in serum. It accounts for approximately 80% of the total serum immunoglobulin. The normal range is 800–1600 mg/dL.

14.
B. The heavy (H) chains divide human immunoglobulin molecules into separate classes and subclasses. The delta (δ) corresponds to IgD. The remaining classes IgA, IgE, IgG, and IgM correspond to α, ε, γ, and μ, respectively.

15.
D. The IgM molecule is a pentamer that contains 10 binding sites. However, the actual valence falls to 5 with larger antigen molecules, probably due to steric restrictions. IgA, IgG, IgD, and IgE monomers each have two antigenic binding sites.

16.
C. IgA is found in sero-mucous secretions as a dimer stabilized by the J-piece. IgA is synthesized locally by plasma cells and dimerized intracellularly. IgM is also held together by a J-piece, but is found as pentamers.

17.
C. Mast cells and basophils have surface receptors (FcεRI) for the Fc portion of IgE. When sensitized mast cells come in contact with the specific allergin they degranulate, producing the symptoms of immediate hypersensitivity. The main function of IgE appears to be the ability to trigger an immune response, thereby recruiting plasma factors and effector cells to areas of trauma or parasite infection.

18.
C. Antigenic analysis of IgG myelomas has revealed four isotypic subclasses of IgG, based on differences in the heavy chains. These subclasses are called IgG1, IgG2, IgG3, and IgG4. All four subclasses are able to cross the placenta and fix complement.

19.
C. In the EMIT a ligand (antigen) in a sample competes with an enzyme-labeled ligand for binding to a specific antibody. The labeled ligand is designed so that following antibody binding, the enzyme is inactive. As the ligand concentration in the test sample increases, more enzyme-labeled ligand remains unbound, resulting in greater enzyme activity.

20.
D. Adjuvants enhance antigenicity nonspecifically. The most common are water-in-oil emulsions. They are not cleared from the injection site as quickly as antigen alone. This gives the immune system a longer time to "see" the antigen and to react. They also seem to activate macrophages, which increases the immune response.

21.
A. Acute glomerulonephritis is caused by the presence of a soluble circulating antigen (Ag) that provokes and combines with antibody (Ab). As these Ag-Ab complexes reach a critical size, they are deposited in the glomerular membranes of the kidney. Upon deposition, an acute inflammatory reac-

tion occurs because of complement activation. As larger particles are formed, they are removed by the mononuclear phagocyte system. Bee-sting allergy and penicillin allergy are examples of Ig-E mediated anaphylactic reactions. Contact dermatitis is mediated by T cells, not antibody.

22.

D. Rheumatoid factors (RF) are immunoglobulins that react with antigenic determinants on the IgG molecule. Although they may be of several types, the one that is easily serologically detectable is IgM. This is because of the agglutination activity of the molecule. RF tests are commonly used in the diagnosis of rheumatoid arthritis.

23.

C. Bone marrow transplants by their nature contain immunologically competent cells—B cell and T cells, in particular. Unless the transplanted marrow is HLA-matched perfectly to the donor, the immunocompetent cells in the transplant will recognize and react against the nonself HLA antigens of the recipient's tissues. This phenomenon is known as graft-*vs.*-host disease, because the graft attempt to reject its host. Acute rejection, chronic rejection, and hyperacute rejection are all examples of graft-*vs.*-host rejection.

24.

D. The MHC class I antigens are described as *serologically defined*. This term means that the genes coding for the class I antigens cause the expression of antigens on the surface of all nucleated cells. The surface antigens can be detected with specific antibodies—hence, the antigens are said to be serologically defined. Mixed lymphocyte cultures are one of the methods for detecting MHC class II antigens—which are not serologically defined. Neither sensitized RBCs nor fluorescent-labeled antigens are employed in identifying class I antigens.

25.

B. The Arthus reaction is a localized reaction that takes place in and around small blood vessels. Circulating IgG reacts with localized antigen to form an immune complex. This complex may be deposited in vessel walls and activate complement to cause an inflammatory reaction.

26.

C. The reaction to bee venom is caused by the presence of an IgE antibody. By injecting doses of allergin, IgG antibody will be stimulated. This IgG blocks the binding of IgE to the allergin (bee venom in this case).

27.

D. The first B cells to respond to antigen stimulation produce IgM antibody. Later in the immune response, stimulated B cells undergo a phenomenon called "class switching" and begin to produce antibodies of the IgG, IgM, and IgE class.

28.

D. Corneas are readily transplanted from one individual to another. This is because the cornea is nonvascularized. Thus the immune system of the host does not "see" the cornea and recognize it as foreign.

29.

D. Identical twins have the same genetic structure. Grafts between them would be isografts or syngeneic grafts. Autografts are transplantations from one site to another in the same individual. Xenograft and heterograft both refer to transplantation between different species. Transplantation between two nonidentical individuals of the same species are called allografts.

30.

D. Bruton's disease is a congenital form of agammaglobulinemia. It is a sex-linked phenomenon that affects males. Since B cells are not produced, the boys have undetectable levels of IgA, IgD, IgE, and IgM by routine assays. IgG may be absent or present at very low levels.

31.

D. Antigens found in tumors produced by chemicals are unique to each individual tumor. In contrast, the tumor antigens found on tumors produced by a virus will be identical in all cases where the same virus induced the tumor. Immune responses to virally induced tumors are generally stronger than immune responses to chemically induced tumors.

32.

B. Lymphokines are soluble messengers that mediate communication between cells. Various lymphokines from different cells have the ability to induce B cell proliferation and differentiation. Interleukin 4 was the first interleukin noted to cause the activation of resting B cells.

33.

D. Interleukin 2 (IL-2) is a lymphokine produced exclusively by activated T lymphocytes. The only known targets of IL-2 are T cells, B cells, and natural killer cells. IL-2 acts on its target cells via the IL-2 receptor. This receptor is not present on resting cells.

34.

C. Staphylococcal protein A binds only the IgG class of immunoglobulin. Binding occurs via the Fc portion of the antibody molecule, leaving the Fab portion available to bind antigen in a testing situation. Binding of the Fab portion to test antigen causes agglutination of the staphylococcal cells (coagglutination).

35.

A. In passive immunization, pre-formed antibody is delivered to the recipient, making the antibody available immediately. In active immunization, a period of days is required before antibody production occurs. Passive immunity is short-lived, in contrast to the possibly live-long persistence of actively induced antibody. Since passive immunization involves the transfer of antibodies, the oral route cannot be used—antibodies are digested in the gastrointestinal tract. The antibodies administered by passive immunization consists largely of IgG class molecules.

36.

B. *Avidity* is used to describe the strength of binding between a multivalent antibody and multivalent antigen. *Affinity* describes the bond between a single antigenic determinant and an individual combining site. *Valence* refers to the number of antigenic determinants on an antigen.

37.

D. The secondary immune response is characterized by the predominance of IgG over IgM. In addition,

due to the formation of memory cells following the primary response, the secondary response occurs much more quickly and much more strongly. This is the basis for immunization as a protection against various infectious diseases.

38.

B. The complement-activation product C5a is chemotactic for neutrophils and macrophages. Neither C1 nor C8 (which occur in the plasma before complement activation) possess such chemotactic properties. IgM antibody, while capable of activating complement by the classical pathway, is not a chemotactic factor for phagocytic cells.

39.

A. Active immunity follows exposure to an antigen that stimulates the recipient to develop his or her own immune response. Vaccines and surviving infections can result in active immunity. Protection is due to the formation of memory cells.

40.

D. Passive immunity results following the injection of antibody synthesized by another individual or animal. This type of immunity is only temporary but may be very important in providing "instant" protection from an infectious agent before the recipient would have time to actively synthesize antibody. The injected antibodies are treated as foreign proteins and are eventually cleared from the body.

41.

D. Tissue is recognized as "self" by the immune system during fetal development. Since sperm does not exist in the fetus, tolerance does not develop. As the individual matures and antigen (sperm) is formed, the possibility for the production of an autoimmune response exists.

42.

B. Prozones occur when an extremely high titer of antibody is present. In the first tubes of the titration, not enough antigen is present to allow for cross-linking and lattice formation. The antibody effectively blocks all the antigen sites present, so agglutination does not occur. Complement is not involved in antibody titration.

43.

B. Anti-nuclear antibody (ANA) is the most consistent feature of systemic lupus erythematosus (SLE). Although renal or nerve pathology may occur, that pathology is secondary to deposition of antigen-antibody complexes and subsequent activation of the complement system. Bone marrow stems cells are not involved in the pathology of SLE.

44.

B. The RPR test uses a cardiolipin antigen. The RPR antigen is similar to the antigen used in the Venereal Disease Research Laboratory (VDRL) test for syphilis. However, in the RPR test, the cardiolipin antigen has been complexed to charcoal particles, allowing the reaction to be read macroscopically.

45.

B. The cardiolipin antigen is particulate, not soluble, in the VDRL test. However, the particles are too small to make macroscopic agglutinates when combined with antibody. This type of reaction is called a flocculation reaction and needs to be read with low power microscopy.

46.

C. Patients with connective tissue disorders such as SLE may show a chronic false positive reaction in the VDRL test. *Treponema pallidum* is the causative agent of syphilis. Other causes of false positives include rheumatic fever, infectious mononucleosis, malaria, and pregnancy.

47.

B. Mg^{2+} is used as a cofactor in the complement cascade, and must be present to activate the series of reactions. If it is not present, these reactions will not proceed. In the presence of Mg^{2+}, C2 can complex with activated C4b. Ca^{2+} helps stabilize C1q, C1r, and C1s.

48.

C. Infectious mononucleosis leads to the production of many antibodies unrelated to infection by the causative agent, Epstein-Barr virus, because the viral infection leads to non-specific stimulation of B cells. Malaria, leprosy, and rheumatoid arthritis may also cause false-positive RPR results. None of the other infections listed are associated with false-positive RPR results.

49.

A. In most infections IgM antibodies will develop first followed by IgG, which develop higher titers and are longer lasting. Anaphylactic reactions are caused by IgE antibody. Delayed hypersensitivity reactions are caused by T cells. Transplacental antibodies belong to the IgG class. IgG antibodies, although they can be detected by CF, do not fix complement efficiently.

50.

A. Testing for antinuclear antibodies (ANA) is commonly performed by the immunofluorescence method—using fluorescein-conjugated antihuman antibody to detect patient antibody bound to nuclear components of test cells. Antistreptolysin O tests are performed with red cells. Heterophile antibodies are detected with various latex or animal cell agglutination reactions. The VDRL test detects flocculation of cardiolipin antigen.

51.

C. The ASO test depends on the ability of antibody in patient serum to prevent lysis of red cells by streptolysin. If the streptolysin (a hemolysin) does not completely lyse the red cells, the test may be interpreted as showing the presence of antibody when there is none. The red cell control contains no hemolysin and so should not show lysis. This lysis does not depend on the presence of complement.

52.

A. The indicator system in an ELISA test consists of an enzyme and its substrate. If the enzyme-labeled antibody has complexed with the immobilized antigen, the addition of substrate will produce a colored end product. Alkaline phosphatase is an enzyme frequently used in ELISA tests. Latex particles, fluorescent dyes, and red cells are not used in ELISA tests but in other test methodologies.

53.

D. Patients infected with the hepatitis C virus (HCV) develop anti-HCV antibody that provides a relatively specific diagnostic tool for this infection. Follow-up testing may involve a form of immunoblotting test or a polymerase chain reaction test. An elevated alanine aminotransferase (ALT), although commonly occurring in HCV infection, is not specific for this infection. Negative tests for antibody to other agents of viral hepatitis do not provide specific diagnostic information. Anti-delta antibody is associated with hepatitis D infection.

54.

D. The major requirements for a substance to be antigenic are that it be foreign to the host (nonself) and be a macromolecule with internal complexity. Compounds with a molecular weight under 10,000 are not ordinarily antigenic by themselves. Although polysaccharides as well as proteins may be antigenic, lipids alone are not.

55.

A. In birds, B cells are produced in the bursa of Fabricius. In humans, although the exact equivalent area of B cell differentiation is not known, the primary sites of B cell differentiation are the fetal liver and (following birth) the bone marrow. T cells mature in the thymus.

56.

B. Light chains are of two distinct types, kappa and lambda. Either type may combine with any of the heavy chains, but in any one molecule, only one type is found. Each immunoglobulin monomer contains two light chains, either kappa or lambda. They extend into the Fab, or antigen-binding, site. This half of the chain is highly variable, whereas the carboxyl terminal portion of the molecule is a constant region.

57.

D. The Fc fragment of an immunoglobulin is produced by papain digestion of an immunoglobulin monomer. The enzyme splits the molecule just above the disulfide molecule joining the heavy chains. Only part of the heavy chain is found in the Fc fragment. The Fab fragment contains the antigen combining sites of both the heavy chains and the light chains.

58.

C. A monoclonal antibody is produced by a single cell or clone. Plasma cells obtained from an immunized animal and subsequently fused with myeloma cells result in a hybrid myeloma or hybridoma that will indefinitely secrete a specific antibody. Hybridomas have been prepared from mouse and human plasma cells fused with myeloma cells. T cells do not produce antibodies.

59.

D. Monoclonal antibodies are produced by the fusion of an antibody-producing cell with a myeloma tumor cell. This hybridoma produces large quantities of highly specific antibody, all molecules of which share class, subclass, and idiotype. Although this material was originally harvested from mouse ascites, today these cells can be grown in tissue culture. Monoclonal antibodies are particularly useful in recognizing cell surface antigens and have been a valuable clinical tool in therapy and in the generation of new diagnostic kits.

60.

B. Skin testing is based upon the presence of T lymphocytes sensitized to antigen. Their activation produces a delayed hypersensitivity reaction, which reaches its peak in about 48 hours. There is no correlation of the amount of the reaction with clinical disease. If the sensitized T cells are transferred from one individual to another, the recipient individual will manifest the same delayed hypersensitivity as the donor.

61.

C. The natural killer (NK) cells destroy target cells through an extracellular nonphagocytic mechanism. Approximately 75% of LGL function is NK cells, and LGL account for the NK activity in mixed cell populations. LGLs make up only about 5% of mononuclear cells of the blood and spleen.

62.

D. Surface immunoglobulins on B cells usually are found with mu and delta heavy chains. They also contain receptors to bind the Fc portion of immunoglobulins. Receptors for C3 have been found on about 75% of B cells. In addition, B cells contain MHC class II antigens, which are involved in T and B cell cooperation.

63.

B. Although helper-T cells are able to modulate the synthesis of antibody by plasma cells, they themselves do not produce antibody. T cells contain receptors for IL-2 and antigens. In addition mature T cells are $CD1^+$.

64.

A. Circulating immune complexes, composed of nuclear antigen and anti-nuclear antibody, deposit in various organ systems, activate complement, and produce organ pathology. T cells are not directly involved in this process. B cells are activated, producing the anti-nuclear antibodies. Neither phagocytosis nor killing of ingested bacteria by neutrophils plays a role in the pathogenic process.

65.

C. Complement protein C3 has a serum concentration of about 1300 μg/mL, which makes it the complement protein present in the greatest concentration. The second highest concentration of complement protein is C4 (600 μg/mL). C3 is cleaved into several fragments including C3a, C3b, and C3c.

66.

C. Immunoglobulin G is referred to as an incomplete antibody. This name is given due to its decreased potential for agglutination compared to IgM. The IgG molecule is a complete immunoglobulin molecule. But IgG does not agglutinate large antigen-bearing particles, such as RBCs, unless conditions are modified by the addition of additional antibodies or by manipulating the protein concentration or ionic strength of the agglutinating medium.

67.

D. The two antigens are not related. There are two different antibodies that are able to react with the two antigens, forming precipitin lines that cross. If the antigens were identical, a smooth curve would have been formed.

68.

B. When two antigens are identical, a smooth curve is formed between them. In the diagram, the antigen in well 2 is identical to one of two antigens in well 1. The same antigen in well 1 is identical to antigen in well 4. It therefore follows that antigens 2 and 4 are identical.

69.

A. The membrane attack complex forms following the binding of C5 to a biologic membrane. The complex is formed by the sequential addition of C6, C7, C8, and C9. When C5-C8 complexes with C9, a tubule is formed that bridges the cell membrane.

70.

D. Contact dermatitis is a cell-mediated hypersensitivity reaction. The offending substance is typically a hapten that combines with a carrier molecule on the skin surface. The hapten-carrier complex is recognized by T cells. The T cells "reject" the cells carrying the hapten-carrier complex, producing the dermatitis. IgE mediates immediate hypersensitivity reactions such as hay fever and some forms of asthma.

71.

B. CRP is an acute phase reactant. Although it is elevated in inflammation, its presence is not diagnostic for any one disease such as rheumatic fever. It does not correlate with antibody levels or with neutrophil phagocytic function.

72.

C. Complement (C) attaches to the Fc part of the antibody molecule. At least two Fc binding sites are required for C1q to attach. The C proteins were named in order of discovery. The correct reaction sequence is C1, 4, 2, 3. As the last step of this reaction sequence, C3 is split into C3a and C3b.

73.

D. The properdin or alternate pathway for complement activation is a more nonspecific defense mechanism, in that it does not require the presence of antibody for activation. It can be activated by a variety of substances, including properdin and the complex polysaccharides found in bacterial cell walls. These materials activate C3 directly. In some hematologic disorders such as sickle cell anemia, this system appears to be deficient.

74.

C. The first response to invading bacteria is mounted by the innate immune system. The innate immune system, while lacking the specificity of the adaptive immune system, is nonetheless effective at handling many invading bacteria. The first response by the innate immune system consists of an influx of neutrophils into the tissue invaded by bacteria. B cells and T cells are part of the adaptive immune response. Macrophages, although phagocytic cells and part of the innate immune system, play only a minor role in the initial response to bacterial invasion.

75.

D. Hereditary angioedema is caused by the lack of an inhibitor to the first reaction in the complement (C) sequence called C1INH. The lack of inhibition causes increased C activity. This activity results in an increase in C2b, which becomes a vasoactive peptide.

76.
B. The fact that the child has a problem with bacterial infection indicates a deficiency in B cells, which are needed to produce antibody. The T cell function appears intact, as evidenced by the T-cell function test and normal lymphocyte count. The normal CH_{50} test indicates the presence and functionality of all complement components. T cells are important in combating intracellular parasites such as fungi.

77.
B. The ELISA system is a method in which an antibody that has been complexed to an enzyme system reacts with an initial antigen-antibody reaction. The enzyme-antibody complex, if bound, reacts with colorless substrate to produce a colored hydrolysis product. ELISA is similar in sensitivity to radioimmunoassay with the substitution of the enzyme system for the radioactive label. The test can be designed to detect either antigen or antibody in patient specimens.

78.
B. Hepatitis B surface antigen (HbsAg) is a marker for active or chronic infection by this virus; it indicates ongoing production of hepatitis B surface antigen. Such a person is infectious; i.e., capable of transmitting the virus. If the person had overcome a past infection, he or she would have antibody to surface antigen but not the surface antigen. Immunization causes formation of anti-surface antigen antibody; the surface antigen is not present in serum.

79.
D. The first step in the complement fixation test, the test system, involves the reaction of antibody in the patient's serum to the corresponding antigen in the presence of guinea pig complement. If antibody-antigen binding occurs, the complement will also bind. The second step is the addition of sensitized sheep red blood cells. If antibody to the test antigen was present, the complement will be bound to the complex, thereby preventing the complement from lysing the sensitized RBCs.

80.
D. The term *idiotype* refers to the variable region of an immunoglobulin molecule. The variable region is the portion of immunoglobulin that binds antigen. Every immunoglobulin with a given antigenic specificity has a unique idiotype.

81.
A. Interferons were discovered by virologists who noticed that individuals suffering from one viral disease rarely contracted another simultaneously. Interferons can be produced by virally infected cells. The interferon is then able to protect nearby uninfected cells. Interferon gamma, also called immune interferon, also stimulates natural killer cells.

82.
B. Following challenge by an antigen, a protective immune response may develop. The transfer of these cells involved, lymphocytes, to a naive (non-immune) host is called adaptive immunity. Adaptive immunity may take some time to be effective, but once active it can last for the life of the host.

83.
C. Under normal circumstances, self-reactive T and B lymphocytes are either anergized (made unresponsive) or deleted (by apoptosis). However, under certain circumstances, self-reactive T and B cells may be activated (i.e., their unresponsiveness may be overcome). If that activation results in a prolonged inflammatory response, additional T and B cells may be recruited by so-called "epitope spreading" to produce autoimmune disease.

84.
B. Group A streptococcus contains antigenic determinants that are similar to antigenic determinants found on heart valve tissue in some individuals. The immune response occurring during the course of a group A streptococcal infection may be extensive enough to include an immune-mediated attack on the heart valves—rheumatic heart disease. *Molecular mimicry* is the term given to this phenomenon whereby an immune response directed against one antigen may be extended to include activity against closely related antigens.

85.
C. Some strains of *Staphylococcus aureus* and Group A streptococcus produce toxins that have the properties of "superantigens." Superantigens react with T cells in a direct way; they stimulate all T cells, rather than stimulating only T cells bearing T-cell re-

ceptors specific for the antigens of the bacterial toxins. The result is a massive T-cell mediated immune response, leading to the disease entities known as toxic shock syndrome (in the case of *Staphylococcus aureus* infection) and toxic shock–like syndrome in the case of Group A streptococcus.

86.

B. An allograft describes a tissue or organ transplanted from an individual of one species to another individual of the same species, where the two individuals are not genetically identical. The result is acute rejection (rejection occurring in days to weeks) caused largely by incompatibility of the transplant's HLA antigens with the recipient's HLA antigens. Under normal circumstances, antirejection immunosuppressive therapy is administered to prevent this rejection. If the two individuals involved were additionally incompatible in terms of the ABO blood group system, the large amount of preformed antibody in the recipient would result in hyperacute rejection (rejection occurring within hours of transplant). Chronic rejection occurs over a period of months of years and is mediated by soluble antigens released from the transplant and stimulating the recipient's immune system.

87.

A. Because the HLA system is extremely polymorphic, the odds are greatly against finding an HLA compatible donor in unrelated individuals. The genes coding for HLA antigens are inherited from one's parents and are expressed co-dominantly. Between an offspring and either parent, there is, statistically, a 25% chance of an HLA match. Between siblings, there is a 50% chance of an HLA match.

88.

B. Exogenous antigens are nonself antigens derived from infectious agents or immunizing preparations. Exogenous antigens are processed for presentation to specific T cells by specialized cells collectively referred to as antigen processing cells (APCs). APCs for exogenous antigens include B cells, macrophages, monocytes, and dendritic cells.

89.

A. T cells recognize antigens for which they have predetermined specificity by encountering peptide

fragments of that antigen complexed to MHC class II molecules on the surface of an antigen presenting cell (APC). The recognition complex on the surface of the T cell is called the T-cell receptor (TCR). T-cell receptors do not respond to their specific antigen on the surface of cells other than APCs, nor do they respond to "free" antigens.

90.

A. Autocrine stimulation of T cells refers to a situation where a given T cell both secretes an interleukin (in this case, IL-2) and responds to the secreted molecule. Paracrine stimulation refers to a situation where a given T cell responds to an interleukin molecule secreted by a different cell. Clonal selection refers to the process whereby an antigenically stimulated lymphocyte undergoes blast transformation and divides to produce a clone of identical cells. T-cell activation refers to the state of a T cell that has encountered the antigen for which it has genetically preprogrammed specificity.

91.

A. The stem cells of the bone marrow give rise to both T cells and B cells, as well as other cells in the blood. Macrophages and monocytes also arise from hematopoietic stem cells but they do not differentiate into lymphocytes. MALT contains mature lymphocytes, particularly B cells, but is not the source of lymphocytes. The fetal liver is a maturation site for B lymphocytes during fetal life but is not the source of those lymphocytes.

92.

D. Contact dermatitis is a delayed-type hypersensitivity reaction mediated by T cells. Antibody is not involved in this type of hypersensitivity so B lymphocytes play no role in it. Neither macrophages nor neutrophils are involved in this type of hypersensitivity either.

93.

B. In the RAST, an allergen is adsorbed onto a solid phase. The patient's serum is allowed to bind to the allergen. This is followed by the addition of labeled anti-human antibody. Therefore, the greater the serum levels of IgE, the greater the binding of the labeled anti-IgE, and the greater the cpm.

94.

C. The results of the immune function tests were normal: the complement (CH$_{50}$ assay), B cell function (immunoglobulin assay), and T cell function (conA stimulation and *Candida* antigen skin test). The WBC count is elevated but the differential was within normal limits. An abnormal NBT test indicates defective neutrophil function, which is consistent with the child's granulomatous disease.

95.

B. The symptoms of fever of unknown origin (FUO), lymphocytosis, and lymphadenopathy suggest EBV or CMV infection and lymphoma or leukemia. Heterophile antibodies become positive later than antibodies to viral core antigen (VCA) of EBV. The IgM titer of 80 for EBV is consistent with acute EBV infection.

96.

D. The case history is typical of a child with X-linked agammaglobulinemia. He presented with chronic and recurrent infections beginning at 5 months of age, when transplacentally acquired IgG had declined. Normal IgG serum level is about 800–1200 mg/dL. The infant had normal T cell function, which rules out combined immunodeficiency and DiGeorge's syndrome. Iatrogenic immunodeficiency refers to an immunodeficiency following therapy prescribed by a physician.

97.

D. The titer of this assay is the reciprocal of the highest dilution demonstrating the desired result. In this case that is tube #8. The dilution is determined as shown below.

Dilution for tube #1:

0.2 mL serum in a total volume of 1.0 mL = 1:5 dilution

Dilutions in succeeding tubes:

0.5 mL diluted serum in a total volume of 1.0 mL = 1:2 dilution

The dilutions in the series of tubes are as follows:

Tube #1, 1:5; tube #2, 1:10; tube #3, 1:20; tube #4, 1:40; tube #5, 1:80; tube #6, 1:160; tube # 7, 1:320; tube #8, 1:640; tube #9, 1:1280; tube #10, 1:2560.

The reciprocal of the dilution in tube #8 (1:640) is 640.

98.

A. An autograft is the transplantation of tissue or an organ from one site to another on the same individual—as is done in skin grafting following thermal burns. Since there is no issue of HLA incompatibility, the transplant will be accepted. Hyperacute rejection occurs within hours of transplantation of tissue to an ABO-incompatible individual. Acute rejection occurs within days to weeks in the case of an allograft transplant without immunosuppressive therapy. Chronic rejection, occurring months to years after an allograft transplant, arises from soluble antigens migrating from the transplant and being recognized by the recipient's immune system.

99.

B. The HLA antigens constitute the "major histocompatibility complex" (MHC). But there are other antigens working against the acceptance of transplanted tissue or organs. These other antigens are referred to collectively as "minor histocompatibility antigens." One of the best studied is an antigen coded for by the Y chromosome and named H-Y antigen. This antigen may cause transplantation problems when tissue or an organ from a male (expressing H-Y antigen) is transplanted to a female who will recognize the H-Y antigen as nonself.

100.

B. The bonds between an antigen and its specific antibody may be electrostatic bonds, hydrogen bonds, or hydrophobic interactions. These bonds are reversible: they may form, dissolve, and then re-form. Covalent bonds, on the other hand, are generally nonreversible. Ionic bonds are not involved in antigen-antibody binding, either, because such bonds do not form readily in the aqueous environment of cells and tissues.

REFERENCES

Murray, P. R., Rosenthal, K. S., Kobayashi, G. S., and Pfaller, M. A. (1998). *Medical Microbiology*, 3rd ed. St. Louis: Mosby.

Roitt, I., Brostoff, J., and Male, D. (1996). *Immunology*, 4th ed. London: Mosby.

Sharon, J. (1998). *Basic Immunology*. Baltimore: Williams & Wilkins.

Turgeon, M. L. (1996). *Immunology and Serology in Laboratory Medicine*, 2nd ed. St. Louis: Mosby.

5 Immunohematology

contents

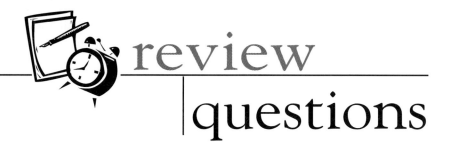

review questions

INSTRUCTIONS Each of the questions or incomplete statements that follow comprises four suggested responses. Select the *best* answer or completion statement in each case.

BLOOD COLLECTION, PRESERVATION, PROCESSING, COMPONENT PREPARATION, AND QUALITY CONTROL

1. A woman wants to donate blood. Her physical examination reveals the following: weight—110 pounds, pulse—73 beats/minute, blood pressure—125/75, hematocrit—35%. Which of the following exclusions applies to the prospective donor?
   A. Pulse too high
   B. Weight too low
   C. Hematocrit too low
   D. Blood pressure too low

2. A potential donor has no exclusions, but she weighs only 95 pounds. What is the allowable amount of blood (including samples) that can be drawn?
   A. 367 mL
   B. 378 mL
   C. 454 mL
   D. 473 mL

3. Donors who have received blood or blood products within 12 months of when they desire to donate are deferred to protect the recipient because the

A. Blood could have transmitted hepatitis (HBV or HCV) or HIV
B. Blood may have two cell populations
C. Donor may not be able to tolerate the blood loss
D. Donor red cell hemoglobin level may be too low

4. Which of the following conditions would contraindicate autologous presurgical donation?
   A. Weight of 100 pounds
   B. Age of 14 years
   C. Hemoglobin of 12 g/dL
   D. Mild bacteremia

5. Which of the following donors would be deferred indefinitely?
   A. History of syphilis
   B. History of gonorrhea
   C. Accutane® treatment
   D. Recipient of human growth hormone

6. Which of the following viruses resides exclusively in leukocytes?
   A. CMV
   B. HIV
   C. HBV
   D. HCV

7. A donor indicates he has taken two aspirin tablets per day for the last 36 hours. The unit of blood
   A. May not be used for pooled platelet concentrate preparation
   B. Should not be drawn until 36 hours after cessation of aspirin ingestion
   C. May be used for pooled platelet concentrate preparation
   D. May be used for red blood cells and fresh-frozen plasma production, but the platelets should be discarded

8. Which of the following best describes what must be done with a unit of blood drawn from a donor who is found to be at high risk of contracting acquired immune deficiency syndrome (AIDS)?
   A. Hold unit in quarantine until donor diagnosis is clarified
   B. Use the blood for research dealing with AIDS
   C. Properly dispose of unit by autoclaving or incineration
   D. Use the plasma and destroy the red blood cells

9. Which of the following is *least* likely to transmit hepatitis?
   A. Cryoprecipitate
   B. RBC
   C. Plasma protein fraction (PPF)
   D. Platelets

10. Which of the following tests is used to confirm a positive screening test for anti-HCV?
    A. Reverse passive hemagglutination (RPHA)
    B. Counterimmunoelectrophoresis (CIE)
    C. Enzyme immunoassay (EIA)
    D. Recombinant immunoblot assay (RIBA)

11. Although cryoprecipitate has primarily been used for treatment of hypofibrinogenemia and hemophilia A, it contains other blood proteins useful in the treatment of coagulopathies. Which of the following is *not* found in cryoprecipitate?
    A. Fibronectin
    B. Factor XIII
    C. Factor VIII:vW
    D. Antithrombin III

12. Fresh-frozen plasma (FFP), when properly collected and stored, provides all the following *except*
    A. Factor V
    B. Factor VIII
    C. Factor IX
    D. Platelets

13. All the following components must be routinely irradiated *except*
    A. RBC for intrauterine transfusion
    B. RBC for exchange transfusion
    C. Platelets for an immunosuppressed patient
    D. Platelets from an HLA compatible donor

14. The addition of adenine in an anticoagulant-preservative formulation aids in
    A. Maintaining ATP levels for red cell viability
    B. Maintaining platelet function in stored blood
    C. Reducing the plasma K^+ levels during storage
    D. Maintaining 2,3-DPG levels for oxygen release to the tissues

15. The pilot tubes for donor unit #3276 break in the centrifuge. You should
    A. Label the blood using the donor's previous records
    B. Discard the unit because processing procedures cannot be performed
    C. Discard the red cells and salvage the plasma for fractionation

D. Remove sufficient segments to complete donor processing procedures

---

Use the following information to answer questions 16 and 17.

A satellite bag containing 250 mL of fresh plasma is selected for quality control of cryoprecipitate production. Cryoprecipitate is prepared according to standard operating procedures. The final product has a total volume of 10 mL. The factor VIII assays are 1 IU/mL before and 9 IU/mL after preparation.

---

16. What is the percent yield of factor VIII in the final cryoprecipitate?
    A. 11%
    B. 25%
    C. 36%
    D. 80%

17. Does this product meet AABB *Standards* for cryoprecipitate production?
    A. Yes
    B. No, the percent recovery is too low
    C. No, the final factor VIII level is too low
    D. Data are insufficient to calculate

Use the following information to answer questions 18–21.

A centrifuge used for platelet preparation has been returned after major repair. A unit of whole blood (450 mL; platelet count 200,000/μL) is selected for calibration of platelet production. The platelet-rich plasma (PRP) contains 250 mL with a platelet count of 300,000/μL. The final platelet concentrate prepared from the PRP contains 50 mL with a platelet count of 900,000/μL.

---

18. What is the percent yield of platelets in the PRP from this unit?
    A. 33%
    B. 45%
    C. 66%
    D. 83%

19. What is the percent yield of platelets in the final product from the PRP?
    A. 30%
    B. 45%
    C. 50%
    D. 60%

20. Does this product meet AABB *Standards* for platelet concentrate production?
    A. Yes
    B. No, the count on the final product is too low
    C. No, the percentage recovery in the PRP is too low
    D. Data are insufficient to calculate

21. The final product was prepared with a PRP spin time of 2 minutes at 2500 rpm. To increase the percent platelet yield in the final product, one would
    A. Increase the time and/or rpm for the first spin
    B. Increase the time and/or rpm for the second spin
    C. Decrease the time and/or rpm for the first spin
    D. Decrease the time and/or rpm for the second spin

22. When 2,3-DPG levels drop in stored blood, which of the following occurs as a result?
    A. Red blood cell K^+ increases
    B. Red blood cell ability to deliver O_2 decreases
    C. Plasma hemoglobin is stabilized
    D. ATP synthesis increases

23. The last unit of autologous blood for an elective surgery patient must be collected no later than _____ hours prior to surgery.
    A. 24
    B. 36
    C. 48
    D. 72

24. Autologous donation is indicated for all the following patients *except* for
    A. Patients with an antibody against a high incidence antigen
    B. Patients with aortic stenosis
    C. Open heart surgery patients
    D. Patients with multiple antibodies

25. It is generally asymptomatic but has a very high carrier rate (70–80% have chronic infections). About 10% of the carriers develop cirrhosis or hepatocellular carcinoma. These statements are most typical of which of the following transfusion-transmitted infections?
    A. HAV
    B. HBV
    C. HCV
    D. HEV

26. Biochemical changes occur during the shelf life of stored blood. Which of the following is a result of this "storage lesion"?
    A. Increase in pH
    B. Increase in plasma K^+
    C. Increase in plasma Na^+
    D. Decrease in plasma hemoglobin

27. It has been determined that a patient has posttransfusion hepatitis and received blood from 8 donors. There is nothing to indicate that these donors may have been likely to transmit hepatitis. What action must be taken initially?
    A. Defer all donors indefinitely from further donations
    B. Repeat all hepatitis testing on a fresh sample from each donor
    C. Notify the donor center that collected the blood
    D. Interview all implicated donors

28. The temperature range for maintaining red blood cells and whole blood during shipping is

A. 0–4 °C
B. 1–6 °C
C. 1–10 °C
D. 5–15 °C

29. Platelets play an important role in maintaining hemostasis. One unit of donor platelets should yield _____ platelets.
    A. 5.5×10^6
    B. 5×10^8
    C. 5.5×10^{10}
    D. 5×10^{10}

30. The pH of four platelet concentrates is measured on the day of expiration. pH and plasma volumes are as follows: pH 6.0, 45 mL; pH 5.5, 38 mL; pH 5.8, 40 mL; pH 5.7, 41 mL. What corrective action is needed in product preparation to meet AABB *Standards* for platelet production?
    A. No corrective action is necessary
    B. Recalibrate pH meter
    C. Increase final plasma volume of platelet concentrates
    D. Decrease final plasma volume of platelet concentrates

31. During preparation of platelet concentrate, the hermetic seal of the primary bag is broken. The red blood cells
    A. Must be discarded
    B. May be labeled with a 21-day expiration date if collected in CPD
    C. Must be labeled with a 24-hour expiration date
    D. May be glycerolized within 6 days and stored frozen

32. The blood bank procedures manual must be
    A. Revised annually
    B. Revised after publication of each new edition of AABB *Standards*
    C. Reviewed prior to a scheduled inspection

D. Reviewed annually by an authorized individual

33. Previous records of patients' ABO and Rh types must be immediately available for comparison with current test results for
   A. 6 months
   B. 12 months
   C. 5 years
   D. Indefinitely

34. Which of the following weak D donor units should be labeled Rh-positive?
   A. Weak D due to transmissible genes
   B. Weak D as position effect
   C. Weak partial D
   D. All the above

35. In order to meet the current AABB *Standards* for leukocyte reduction to prevent HLA alloimmunization or CMV transmission, the donor unit must retain at least _____ of the original red cells and leukocytes must be reduced to less than _____.

   A. 85%, 5×10^8
   B. 80%, 5×10^6
   C. 75%, 5×10^5
   D. 70%, 5×10^4

36. All the following tests must be performed during donor processing *except*
   A. ABO and Rh grouping
   B. HB_sAg
   C. HIV-1-Ag
   D. HB_sAb

37. A 70-kg man has a platelet count of 15,000/μL and there are no complicating factors such as fever or HLA sensitization. If he is given a platelet pool of 6 units, what would you expect his posttransfusion count to be?

A. 21,000–27,000/μL
B. 25,000–35,000/μL
C. 45,000–75,000/μL
D. 75,000–125,000/μL

38. Which of the following tests on donor red blood cells must be repeated by the transfusing facility when the blood was collected and processed by a different facility?
   A. Confirmation of ABO group and Rh type of blood labeled D-negative
   B. Confirmation of ABO group and Rh type
   C. Weak D on D-negatives
   D. Antibody screening

INSTRUCTIONS: Each numbered group of incomplete statements (questions 39–63) is followed by four suggested responses. Select the *best* answer or completion statement in each case. Lettered responses may be used once, more than once, or not at all.

For the following components prepared from whole blood (questions 39–43), indicate the required storage temperature.

39. Red blood cells (RBC), liquid

40. Red blood cells, frozen

41. Fresh-frozen plasma

42. Cryoprecipitate

43. Platelet concentrate
   A. 1–6 °C
   B. 20–24 °C
   C. −18 °C or colder
   D. −65 °C or colder

For the following components prepared from whole blood (questions 44–48), indicate the shelf life.

44. Red blood cells in CPDA-1

45. Fresh-frozen plasma

46. Cryoprecipitate

47. Fresh-frozen plasma, thawed

48. Platelet concentrate in PL-732 (with agitation)
    A. 24 hours
    B. 5 days
    C. 35 days
    D. 1 year

Using the specified anticoagulant/preservative (questions 49–52), indicate the allowable shelf life for blood for transfusion therapy.

---

49. CPD (citrate phosphate dextrose)

50. CPDA-1 (citrate phosphate dextrose adenine)

51. AS-1 (Adsol®)

52. EDTA
    A. 21 days
    B. 35 days
    C. 42 days
    D. Not an approved anticoagulant

For the following situations (questions 53–59), indicate whether the individual volunteering to donate blood for allogeneic transfusion should be accepted or deferred. Assume results of the physical examination to be acceptable unless noted.

---

53. A 65-year-old man whose birthday is tomorrow

54. A 45-year-old woman who donated a unit during a holiday appeal 54 days ago

55. A 50-year-old physician who just returned from a country endemic for malaria but did not take prophylactic medicine or have malaria symptoms

56. A 25-year-old man who says he had yellow jaundice right after he was born

57. An 18-year-old with poison ivy on his hands and face

58. A woman who had a baby two months ago

59. A 35-year-old runner (pulse 46)
    A. Defer temporarily
    B. Defer for 12 months
    C. Defer permanently
    D. Accept

For the following patients (questions 60–63), indicate the component of choice for transfusion therapy.

---

60. Patients with warm autoimmune hemolytic anemia (AIHA) due to α-methyldopa (Aldomet®) with hemoglobins of 8.5 g/dL or above

61. Patients requiring transfusion with RBC that will not transmit cytomegalovirus (CMV)

62. Patients with normovolemic anemia

63. Patients who are thrombocytopenic secondary to the treatment of acute leukemia
    A. Platelet concentrate
    B. RBC
    C. Leukocyte-reduced RBC
    D. Transfusion not indicated

BLOOD GROUPS, GENETICS, SEROLOGY

64. Most blood group antibodies are of what immunoglobulin classes?
    A. IgA and IgD
    B. IgA and IgM
    C. IgE and IgD

D. IgG and IgM

65. In each individual there is one pair of sex chromosomes. The remaining 22 pairs of chromosomes are called
    A. Allosomes
    B. Antisomes
    C. Autosomes
    D. Isosomes

66. Which of the following blood groups reacts *least* strongly with an anti-H produced in an A_1B individual?
    A. Group O
    B. Group A_2B
    C. Group A_2
    D. Group A_1

67. How many genes encode the following Rh antigens: D, C, E, c, e?
    A. One
    B. Two
    C. Three
    D. Four

68. A Bombay (O_h) individual's blood specimen can be differentiated from blood specimens of normal group O persons by the
    A. Cells giving a negative reaction with anti-A,B
    B. Serum containing anti-H
    C. Cells giving a positive reaction with *Ulex europaeus*
    D. Cells giving a negative reaction with *Dolichos biflorus*

69. The secretor locus is linked to which blood group locus?
    A. Duffy
    B. Kell
    C. Lewis
    D. Lutheran

70. If a person has the genetic makeup *Hh, AO, LeLe, sese*, what substance will be found in the secretions?
    A. A substance
    B. H substance
    C. Le^a substance
    D. Le^b substance

71. The following results were obtained when typing a patient's blood sample.

Cell Typing Results		Serum Typing Results	
anti-A	anti-B	A_1 cells	B cells
4+	2+	0	4+

The tech suspects that this is a case of an acquired B antigen. Which of the following would support this suspicion?
    A. A positive autocontrol test
    B. Secretor studies show that the patient is a nonsecretor
    C. A patient diagnosis of leukemia
    D. The patient's red cells give a negative result with a monoclonal anti-B reagent lacking the ES-4 clone

72. Which of the following lectins differentiates A_1 from A_2 cells?
    A. *Dolichos biflorus*
    B. *Glycine soya*
    C. *Salvia sclarea*
    D. *Ulex europaeus*

73. Which of the following sugars must be present on a precursor substance for A and B antigenic activity to be expressed?
    A. D-Galactose
    B. *N*-Acetylgalactosamine
    C. Glucose
    D. L-Fucose

74. An antigen-antibody reaction alone does not cause hemolysis. Which of the following is required for red blood cell lysis?
    A. Albumin
    B. Complement
    C. Glucose-6-phosphate dehydrogenase
    D. Anti-human globulin

75. A white female's red blood cells gave the following reactions upon phenotyping: D+ C+ E− c+ e+. Which of the following is the most probable Rh genotype?
    A. *DCe/Dce*
    B. *DCe/dce*
    C. *DCe/DcE*
    D. *Dce/dCe*

76. A black patient has the following Rh phenotype: D+ C+ E+ c+ e+. Which of the following genotypes is the *least* probable?
    A. *DCE/dce*
    B. *DCe/DcE*
    C. *DCe/dcE*
    D. *DcE/dCe*

77. An individual of the *dce/dce* genotype given *dCe/dce* blood has an antibody response that appears to be anti-C and anti-D. The most likely explanation for this is
    A. The antibody is anti-G
    B. The antibody is anti-partial D
    C. The antibody is anti-Cw
    D. An incorrect reading of the agglutination reactions

78. If a patient has the Rh genotype *DCe/DCe* and receives a unit of red blood cells from a *DCe/dce* individual, what Rh antibody might the patient develop?
    A. Anti-C
    B. Anti-c
    C. Anti-d
    D. Anti-LW

79. The LW antigen is associated with the Rh system in what way?
    A. The LW gene is linked to the Rh gene
    B. More D antigen is present on LW-positive cells than on LW-negative cells
    C. The LW antigen is present only when the D antigen is present
    D. More LW antigen is present on D-positive cells than on D-negative cells

80. If a group *DCe/dce* man marries a *dce/dce* woman, what percentage of their offspring can be expected to be D-negative?
    A. 0%
    B. 25%
    C. 50%
    D. 75%

81. The following results were obtained when testing the individuals below:

| | Anti- | | | | | Test for |
	D	C	E	c	e	Weak D
HUSBAND	0	+	0	+	+	+
WIFE	0	0	0	+	+	0
INFANT	+	0	0	+	+	N/A

Which of the following conclusions is most likely?
    A. The husband is not the infant's father
    B. The husband is proved to be the infant's father
    C. The husband cannot be excluded from being the infant's father
    D. The D typing on the infant is a false positive

82. If a D-positive person makes an anti-D, this person is probably
    A. Partial D
    B. D-negative
    C. Weak D as position effect
    D. Weak D due to transmissible genes

83. A serum containing anti-k is not frequently encountered. This is because
   A. People who lack the k antigen are rare
   B. People who possess the k antigen are rare
   C. The k antigen is not a good immunogen
   D. Kell$_{null}$ people are rare

84. How many genetic circumstances can produce the Lu(a−b−) phenotype?
   A. One
   B. Two
   C. Three
   D. There is no Lu(a−b−) phenotype

85. Which of the following is a characteristic of the Xg^a blood group system?
   A. The Xg^a antigen has a higher frequency in women than in men
   B. The Xg^a antigen has a higher frequency in men than in women
   C. The Xg^a antigen is enhanced by enzymes
   D. Anti-Xg^a is usually a saline-reacting antibody

86. Which of the following antigens is a low-incidence antigen, usually not present on antibody screening or panel cells?
   A. I
   B. LW
   C. P
   D. Wr^a

87. Which of the following is a characteristic of Kidd antibodies?
   A. Usually IgM antibodies
   B. Corresponding antigens are destroyed by enzymes
   C. Usually strong and stable during storage

   D. Often implicated in delayed hemolytic transfusion reactions

88. All the following statements are true of anti-Fy^a and anti-Fy^b *except*
   A. Are clinically significant
   B. React well with enzyme-treated panel cells
   C. Cause hemolytic transfusion reactions
   D. Cause a generally mild hemolytic disease of the newborn

89. Which of the following antigens are associated with "high-titered, low-avidity" antibodies?
   A. Ch^a and Fy^a
   B. Ch^a and Rg^a
   C. Co^a and Rg^a
   D. Do^a and Js^b

90. All the following statements about anti-U are correct *except*
   A. Is clinically significant
   B. Is only found in black individuals
   C. Only occurs in S−s− individuals
   D. Only occurs in Fy(a−b−) individuals

91. A patient had an anti-E identified in his scrum 5 years ago. His antibody screening test is now negative. To obtain suitable blood for transfusion, the best procedure is to
   A. Type the patient for the E antigen as an added part to the crossmatch procedure
   B. Type the donor units for the E antigen and crossmatch the E-negative units
   C. Crossmatch donors with the patient's serum and release the compatible units for transfusion
   D. Perform the crossmatch with enzyme-treated donor cells, since enzyme-treated red cells react better with Rh antibodies

92. A patient's red blood cells are being typed for the Fyᵃ antigen. Which of the following is the proper cell type of choice for a positive control of the anti-Fyᵃ reagent?
    A. Fy(a+b−)
    B. Fy(a+b+)
    C. Fy(a−b+)
    D. Fy(a−b−)

93. Which of the following antibodies has been clearly implicated in transfusion reactions and hemolytic disease of the newborn?
    A. Anti-I
    B. Anti-K
    C. Anti-Leᵃ
    D. Anti-N

94. The phenotype Jk(a−b−) is very rare. In which ethnic background is there a much higher incidence?
    A. Arabian
    B. East Asian
    C. Irish
    D. Scandinavian

95. The phenotype Fy(a−b−) is very prominent among blacks (nearly 100% in some areas of Africa). What special trait accompanies those individuals who are Fy(a−b−)?
    A. Resistance to typhoid fever
    B. Resistance to malaria
    C. Resistance to botulism
    D. Cells are usually Rh-negative

96. Enzymes are often used to aid in the identification of antibodies. Which of the following antibodies is primarily IgG, is best detected at the AHG phase, can cause hemolytic transfusion reactions and hemolytic disease of the newborn, and the corresponding antigen is destroyed by proteolytic enzymes?
    A. Anti-D
    B. Anti-S

C. Anti-K
D. Anti-Jkᵃ

97. Often when trying to identify a mixture of antibodies, it is useful to neutralize one of the known antibodies. Which one of the following antibodies is neutralizable?
    A. Anti-D
    B. Anti-Jkᵃ
    C. Anti-Leᵃ
    D. Anti-M

98. Which of the following antibodies does *not* match the others in terms of optimal reactive temperature?
    A. Anti-Fyᵃ
    B. Anti-Jkᵇ
    C. Anti-N
    D. Anti-U

99. Which of the following antigens is destroyed by proteolytic enzymes?
    A. E
    B. Leᵃ
    C. K
    D. M

100. The antiglobulin test does not require washing or the addition of IgG coated cells in which of the following antibody detection methods?
    A. Solid-phase red cell adherence assays
    B. Gel test
    C. Affinity column technology
    D. Polyethylene glycol (PEG) technique

101. Which set of antibodies could you possibly find in a patient with no history of transfusion or pregnancy?
    A. Anti-I, anti-s, anti-P₁
    B. Anti-Leᵇ, anti-A₁, anti-D
    C. Anti-M, anti-c, anti-B
    D. Anti-P₁, anti-Leᵃ, anti-I

102. The mixed lymphocyte culture (MLC) or reaction is primarily used to recognize foreign _____ region antigens.
  A. HLA-A
  B. HLA-B
  C. HLA-C
  D. HLA-D

103. In which of the following instances may mixed-field (mf) agglutination be observed?
  A. Direct antiglobulin test (DAT) result of patient undergoing delayed hemolytic transfusion reaction
  B. Indirect antiglobulin test (IAT) result of patient who has anti-Le^a
  C. DAT result of patient on high doses of α-methyldopa
  D. Typing result with anti-A of patient who is A$_2$ subgroup

104. The antibody produced during the secondary response to a foreign antigen is usually
  A. IgM
  B. A product of T lymphocytes
  C. Produced a month or more after the second stimulus
  D. Present at a higher titer than after a primary response

105. The ABO serum grouping may *not* be valid when
  A. The patient has hypogammaglobulinemia
  B. IgM alloantibodies are present
  C. Cold autoantibodies are present
  D. All the above

106. A group A, D-negative obstetric patient with anti-D (titer 256) is carrying a fetus who needs an intrauterine transfusion. Which of the following units should be chosen?
  A. Group A, D-negative RBC
  B. Group A, D-negative whole blood
  C. Group O, D-negative RBC
  D. Group O, D-negative whole blood

107. Which of the following is generally detected at the indirect antiglobulin phase of testing?
  A. Anti-Jk^a
  B. Anti-M
  C. Anti-P$_1$
  D. Anti-I

108. Which of the blood group systems is associated with antibodies that are generally IgM?
  A. Rh
  B. Duffy
  C. Kell
  D. Lewis

109. Some antigens that are primarily found on white blood cells can occur on erythrocytes. Which of the following are the red blood cell equivalents of human leukocyte antigens (HLA)?
  A. Le^a, Le^b
  B. Bg^a, Bg^b, Bg^c
  C. Kp^a, Kp^b, Kp^c
  D. Do^a, Do^b

110. The following phenotypes resulted from blood typing a mother, 6-month-old baby, and alleged father in a case of paternity testing.

	ABO	Rh	HLA
MOTHER	A	ce	A2, A29, B12, B17
BABY	O	ce	A2, A3, B12, B15
ALLEGED FATHER	A	DCce	A3, A9, B5, B27

Which of the following statements is true? The alleged father
  A. Is excluded by the ABO system
  B. Is excluded by the Rh system
  C. Is excluded by the HLA system
  D. Can't be ruled out

INSTRUCTIONS: Each numbered group of incomplete statements (questions 111–123) is followed by four suggested responses. Select the *best* answer in each case. Lettered responses may be used once, more than once, or not at all.

Eight blood samples are received in the laboratory for ABO grouping. For each patient (questions 111–118), indicate the most likely cell and serum reactions selected from the lettered reaction matrix.

111. A patient with an acquired antigen due to infection with gram-negative bacteria

112. A patient with multiple myeloma

113. A newborn

114. An A_2 individual making an anti-A_1

115. A patient with antibodies to acriflavin (a yellow dye)

116. A patient who is immunodeficient

117. A *cis-AB* individual

118. A patient with cold hemagglutinin disease (CHD)

	Cell Typing Results		Serum Typing Results		
	anti-A	anti-B	A_1 cells	B cells	O cells
A.	+	+	+	+	+
B.	+	0	+	+	0
C.	+	+	0	+	0
D.	0	+	0	0	0

For the following items (questions 119–123), select the answer that most closely corresponds to the description.

119. Found predominantly in whites

120. Associated with weak Kell system antigenic expression

121. Associated with the presence of chronic granulomatous disease

122. Linked with *MN*

123. A rare allele of *M* and *N*
   A. McLeod phenotype
   B. M^g
   C. Kp^a
   D. *Ss*

ANTIBODY IDENTIFICATION, TRANSFUSION THERAPY, TRANSFUSION REACTIONS

For questions 124–132, refer to the red cell panel chart on page 247.

124. The racial origin of the donor of Cell #3 is most likely
   A. Black
   B. Eskimo
   C. Oriental
   D. White

125. The donor of Cell #5 is homozygous for which combination of the following genes?
   A. $Ce, P_1, M, s, k, Jk^a, Fy^a, Le^b$
   B. $Ce, P_1, s, k, Jk^a, Fy^a, Le^b$
   C. $Ce, s, k, Jk^a, Fy^a, Le^b$
   D. Ce, s, k, Jk^a, Fy^a

126. After testing a patient's serum with the panel, one observes there are no reactions at IS or 37 °C with Cells #1–8. There is a 1+ anti-human globulin (AHG) reaction with Cells #1 and #6 and a 3+ AHG reaction with Cells #4 and #5. All other Cells, #2, #3, #7, and #8, are negative at AHG. Which of the following statements is true?
   A. Anti-Fy^a appears to be present
   B. Anti-Fy^a is present as well as an antibody that is reacting with an undetermined antigen on Cells #4 and #5
   C. Ficin will enhance the reactions of the antibody(ies) present
   D. Anti-Fy^a is present but can be ignored, as most people are Fy(a−b−)

Red Cell Panel Chart

Cell#	D	C	E	c	e	M	N	P_1	S	s	K	k	Jk^a	Jk^b	Fy^a	Fy^b	Lu^a	Le^a	Le^b	Xg^a
1	+	+	0	+	+	+	+	+	0	+	+	+	0	+	+	+	0	0	+	0
2	+	+	0	0	+	0	+	0	+	+	0	+	0	+	0	+	0	0	+	+
3	+	+	0	+	+	+	0	+	+	0	0	+	+	+	0	0	0	+	0	+
4	+	0	+	+	0	+	+	0	+	0	0	+	+	0	+	0	0	0	+	0
5	0	+	0	0	+	+	+	+	0	+	0	+	+	0	+	0	0	0	+	0
6	0	0	+	+	0	+	0	+	+	+	0	+	0	+	+	+	0	0	0	0
7	0	0	0	+	+	0	+	+	+	0	+	0	+	+	0	+	+	0	+	+
8	0	0	0	+	+	+	+	0	+	+	0	+	+	0	0	+	0	+	0	+

127. The serum of a patient tested with the reagent red cell panel using a low ionic salt solution (LISS) additive demonstrates 3+ reactivity with Cells #1–8 at the indirect antiglobulin phase. The autocontrol is negative. This pattern of reactivity is most likely due to

    A. Rouleaux formation

    B. Warm autoantibody

    C. Alloantibody directed against a high-frequency antigen

    D. Antibody directed against a preservative present in LISS

128. A patient's serum reacts with all the panel cells except Cell #7 at the antiglobulin phase only. Which of the following techniques would be most helpful at this point?

    A. Treat the panel cells with a proteolytic enzyme and repeat the panel with untreated serum

    B. Treat the panel cells with dithiothreitol (DTT) and repeat the panel with untreated serum

    C. Treat the patient's serum with dithiothreitol (DTT) and repeat the panel with treated serum

    D. Treat the patient's serum with a proteolytic enzyme and repeat the panel with treated serum

---

In addition to the red cell panel chart above, use the following information to answer questions 129–131.

The patient is group A, D-negative and has not been recently transfused. Cells #5, #6, and #7 are negative in all phases with this patient's serum. The autocontrol is negative. Other cell results are as follows:

Cell#	IS (Immediate Spin)	37 °C LISS	AHG
1	0	1+	4+
2	0	1+	4+
3	2+	1+	4+
4	0	1+	4+
8	2+	0	0

129. From the reactions given it appears that there is (are)

    A. One antibody reacting

    B. One antibody reacting that shows dosage

    C. "Cold" and "warm" antibodies reacting

    D. Two "warm" antibodies reacting

130. The antibody that reacts at immediate spin is

    A. Anti-D

    B. Anti-P_1

    C. Anti-Le^a

    D. Anti-Le^b

131. The antibody that reacts at 37 °C and with anti-human globulin (AHG) is
    A. Anti-C
    B. Anti-D
    C. Anti-CD
    D. Anti-K

132. To confirm that an antibody identification is correct
    A. Make an eluate
    B. Do saliva testing
    C. Run an additional panel
    D. Type the patient's cells for the corresponding antigens

133. The following results were obtained upon testing a specimen of a patient, being admitted after a car accident, who had no recent history of transfusion or medical problems.

    ABO group: A
    Rh type: D-positive
    Antibody screening test: positive, one screening cell only
    Direct antiglobulin test: negative
    Antibody identification: anti-K identified
    Patient's cell phenotyping: K+

    Which of these results seem in doubt?
    A. ABO grouping
    B. Rh grouping
    C. Antibody identification
    D. Cell phenotyping for K antigen

134. False-negative results at the indirect antiglobulin phase of an antibody screening test are most likely due to
    A. Excessive washing of the red cells
    B. Inadequate washing of the red cells
    C. Warm autoantibody present in the patient's serum
    D. Failure to allow the blood to clot properly

135. What is the process of removing an antibody from the red blood cell membrane called?
    A. Absorption
    B. Adsorption
    C. Elution
    D. Immunization

136. At the end of an antiglobulin test, IgG-coated control cells are added to the negative tests and centrifuged. If agglutination occurs, this means the
    A. Test is valid
    B. Antiglobulin reagent was neutralized
    C. Cells were not washed thoroughly
    D. Control cells are contaminated

137. The major crossmatch is performed using
    A. Donor's serum and recipient's red cells
    B. Donor's red cells and recipient's serum
    C. Donor's serum and reagent red cells
    D. Recipient's serum and reagent red cells

138. A male trauma victim whose blood type is group AB, D-negative has a negative antibody screening test. He has been transfused with both of the group AB, D-negative units (U) in inventory within the last hour. He is now in surgery and expected to need large amounts of blood. Of the following available U in inventory, which type should be given next?
    A. 30 U of group O, D-positive
    B. 26 U of group A, D-positive
    C. 10 U of group O, D-negative
    D. 5 U of group A, D-negative

139. Which of the following will the major crossmatch do?
    A. Prevent immunization
    B. Prevent delayed transfusion reactions
    C. Guarantee normal survival of the red blood cells
    D. Frequently verify donor ABO compatibility

140. Given that a patient's antibody screening test is negative, which of the following may cause a false-positive result in a major compatibility test?
   A. Incorrect ABO typing of the donor or patient
   B. An alloantibody against a low-frequency antigen on the donor cells
   C. Prior coating of IgG antibody on the donor cells
   D. All the above

141. Which of the following will be incompatible in the major crossmatch?

	Donor	Recipient
A.	Group A, D-negative	Group A, D-positive
B.	Group O, D-positive	Group A, D-positive
C.	Group AB, D-positive	Group A, D-positive
D.	Group A, D-positive	Group A, D-negative

142. A resident physician hand-delivers a blood sample, drawn by the attending physician, for pretransfusion testing from a patient who is difficult to draw. The sample is unlabeled. One should
   A. Discard the sample and request that the resident obtain a new sample, adhering to proper guidelines for labeling
   B. Label the specimen with the information the resident provides
   C. Label the specimen with information from the accompanying transfusion request form
   D. Request the sample be returned to the nursing station to be labeled

143. A specimen of blood is received in the blood bank with request slips for transfusion. The tube has the patient's first and last name and medical records identification number on the label. What else must be on the tube label as required by AABB *Standards*?
   A. Patient's room number
   B. Date of phlebotomy
   C. Initials of phlebotomist
   D. Attending physician's name

144. A physician calls the blood bank and wants an additional unit of RBC cross-matched for a patient. Several specimens from that patient are identified that have been drawn over the past month. Which of the following is the oldest acceptable specimen to be used for crossmatching?
   A. 1 day old
   B. 4 days old
   C. 1 week old
   D. 1 month old

145. A patient has a hemoglobin of 8.1 g/dL. The surgeon wants to raise the hemoglobin to 10 g/dL before surgery. How many units of RBC need to be administered to this patient to raise the hemoglobin to the required level?
   A. 1
   B. 2
   C. 3
   D. 4

146. A patient with an anti-K and an anti-Jk^a in her plasma needs 2 units of RBC for surgery. How many group-specific units would need to be screened to find 2 units of RBC? The frequency of Jk(a+) is 77%; the K+ frequency is 10%.
   A. 6
   B. 10
   C. 20
   D. 36

Use the following information to answer questions 147 and 148.

A postpartum female is bleeding because of disseminated intravascular coagulation (DIC). The attending physician orders cryoprecipitate for fibrinogen replacement. The freezer inventory contains the following cryoprecipitate: 6 bags Group A, 8 bags Group O, 6 bags Group AB, 12 bags Group B.

---

147. How many bags (units) should be thawed and pooled to provide 2 g of fibrinogen?
    A. 2
    B. 4
    C. 8
    D. 10

148. The patient is group A. Which cryoprecipitate units would most appropriately be used to treat this patient?
    A. Group A only
    B. Group AB only
    C. Group A and Group O
    D. Group A and Group AB

149. If 98% of the red blood cells are viable in a unit of RBC at the time of transfusion, what percentage of red cells will remain viable 28 days posttransfusion?
    A. 10%
    B. 30%
    C. 50%
    D. 70%

150. What is the component of choice for someone who needs a red blood cell (RBC) transfusion when there is a history of febrile transfusion reactions?
    A. RBC less than 5 days old
    B. Leukocyte-reduced RBC
    C. RBC 30 to 35 days old
    D. Frozen RBC that have been thawed and deglycerolized

151. Which of the following is the component of choice when a physician is concerned about restoring or maintaining oxygen-carrying capacity?
    A. Albumin
    B. Cryoprecipitate
    C. Whole blood
    D. Red blood cells

152. The serum of a patient contains an antibody that reacts with all random donor cells and panel cells that have been tested. The best possibility to find compatible blood would be to test
    A. Grandparents
    B. Parents
    C. Siblings
    D. Spouse

153. A resident physician on the trauma team runs a pretransfusion blood sample from a male trauma victim to the blood bank and wants 6 units (U) of uncrossmatched blood to be issued immediately. The resident says the victim has a donor card in his wallet indicating a group B, D-positive blood type. One should
    A. Issue 6 U of uncrossmatched group B, D-positive whole blood
    B. Check patient and donor records to confirm the blood type, then issue 6 U of uncrossmatched group B, D-positive blood
    C. Withhold blood until ABO and compatibility testing are completed
    D. Issue 6 U of group O RBC

154. Four units of fresh-frozen plasma have been ordered to correct factor V deficiency in a group O patient. One should thaw and issue _____ plasma.
    A. Group O
    B. Group A
    C. Group B
    D. Any blood group available

155. Which of the following is acceptable to be given intravenously with a blood transfusion?

A. 5% dextrose in water

B. Physiologic saline

C. Ringer's solution

D. Dextran

156. Hemolytic transfusion reactions are the most serious type of reactions to blood transfusion. The majority of hemolytic transfusion reactions are caused by _____ errors.

    A. Blood typing

    B. Antibody identification

    C. Clerical

    D. Crossmatching

157. What type of transfusion reaction is often diagnosed by a positive DAT and a gradual drop in the patient's hemoglobin level?

    A. Anaphylactic

    B. Febrile

    C. Delayed hemolytic

    D. Acute hemolytic

158. What antibody, that is labile in both stored serum and the patient's plasma, is a frequent cause of delayed hemolytic transfusion reactions?

    A. Anti-A

    B. Anti-D

    C. Anti-Jk^a

    D. Anti-K

159. Occasionally patients have an anaphylactic reaction to a specific immunoglobulin class during a transfusion. Which immunoglobulin class is most often implicated?

    A. IgA

    B. IgD

    C. IgE

    D. IgG

160. A transfusion of which of the following is *least* likely to transmit HIV, HCV, or HBV?

    A. Pooled Plasma, Solvent/Detergent-Treated

    B. Cryoprecipitate

    C. Leukocyte-reduced RBC

    D. Platelets

161. Antiglobulin reagent can be neutralized by all the following *except*

    A. Human serum

    B. RhIG

    C. Bovine albumin

    D. Cryoprecipitate

162. Which of the following is required in an antibody detection test?

    A. Immediate spin

    B. Antiglobulin test

    C. Autologous control

    D. All the above

163. Advantages of autologous blood transfusions generally include the avoidance of all the following *except*

    A. Transmission of disease

    B. Clerical error

    C. Allergic reactions

    D. Graft-*vs.*-host disease

164. Before blood is issued for transfusion, a patient's previous blood bank records must be reviewed for all the following *except*

    A. ABO group and Rh type

    B. Clinically significant antibodies

    C. Serious adverse reactions

    D. Hepatitis testing

165. A positive hemagglutination reaction in the major crossmatch may be caused by all the following *except*

    A. Incorrect ABO grouping of the donor

    B. Unexpected antibodies in the recipient serum

    C. A positive DAT on the recipient red cells

    D. A positive DAT on the donor red cells

166. Which of the following blood types necessitates that a separate Rh control tube be set up when using a monoclonal anti-D reagent?
    A. Group O, D-positive
    B. Group A, D-positive
    C. Group B, D-positive
    D. Group AB, D-positive

167. Six units of blood were ordered stat for a young female patient who has the following tube typing results using a washed red cell suspension with monoclonal reagents. The physician has just called requesting emergency release of 2 units of RBC.

Cell Typing Results				Serum Typing Results	
anti-A	anti-B	anti-D	Rh control	A₁ cells	B cells
2+	4+	3+	2+	4+	4+

Which of the following should be done first?
    A. Perform a DAT on the patient's red cells
    B. Tell the physician that no blood can be released until a full work up has been done
    C. Begin the antibody screening test
    D. Select 2 units of group O, D-negative RBC for emergency release

168. Referring to the tube typing results in Question 167, the most probable cause of the patient's positive Rh control test is that the patient has
    A. A positive DAT result with anti-IgG
    B. A cold autoantibody
    C. Leukemia
    D. Multiple myeloma

169. A patient experiences severe rigors and goes into shock after receiving part of a unit of RBC. The patient's temperature, which was 37.5 °C pretransfusion, is now 40.0 °C. Which of the following is the most likely type of reaction?
    A. Hemolytic
    B. Anaphylactic
    C. Septic
    D. Embolic

170. Referring to the reaction described in Question 169, the incidence of this type of reaction is highest with which of the following components?
    A. RBC
    B. FFP
    C. Cryoprecipitate
    D. Platelets

171. The minor crossmatch is seldom performed and the primary reason is
    A. That a false-positive incompatibility is seen when the donor has a positive DAT
    B. Donor units have been screened for the presence of clinically significant antibodies
    C. Donor antibodies cannot harm a patient
    D. It will not pick up ABO incompatibilities

172. The serum of a patient transfused 2 weeks ago reacts 3+ on immediate spin and 1+ at the indirect antiglobulin phase of testing with all reagent red cells except for the cord cell. The autocontrol reacts similarly to the panel cells. In order to crossmatch this patient one should
    A. Use autoadsorbed serum
    B. Use the prewarmed technique
    C. Identify the antibody and obtain blood from the rare donor file
    D. Use a LISS additive

INSTRUCTIONS: Each numbered set of test results or conditions (questions 173–183) is followed by four or five lettered responses. Select the *best* answer in each case. Lettered responses may be used once, more than once, or not at all.

Six units of blood from volunteer donors are tested for ABO group, Rh type, and unexpected antibodies. For each set of test results (questions 173–178), indicate the final disposition of the donated unit. Assume additional FDA required testing is nonreactive, unless noted.

	Cell Typing Results			Serum Typing Results		
anti-A,B	anti-A	anti-B	anti-D	A$_1$ cells	A$_2$ cells	B cells
173. 0	0	0	3+	4+	3+	4+
174. 0	0	0	0	4+	4+	4+

Weak D test = 3+, DAT = 0

175. 0	0	0	0	4+	4+	4+

Weak D test = 1+, DAT = 1+

176. 2+	0	0	3+	2+	0	4+
177. 0	0	0	3+	0	0	4+
178. 0	0	0	3+	4+	4+	4+

Antibody screen = positive,
Antibody identification = anti-Fy^a

A. Label group O, D-positive
B. Label group O, D-negative
C. Label the RBC group O, D-positive; do not use the plasma
D. Perform additional testing
E. Discard the unit

For the following conditions (questions 179–183), select the blood component of choice for treatment.

179. von Willebrand's disease

180. Hypofibrinogenemia

181. Factor V deficiency

182. Liver disease

183. Hemorrhagic episode during intensive chemotherapy
A. Platelet concentrate
B. RBC
C. Cryoprecipitate
D. Fresh-frozen plasma

HEMOLYTIC DISEASE (HEMOLYTIC DISEASE OF THE NEWBORN, IMMUNE HEMOLYTIC ANEMIA)

184. Routine testing early in a pregnancy should include all the following *except*
A. ABO and Rh testing
B. Antibody screening
C. Amniocentesis
D. Weak D testing on apparent Rh-negative patients

185. In which of the following blood group systems may the red blood cell typing change during pregnancy?
A. P
B. MNS
C. Lewis
D. Duffy

186. Hemolytic disease of the newborn (HDN) may be predicted before delivery of the infant when due to all the following *except*
A. Anti-A
B. Anti-D
C. Anti-Fy^a
D. Anti-U

187. Which is the class of immunoglobulin uniquely associated with hemolytic disease of the newborn (HDN)?
A. IgA
B. IgD
C. IgE
D. IgG

188. A neonate with a positive direct antiglobulin test (DAT) indicates that there was an incompatibility between a mother and her fetus. The system that is most commonly associated with an incompatibility is
    A. ABO
    B. Rh
    C. Kell
    D. Kidd

189. The cord blood of an infant of a D-negative mother with anti-D, titer 2048, is submitted to the laboratory along with a sample of maternal blood with a request to select blood for possible exchange transfusion. The neonate appears to be D-negative. The weak D status cannot be determined, since the DAT result is positive (4+). The most likely explanation is
    A. Wharton's jelly contaminated the sample
    B. The baby has ABO HDN
    C. The baby has a "blocked D" antigen
    D. A different antibody is causing the positive DAT

190. A newborn is group O, D-positive and has a 3+ direct antiglobulin test (DAT). The mother's antibody screening test is negative. Assuming the antibody detection test is valid, one should consider hemolytic disease of the newborn (HDN) due to an antibody directed against
    A. Fy^b antigen
    B. K antigen
    C. Low-incidence antigen
    D. A or B antigen

191. The most conclusive way to demonstrate the antibody that is causing a positive DAT in a newborn is to perform an antibody
    A. Titration using the mother's serum
    B. Panel using the mother's serum
    C. Panel using an eluate from the mother's red cells
    D. Panel using an eluate from the baby's red cells

192. Which two of the following conditions are the most serious immediate consequences of HDN?
    A. Anemia and a positive DAT
    B. Hyperbilirubinemia and anemia
    C. Hyperbilirubinemia and jaundice
    D. Hyperbilirubinemia and kernicterus

193. A premature infant with *hydrops fetalis* and a bilirubin of 20 mg/dL is referred to an intensive care unit. The neonatologist wants to perform an exchange transfusion to correct anemia and prevent kernicterus. No blood specimen from the mother is available. The infant's serum has a positive antibody screen. The DAT is 4+. The best approach would be to
    A. Identify the antibody in the serum and crossmatch blood negative for the offending antigen, using the serum in a major crossmatch
    B. Issue group O, D-negative blood for the exchange
    C. Refuse to issue blood for exchange until a sample can be obtained from the mother
    D. Identify the antibody in the serum and eluate and crossmatch blood negative for the offending antigen, using both the serum and eluate in a major crossmatch

194. Which of the following is *not* true of an exchange transfusion when an infant is suffering from HDN?
    A. Removes unconjugated bilirubin
    B. Reduces the amount of incompatible antibody in the baby's circulation
    C. Removes antibody coated red blood cells
    D. Provides red blood cells of the baby's type

195. A massive fetomaternal hemorrhage in a D-negative woman who had a D-positive infant should be suspected if the

A. Infant is premature

B. Infant has a positive acid elution slide test

C. Mother requires a transfusion following delivery

D. Weak D test on the maternal blood shows a mixed-field reaction microscopically

196. A D-negative woman who received antepartum RhIG delivered a D-positive infant and received one vial of RhIG the same day. Because of postpartum hemorrhage her physician ordered two units of RBC for her two days later. The antibody screening test was positive but the crossmatches were both compatible. The most likely cause for the positive antibody screening test was the presence of a(n)

A. Clinically significant anti-K

B. Actively acquired anti-D

C. Passively acquired anti-D

D. Rh antibody other than anti-D

197. The principle of the Kleihauer-Betke stain is that

A. Fetal hemoglobin is more resistant to alkaline buffer than adult hemoglobin

B. Adult hemoglobin is more resistant to alkaline buffer than fetal hemoglobin

C. Fetal hemoglobin is more resistant to erythrosin and hematoxylin staining than adult hemoglobin

D. Adult hemoglobin is more soluble in acid buffer than fetal hemoglobin

198. Which of the following antibodies present in a multitransfused obstetric patient would be most likely to cause HDN in her infant?

A. Anti-Le^a

B. Anti-c

C. Anti-P$_1$

D. Anti-K

Use the following information to answer questions 199 and 200.

A Kleihauer-Betke acid elution stain for postpartum fetomaternal hemorrhage (FMH) is reported to be 1.3%.

199. What is the total volume of FMH?

A. 6.5 mL

B. 13 mL

C. 26 mL

D. 65 mL

200. How many vials of a standard dose of RhIG should be administered within 72 hours to the mother with this amount of FMH? (Presume the infant to be D-positive.)

A. 1

B. 2

C. 3

D. 4

201. Which of the following is *not* a characteristic of polyagglutinable cells?

A. Agglutinated by most human serums

B. Agglutinated by cord serums

C. Caused by bacterial enzymes

D. Classified by lectins

202. To demonstrate whether antibodies have become attached to a patient's red blood cells *in vivo,* which of the following tests would be most useful?

A. Direct antiglobulin test

B. Complement fixation test

C. Elution procedure

D. Indirect antiglobulin test

203. All the following are true concerning warm autoimmune hemolytic anemia (WAIHA) *except*

A. It occurs only in elderly patients

B. It is usually associated with IgG antibodies

C. Splenomegaly is common

D. It can occur during α-methyldopa therapy

204. The specificity of the antibody in warm autoimmune hemolytic anemia (WAIHA) is most often associated with which of the following blood group systems?
    A. ABO
    B. Kell
    C. Kidd
    D. Rh

205. What is the most important consideration in patients suffering from life-threatening anemia and whose serum contains warm autoantibodies?
    A. Determine the specificity of the autoantibody
    B. Determine the immunoglobulin class of the autoantibody
    C. Exclude the presence of alloantibody(ies)
    D. Avoid transfusion

206. The serum and eluate from a male patient with a 3+ DAT on α-methyldopa therapy demonstrates anti-e specificity. The patient denies knowledge of having received blood transfusions. To determine whether the anti-e is an auto- or alloantibody, one should
    A. Type the patient's red cells with a low protein anti-e reagent
    B. Adsorb the serum with the patient's red cells
    C. Adsorb the eluate with R_2R_2 red cells
    D. Adsorb the eluate with rr red cells

207. A patient has a 2+mf DAT with anti-IgG. He was transfused 1 week ago with 2 units of RBC during surgery. His eluate would most likely contain
    A. No antibody
    B. Autoantibody
    C. Alloantibody
    D. Drug-related antibody

208. Anti-I is the most common antibody found in cold hemagglutinin disease (CHD). Occasionally anti-Pr is the offending antibody. How can anti-Pr be differentiated from anti-I?
    A. Pr antigen is destroyed by enzymes
    B. I antigen is destroyed by enzymes
    C. Pr antigen is a low-incidence antigen
    D. There is no way to differentiate the two antigens

209. How is cold hemagglutinin disease (CHD) different from paroxysmal cold hemoglobinuria (PCH)?
    A. PCH is a common form of cold autoimmune anemia while CHD is rare
    B. PCH is a warm autoimmune hemolytic anemia
    C. The offending antibody in PCH is an IgG antibody unlike the IgM antibody in CHD
    D. The offending antibody in PCH is an IgM antibody while an IgG antibody is common in CHD

210. If during a Donath-Landsteiner test there is hemolysis in both a test and control tube at the conclusion of the test, this indicates that the test is
    A. Positive
    B. Negative
    C. Invalid
    D. False-negative

211. A patient has a positive DAT due to cephalosporin therapy and a negative antibody screening test result. Two units of RBC have been ordered. In order to crossmatch this patient, one should crossmatch with
    A. The eluate from the patient's red cells
    B. Autoadsorbed patient's serum
    C. Untreated patient's serum
    D. Cephalosporin treated donor cells and untreated patient's serum

212. A patient recuperating from a *Mycoplasma pneumoniae* infection has a potent antibody reacting on immediate spin with all reagent red cells except the cord cell. The most likely specificity is
    A. Auto anti-I
    B. Auto anti-Pr
    C. Allo anti-I
    D. Allo anti-i

213. A patient being treated with α-methyldopa has a 4+ DAT result. You would expect an eluate from his red cells to most likely react with
    A. All the untreated panel cells tested
    B. Just the untreated D-positive cells tested
    C. All panel cells treated with α-methyldopa
    D. All panel cells when α-methyldopa is added to the eluate

214. A patient with drug-induced hemolytic anemia has the following DAT results:

    Polyspecific AHG = 3+
    Anti-IgG = 3+
    Anti-C3d = 0

    Which of the following drugs is most likely to be the cause?
    A. Phenacetin
    B. Quinidine
    C. Penicillin
    D. Tolmetin

215. A patient with cold hemagglutinin disease (CHD) has a positive DAT when tested with a polyspecific AHG. Which of the following would most likely be detected on her red cells?
    A. IgM
    B. IgG

C. IgA
D. C3

216. If a patient's red blood cells are DAT+ due to penicillin antibody the
    A. Serum will react if penicillin is added to the test system
    B. Serum will react with all red cells
    C. Eluate will react with penicillin-coated red cells
    D. Eluate will react with all red cells

217. A patient's preoperative antibody screening test is negative, but the autocontrol is positive. A DAT performed on his red cells is 2+ with anti-IgG. His last transfusion was 9 months ago and he has a negative drug history. Which of the following would most likely be present in his eluate?
    A. No antibody
    B. Alloantibody
    C. Alloantibody and autoantibody
    D. Autoantibody

218. The likelihood of finding autoantibody in the serum of a patient with WAIHA is
    A. Extremely rare since autoantibody should be on the patient's red cells
    B. About 25% if enzyme treated panel cells are used
    C. About 50% by saline antiglobulin technique
    D. 100% by any antiglobulin technique

For the following situations (questions 219–226), indicate whether the women are candidates for Rh immune globulin (RhIG) prophylaxis. Assume D-negative mothers have a negative test for weak D and a nonreactive antibody screening test unless noted.

219. Mother D-negative; infant weak D

220. Mother weak D (strong); infant D-positive

221. Mother D-negative; twin #1 D-negative, twin #2 D-positive

222. Mother D-negative with anti-Fy^a; infant D-positive

223. Mother group O, D negative; infant group A, DAT = 2+, monoclonal anti-D negative at immediate spin, weak D test not performed

224. Mother D-negative, with anti-D, titer 2, history of RhIG injection postamniocentesis procedure at 30 weeks; infant D-positive

225. Female D-negative; miscarriage at 11 weeks

226. Mother D-negative; infant D-positive; rosette test = 1–2 rosettes per field
   A. Yes, 50 μg dose
   B. Yes, 300 μg dose
   C. Yes, additional testing necessary to determine dose
   D. RhIG is not indicated

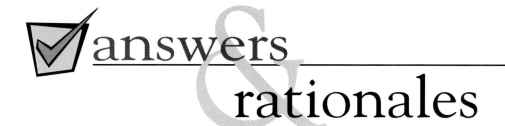

BLOOD COLLECTION, PRESERVATION, PROCESSING, COMPONENT PREPARATION, AND QUALITY CONTROL

1.

C. Some potential donors are rejected to protect the recipient and others are rejected to protect themselves. In this case, the woman meets the criteria except that her hematocrit is too low and the loss of a unit of blood may have a detrimental effect on her. The minimum acceptable hematocrit is 38%.

2.

C. Donors are allowed to donate no more than 10.5 mL/kg of their body weight. This amount includes the samples used for testing drawn at the time of collection. The calculation for a 95-lb donor is

95 lb ÷ 2.2 lb/kg = 43.2 kg
43.2 kg × 10.5 mL/kg = 453.6 mL

If less than 300 mL is to be collected, the anticoagulant must be reduced proportionately.

3.

A. Hepatitis viruses and HIV have extended incubation periods in which exposure has occurred but neither serological nor clinical manifestations of the disease are evident. The current screening tests, although quite sensitive, are unable to detect the viruses if testing is performed during this incubation period. To safeguard against the possibility that the donor received blood or blood products collected during the incubation period, a 12-month deferral is incurred to allow for fulmination of the disease.

4.

D. During autologous presurgical donation a different set of criteria is used for donor acceptability. All the conditions listed are acceptable with the exception of the bacteremia. The bacteria may proliferate in the stored blood and be reinfused into the donor (patient) during or after the surgery. Even treatment for a suspected bacteremia is a contraindication for autologous donation.

5.

D. Recipients of human growth hormone are deferred indefinitely because of the risk of transmission of Creutzfeldt-Jakob disease. Recipients of recombinant growth hormone incur no deferral. A history of either syphilis or gonorrhea causes a deferral of 12 months from completion of treatment. Accutane®, a drug used to treat acne, may be a teratogen and requires a 1-month deferral after receipt of the last dose.

6.

A. Of the viruses listed, CMV is the only one that resides exclusively in leukocytes. Although CMV transmission is not a problem for most patients, it can cause serious disease in low-birth-weight neonates of CMV-negative mothers and immunocompromised patients. These patients should be transfused with CMV seronegative or leukocyte-reduced cellular components.

7.

C. Donors who have ingested aspirin within 36 hours of donation need not be excluded for whole blood donation. The platelets prepared from such donors should be labeled and may be used in a multiple pool prepared for adult transfusion. Because aspirin affects platelet function, a single unit of platelet concentrate from this donor should not be used for platelet therapy for infants and neonates. This donor should not be the soul source of platelets and therefore would be temporarily deferred as a plateletpheresis donor.

8.

C. Under no circumstances should any blood component from these donors be released from the donor center to a transfusion unit. Donors in high risk groups for AIDS must be deferred from donating. If high-risk activity becomes known retrospective to blood donation (such as in the self-exclusion process), the blood components from the donation must be retrieved and destroyed.

9.

C. Plasma protein fraction (PPF) and albumin preparations (5% and 20%) provide colloid replacement and volume expansion with virtually no risk of viral transmission. These are pooled products and are pasteurized by heating to 60 °C for 10 hours. Other products such as clotting factor concentrates are usually treated by solvent-detergent method to inactivate viruses with lipid envelopes such as HBV, HCV, HIV, and HTLV-I.

10.

D. The screening test for anti-HCV is an EIA test. This test has a high rate of false-positive results. A donor who is confirmed positive by RIBA is considered to truly have anti-HCV.

11.

D. Cryoprecipitate provides the only known concentrated source of fibronectin, useful in the phagocytic removal of bacteria and aggregates by the reticuloendothelial system. It also contains factors VIII:C, VIII:vW, and XIII. Antithrombin III (AT III), necessary to prevent a thromboembolic disorder, is depleted in DIC and liver disease. Transfusion sources of AT III are fresh frozen plasma (FFP) and commercial concentrates.

12.

D. Fresh-frozen plasma (FFP) contains all the plasma clotting factors. FFP's primary use is for patients with clotting factor deficiencies for which no concentrate is available and patients who present multiple factor deficiencies such as in liver disease. Platelets are not a plasma clotting factor, and they must be maintained at 20–24 °C with continuous gentle agitation to maintain their viability.

13.

B. The AABB *Standards* requires that when a patient is likely at risk for graft-*vs.*-host disease (GVHD) all cellular blood components be irradiated before transfusion. This includes components for patients who are immunodeficient or immunoincompetent such as a patient on immunosuppressive therapy and a fetus who receives intrauterine transfusion. Irradiation of RBC for exchange transfusion is not required by AABB *Standards* although many hospital transfusion services do so. Immunocompetent individuals require irradiated components if they are to receive cellular components from someone who may be homozygous for a shared HLA haplotype such as a blood relative or an HLA matched donor. Gamma irradiation of cellular components is the *only* way to prevent transfusion-associated GVHD that occurs when immunocompetent donor T cells survive in the patient's circulation and mount an immune response against the host cells. A minimum of 25Gy delivered to the midplane of the container and at least 15Gy to all other areas will prevent GVHD.

14.

A. The limiting criterion for *in vitro* storage of blood is the survival in the recipient of at least 70% of the transfused red cells for at least 24 hours after transfusion. Additional adenine in an anticoagulant-preservative formulation provides a substrate for the continued generation of ATP *in vitro*. The overall effect is improved viability.

15.

D. Donor blood may not be labeled according to test results obtained from previous donations. Several segments removed from the donor unit will provide sufficient sample for all required testing but will limit the number of segments available for crossmatching. After centrifugation, the plasma may be removed from the segments and clotted with calcium chloride or a similar commercial product for use in test procedures requiring serum. Alternatively, institutions with sterile connecting devices may attach a small bag and remove an aliquot sufficient for testing.

16–17.

(16:C, 17:A) *In vitro* recovery of factor VIII must be assayed monthly to ensure proper control of conditions during cryoprecipitate production. A minimum of 80 international units (IU) per container must be present in the final product. One international unit is defined as the clotting activity of 1 mL of fresh plasma. The total number of factor VIII units is calculated from the formula:

Factor VIII IU/mL $\times$ volume in mL
$$= \text{Total IU Factor VIII}$$

In this case 9 IU/mL $\times$ 10 mL = 90 IU per container in the final product. This exceeds the required 80 IU/container and so meets AABB *Standards*.

Although there is no existing standard for percent recovery of factor VIII during production, this information may be helpful in monitoring various stages of production when the monthly quality control assays fall below the acceptable standard. Recovery can be calculated by the formula:

$$\frac{\text{Post (F VIII IU/mL} \times \text{volume in mL)}}{\text{Pre (F VIII IU/mL} \times \text{volume in mL)}} \times 100$$
$$= \% \text{ Factor VIII recovery}$$

In this instance:

$$\frac{9 \text{ IU/mL} \times 10 \text{ mL}}{1 \text{ IU/mL} \times 250 \text{ mL}} \times 100$$
$$= 36\% \text{ Factor VIII recovery}$$

18–21.

(18:D, 19:D, 20:B, 21:B) Each centrifuge used for platelet production must be calibrated upon receipt or after major repair. Calculating percent recovery during various stages of platelet production is a valuable troubleshooting tool when monthly quality control assays consistently fall below the minimum standard of 5.5×10^{10} platelets per platelet concentrate. In this exercise the first spin gives an 83% platelet yield, and the second spin produces a 60% yield from the PRP. Increasing the time or rpm of the PRP will result in a greater percent

yield for the platelet concentrate. Yield is calculated from the following formulas:

Platelet count/μL $\times$ 1000 μL/mL
$$\times \text{ Volume in mL} = \text{Total count in component}$$

$$\frac{\text{Total count in PRP}}{\text{Total count in whole blood}} \times 100$$
$$= \% \text{ yield from whole blood}$$

$$\frac{\text{Total count in platelet concentrate}}{\text{Total count in PRP}} \times 100$$
$$= \% \text{ yield from PRP}$$

In the example above the total count in PRP would be

300,000/μL $\times$ 1000 μL/mL $\times$ 250 mL
$$= 7.5 \times 10^{10} \text{platelets}$$

The total count in whole blood is

200,000/μL $\times$ 1000 μL/mL $\times$ 450 mL
$$= 9 \times 10^{10} \text{ platelets}$$

The percent yield from whole blood is

$$\frac{7.5 \times 10^{10}}{9 \times 10^{10}} \times 100 = 83\%$$

The total count in the platelet concentrate is

900,000/μL $\times$ 1000 μL/mL $\times$ 50 mL
$$= 4.5 \times 10^{10} \text{ platelets}$$

The percent yield from PRP is

$$\frac{4.5 \times 10^{10}}{7.5 \times 10^{10}} \times 100 = 60\%$$

At least 75% of prepared platelet packs must contain a minimum of 5.5×10^{10} cells. Since there are only 4.5×10^{10} cells in this platelet concentrate, it would be considered too low.

22.

B. A low red blood cell concentration of 2,3-DPG increases red cell affinity for O_2 causing less O_2 to be released to the tissues. As blood is stored, 2,3-DPG levels fall. Once the blood is transfused, red cells regenerate 2,3-DPG and ATP, which are fully restored in about 24 hours. Other metabolic changes that occur as blood is stored are an increased plasma K^+ as red cells leak K^+, an increase in plasma hemoglobin, and a decrease in ATP.

23.

D. Autologous blood may not be drawn later than 72 hours prior to surgery. The reason is to allow time for adequate volume repletion. However, the medical director may decrease this time if the patient's condition warrants it.

24.

B. Preoperative autologous donation is commonly done for orthopedic surgery, radical prostatectomy, and open heart surgery. Patients with unstable angina or severe aortic stenosis are considered poor risk. Because it is difficult to find donors for patients with multiple antibodies or an antibody to a high incidence antigen, these individuals are encouraged to donate if able and their cells are frozen for later use.

25.

C. Hepatitis C virus (HCV) is transfusion transmitted. Since anti-HCV testing is done on all donor samples there is only a small risk (< 1 in 100,000) of transmission from tested donors. The acute phase of the disease is frequently asymptomatic, but most of these patients become chronic carriers with 70–80% having persistent infections. About 10% of those chronically infected eventually develop cirrhosis and/or hepatic carcinoma.

26.

B. Red blood cells continue to metabolize, albeit at a slower rate during storage at 1–6 °C. Decreased ATP levels result in loss of RBC viability. Plasma hemoglobin, ammonia, and K^+ levels increase, whereas plasma Na^+ and pH and 2,3-DPG levels decrease. These biochemical changes are collectively referred to as the "storage lesion" of blood.

27.

C. Since the patient received 8 units of blood and none of the donors has been implicated in other cases of hepatitis, none of these donors would be deferred. The donor center should be immediately notified so they can enter in each donor's record that he/she has been implicated in a case of transfusion transmitted hepatitis. After a second implication the donor would be indefinitely deferred. If only one donor had been implicated, he/she would have been indefinitely deferred.

28.

C. Red blood cells and whole blood must be stored at between 1 and 6 °C in a monitored refrigerator with a recording thermometer and audible alarm system. During transportation between collection and transfusion facilities, blood must be packed in well-insulated containers designed to maintain a temperature range of 1–10 °C. Wet ice in a leak-proof plastic bag is placed on top of the blood. The amount of ice to be used is dictated by the transportation time, number of units packed, and the ambient outside temperature.

29.

C. In addition to the minimum number of platelets that should be present, 5.5×10^{10}, the pH of the unit must be 6.2 or higher in at least 75% of the units. The units should be assayed at the end of the allowable storage period. A donor who has taken aspirin should not be the sole donor of platelets for a patient. Aspirin has an adverse effect on platelet aggregation.

30.

C. Platelets must be stored in sufficient plasma volume to prevent the pH from falling below 6.2 at the time of expiration. Lactic acid is a by-product of anaerobic glycolysis during platelet storage, causing a drop in plasma pH and a loss of discoid shape, hence viability. Second generation platelet bags allow better gas exchange, permitting platelets to be stored for longer periods of time at a favorable pH.

31.

C. Red blood cells expire 24 hours from the time the hermetic seal is broken, provided they are maintained at 1–6 °C during the storage period. The new expiration date and time must be placed on the label and in the appropriate records. An open system exposes the blood to possible bacterial contamination. Blood may be frozen for up to 6 days after collection when maintained at 1–6 °C in a closed system. If the seal is inadvertently broken on a rare unit during component preparation, the red cells may be salvaged by glycerolization and freezing, providing this is accomplished within the 24-hour restriction.

32.

D. The AABB *Standards* requires that an authorized individual (such as a supervisor or medical director) review the standard operating procedures (SOPs), policies, and process annually and document the review. The SOPs should be reviewed and revised as needed to reflect the techniques used by the laboratory. It is prudent to conduct a review prior to a scheduled inspection and following publication of each new edition of AABB *Standards* to ensure conformance with new requirements.

33.

B. Previous ABO and Rh records of patients must be retained for 5 years and be immediately available for 12 months as a check to confirm the identity of the current pretransfusion sample. Records of unexpected antibodies identified in the serum of intended recipients and of serious adverse reactions to blood components must be retained indefinitely. Consulting records may prevent a delayed hemolytic transfusion reaction when the antibody is no longer demonstrable.

34.

D. In the United States the weak D test is performed routinely when a donor appears to be Rh-negative, and all weak D donor units are labeled Rh-positive. Weak D units are much less immunogenic than normal D units. In many countries neither donors nor recipients are tested for weak D.

35.

B. In order to meet the current AABB *Standards* for leukocyte reduction to prevent HLA alloimmunization or CMV transmission, the donor unit must retain at least 80% of the original red cells and the leukocytes must be reduced to less than 5×10^6. Leukocyte reduction may also prevent febrile reactions in two ways. By reducing the number of leukocytes in the component to a low enough level one can prevent febrile reactions when patients have leukocyte antibodies. Cytokines are also known to cause febrile reactions. If prestorage leukocyte-reduction is done cytokine generation should be prevented.

36.

D. ABO grouping must be determined by doing both cell and serum grouping. The Rh type must be determined by direct agglutination with anti-D; if negative, the test is incubated and converted to the indirect antiglobulin test to detect weak D phenotypes. Performing an antibody screening test on the serum or plasma of a donor is required when the donor has a history of transfusion or pregnancy. For practical purposes most donor centers screen all donors for clinically significant antibodies. The absence of hepatitis B surface antigen (HB$_s$Ag) must be confirmed using a method currently licensed by the FDA. The test for hepatitis B surface antibody (HB$_s$Ab) is not required.

37.

C. In the average size adult (70 kg) a unit of platelet concentrate should raise the platelet count by 5000–10,000/µL if there are no other complicating factors to cause decreased survival. Complicating factors include fever, sepsis, disseminated intravascular coagulation (DIC), and HLA sensitization. One apheresis platelet unit is equivalent to 6–8 units of pooled platelet concentrate and has the advantage of decreased donor exposure.

38.

A. The ABO group and the Rh type on all D-negatives must be repeated by the transfusing facility for units of RBC or whole blood collected and processed at another facility. This is generally accomplished by repeating the cell grouping only. To save time and reagent cost, it is convenient to test units labeled Group O with anti-A,B only. Confirmatory testing for weak D is not required. The Rh type of units labeled D-positive need not be confirmed. Repeat antibody screening and viral testing are not required.

39–43.

(39:A, 40:D, 41:C, 42:C, 43:B) The storage temperature for whole blood, modified whole blood and red blood cells (RBC), including leukocyte-reduced and deglycerolyzed products, is between 1 and 6 °C. This range may be extended to 10 °C during brief periods of transport. RBCs are frozen in a glycerol solution. These units must be stored at −65 °C or lower. Fresh-frozen plasma (FFP) and cryoprecipitate are stored at −18 °C or colder with a one-year expiration. Although this temperature meets AABB *Standards*, optimal storage temperature is −30 °C or below. In fact FFP expiration may be extended to 7 years if kept at −65 °C or lower.

Frozen storage at low temperatures maintains optimum levels of the labile coagulation factors V and VIII in FFP and VIII in cryoprecipitate. Plasma should be frozen within 8 hours of collection when collected in CPD or CPDA-1. Platelet concentrates are stored at room temperature (20–24 °C). They need to be agitated during storage.

44–48.

(44:C, 45:D, 46:D, 47:A, 48:B) Whole blood and RBC may be stored up to 35 days when collected in CPDA-1, as long as the hermetic seal remains unbroken. Adenine added to the anticoagulant increases the viability of the cells. Cells stored only in CPD have a shorter allowable storage of 21 days. Fresh-frozen plasma (FFP) and cryoprecipitate expire 12 months from the date of collection if stored at −18 °C or colder. The expiration time for these components is based on the deterioration of the labile factor VIII. Units stored beyond 12 months may have reduced levels of factor VIII unless stored at much lower temperatures. Recently FFP has been approved for 7-year storage if kept at −65 °C or lower. Once thawed, FFP expires in 24 hours when stored at 1–6 °C. The type of plastic used in the manufacture of the bag affects the allowable storage time for platelets. The older type of bag (polyvinylchloride) does not allow as effective a gas exchange as the newer types of plastic. Platelet concentrates, prepared in PL–732 bags and stored at 20–24 °C with agitation, expire 5 days from the date and time of collection.

49–52.

(49:A, 50:B, 51:C, 52:D) Blood cells continue to metabolize *in vitro*. Plasma glucose and ATP are depleted. Intermediary metabolites are generated. These may interfere with the production of energy via glycolysis. This results in a gradual loss of red blood cell viability. Storage at lowered temperatures (1–6 °C) slows metabolism. ACD and CPD solutions contain sufficient glucose to support RBC viability for 21 days. CPDA-1 also contains adenine, which allows extension of the shelf life to 35 days. Adenine maintains viability by ATP regeneration. Red blood cells prepared with additive solutions such as AS-1 have a shelf life of 42 days. EDTA is not an approved solution for the storage of blood for transfusion.

53–59.

(53:D, 54:A, 55:B, 56:D, 57:D, 58:D, 59:D) Donors may be accepted after age 17 provided all results of the physical examination are normal. There is no upper age limit. Elderly donors may participate in a blood program at the discretion of the local blood bank physician. Many senior citizens obtain written permission from their personal physicians and present approval at the time of donation. The interval between donation of blood for allogeneic transfusion is 8 weeks, or 56 days. This time period is designed to protect the health of the donor. Exceptions at the discretion of the blood bank and personal physician may be made if the blood is intended for autologous use. Individuals who have traveled to countries endemic for malaria (as determined by the World Health Organization) but have not had malaria symptoms must be deferred for 12 months whether or not antimalarial medication was taken as a preventive measure. When the individual returns for donation in 12 months, blood may be drawn, provided that other donor criteria, including temperature, blood pressure, pulse, and hemoglobin, are within acceptable limits. A history of jaundice in the first days of life is indicative of hemolytic disease of the newborn and is not a cause for deferral. A mild skin rash caused by acne, poison ivy, psoriasis, or other allergies is not a cause for donor deferral, as long as the disorder does not extend into the antecubital area at the venipuncture site. Final acceptance or deferral may be made at the phlebotomist's discretion, dependent upon whether the arm can be properly prepared to maintain sterility of the product without undue discomfort to the donor. A woman who has been pregnant is deferred until 6 weeks following conclusion of the pregnancy unless her blood is needed for her infant and the donation is physician approved.

The acceptable limits of the physical examination include:

Temperature: 37.5 °C (99.5 °F) or less

Pulse: 50–100

Blood pressure: ≤180 systolic, ≤100 diastolic

Runners or other athletes may be accepted when the pulse rate is less than 50, as long as no irregularity in beats is detected. These parameters are incorporated in the AABB *Standards* for the safety of the donor and are in general use by all blood-collecting facilities. For donor suitability, the FDA and AABB require only that the hemoglobin level be no less than 12.5 g/dL (with no sex differentiation) and that the temperature and blood pressure be within normal limits as determined by a qualified physician or by persons under his or her supervision.

60–63.

(60:D, 61:C, 62:B, 63:A) Patients with warm autoimmune hemolytic anemia (AIHA) secondary to α-methyldopa respond rapidly following cessation of the drug. They can usually be managed without transfusion. The DAT (direct antiglobulin test) may not revert to negative for up to six months or even longer. Leukocyte-reduced blood components ($\leq 5 \times 10^6$) are indicated in order to avoid repeated febrile episodes, CMV transmission, and alloimmunization to leukocytes. Leukocytes can be removed by filtration, centrifugation, or washing. Currently, the preferred and most efficient method is filtration with commercially available adsorption filters capable of reducing leukocytes to the required level. Patients with normovolemic anemia should be transfused with RBC, which provide the red blood cells needed to correct the anemia in the smallest volume. These patients may not be able to tolerate whole blood because of the volume increase. It is not necessary to use leukocyte-reduced RBC for patients with normovolemic anemia. Thrombocytopenia means there is a lack of platelets. Often platelet counts drop in acute leukemia and during the subsequent treatment. Platelet counts below 20,000/μL are not uncommon under the circumstances, and the patient is considered to have severe thrombocytopenia. Leukocyte-reduced platelets will lower the chance of alloimmunization and are routinely given prophylactically to leukemia patients.

BLOOD GROUPS, GENETICS, SEROLOGY

64.

D. The body makes five different immunoglobulins: IgA, IgD, IgE, IgG, and IgM. IgG makes up about 80% of the total serum immunoglobulin. Although IgA is more abundant than IgM (13% *vs.* 6%), IgM is more common as a blood group antibody.

65.

C. There are 46 chromosomes in normal individuals. There are 22 pairs of autosomes and one pair of sex chromosomes. The X and Y chromosomes determine the sex of an individual. They may be the same, XX as in the female, or different, XY as in the male.

66.

D. All red blood cells contain some amount of H substance. The only exception is the very rare O_h (Bombay) individual because these persons lack the H gene that codes for H substance. Group O cells contain the most H substance, and A₁B cells contain the least amount of H substance. The order of decreasing reactivity with anti-H is: O>A₂> A₂B>B>A₁>A₁B.

67.

B. Two genes control Rh antigen activity. *RHD* controls the expression of D antigen and *RHCE* determines the C, E, c, and e antigens. *RHD* is absent or inactive in D-negative individuals. Alleles of *RHCE* are *RHcE, RHcE,* and *RHce*. The RH is often dropped (for example *CE, Ce, cE, ce*).

68.

B. Bombay individuals' red blood cells not only lack A and B substances, but they also lack H substance. Bombays are genetically *hh* and therefore are unable to produce the precursor H substance upon which the A and B transferases act to produce A and B substances. In their serum they will have anti-A, anti-B, anti-A,B and an equally strong anti-H, which will react with normal group O cells. Bombay red blood cells also give a negative reaction with *Ulex europaeus* (anti-H lectin) while O cells are positive. Neither O nor O_h red blood cells react with anti-A,B or *Dolichos biflorus* lectin (anti-A₁) thus giving no point of differentiation.

69.

D. The Lutheran and secretor loci are close together on the same chromosome. This was the first autosomal linkage discovered. Another locus linked to Se and Lu is that for the disease myotonic dystrophy.

70.

C. The *Le* gene codes for a transferase enzyme, L-fucosyl transferase, that attaches fucose to the subterminal sugar on the Type 1 precursor substance producing Leᵃ substance. This occurs independently of the ABH secretor status. For Leᵇ as well as ABH substances to be present in the secretions both the *Se* gene and the *Le* gene must be present.

The *Se* gene produces a transferase that attaches a fucose to the terminal sugar on precursor substance forming H substance in the secretions. Type 1H and Type 2H are the precursors for A and B substance. The *Le* gene can act upon Type 1H as well to form Le^b substance; therefore, a nonsecretor who has an *Le* gene will only secrete Le^a, while a secretor will secrete a little Le^a and a lot of Le^b substance.

71.

D. Monoclonal reagents containing the ES-4 clone react well with acquired B cells and those lacking that clone do not react. Most human anti-B will react, but not the individual's own anti-B. Acquired B antigens are often associated with carcinoma of the colon, gram-negative infection, and intestinal obstructions. Also, B substance will not be found in the saliva if the patient is an ABH secretor. Acquired B occurs in group A people when microbial enzymes deacetylate the A determinant sugar (*N*-acetylgalactosamine) so that it resembles the B sugar (D-galactose).

72.

A. A$_1$ lectin is a saline extract prepared from seeds. *Dolichos biflorus* reagent will react only with cells containing A$_1$ antigen. Those group A cells not agglutinated by *D. biflorus* reagents are generally classified as A$_2$ cells. About 20% of group A individuals' red blood cells will not be agglutinated by *D. biflorus*. *Ulex europaeus* is another lectin commonly used in blood banking; it detects the H antigen.

73.

D. The sugar L-fucose is attached to the terminal sugar of precursor substance by a fucosyl transferase. The fucosyl transferase is coded on the red cells by the *H* gene or in the secretions by the *Se* gene, and the resulting configuration is called H substance. Without H substance present, the sugars giving A or B antigenic activity cannot attach.

74.

B. IgM is the immunoglobulin that most readily activates complement. The IgG immunoglobulins can activate complement to a lesser extent. IgG3 activates complement more efficiently than the other IgG subclasses. The last stages of the complement cascade ultimately lead to red blood cell lysis.

75.

B. The answer is based upon the frequencies of genes. The genes that code for the haplotypes *DCe* and *dce* are high in the white population. A *DCe/dce* genotype has a frequency of approximately 31.1% in the general white population. The other two possible choices among the answers that would fit the typing results are *DCe/Dce* and *Dce/dCe* and have frequencies of approximately 3.4% and 0.2%, respectively. *DCe/DcE* is incorrect because the typing does not indicate that the E antigen is present.

76.

A. These genotypes all have a low frequency in the black population. *DCE/dce* is the rarest with a frequency of < 0.05%. *DCe/DcE* is the most frequent with an occurrence of 3.7%.

77.

A. Red blood cells that have either the C or D antigen also have the G antigen. When anti-G is made, it is capable of reacting with the G antigen on both C-positive and D-positive red blood cells, therefore appearing to be anti-CD. In the stated case, the immunizing red blood cells were D-negative and C-positive. Therefore, what appears to be a combination of anti-D and anti-C is anti-G or a combination of anti-C and anti-G.

78.

B. The unit from the *DCe/dce* donor has the c antigen which the patient lacks. This antigen is a good immunogen. Remember, "d" simply implies the absence of D and is not an antigen. Both donor and patient are likely to have the high incidence antigen LW that, although associated with the Rh system, is not an Rh antigen.

79.

D. The LW antigen occurs in nearly every individual but in varying amounts. More LW is present on D-positive cells than D-negative cells. Persons with very little LW antigen can make an anti-LW, which will react with those cells with a large amount of LW antigen. The *LW* and *Rh* genes segregate independently.

80.

C. Fifty percent of the children can be expected to be D-positive (*DCe/dce*) and 50% can be expected to be D-negative (*dce/dce*). The following chart clearly illustrates how the percentages were determined. The mother can pass on only *dce* haplotype, whereas the father can pass on *DCe* or *dce*.

Father

Mother	DCe	dce
dce	*DCe/dce*	*dce/dce*
dce	*DCe/dce*	*dce/dce*

81.

C. The husband's genotype is most likely *Dce/dCe*. He is weak D because of position effect and has a normal *D* gene. The *C* in transposition to a normal *D* gene often causes a weakened expression of D antigen. The infant has inherited the father's normal *D* gene, but does not have *C* in transposition, and therefore has a normal D antigen expression. Thus the husband is not excluded and is probably the father.

82.

A. Occasionally, D-positive people make an apparent anti-D. The D antigen is made up of several determinants, and those missing one or more determinants are called partial D. When individuals lack one of these determinants, they can make an antibody, after appropriate stimulation, against the determinant that they lack. Therefore, a D-positive or weak D person appears to make an anti-D.

83.

A. The k antigen is a high-frequency or "public" antigen present in greater than 99% of the random population. The probability of encountering an individual who is k-negative and capable of producing the corresponding antibody after red blood cell stimulation is very low. Kell system antigens are good immunogens, second only to those of the Rh system.

84.

C. Three mechanisms can lead to the Lu(a−b−) phenotype, one in which a person is homozygous for an amorphic Lutheran allele (*LuLu*) and in the second a dominant suppressor gene, usually denoted *In(Lu)* is inherited. This gene suppresses the expression of the Lu antigens even in the presence of normal Lutheran genes. The *In(Lu)* gene also affects the expression of the P₁, i, and Auᵃ antigens but not to the extent the Lu antigens are affected.

The third is due to an X-borne recessive suppressor gene.

85.

A. The Xgᵃ antigen is produced by a gene on the X chromosome. Since women inherit two X chromosomes, there is a higher incidence of the antigen in females. The antibody is usually detected by an indirect antiglobulin test, and the antigenic activity is depressed by enzymes.

86.

D. Of the choices listed, LW, I, and P should be readily recognizable as high-incidence antigens. On the other hand, Wrᵃ is found in approximately 1 out of 1000 samples tested. The low-incidence antigens usually do not play a significant role in routine blood banking.

87.

D. Kidd antibodies are often weak and deteriorate during storage. They are usually IgG, antiglobulin reactive only, and complement dependent. Reactions are enhanced when enzyme-treated panel cells are used. Kidd antibodies also show dosage and the titer may drop to undetectable levels after the primary response. For this reason they are often implicated in delayed hemolytic transfusion reactions when there is no previous record of the presence of the antibody. A Kidd antibody rarely occurs singly in a patient's serum but is often seen accompanying other antibodies.

88.

B. Enzymes denature the Fyᵃ and Fyᵇ antigens and render panel cells Fy(a−b−). Therefore, anti-Fyᵃ and -Fyᵇ will not react with enzyme-treated red cells. These Duffy antibodies are clinically significant. They can cause hemolytic transfusion reactions and mild hemolytic disease of the newborn. They are usually IgG antibodies and are best detected by the indirect antiglobulin test.

89.

B. Chido and Rodgers are antigens that are associated with "high-titer, low-avidity" (HTLA) antibodies. HTLA means that the antibodies have a relatively high titer with a low avidity for the corresponding antigen, often not stronger than a 1+ agglutination. Clinically, these antibodies are usually not significant. They are IgG and are detected by the indirect antiglobulin test.

answers & rationale

90.

D. Anti-U is a clinically significant IgG antibody causing hemolytic transfusion reactions and hemolytic disease of the newborn. All white people are U+. However, about 99% of blacks are U+ and 1% are U−. Those people who are U− are also S−s− except for very rare genetic mutations.

91.

B. Although the patient's antibody screening is negative at this time, previous records show the patient had an anti-E. Anti-E is a significant IgG antibody; only blood negative for the E antigen should be transfused to the patient. Failure to give E-negative blood could result in a serious delayed transfusion reaction due to an anamnestic response.

92.

B. For control purposes the cell should have the weakest expression of the antigen in question; that would be an Fy(a+b+) cell. A weaker cell from a heterozygote is used because a weak antiserum might detect an antigen from a homozygote but not from a heterozygote (dosage effect). If this should happen, then red blood cells might be mistyped as Fy(a−) when in fact the cells are Fy(a+).

93.

B. Most antibodies in the Kell system are red blood cell stimulated. They are generally IgG antibodies and usually detected in the antiglobulin phase of testing. Because of their nature, they have been implicated in both transfusion reactions and hemolytic disease of the newborn. The other choices are usually IgM antibodies that cannot cross the placenta and are rarely involved in transfusion reactions.

94.

B. The lack of Kidd antigens results in the Jk(a−b−) phenotype, which is extremely rare. This lack may be caused by an inhibitor mechanism or by a silent allele at the Kidd locus. The Jk(a−b−) people who have been found are predominantly East Asians, particularly from the Pacific Islands.

95.

B. It appears that the Fy^a and/or the Fy^b antigens need to be present on the red blood cell for *Plasmodium vivax* or *knowlesi* (malaria parasites) to enter the cell. In Africa where malaria is endemic, African blacks who are predominantly Fy(a−b−) have resistance to malaria, probably acquired through natural selection. In American blacks the frequency of Fy(a−b−) is much lower than in Africa due to interracial mating and lack of the disease malaria.

96.

B. All the antibodies listed fit one or more of the descriptions. For example, anti-D fits all the descriptions except that anti-D is enhanced with enzyme-treated cells. Only anti-S fits all the categories.

97.

C. Anti-Le^a, -Le^b, and -P_1 may all be neutralized by commercially available soluble substances. Alternatively, when performing an antibody identification on a patient that has one of the above antibodies, it may be helpful to use antigen-negative cells to exclude/include other antibodies. Of course this is dependent upon having access to these cells.

98.

C. Anti-N is the only antibody listed which is generally a room temperature saline agglutinin. The remaining choices, anti-Fy^a, anti-Jk^b, and anti-U, are best detected at the antiglobulin phase. Remember, this is where these antibodies are optimally reactive; it does not mean they will never react anywhere else. Some antibodies just don't read the books!

99.

D. The M and N antigen basic structure (glycophorin A) has a large amount of sialic acid (*N*-acetylneuraminic acid) incorporated into it. Sialic acid is susceptible to the action of the proteolytic enzymes such as papain and ficin. The enzyme cleaves off that part of the structure that contains the M and N antigens. Enzymes are useful in antibody identification when one may be dealing with a mixture of antibodies.

100.

B. Solid-phase red cell adherence assays, the gel test, and affinity column technology are all third-generation antibody detection methods. They have equal or greater sensitivity for clinically significant antibodies than first and second generation techniques. In general they have the following advantages: less hands-on time, smaller sample size, improved safety, stable end points, and they can be automated. In the gel test, the antiglobulin test does not require washing or the addition of IgG coated cells, since unbound globulins are trapped in the viscous barrier at the top of the gel column. Upon centrifugation, the anti-IgG in the column traps red cells that have been coated with IgG during the incubation period. In affinity column technology the viscous barrier traps unbound IgG, but *Staphylococcus aureus* derived Protein A and Protein G are in the column instead of anti-IgG and react with the Fc portion of IgG coated red cells. The other two techniques, solid-phase red cell adherence and polyethylene glycol, require a washing step.

101.

D. The three antibodies, anti-P_1, anti-Le^a, and anti-I, are generally naturally occurring (non-red-cell-immune) IgM antibodies. Each of the other answers has at least one antibody that is generally considered an immune antibody; that is, one that needs to be stimulated by exposure to the corresponding red cell antigen. One must keep in mind that on occasion, antibodies that are usually naturally occurring can be stimulated.

102.

D. HLA-D typing is done by mixed lymphocyte culture (MLC). HLA-A, HLA-B, and HLA-C antigens are serologically defined and are identified by microlymphocytotoxicity tests. Many laboratories now perform HLA typing by DNA hybridization techniques.

103.

A. Mixed-field agglutination refers to an agglutination pattern where there are two distinct cell populations, one agglutinated and one not. The appearance is clumps of cells among many unagglutinated cells. In a delayed hemolytic transfusion reaction, surviving donor cells will be coated with patient antibody and the patient's own cells will not, yielding a mixed field DAT result. Other examples of mixed-field agglutination are seen in patients who have been transfused with blood of another ABO group, patients with Lutheran antibodies, and in D-negative mothers with D-positive infants where there was a large fetomaternal bleed. Also, A_3 subgroup may demonstrate a mixed-field reaction with anti-A.

104.

D. The first antibody to become detectable in a primary immune response to a foreign blood group antigen is IgM followed by IgG, usually detectable from less than a week to several months after immunization. After secondary exposure to the same antigen, the antibody titer usually increases rapidly within several days. The antibody produced by the B lymphocytes in the secondary response is IgG.

105.

D. All the conditions listed affect the agglutination of A and B cells in serum grouping. The gamma globulin fraction of the serum contains the immunoglobulins. When it is reduced, there will be fewer molecules of blood group antibodies, leading to weakened or negative reactions. Both cold autoagglutinins and cold reactive IgM alloantibodies, which will react at room temperature (such as anti-M), may agglutinate the cells used due to the presence of the corresponding antigen on the group A and/or B red blood cells. Cold auto- and alloantibodies are the most common causes of ABO discrepancies.

106.

C. Blood for intrauterine transfusion should be group O, D-negative (since the fetus's blood group is unknown) and negative for the antigen corresponding to any other IgG antibody in the maternal serum. It should be recently drawn and administered as RBC (Hct 75–85%) to minimize the chance of volume overload. It should be irradiated, CMV safe, and known to lack hemoglobin S.

107.

A. Anti-Jk^a is an IgG antibody and is nearly always detected in the indirect antiglobulin test. Rarely it can be detected at the 37 °C phase of testing. Anti-M, anti-P_1, and anti-I are generally IgM antibodies and react at room temperature and below by direct agglutination.

108.

D. Lewis antibodies are generally IgM. Antibodies in the Rh, Duffy, and Kell systems are generally IgG. There may be rare IgM exceptions.

109.

B. Bg antibodies react with the red blood cell equivalents of HLA antigens. Bg^a corresponds with HLA-B7, Bg^b with HLA-B17, and Bg^c with HLA-A28. These antibodies can be frustrating in that few panel cells will react and their Bg type is often not listed.

110.

C. There is no ABO exclusion. Although the alleged father and mother are group A, they could both be heterozygous (*AO*) with the baby inheriting the *O* gene from each parent. The child appears to be of the Rh genotype *dce/dce*. One of these haplotypes is inherited from the mother. It is feasible for the alleged father to be *DCe/dce*. He could then contribute the second haplotype. The baby can inherit the *A2B12* haplotype from the mother. Although *A3* can come from the alleged father, *B15* cannot and, therefore, there is a direct HLA exclusion.

111–118.

(111:C, 112:A, 113:D, 114:B, 115:C, 116:D, 117:C, 118:A)
Discrepancies in ABO blood grouping may occur for numerous reasons. Any discrepancy between cell and serum grouping must be resolved before blood is identified as belonging to a particular ABO group. The presence of an acquired B antigen on cells that are normally group A can be found in some disorders, where gram-negative bacteria have entered the circulation. The serum will contain an anti-B, which will not agglutinate the patient's own cells which have the acquired B antigen. The red cell reaction with anti-B reagent may be weaker than usual. Protein abnormalities of the serum such as are present in multiple myeloma may cause the presence of what appear to be additional antibodies. The rouleaux of the red blood cells caused by the excess globulin may appear to be agglutination. Saline replacement of the serum and resuspension of the cells will usually resolve the problem in the serum grouping. Washed red blood cells should be used for the cell grouping. Infants do not begin making antibodies until they are 3 to 6 months of age. Newborns therefore will not demonstrate the expected antibody(ies) on reverse grouping. The antibody that is present is probably IgG from the mother that has crossed the placenta. An A_2 individual has the ability to make an antibody that agglutinates A_1 red cells. This anti-A_1 will cause a

serum grouping discrepancy, but the antibody is almost always naturally occurring and clinically insignificant. A patient's serum may have antibodies to the yellow dye used to color anti-B reagents. If serum or plasma suspended red cells are used in the cell grouping, a false positive reaction may occur. Using washed cells will eliminate the problem. Patients who are immunodeficient may have such depressed immunoglobulins that their serum does not react with the expected A and B reagent red cells. *Cis-AB* individuals usually have a weaker than normal B antigen and anti-B in their serum, which does not react with their own red cells. *Cis-AB* may arise from unequal crossing over resulting in an A and B gene residing on the same chromosome. A patient with cold hemagglutinin disease (CHD) may have a discrepancy affecting both cell and serum groupings. The red blood cells should be washed with warm saline before typing; the serum and reagent A and B cells should be prewarmed before mixing and testing and converted to the antiglobulin test if necessary.

119–123.

(119:C, 120:A, 121:A, 122:D, 123:B) The Kell System has a number of antigens, among which is Kp^a (Penney). This antigen has not been reported in blacks. The corresponding antibody is very rare because so few individuals have the antigen that stimulates its production. When it is present, it is not a serious problem because Kp(a−) blood is easily found. The McLeod phenotype is one in which all the Kell-associated antigens are expressed only weakly. McLeod cells are missing a precursor substance called Kx. Kx is coded for by a gene present on the X chromosome. Some of the male children afflicted with chronic granulomatous disease are of the McLeod phenotype, but exactly how the two are associated is not clear. The *Ss* locus is closely linked with the *MN* locus and they are considered part of the same blood group system. M^g (Gilfeather) is a rare allele in the MN system. When the M^g antigen is present it can cause typing difficulties, since it will not react with either anti-M or anti-N. Because the MN antigens are well developed at birth, they were often used in paternity testing. The presence of an M^gM or M^gN combination can look like a homozygous *M* or *N* leading to a second order (indirect) exclusion unless the red cells are tested with anti-M^g. The presence of the M^g antigen on the red blood cells of the alleged father and child practically proves paternity. Currently most paternity testing is done by DNA analysis, not by red cell antigen testing.

ANTIBODY IDENTIFICATION, TRANSFUSION THERAPY, TRANSFUSION REACTIONS

124.
A. The racial origin of this donor is probably black. This origin can be determined by looking at the Duffy (Fy) phenotype. About 70% of American blacks are Fy(a−b−). The phenotype is extremely rare in whites.

125.
D. Donor 5 is homozygous for the following genes: *Ce, s, k, Jk^a, Fy^a*, since the corresponding antigen is produced and the antithetical antigen is not being produced by an allele (for example C+c− implies homozygosity: *CC*). The donor cannot be homozygous for *M*, since its allele is producing N antigen. There is no way to tell whether P_1 is homozygous, since it lacks a co-dominant allele and P_1 does not show dosage. There is no *Le^b* gene. The antigen is produced by the action of the *Le* gene on Type 1 H. The Lewis genes are *Le* and the amorph *le*, and dosage is not observed.

126.
A. Anti-Fy^a can be identified by eliminating specificities where the corresponding antigens appear on the panel cells that do not react. The differences in the strength of reactivity can be explained by the fact that the Duffy antigens show dosage (react stronger with cells from homozygotes). Cells #1 and #6 are from *Fy^a* heterozygotes [Fy(a+b+)]. Cells #4 and #5 are from *Fy^a* homozygotes [Fy(a+b−)]. When eliminating an antibody specificity known to show dosage, it is best to have a negative reaction with a panel cell from a donor who is homozygous for the corresponding gene. Fy^a and Fy^b antigens are destroyed by enzymes. Although the Fy(a−b−) type is common in blacks, the frequency of Fy^a in whites is about 66%. Anti-E and anti-s should be ruled out with Fy(a−) cells from individuals who are homozygous for *E* and *s* (in other words, E+e− and S−s+).

127.
C. Serum must be present to cause pseudoagglutination; it should not occur at the antiglobulin phase of testing when the rouleaux-producing properties have been removed by washing. Warm and cold autoantibodies result in a positive autocontrol, usually equal in strength to reactivity observed with reagent red cells. Antibodies directed against preservatives in potentiating media should also react in the autocontrol. When the autocontrol is nonreactive and all panel cells are uniformly positive, one should suspect the presence of an alloantibody directed against a "public," or high-frequency, antigen. A selected panel of red cells, each lacking a different high-frequency antigen, should be tested until a compatible cell is found. The patient's red cells may be typed for a variety of high-frequency antigens. If such an antigen is found to be missing on the red cells, the corresponding serum antibody is likely that specificity.

128.
B. Cell #7 is negative for the high-frequency antigen k (cellano). Many other specificities cannot be ruled out since there is only one negative reaction. Treating the panel cells with dithiothreitol (DTT) destroys Kell system antigens. If no reactions are seen when the panel is repeated with DTT treated cells, then many other clinically significant antibodies can be ruled out and the presence of anti-k would be supported. If the patient has not recently been transfused, his cells should be typed with anti-k and would be expected to be k-negative. Proteolytic enzymes neither destroy Kell system antigens nor enhance their reactions with Kell system antibodies. Treating serum with DTT will destroy IgM antibodies by cleaving disulfide bonds of the pentamer and would not be helpful since anti-k is generally IgG.

129.
C. From the presence of positive reactions taking place at two different temperatures, it appears that there are two different antibodies reacting. There is a cold antibody reacting with Cells #3 and #8 at immediate spin and a warm antibody reacting with Cells #1, #2, #3, and #4. It is unlikely that the cold antibody is carrying over to a warmer phase, since there is no 37 °C reaction with Cell #8.

130.

C. Anti-Le^a, -Le^b, and -P$_1$ are antibodies that react at immediate spin (room temperature or below). Of these, P$_1$ and Le^b antigens are present on Cell #7, which shows negative reactivity. This eliminates them from consideration. Le^a antigen is present on Cells #3 and #8, both of which show a positive immediate spin reaction.

131.

B. All the antibodies listed react at warm temperatures. Anti-K and anti-k do not usually react without the addition of AHG. Anti-C and -D may react at 37 °C without AHG, but usually only if albumin or enzymes are used as potentiators. Anti-C and -D are often found together. In this instance, however, there would be a positive reaction with Cell #5 if anti-C were present as well as anti-D.

132.

D. A patient's red blood cells should be negative for the antigen corresponding to the antibody identified as long as the autocontrol is also negative. In this case, one already knows that the patient is group A, D-negative (does not have D antigen). A standard approach has been to require 3 antigen-positive cells that react and 3 antigen-negative cells that do not for each antibody identified to establish probability that the antibody(ies) has (have) been correctly identified. There are only two Le(a+) donor cells on this panel. The anti-Le^a reacts only at immediate spin (IS) and the anti-D does not. Presumably the screening cells have an additional Le(a+) cell. Since this antibody appears to be clinically insignificant, many would simply ignore it by eliminating the IS. At any rate, it would certainly not be necessary to run another panel.

133.

D. When an antibody is identified, the patient's cells should be checked to see if in fact they are negative for the corresponding antigen. One would expect this patient to be K−k+. The patient's positive antibody screening test is consistent with an anti-K, and this is what was identified in the antibody identification. Three K antigen-positive and three K antigen-negative cells were tested and reacted appropriately. The antibody identification could have been misinterpreted, but it seems more likely the phenotyping may be wrong. This would

be the easiest and quickest part of the workup to double-check, preferably using a different anti-K reagent. Also, given the history, there is no reason to doubt the validity of the direct antiglobulin test, which also functions as a control for typings by indirect antiglobulin technique.

134.

B. Although there are many potential sources for error in performing an indirect antiglobulin test, the most common error leading to a false-negative reaction is the failure to wash adequately the red blood cells prior to addition of antiglobulin reagent (AHG). Traces of free human globulin can neutralize the AHG reagent. Red cells known to be coated with IgG antibody (Coombs' control cells, check cells) are added to all negative tests. Agglutination of these control cells confirms that AHG was present in the system and that proper washing procedures were performed.

135.

C. Elution is a process in which bound antibody is released from red blood cells. The eluate produced can then be further tested to identify the specificity of the antibody. Some elution methods use temperature, chemicals, or manipulation of the pH to dissociate antibodies from red cells.

136.

A. If the antiglobulin test was performed properly and the antiglobulin reagent is working properly, the IgG-coated control red blood cells should be agglutinated; thus, the test is valid. If they are unagglutinated, this could mean the antiglobulin reagent has been neutralized or may have been omitted. The test should be repeated if this happens.

137.

B. The major crossmatch is performed by testing the serum of the recipient with a suspension of the donor's red blood cells. The serum and red cells are usually tested at the immediate spin (IS), 37 °C, and indirect antiglobulin phases to detect both ABO mismatches and the presence of clinically significant antibodies. Since clinically significant antibodies (other than anti-A and anti-B) are almost always detected during the antibody screening test, AABB *Standards* sanctions performing only the immediate spin crossmatch (for ABO compatibility) when the patient has a negative antibody screening test. An antiglobulin crossmatch *must be performed* when a patient has a positive antibody screening test due to a clinically significant antibody, or if the patient has a history of a clinically significant antibody. Compatible units must also be phenotyped for the corresponding antigen and shown to be negative. When an antiglobulin crossmatch is performed, potentiating media such as albumin, polyethylene glycol (PEG), or low-ionic strength saline solutions (LISS) may be added to the test system to enhance sensitivity and/or decrease incubation time.

138.

B. A group AB individual can receive red blood cells from donors of all ABO groups. Since the patient does not have anti-D it would be best to next select group A, D-positive units (U) because the need for large amounts of blood is anticipated. These Us should be given as red blood cells (RBC), since the plasma has anti-B. If necessary the patient may be later switched to group O, D-positive RBC. It would not be wise to deplete the D-negative supply, since D-negative women of child-bearing age may need blood and should not be exposed to the D antigen. The decision to transfuse D-positive blood to a D-negative patient must be approved by the physician in charge of the transfusion service.

139.

D. The major crossmatch, which is the recipient's serum with the donor's cells, will reveal only if the patient has a detectable antibody against some antigen on the donor cells. In the presence of a negative antibody screening test, an incompatible crossmatch at the immediate spin phase will most likely be due to an ABO mismatch between the recipient's serum and the donor's cells. For this reason, AABB *Standards* mandates performing only the immediate spin crossmatch when the patient has a negative antibody screening test and no history of clinically significant antibodies. The major crossmatch will not guarantee *in vivo* response to the transfused red blood cells. Also, it will not detect all ABO typing errors, and it will not detect most Rh typing errors.

140.

C. A false-positive crossmatch could occur if the donor has a positive direct antiglobulin test (DAT). A DAT should be done on the donor cells and if positive, the unit should be removed from inventory. Another possible cause of a false-positive crossmatch could be

contaminants in dirty glassware causing clumping of red cells. The other responses are true-positives. If a strong incompatibility is immediately present, one should check the ABO type of the patient and the donor. If the antibody screening test was negative, one might suspect an antibody against a low-incidence antigen on the donor's cells.

141.

C. The major crossmatch consists of testing donor cells with recipient serum. A group A individual will have anti-B in his serum, which will agglutinate AB cells. D-positive cells given to a D-negative person will cause antibody stimulation, but there will not be a visible reaction without a preformed antibody.

142.

A. The most critical step to ensuring safe transfusion is obtaining a properly labeled blood sample from the correct patient. Transfusion accidents due to ABO mismatches are usually the result of a patient receiving the wrong blood. The identity of the patient must be verified, both verbally and by comparison of the wristband with the transfusion request form. Tubes must be labeled properly at the bedside with the full name, another acceptable identifier such as the medical record number, and the date.

143.

B. Sufficient information for unique identification of the patient (including two independent identifiers) and the date of sample collection must be on the label. The phlebotomist's signature or initials must appear on either the tube of blood or on the request slips. It is not necessary for both to be signed. The physician's name, the patient's room number, and the time of the phlebotomy may be helpful but are not required by AABB *Standards*.

144.

A. According to AABB *Standards*, specimens used for antibody screening and crossmatching must be less than 3 days old if the patient has been transfused or pregnant within the past 3 months. Either serum or plasma may be used. The specimen must be labeled properly at the bedside at the time of collection. Specimens are required to be retained for only 7 days posttransfusion.

145.

B. In general, one unit of red blood cells should raise a patient's hemoglobin by 1 g/dL. In this instance a 2 g/dL rise is required, so two units would need to be given. This rule is true for patients of average size. A very large or heavy individual with an expanded blood volume may require additional units to attain the same level. Conversely, a pediatric patient may require less.

146.

B. The percentage of compatible blood is obtained by multiplying the frequencies of antigen-negative. In this instance one wants to find Jk(a−), K− blood. The incidence of Jk(a+) blood is 77%; therefore, the incidence of Jk(a−) blood is 23%. Likewise, K+ incidence is 10%; K− would be 90%. Multiply these two frequencies together to get the frequency for Jk(a−), K− units: $0.23 \times 0.90 = 0.21$, or an incidence of 21 units in 100. Divide 2 by this figure since 2 units are needed: $2/0.21 = 9.5$, or 10 units must be screened to find 2 compatible units.

147.

C. Cryoprecipitate provides a source of fibrinogen and fibronectin in addition to factors VIII and XIII. This component is indicated for use in bleeding disorders associated with hypofibrinogenemia, such as DIC, when excessive fibrinogen consumption is occurring. Each unit contains an average of 250 mg of fibrinogen or 0.25 g. The AABB *Standards* requires a minimum of 150 mg per individual collection. The amount of pooled product to administer is calculated by the formula:

$$\frac{\text{Total grams desired}}{0.25 \text{ g/unit}} = \begin{array}{l}\text{Total number of}\\\text{cryoprecipitate units}\\\text{to administer}\end{array}$$

Example:

$$\frac{2 \text{ g}}{0.25 \text{ g/unit}} = 8 \text{ Units}$$

148.

D. Plasma compatible with the recipient's ABO group is preferred when large volumes are transfused. Both group O and group B plasma contain anti-A that can cause a positive direct antiglobulin test (DAT) when infused into either group A or AB recipients. Compatibility testing is not required prior to cryoprecipitate administration. Plasma compatibility is not as important with cryoprecipitate as with platelet concentrates. Approximately 10 mL of plasma is in a cryo unit and 50 mL in a single platelet concentrate.

149.

D. Approximately 1% of transfused red cells are cleared daily from the circulation of a recipient. The clearance rate may be increased in patients with autoimmune hemolytic anemia, pernicious anemia, aplastic anemia, hemorrhage, splenomegaly, and fever. Transfused cells survive normally in patients with anemia due to intrinsic red cell enzyme defects, spherocytosis, and paroxysmal nocturnal hemoglobinuria.

150.

B. Febrile reactions are brought about by the interaction of antibodies in the recipient directed against antigens on donor leukocytes or by cytokines secreted by leukocytes. The antigens involved are both the HLA and granulocyte-specific antigens. Leukocyte-reduced RBC are the component of choice for a patient with repeated febrile transfusion reactions. Although frozen RBC that have been thawed and deglycerolized are considered leukocyte-reduced, the cost and time involved in preparation makes them an unpractical choice.

151.

D. Red blood cells are the component of choice to maintain or restore oxygen-carrying capacity. This component has the least effect on blood volume and the maximum effect on the oxygen-carrying capacity of all the products available for transfusion. In some patients, increasing the total blood volume more than what is absolutely necessary could have a detrimental effect. Examples are patients with chronic anemia or congestive heart failure.

152.

C. Children inherit half their genetic characteristics from each parent. Unless the parents are identical in antigen composition (a situation only found in identical twins), the child cannot be totally compatible with either parent. Siblings, however, have access to the same genetic material from each parent and so may have identical genes and antigens. A spouse genetically would be equivalent to a random donor.

153.

D. Because time is of the essence when a trauma victim is severely hemorrhaging, blood bank personnel must respond promptly. Group-specific blood may not be issued on the basis of previous patient or donor records. If the situation is so urgent as to preclude performing an ABO and Rh typing, or when a blood sample cannot be obtained, group O red blood cells (RBC) may be issued. The decision as to whether group O, D-positive or O, D-negative RBC should be used will depend upon inventory and the age and sex of the trauma victim. Blood banks located in a trauma center should have a written procedures manual with well-defined criteria. All staff must be familiar with these guidelines.

154.

D. Large volumes of transfused plasma should be ABO compatible with the recipient's red blood cells. Isoagglutinins present in the plasma will attach to the corresponding antigen on the patient's red cells *in vivo* and cause a positive DAT and perhaps hemolysis. Plasma of any blood group can be given to a group O patient, since his red cells will not be agglutinated by anti-A or anti-B in donor plasma.

155.

B. Physiologic saline is the only generally acceptable solution allowed to be added to blood or blood components. Ringer's solution causes small clots to develop in anticoagulated blood and 5% dextrose causes red cell lysis. Other solutions and medication should not be added to blood unless they have been proved safe and are sanctioned by the FDA.

156.

C. The majority of deaths due to hemolytic transfusion reactions are caused by clerical errors, not laboratory errors. Patients, blood samples, and lab records, if misidentified, may lead to the wrong ABO type blood being administered to the patient. These deaths most often occur in areas of high stress such as in emergency rooms and surgical suites.

157.

C. A delayed hemolytic transfusion reaction is generally the result of a patient's second exposure to an antigen present on donor red blood cells. The patient sometime previously had been exposed to the antigen, and this is his or her anamnestic response. It usually occurs from 3 to 14 days after transfusion and is accompanied by extravascular red blood cell destruction. Often the patient is asymptomatic.

158.

C. Kidd antibodies are generally IgG, complement dependent, and warm reacting. However, they are usually weak and labile. Because of this, they may go undetected in pretransfusion testing and the patient may inadvertently be transfused with antigen-positive blood, leading to a delayed transfusion reaction.

159.

A. Some people are genetically deficient in IgA. If these people have anti-IgA, they may suffer a severe anaphylactic reaction when subsequently exposed. Once these people are identified, they must receive IgA-deficient components such as multiple-washed or frozen-thawed RBC or components drawn from IgA-deficient donors.

160.

A. Viral inactivation methods such as the use of a solvent/detergent combination have eliminated the risk of transmission of viruses with a lipid envelope in clotting factor concentrates. This method has recently been applied to group specific frozen plasma. Pooled Plasma, Solvent/Detergent-Treated is much safer than the other components listed from the standpoint of HIV, HBV, and HCV, since the process destroys lipid-enveloped viruses. It does not destroy nonlipid-enveloped viruses such as parvovirus B19. Another approach to safety is "FFP-Donor Retested," which means that the FFP (fresh-frozen plasma) has been held for 90 days or more and released only after the donor has been retested negative for infectious disease markers. It is not a pooled product. The retesting should show that the donor was not in an infectious window period when the plasma was drawn.

161.

C. Antiglobulin reagent (AHG) is prepared by injecting animals (most commonly rabbits) with human globulin, causing the animal to produce antibodies directed against this human protein. AHG will detect globulin bound to red blood cells in an agglutination reaction. Free globulin present in the system will neutralize AHG, resulting in false-negative reactions. Cryoprecipitate, serum, and Rh immune globulin (RhIG) contain human globulins while bovine albumin does not. Positive reactions obtained when IgG-coated red blood cells are added to nonreactive tests is a quality control measure used to ensure that the washing step was properly performed and the AHG reagent was not neutralized.

162.

B. Of the choices provided, only the antiglobulin test is required. This is usually preceded by an incubation at 37 °C. An enhancement medium such as albumin, a low-ionic strength saline solution (LISS), or polyethylene glycol (PEG) may also be used. An immediate spin can be done to rule out strong IgM antibodies, but this is not required. Although some laboratories routinely include an autologous control, it has never been required by AABB *Standards* and is not considered cost effective by many laboratories.

163.

B. Autologous transfusions are the safest form of transfusion available, although they are not always the most practical. When administered properly they eliminate disease transmission, immunization to foreign antigens, and allergic and graft-*vs.*-host reactions. Clerical error is still a significant risk. An AABB survey revealed that 1.2% of respondents reported an erroneous autologous transfusion. While preoperative autologous collection is feasible for elective surgery, this form of autologous transfusion is not possible in cases of unexpected or massive blood loss. Intraoperative blood collection is another form of autologous transfusion used during operations where the estimated blood loss is great. Another advantage of autologous transfusions is that allogeneic donor blood is available for other patients.

164.

D. Reviewing the previous records of a patient may help to confirm the identity of the current pretransfusion sample. Records should be checked for ABO group and Rh type, clinically significant antibodies that were present but may no longer be detectable, and adverse reactions to previous units transfused. ABO records from the past 12 months must be immediately available and retained for 5 years; antibody and adverse reaction records must be available indefinitely for review before issuing blood for transfusion. It is not necessary to check hepatitis records of the patient.

165.

C. The major crossmatch is performed using the recipient's serum and the donor's red blood cells. Therefore, a positive DAT on the recipient's cells will not affect the crossmatch results. A positive reaction may be obtained when the recipient has an antibody directed against a corresponding antigen on the donor's red cells. If this is a low-frequency antigen, the crossmatch may be incompatible and the antibody screening result negative. A positive reaction may also indicate that the donor's red cells are coated with human globulin. This can be confirmed by performing a direct antiglobulin test (DAT) on the donor's red cells. Units of blood demonstrating a positive DAT should be returned to the collecting facility.

166.

D. Monoclonal anti-D reagents are low protein reagents, therefore, a negative reaction with anti-A and/or anti-B (also low protein) serves as a control. When the patient appears to be group AB, D-positive, it is necessary to set up a separate control. A drop of the patient's cell suspension with his own serum (autocontrol) or with 6–8% albumin makes a suitable control.

167.

D. Both the ABO grouping and Rh typing are in question. Since the transfusion need is urgent, group O, D-negative donor units should be selected initially for this young woman of child-bearing age. They should be transfused, if necessary, before the problem has been resolved or crossmatching performed. In some cases, the risk of withholding transfusion is far greater than the risk of a transfusion reaction in a patient with an unresolved antibody problem. The physician must sign an emergency release form indicating the clinical situation was such to warrant the release of blood.

168.

B. The patient most likely has a potent cold autoagglutinin. The antibody screening test and crossmatches with group O, D-negative donor units should be set up as soon as possible by prewarmed technique. In the past when Rh typing was primarily done with high-protein reagents, an Rh control, containing all the potentiating ingredients found in the Rh reagent except for the anti-D, was tested in parallel. The most likely cause of a positive Rh control with a high-protein reagent is a strongly positive DAT result. This would not be the cause in this case because monoclonal anti-D is a low-protein reagent. The usual cause of false-positive reactions with low-protein reagents is a potent cold autoagglutinin. A single wash may not remove all the antibody from the patient's red cells. The cells should be washed with warm saline; and if they are still autoagglutinated, antibody can be removed by 45 °C heat elution or treatment with a sulfhydryl reagent such as dithiothreitol (DTT), which destroys IgM antibodies. Since washed red cells were used for typing the patient's red cells, multiple myeloma could not be the cause of the false-positive, since the abnormal protein causing the pseudo-agglutination (rouleaux) would have been washed away.

169.

C. Although rigors and shock may be caused by hemolytic or anaphylactic reactions, bacterial sepsis is the most likely cause in this case. The sudden rise of the patient's temperature from normal to 40 °C or above is typical. Bacterial sepsis is an important cause of transfusion reactions, with about one-fourth of these reactions resulting in death.

170.

D. The incidence of bacterial sepsis is highest with platelet components. It is higher with pooled platelets than platelets collected by apheresis. Pooled platelets usually involve 6 or more donations from different donors, multiplying the chance of contamination. Most bacteria grow better at room temperature (the normal storage temperature for platelets) than refrigerator temperature. Sepsis from RBC is usually due to *Yersinia enterocolitica,* which grows well at refrigerator temperature.

171.

B. Donor centers routinely perform antibody screening tests during the processing of donor units from individuals who may have formed a clinically significant antibody, precluding the necessity for performing a minor crossmatch. A false-positive at the AHG phase of the minor crossmatch is caused by the patient's red cells having a positive DAT. Although donor antibodies, which become diluted

in the patient's circulation, seldom cause hemolytic transfusion reactions if the corresponding antigens are on the patient's red cells, decreased cell survival may occur.

172.

B. The reactions are most likely all caused by the cold autoagglutinin anti-I. The I antigen is not well developed on cord cells. Autoadsorption of the patient's serum with his/her own cells should not be performed following recent transfusion. Alloantibody may be adsorbed onto circulating donor red cells, resulting in false-negative reactions with repeat testing of the autoadsorbed serum and reagent red cells. The weak reactions at antiglobulin (AHG) phase of testing are most likely due to complement being bound at room temperature by the cold autoantibody reacting with the anti-C3d in polyspecific AHG reagent. A prewarmed technique, where the donor's cells and patient's serum are warmed separately to 37 °C before combining, is commonly used to eliminate interference from cold agglutinins. Many transfusion services use an anti-IgG reagent, instead of a polyspecific reagent that contains anti-IgG and anti-C3d, in order to avoid such problems, but the prewarmed crossmatch should eliminate complement from being bound. Since the patient was recently transfused, there is a slight possibility that the reactions at AHG could be caused by a high incidence alloantibody causing delayed hemolysis. Such an antibody would still react by prewarmed technique.

173–178.

(173:A, 174:A, 175:E, 176:D, 177:D, 178:C) The ABO group and Rh type must be determined by the blood-collecting facility with every donation. The unit must be labeled using the interpretation of current testing, not with previous donor records from repeat donors. When the immediate spin (IS) reaction of the donor red cells is positive with anti-D (with a negative Rh control), the unit may be labeled D-positive. If the red cells fail to agglutinate anti-D directly, the test must be incubated and converted to the indirect antiglobulin test to detect weak D phenotype. All units tested with anti-D that are IS negative but are found to be weak D must be labeled D-positive to avoid sensitizing an intended D-negative recipient to the D antigen. A direct antiglobulin test (DAT) should be performed as a control along with the weak D test. For the test to be valid the DAT must be negative.

If DAT-positive the weak D status cannot be interpreted because the donor's red cells are coated with antibody prior to the incubation with anti-D. DAT positive units of blood should be discarded. Two different test methods, a cell grouping and a serum grouping, must be used for ABO grouping; the results of these methods must be in agreement before a label is applied to the unit. Although testing the red cells with anti-A,B and testing the serum with A_2 red cells is not required, many collecting facilities incorporate these additional reagents to detect discrepancies due to subgroups of A or B. When the cell and serum groupings are not in agreement, additional testing to resolve the discrepancy is required. Weak or missing red-cell reactions with anti-A,B or anti-A, or both, accompanied by serum reactions with A_1 cells, but not A_2 cells, are an indication that the donor may be a subgroup of A with anti-A_1. Extended incubation of the cell grouping, testing with additional A_1 cells, A_2 cells and anti-A_1 lectin, and adsorption/elution/titration/secretor studies are techniques used to resolve discrepancies due to subgroups. Donor units found to contain unexpected antibodies should be processed into RBC with small amounts of plasma. They should be labeled to indicate the antibody specificity. It is helpful to attach a tie tag with this information to the RBC. Transfusing large amounts of antibody containing plasma (such as anti-Fy^a) into a Fy(a+) recipient may cause decreased red cell survival and, therefore, is not used for individual transfusion to patients. Plasma from units with antibodies may be salvaged for reagent use or source plasma.

179–183.

(179:C, 180:C, 181:D, 182:D, 183:A) There are three parts to the factor VIII molecule: F VIII:C, F VIII:Ag, and F VIII:vW. Individuals manifesting the X-linked (gene carried on the X chromosome) disorder known as hemophilia A are deficient in F VIII:C. The clinical severity, resulting in hemorrhage either spontaneously or following trauma, depends upon the level of F VIII:C present. Deficiency in F VIII:vW is known as von Willebrand's disease. It is not X-linked and is the most common inherited coagulopathy. Deficiency in F VIII:vW results in impaired platelet adhesion and aggregation, leading to prolonged bleeding. Cryoprecipitate contains both F VIII:C and F VIII:vW and may be used for treatment of these disorders, although it is not the preferred treatment. F VIII

concentrates have become safer with improved viral inactivation processes, and some now have therapeutic amounts of F VIII:vW as well. Cryoprecipitate also contains an average of 250 mg of fibrinogen per unit, as well as Factor XIII and fibrinectin, and currently it is primarily used to treat hypofibrinogenemia. Although Factor V deficiency is rare, it can present severe manifestations leading to hemarthrosis. Treatment of choice is fresh-frozen plasma (FFP) because F V is a labile factor not found in cryoprecipitate. FFP can be used to correct the factor deficiencies found in liver disease (factors II, VII, IX, and X). Since all these are stable factors, the plasma need not be fresh even though FFP is commonly used. Platelet concentrates are used to correct thrombocytopenia following chemotherapy. Fresh whole blood is seldom available. Specific components are instead provided to give the patient exactly what is needed and conserve blood resources.

HEMOLYTIC DISEASE (HEMOLYTIC DISEASE OF THE NEWBORN, IMMUNE HEMOLYTIC ANEMIA)

184.

C. ABO testing, Rh testing (for weak D when applicable), and antibody screening should all be performed early in a pregnancy. Amniocentesis should be done only when clinically indicated. Furthermore, amniocentesis generally is not done before the third trimester although in recent years the procedure has been done as early as 14 weeks.

185.

C. The Lewis typings of a pregnant woman may appear to be Le(a−b−), even though the original typing may have been Le(a−b+). When women are pregnant they have an increased plasma volume and increased amount of lipoprotein in relation to red blood cell mass. Since Lewis antigens are adsorbed onto red cells and lipoprotein from plasma, the dilutional effect and greater lipoprotein mass would lead to less adsorption of Le^b onto red cells. After the pregnancy, the woman will return to her original type.

186.

A. Prenatal testing for all pregnant women should include ABO, Rh, and antibody screening to exclude the presence of antibodies with the potential for causing hemolytic disease of the newborn (HDN). The presence of an antibody does not indicate that the infant will be affected. Testing the red blood cells of the father, to determine whether the corresponding antigen is expressed and, if so, whether he is a homozygote or heterozygote, should indicate the probability for the presence of the antigen on infant cells. ABO-HDN is not predicted until postpartum when the blood type of the infant is determined.

187.

D. IgG is the only immunoglobulin that is transported across the placenta. It does not cross the placenta because of low molecular weight or simple diffusion, as evidenced by higher concentrations of antibody present in cord than in maternal serum. IgG molecules are actively transported via the Fc portion beginning in the second trimester. Therefore, potentially any IgG blood group antibody produced by the mother could cause hemolytic disease of the newborn (HDN), if the fetus possesses a well developed corresponding antigen. The disease varies widely in severity being dependent on multiple factors.

188.

A. Although the ABO system is most often implicated in fetomaternal incompatibilities, it very rarely causes clinical symptoms. ABO-HDN generally occurs in group O mothers who have group A or B children. Although Rh-HDN can be prevented, there is no prevention for ABO-HDN, and generally there is none needed since exchange transfusion is rarely necessary.

189.

C. When D+ red blood cells are sufficiently coated with antibody, leaving no or few remaining sites to react with D antiserum, the cells are referred to as having a "blocked D" and may react weakly or not at all with a low protein anti-D reagent. One may suspect this phenomenon, confirmed by elution of anti-D from the red cells, when the DAT is strongly positive. Enough antibody may be removed with a gentle heat elution (45 °C) to permit accurate D typing of the coated red cells.

190.

C. Given that all prenatal and neonatal testing is valid, one should consider an antibody against a low-incidence antigen. The low-incidence antigen

was of paternal origin, and it stimulated the mother to form an IgG antibody. To prove this theory, an eluate from the baby's cells should be tested with the father's cells. Also, the mother's serum and the baby's eluate could be tested with a panel of low-incidence antigens to identify the specificity of the antibody.

191.

D. An antibody panel performed on an eluate made from the baby's red blood cells is the most conclusive way to identify positively the antibody causing the positive DAT. This would be especially helpful in a case where the mother has several antibodies that could cause hemolytic disease of the newborn. However, RBC for transfusion in the neonatal period should be negative for any antigen corresponding to any IgG antibody that crossed the placenta.

192.

B. During the first few hours of life, the primary risk to a baby with hemolytic disease of the newborn is heart failure caused by severe anemia. After the first 24 hours, in which the anemia can be compensated, the highest risk to the infant comes from hyperbilirubinemia. Kernicterus, which is brought on by hyperbilirubinemia (generally >18 mg/dL of unconjugated bilirubin) in a full-term infant in the first days of life, can cause irreversible brain damage. Depending on the severity of the hyperbilirubinemia, one or more exchange transfusions may be needed.

193.

D. A positive DAT on the infant's red blood cells indicates that IgG antibody has crossed the placenta and coated the neonate's red cells. Identification of the antibody in the maternal serum and elution of the same antibody from the infant's red cells confirms the specificity of the offending antibody. In lieu of a maternal blood sample, the identity of the antibody may be confirmed by testing the infant's eluate and serum. The eluate contains the antibody(ies) responsible for the clinical HDN; the serum may contain additional maternal antibody(ies) directed against antigens absent on the infant's cells but present on the donor's cells. Blood compatible with both serum and eluate should be prepared for exchange transfusion.

194.

D. Providing blood of the baby's type is exactly what one does not want to do. This would defeat the purpose of the exchange transfusion. For example, if an infant was suffering from HDN due to an anti-D, by transfusing D-positive cells, these cells would be coated with anti-D and would have decreased survival.

195.

D. A mixed-field weak D test on maternal blood indicates the presence of D-positive baby cells circulating with the mother's D-negative cells, suggestive of a large fetomaternal hemorrhage. If a mother does demonstrate a positive weak D test when previously it was negative, a Kleihauer-Betke acid elution test should be done on the mother's red blood cells. This test is used to quantify the amount of the fetal blood that has entered the mother's circulation. The results of the test will determine how many vials of Rh immune globulin should be administered to the patient. One vial will protect against approximately 30 mL of fetal blood (or 15 mL of red cells) that have entered the mother's circulation. A more sensitive method to identify fetomaternal hemorrhage (FMH) than the test for weak D is the rosette test. A maternal red cell suspension is incubated with an anti-D of human source, allowing antibody to coat D+ fetal cells. D+ indicator cells are added which bind to the coated D+ cells forming rosettes. This is a qualitative test and must also be followed by a quantitative test.

196.

C. The most likely cause for the positive antibody screening test is the presence of a passively acquired anti-D. Since the mother received antepartum Rh immune globulin (RhIG), anti-D from that injection may still be present at delivery. Depending on how the RhIG was injected postpartum, the anti-D could already be present in the patient's serum. Since antepartum RhIG was given, it is unlikely that active immunization has occurred. Passively acquired anti-D rarely has an antiglobulin titer above 4 and should be entirely IgG. When in doubt about whether anti-D is passive or represents active immunization, it is always better to administer RhIG at the appropriate time. The crossmatches are compatible because D-negative RBC would have been chosen for transfusion.

197.

D. The Kleihauer-Betke acid elution stain is used to quantify the amount of fetal cells present in the maternal circulation postpartum to calculate the correct dose of RhIG to administer. Adult hemoglobin is soluble in acid buffer, whereas fetal hemoglobin is resistant to acid elution. A thin blood smear is subjected to acid elution, pH 3.2, then stained with erythrosin B and Harris hematoxylin. Normal adult cells appear as pale ghosts microscopically; fetal cells are bright pink. The number of fetal cells in 2000 maternal cells is calculated. The volume of fetal hemorrhage is calculated as follows:

$$\frac{\text{Number of fetal cells}}{\text{Number of maternal cells}} \times \frac{\text{maternal blood}}{\text{volume (estimate 5000 mL)}} = \text{fetal bleed}$$

This is equivalent to: Fetal cells expressed as a percentage of maternal cells × 50 = mL of fetal whole blood. One vial of a standard 300 μg dose protects the D-negative mother against sensitization to the D antigen for a 30 mL bleed. Therefore, the fetal hemorrhage volume is divided by 30 to determine the number of vials.

198.

B. Neither anti-P_1 nor anti-Le^a is likely to cause hemolytic disease of the newborn (HDN). They are almost exclusively IgM antibodies (cannot cross the placenta), and the corresponding antigens are not well developed on neonatal red blood cells. Both anti-K and anti-c are almost exclusively IgG antibodies and are capable of causing serious HDN. However, the K antigen has a much lower frequency (<10%) in the population than the c antigen (>80%), so the infant is much more likely to be c+.

199.

D. The Kleihauer-Betke acid elution stain is used to estimate the amount of fetal red blood cells present in the circulation of a D-negative mother postpartum. Failure to quantify the FMH may result in the administration of insufficient Rh immune globulin. Sensitization to the Rh antigen may occur, leading to HDN in subsequent pregnancies. The fetal bleed is calculated using the formula: KB% × 50 = milliliters fetal blood present or 1.3 × 50 = 65 mL.

200.

C. One standard dose of Rh immune globulin (300 μg) protects the mother from a 30 mL bleed. Because the precision of a Kleihauer-Betke stain is poor, a margin of safety is employed to prevent RhIG prophylaxis failure. The total bleed in milliliters is divided by the level of protection in one dose (30 mL). For decimals less than five, round down and add one dose (e.g., 2.3 rounds down to 2 + 1 dose = 3 vials total dose); for decimals five or greater, round up and add one dose (e.g., 2.6 rounds up to 3 + 1 dose = 4 vials total dose).

Example:

$$\frac{65 \text{ mL bleed}}{30 \text{ mL}} = 2.2; \text{ give 3 vials RhIG}$$

201.

B. Polyagglutination is a condition of an individual's red blood cells that causes them to be agglutinated by most adult human sera but not by their own. A distinguishing characteristic is that polyagglutinable cells are not agglutinated by cord serum. The antibodies that react with polyagglutinable cells are naturally occurring IgM antibodies that are not present at birth but develop in infants in the same manner as anti-A and anti-B. Polyagglutination is classified by testing the cells against a battery of lectins.

202.

A. The direct antiglobulin test (DAT) is the easiest and the quickest way to detect *in vivo* sensitization of red blood cells. The indirect antiglobulin test is used to detect *in vitro* sensitization of red blood cells and is most commonly used in antibody detection tests and crossmatching. Uses of the direct antiglobulin test include investigation of hemolytic disease of the newborn, autoimmune hemolytic anemia, transfusion reactions, and drug-induced sensitization of red blood cells.

203.

A. Cold hemagglutinin disease (CHD) with immune hemolysis often occurs in elderly patients. Warm autoimmune hemolytic anemia (WAIHA) causing immune hemolysis may be secondary to another clinical disease or idiopathic and occurs at any age. Reticulocytosis and splenomegaly are associated with increased removal of red blood cells from the circulation. Approximately 15–20% of patients on α-methyldopa therapy demonstrate a positive DAT, but less than 1% of the DAT+ individuals develop a hemolytic episode.

204.

D. Most antibodies in WAIHA have specificity directed toward the Rh blood group system antigens. Sometimes the antibody has a simple specificity; anti-e is the most common warm autoantibody of simple specificity. Usually the antibody has a broad specificity, reacting with blood cells of most Rh phenotypes except for rare phenotypes such as Rh$_{null}$. In addition, there are mimicking or relative specificities—for example, an apparent auto anti-e that can be adsorbed onto e-negative red cells.

205.

C. Although it is best to avoid transfusing patients with warm autoantibodies, life-threatening anemia may develop, which necessitates them to receive blood. The primary concern in patients demonstrating serum warm autoantibody is to detect and identify the presence of underlying alloantibodies that may be masked by the reactions of the autoantibody. One must be certain to differentiate between auto- and alloantibodies. If the autoantibody appears to have a simple specificity such as anti-e, alloantibody identification can be accomplished by testing reagent red cells that are e-negative and antigen positive for the alloantibodies to be excluded. Alternatively, when sufficient e-negative panel cells are not available to do a thorough rule out, autoadsorption of the serum with the untransfused patient's red cells will remove autoantibody but not alloantibody.

206.

A. Autoantibodies are directed against antigens present on the patient's own red blood cells. The easiest way to determine whether the anti-e is auto or allo when the patient has not been recently transfused is to type the patient's red cells with a low-protein anti-e reagent. A high-protein reagent should not be used, since a false positive reaction is likely to occur. The preparation of an eluate when patients have no history of recent transfusion is not necessary; it is presumed that the eluate contains only autoantibody.

207.

C. When a patient has been recently transfused, a positive DAT may indicate the presence of clinically significant alloantibody attached to circulating donor's cells. A positive DAT may also reflect autoantibody attached to patient's or donor's cells, either because of drug sensitivity or secondary to clinical disease which is less likely in this case. It is important to obtain information including diagnosis, clinical condition, medication history, and laboratory data such as hematocrit, bilirubin, haptoglobin and reticulocyte count, both pre- and posttransfusion to determine whether a delayed hemolytic transfusion reaction (DHTR) has occurred. A DHTR commonly demonstrates a mixed-field DAT result.

208.

A. Cold hemagglutinin disease (CHD) is characterized by IgM antibodies, usually anti-I but occasionally anti-Pr. The Pr antigen is a high-frequency antigen that is destroyed by enzymes, whereas the reaction between anti-I and the I antigen is enhanced by enzyme treatment. Anti-I and anti-i are differentiated by titrating the serum against adult I cells and cord cells. The anti-I will have a higher titer against the adult cells, and the anti-i will have a higher titer against the cord cells.

209.

C. Paroxysmal cold hemoglobinuria (PCH) is the rarest form of cold autoimmune hemolytic anemia. It is characterized by an IgG antibody usually exhibiting anti-P specificity. A diagnostic test used to aid in the identification of PCH is the Donath-Landsteiner test. CHD is usually caused by anti-I, which is IgM.

210.

C. The Donath-Landsteiner (D-L) test is a diagnostic test for PCH. A characteristic of the antibody involved is that it will bind to red blood cells at cold temperatures; at 37 °C it will cause red blood cell lysis. In the D-L test a tube with the patient's serum and test cells is incubated at 4 °C while a control tube is incubated at 37 °C. After the 4 °C incubation the tube is placed in the 37 °C incubator. After incubation the tubes are centrifuged and examined for hemolysis. If there is hemolysis noted in the test and none in the control, the test is positive. If no hemolysis is noted in either tube,

the test is negative, and if hemolysis is present in both tubes, the test is invalid.

211.

C. Cephalosporin antibodies will generally *not* react with red blood cells unless they have been treated with the drug. The negative antibody screening test indicates that crossmatches will be similarly compatible. An eluate from the patient's red cells would be expected to be nonreactive as well. An eluate would not be prepared unless the patient had been recently transfused and a delayed hemolytic transfusion reaction (DHTR) was suspected.

212.

A. It is believed that anti-I found in the serum of patients with *Mycoplasma pneumoniae* infection is a response to an antigen on the organism that cross-reacts with the I antigen found almost universally on red cells; therefore, we would expect to find a positive autocontrol. Anti-Pr and anti-i are also cold autoagglutinins. Anti-i usually reacts well with cord cells but not adult cells, unless of extremely high titer, and is found in individuals with infectious mononucleosis. Cold autoagglutinins found in the serum of most people can be a nuisance when they interfere with serum testing for clinically significant alloantibodies. Prewarming the cells and serum at 37 °C before mixing and washing with 37 °C saline before the IAT reading may eliminate interference. If the patient has not been recently transfused, the serum may alternatively be adsorbed with autologous red cells at 4 °C to remove cold autoantibody. Pretreating autologous cells with enzymes may result in more efficient removal of the autoantibody unless the autoantibody is anti-Pr.

213.

A. The drug α-methyldopa, a blood pressure medication that is no longer frequently used, induces autoantibody formation that is indistinguishable from antibody produced in WAIHA. The antibody produced usually reacts with all panel cells tested. Some of the other drugs that induce autoantibody formation are L-dopa, procainamide, and some nonsteroidal anti-inflammatory drugs.

214.

C. Of the drugs listed only penicillin has the observed DAT profile. IgG alone is also generally seen when α-methyldopa and cephalosporins are the implicated drugs. When phenacetin, quinidine, and tolmetin are the drugs in question, only C3 (complement) is usually detected on the patient's red cells.

215.

D. Although the cold autoagglutinin is generally IgM, complement is usually the only protein detected on the red blood cells. The IgM antibody binds complement at lower temperatures in the extremities (such as fingers exposed to cold temperatures) and then dissociates when the red cells circulate. The polyspecific AHG is not required to have anti-IgM but must have anti-IgG and anti-C3d.

216.

C. Antibody directed against drugs may be suspected if patients present a positive DAT with a nonproductive eluate. The eluate and serum antibody may demonstrate reactivity only with reagent red cells coated with the appropriate drug and not with uncoated red cells. A current medication history and demonstration of eluate reactivity against the appropriate drug-coated red cells confirms the cause of the positive DAT. Drug-related antibodies are seldom clinically significant, and elaborate testing usually is not performed unless the patient shows symptoms of active hemolysis.

217.

D. Autoantibody(ies) directed against self-antigens may attach to a patient's own red blood cells *in vivo,* resulting in a positive DAT. A variety of elution techniques can remove this antibody from the red cells for testing. When a patient has not been transfused recently (within 3 to 4 months), it may be presumed that autoantibody only is present in the eluate. If recently transfused, donor's cells may be present in the patient's circulation. Alloantibody may be attached to donor cells, and autoantibody may be attached to patient's or donor's cells. When this is the case, alloantibody and autoantibody both could be recovered in the eluate.

218.

C. If the autoantibody has a high binding constant, the patient's plasma may not appear to contain free antibody. About 50% of patients with WAIHA will have autoantibody detectable by saline antiglobulin technique. If the test cells are enzyme-treated

or certain enhancement techniques are used, as many as 90% of the patients will demonstrate free autoantibody.

219–226.

(219:B, 220:D, 221:B, 222:B, 223:B, 224:B, 225:A, 226:C)

Mothers who are not candidates to receive Rh immune globulin (RhIG) are (1) D-positive, (2) D-negative delivering a D-negative infant, or (3) D-negative who have produced alloanti-D. For purposes of determining RhIG candidacy, the weak D phenotype is considered to be D-positive. If the mother is D-negative and has not made anti-D, she must receive RhIG when delivering a D-positive or weak D phenotype infant. When only one of the infants in a multiple birth is D-positive and the other(s) is (are) D-negative, the mother is a candidate for RhIG. The presence of antibodies other than anti-D in the pre- or postpartum serum does not preclude a D-negative woman from receiving RhIG. When the infant's red cells are DAT+, it may be difficult to determine the correct Rh status. Since RhIG is a low risk product, experts recommend a fail-safe approach and give RhIG when in doubt. Most obstetricians routinely inject RhIG at 28 weeks antenatally to prevent sensitization during a third-trimester fetal bleed. This injected anti-D is sometimes detectable postpartum and does not preclude additional administration of RhIG at delivery. Whenever doubt exists as to the weak D status of the infant or the origin of the anti-D postpartum, RhIG should be administered. The preferred method, which is more sensitive than a microscopic weak D test for determining fetomaternal hemorrhage (FMH), is the rosette test, which will detect FMH of >10 mL. A positive test would show one or more rosettes per field when an enhancing medium is used. Additional testing must be performed to quantify the amount of FMH to prevent sensitization to the D antigen. The Kleihauer-Betke acid elution stain is the standard technique available to determine whether a bleed of more than 15 mL red cells (30 mL whole blood) occurred, necessitating additional 300 μg doses beyond the standard 1-vial dose. Other methods include the enzyme-linked antiglobulin test (ELAT) and flow cytometry. The 50 μg dose of RhIG is used only when a female of 12-weeks gestation or less suffers a miscarriage. It is not intended for administration postpartum or for injection antenatally, either at 28 weeks or after amniocentesis.

answers & rationale

REFERENCES

Harmening, D. M. (1999). *Modern Blood Banking and Transfusion Practices,* 4th ed. Philadelphia: F. A. Davis.

Menitove, J. (Ed.) (2000). *Standards for Blood Banks and Transfusion Services,* 20th ed. Bethesda, MD: American Association of Blood Banks.

Mollison, P. L., Engelfield, C. P., and Contreras, M. (1997). *Blood Transfusion in Clinical Medicine,* 10th ed. Malden, MA: Blackwell Science.

Quinley, E. D. (1998). *Immunohematology-Principles and Practice,* 2nd ed. Philadelphia: Lippincott-Raven.

Vengelen-Tyler, V. (Ed.) (1999). *Technical Manual,* 13th ed. Bethesda, MD: American Association of Blood Banks.

6 Microbiology

contents

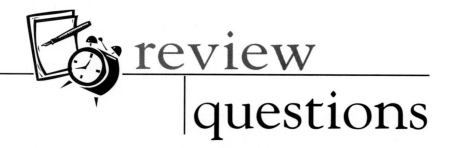

review questions

INSTRUCTIONS Each of the questions or incomplete statements that follow comprises four suggested responses. Select the *best* answer or completion statement in each case.

AEROBIC BACTERIA

1. In suspected cases of brucellosis the optimal specimen to be collected for the isolation of the etiologic agent is
   A. Blood
   B. Nasopharyngeal exudates
   C. Transtracheal aspirate
   D. Cerebrospinal fluid

2. The vast majority of clinical isolates of *Klebsiella* are
   A. *K. ozaenae*
   B. *K. pneumoniae*
   C. *K. aerogenes*
   D. *K. oxytoca*

3. Organisms that have a cell wall containing large amounts of lipid material belong to the genus
   A. *Chlamydia*
   B. *Mycobacterium*
   C. *Mycoplasma*
   D. *Leptospira*

4. The enterotoxins of both *Vibrio cholerae* O1 and noninvasive (toxigenic) strains of *Escherichia coli* produce serious diarrhea by what mechanism?

   A. Stimulation of adenylate cyclase, which gives rise to excessive fluid secretion by the cells of the small intestine
   B. Penetration of the bowel mucosa
   C. Stimulation of colicin production
   D. The elaboration of a dermonecrotizing toxin

5. *Chlamydia trachomatis* causes which of the following?
   A. Trachoma, a major cause of preventable blindness in the world
   B. Zoonosis in birds and the cause of parrot fever in humans
   C. A skin disease found predominantly in tropical areas
   D. Rat-bite fever

6. Colonies of *Neisseria* sp. turn color when a redox dye is applied. The color change is indicative of the activity of the bacterial enzyme
   A. Beta-galactosidase
   B. Urease
   C. Cytochrome oxidase
   D. Phenylalanine deaminase

7. A test for the hydrolysis of esculin in the presence of bile is especially useful in identifying species of the genus

A. *Haemophilus*

B. *Enterococcus*

C. *Brucella*

D. *Staphylococcus*

8. The species of *Mycobacterium* that would be most commonly associated with contamination of the hot water system in large institutions such as hospitals is

A. *M. xenopi*

B. *M. ulcerans*

C. *M. marinum*

D. *M. haemophilum*

9. All the following statements about *Shigella sonnei* are true *except*

A. Large numbers of organisms must be ingested to produce disease

B. The organism produces an inflammatory condition in the large intestine with bloody diarrhea

C. The organism produces disease most commonly in the pediatric population

D. The organism tolerates an acid environment

10. An environmental sampling study of respiratory therapy equipment produced cultures of a yellow, nonfermentative, gram-negative bacillus from several of the nebulizers, which would most likely be species of

A. *Chryseobacterium*

B. *Alcaligenes*

C. *Pseudomonas*

D. *Moraxella*

11. Which one of the following microorganisms cannot be cultivated on artificial cell-free media?

A. *Francisella tularensis*

B. *Helicobacter pylori*

C. *Actinobacillus lignieresii*

D. *Mycobacterium leprae*

12. *Mycobacterium fortuitum,* a rapid-growing *Mycobacterium,* grows on MacConkey agar in 5 days. Which other species of *Mycobacterium* is able to demonstrate growth within the same time period on MacConkey agar?

A. *M. chelonei*

B. *M. tuberculosis*

C. *M. bovis*

D. *M. kansasii*

13. The characteristics of being lactose negative, citrate negative, urease negative, lysine decarboxylase negative, and non-motile best describe which organism?

A. *Proteus vulgaris*

B. *Yersinia pestis*

C. *Aeromonas hydrophila*

D. *Shigella dysenteriae*

14. The organism associated with a disease characterized by the presence of a pseudomembrane in the throat and the production of an exotoxin that is absorbed into the system with a lethal effect is

A. *Clostridium difficile*

B. *Vibrio cholerae*

C. *Staphylococcus aureus*

D. *Corynebacterium diphtheriae*

15. Enterotoxin produced by *Staphylococcus aureus* is responsible for causing

A. Carbuncles

B. Enterocolitis

C. Scalded skin syndrome

D. Toxic shock syndrome

16. A fermentative gram-negative bacillus that is oxidase positive, motile, grows well on MacConkey agar is

A. *Aeromonas hydrophila*

B. *Pseudomonas aeruginosa*

C. *Xanthomonas maltophilia*

D. *Yersinia enterocolitica*

17. Fecal cultures are inoculated on thiosulfate citrate bile salts sucrose agar specifically for the isolation of
    A. *Shigella* species
    B. *Vibrio* species
    C. *Campylobacter* species
    D. *Salmonella* species

18. The K antigen of the family *Enterobacteriaceae* are
    A. The somatic antigens
    B. Heat labile
    C. The antigens used to group *Shigella*
    D. Located on the flagellum

19. The etiologic agent of primary atypical pneumonia is
    A. *Chlamydia psittaci*
    B. *Streptococcus pneumoniae*
    C. *Corynebacterium diphtheriae*
    D. *Mycoplasma pneumoniae*

20. *Abiotrophia* formerly known as nutritionally variant streptococci (NVS) will not grow on routine blood or chocolate agars because they are deficient in
    A. Vitamin B_{12}
    B. Pyridoxal
    C. Hemin
    D. Thiophene-2-carboxylic hydrazide

21. Exfoliatin produced by *Staphylococcus aureus* is responsible for causing
    A. Toxic shock syndrome
    B. Enterocolitis
    C. Scalded skin syndrome
    D. Staphylococcal pneumonia

22. A slow-growing, orange-pigmented, acid-fast bacillus was isolated from a cervical lymph node of a child with symptoms of cervical adenitis. The most likely etiologic agent in this case would be

    A. *Mycobacterium avium-intracellulare*
    B. *Mycobacterium fortuitum*
    C. *Mycobacterium scrofulaceum*
    D. *Mycobacterium chelonei*

23. The classic presumptive test for the identification of respiratory disease caused by *Mycoplasma pneumoniae* is the
    A. Cold agglutinin test
    B. Weil-Felix test
    C. ASO test
    D. Capsular swelling test

24. *Streptococcus pyogenes* (group A) organisms are best presumptively identified using
    A. Bacitracin disk
    B. ONPG disk
    C. PYR disk
    D. Optochin disk

25. The causative agent of melioidosis is
    A. *Burkholderia cepacia*
    B. *Burkholderia pseudomallei*
    C. *Moraxella catarrhalis*
    D. *Stenotrophomonas maltophilia*

26. Which microorganism will grow only on a culture media that has been supplemented with either cysteine or cystine?
    A. *Bartonella bacilliformis*
    B. *Kingella kingae*
    C. *Actinobacillus lignieresii*
    D. *Francisella tularensis*

27. A gram-positive coccus that is catalase positive, nonmotile, lysostaphin resistant, bacitracin sensitive, furazolidine resistant, and modified oxidase positive is best identified as a member of the genus
    A. *Micrococcus*
    B. *Lactococcus*
    C. *Veillonella*
    D. *Staphylococcus*

28. The identification of *Mycobacterium malmoense* and *Mycobacterium szulgai* has been aided by the use of thin-layer chromatography, which profiles their characteristic _____ extracted from their cell walls.
    A. Mucopolysaccharides
    B. Teichoic acid
    C. Lipids
    D. Lipopolysaccharides

29. A culture of a decubitus ulcer grew a gram-negative facultative bacillus. On TSI it produced an acid slant, acid butt, and gas from glucose fermentation. Test reactions in other media were as follows:

Citrate	negative
Indole	positive
Urease	negative
ONPG	positive
Voges-Proskauer	negative

    The organism was identified as
    A. *Enterobacter cloacae*
    B. *Escherichia coli*
    C. *Citrobacter (diversus) koseri*
    D. *Providencia stuartii*

30. An example of an oxidase-positive, glucose nonfermenting organism is
    A. *Enterobacter* sp.
    B. *Escherichia coli*
    C. *Klebsiella* sp.
    D. *Pseudomonas aeruginosa*

31. A fastidious gram-negative bacillus was isolated from a case of periodontal disease, which upon dark-field examination was noted to have a gliding motility. The most likely identification of this etiologic agent would be
    A. *Capnocytophaga*
    B. *Kingella*

C. *Plesiomonas*
D. *Chromobacterium*

32. The species of *Vibrio* closely associated with rapidly progressing wound infections seen in patients with underlying liver disease is
    A. *Vibrio alginolyticus*
    B. *Vibrio cholerae*
    C. *Vibrio vulnificus*
    D. *Vibrio parahaemolyticus*

33. Severe disseminated intravascular coagulation often complicates cases of
    A. Pneumococcemia
    B. Gonococcemia
    C. Streptococcemia
    D. Meningococcemia

34. The recommended culture medium for the recovery of *Chlamydia* from clinical specimens is
    A. McCoy cells
    B. Charcoal yeast extract medium
    C. Fletcher semisolid media
    D. WI–38 cells

35. *Chlamydia psittaci* infections in humans most commonly result after exposure to infected
    A. Mammalian species
    B. Arthropod species
    C. Amphibian species
    D. Avian species

36. *Nocardia asteroides* infections in humans characteristically produce
    A. Draining cutaneous sinuses
    B. Carbuncles
    C. Septic shock
    D. Serous effusions

37. The predominant serotype of *Haemophilus influenzae* implicated in meningeal infection is
    A. Serotype a
    B. Serotype b
    C. Serotype c
    D. Serotype d

38. *Erysipelothrix* infections in humans characteristically produce
    A. Pathology at the point of entrance of the organism
    B. Central nervous system pathology
    C. The formation of abscesses in visceral organs
    D. Pathology in the lower respiratory tract

39. The potentially lethal intoxication type of food poisoning associated with improperly canned food is caused by
    A. *Bacillus cereus*
    B. *Clostridium botulinum*
    C. *Clostridium perfringens*
    D. *Staphylococcus aureus*

40. When clinical specimens are being processed for the recovery of *Mycobacterium tuberculosis,* the generally recommended method for digestion and decontamination of the sample is
    A. 6% NaOH
    B. HCl
    C. NALC-NaOH
    D. TSP

41. *Salmonella typhi* exhibits a characteristic biochemical activity pattern, which differentiates it from the typical *Salmonellae* reactions. All the following reactions are produced by *S. typhi, except*
    A. Large amounts of H$_2$S are produced in TSI agar
    B. Anaerogenic
    C. Citrate negative
    D. Agglutination in Vi grouping serum

42. In the CAMP test a single streak of a beta-hemolytic streptococcus is placed perpendicular to a streak of beta-lysin-producing *Staphylococcus aureus*. After incubation a zone of increased lysis in the shape of an arrowhead is noted, which indicates the presumptive identification of
    A. *S. bovis*
    B. *S. agalactiae*
    C. *S. pyogenes*
    D. *S. equinus*

43. Direct molecular detection using a DNA probe is clinically useful for the detection of slow-growing microorganisms such as
    A. *Capnocytophaga gingivalis*
    B. *Eikenella corrodens*
    C. *Staphylococcus aureus*
    D. *Mycobacterium tuberculosis*

44. *Staphylococcus saprophyticus*, a recognized pathogen of young females, is a cause of
    A. Impetigo
    B. Urinary tract infections
    C. Furuncles
    D. Otitis media

45. The sexually acquired disease characterized by genital ulcers and tender inguinal lymphadenopathy, which is caused by a small, gram-negative bacillus, is known as
    A. Chancroid
    B. Lymphogranuloma venereum
    C. Trachoma
    D. Granuloma inguinale

46. Color Plate 26 shows the Gram stain of a blood culture on a 23-year-old pregnant woman who presented with fever and flulike symptoms in her ninth month. The isolate on blood agar produced small, translucent beta hemolytic colonies, which were catalase positive and motile. Which of the following is the most likely etiologic agent in this case?

A. *Propionibacterium acnes*

B. *Listeria monocytogenes*

C. *Haemophilus influenzae*

D. *Escherichia coli*

47. A purulent aspirate of joint fluid from a 40-year-old female seen in the arthritis clinic was sent for microbiologic examination. The Gram stain of this sample revealed many polymorphonuclear cells with intracellular and extracellular gram-negative diplococci. Given the specimen type and microscopic findings, the appropriate selective medium for primary isolation would be

A. Mannitol salt agar

B. Potassium tellurite agar

C. Thayer-Martin agar

D. Cary-Blair agar

48. The etiologic agent of Hansen's disease is

A. *Mycobacterium bovis*

B. *Mycobacterium tuberculosis*

C. *Mycobacterium leprae*

D. *Mycobacterium fortuitum*

49. *Campylobacter* species are associated most frequently with cases of

A. Osteomyelitis

B. Gastroenteritis

C. Endocarditis

D. Appendicitis

50. The etiologic agent commonly associated with septicemia and meningitis of newborns is

A. *Streptococcus pyogenes*

B. *Streptococcus pneumoniae*

C. *Streptococcus agalactiae*

D. *Streptococcus bovis*

51. An organism frequently misidentified as an enteric pathogen because it produces a large amount of H_2S is

A. *Shewanella putrefaciens*

B. *Pseudomonas putida*

C. *Burkholderia cepacia*

D. *Burkholderia pseudomallei*

52. *Arizona* isolates formerly were considered a separate genus. These organisms, because of their characteristics, are now considered members of the genus

A. *Tatumella*

B. *Citrobacter*

C. *Salmonella*

D. *Cedecea*

53. Which of the following is the most commonly isolated species of *Bacillus* in opportunistic infections such as bacteremia, post-traumatic infections of the eye, and endocarditis?

A. *B. subtilis*

B. *B. licheniformis*

C. *B. cereus*

D. *B. circulans*

54. The etiologic agent of whooping cough is

A. *Brucella suis*

B. *Haemophilus ducreyi*

C. *Francisella tularensis*

D. *Bordetella pertussis*

55. Loeffler's serum medium is recommended for the cultivation of

A. *Haemophilus ducreyi*

B. *Bordetella pertussis*

C. *Campylobacter jejuni*

D. *Corynebacterium diphtheriae*

56. Enriched media, such as blood cysteine glucose agar, are used for the isolation of

A. *Bordetella pertussis*

B. *Haemophilus ducreyi*

C. *Francisella tularensis*

D. *Pasteurella multocida*

57. An important characteristic of *Neisseria gonorrhoeae* or the infection it produces is:
    A. A Gram stain of the organism shows Gram-positive diplococci
    B. Asymptomatic infections are common in males
    C. Gonorrhea is a disease of humans and domestic animals
    D. Nonpiliated strains are avirulent

58. On Tinsdale agar, colonies of *Corynebacterium diphtheriae* are differentiated by the observance of
    A. Liquefaction of the agar surrounding the colonies present on the medium
    B. Opalescent colonies with a white precipitate in the surrounding agar
    C. Black colonies present on the culture medium, which are surrounded by brown halos
    D. Pitting of the agar medium surrounding the colonies that are present

59. Which of the following organisms would most likely produce the biochemical reactions shown in Color Plate 27?
    A. *Salmonella enteritidis*
    B. *Citrobacter freundii*
    C. *Proteus mirabilis*
    D. *Providencia rettgeri*

60. A gram-negative, "kidney bean" cellular morphology is a distinguishing characteristic of
    A. *Neisseria* species
    B. *Yersinia* species
    C. *Bartonella* species
    D. *Actinobacter* species

61. Precipitates of diphtheria toxin and anti-toxin formed in agar gels are an in vitro means for detecting toxigenic strains of *Corynebacterium diphtheriae*. The name of this test procedure is the

    A. Anton test
    B. Schlicter test
    C. Ascoli test
    D. Elek test

62. The etiologic agent of the disease erysipelas is
    A. *Bartonella bacilliformis*
    B. *Streptobacillus moniliformis*
    C. *Streptococcus pyogenes*
    D. *Erysipelothrix rhusiopathiae*

63. *Enterococcus* sp., when present, could most likely be recovered from a stool sample if the primary plating agars included a
    A. Phenylethyl alcohol plate
    B. Xylose lysine desoxycholate agar
    C. Thiosulfate citrate bile salts sucrose agar
    D. Bismuth sulfite

64. The finding of five to six acid-fast bacilli per field ($\times$ 800 to $\times$ 1000) in a fuchsin smear of expectorated sputum should be reported as
    A. Negative for acid-fast bacilli (AFB)
    B. Few AFB (2+)
    C. Many AFB (3+)
    D. Numerous AFB (4+)

65. Which of the following nonfermenters is rarely isolated in the U.S.?
    A. *Pseudomonas aeruginosa*
    B. *Stenotrophomonas maltophilia*
    C. *Burkholderia pseudomallei*
    D. *Burkholderia cepacia*

66. The most common normal flora organisms of the upper respiratory tract are
    A. *Lactobacillus* sp.
    B. *Staphylococcus aureus*
    C. *Propionibacterium* sp.
    D. Viridans streptococci

67. The most common manifestation of neonatal gonorrhea is

A. Conjunctivitis

B. Arthritis

C. Vulvovaginitis

D. Bacteremia

68. *Neisseria lactamica* closely resembles *Neisseria meningitidis* but can be differentiated from it by its ability to degrade

A. Maltose

B. Lactose

C. Glucose

D. Sucrose

69. A causative agent of the form of conjunctivitis known as pinkeye is

A. *Haemophilus influenzae* biotype III

B. *Moraxella lacunata*

C. *Chlamydia trachomatis*

D. *Listeria monocytogenes*

70. The single species in the genus *Hafnia* is

A. Tarda

B. Gergoviae

C. Ruckeri

D. Alvei

71. *Acinetobacter* species are similar to *Neisseriaceae* with the notable exception that they are

A. Gram-negative coccoid organisms

B. Grown on blood and chocolate agars

C. Oxidase negative

D. Glucose positive

72. *Legionella pneumophila* is the etiologic agent of both Legionnaires' disease and

A. Pontiac fever

B. Swine fever

C. Rift Valley fever

D. San Joaquin Valley fever

73. A species of *Brucella* that did not require increased carbon dioxide for growth and produced hydrogen sulfide was isolated from an abattoir worker. The dye inhibition test showed growth in the presence of thionine and fuchsin and the urease test was positive in 2 hours. The species identification made as a result of this information was

A. *B. canis*

B. *B. suis*

C. *B. ovis*

D. *B. melitensis*

74. Hemolytic uremic syndrome (HUS) is a complication after infection with:

A. *E. coli* O157: H7

B. *Shigella sonnei*

C. *Vibrio cholerae* O1

D. *Salmonella typhi*

75. Identify the fermentative agent that may infect reptiles or fish as well as humans when they are exposed to contaminated soil or water.

A. *Edwardsiella*

B. *Aeromonas*

C. *Chromobacterium*

D. *Chryseobacterium*

76. *Campylobacter jejuni* is:

A. Nonmotile

B. Microaerophilic

C. Oxidase negative

D. A straight gram negative bacillus

77. Streptococci obtain all their energy requirements from the fermentation of sugars to

A. Succinic acid

B. Formic acid

C. Lactic acid

D. Valeric acid

78. Streptococci are unable to protect themselves from the killing effects of H_2O_2 because they cannot synthesize the enzyme

A. Coagulase

B. Hyaluronidase

C. Lipase

D. Catalase

79. The beta hemolysis produced by streptococci that is seen on the surface of a blood agar plate is primarily the result of streptolysin
A. O
B. H
C. S
D. M

80. Which of the following has a negative oxidase test?
A. *Aeromonas*
B. *Hafnia*
C. *Vibrio*
D. *Pseudomonas*

81. Dental caries are particularly associated with a bacterial infection containing
A. *Staphylococcus saprophyticus*
B. *Streptococcus agalactiae*
C. *Moraxella (Branhamella) catarrhalis*
D. *Streptococcus mutans*

82. All the following are correct about *Neisseria gonorrhoeae, except*
A. Adversly affected by drying and fatty acids
B. No capsule on outer surface
C. Fastidious in growth requirement
D. Serotying exploits antigenic variation of Por proteins

83. All the following are true about gonorrhea *except*
A. Primary site of infection in males is urethra
B. Transmitted by sexual contact
C. Primary site of infection in females is cervix
D. Mediated penicillin resistance not seen

84. When a case of nocardiosis is suspected, isolates of *Nocardia asteroides* can be separated from other bacteria by

A. Cold shocking of the culture
B. Incubating the culture at greater than 37 °C
C. Drying the specimen before inoculating the culture media
D. Heat shocking the culture

85. A 21-year-old sexually active woman came to the university student health service with a 2-day history of urinary frequency with urgency dysuria and evidence of blood. She had no history of prior urinary tract infection. Laboratory test showed a slightly elevated white blood cell count of 10,500/μl. The urine sediment contained innumerable white cells, suggestive of urinary tract infection. Cultures yielded more than 10^5 colony-forming units of a lactose fermenting gram-negative rod. The most likely etiologic agent in this case is
A. *Proteus mirabilis*
B. *Klebsiella pneumoniae*
C. *Escherichia coli*
D. *Morganella morganii*

86. The method of typing *Klebsiella* most commonly used in the clinical laboratory is based on
A. O antigens
B. Bacteriocins
C. H antigens
D. K antigens

87. The symptom of diffuse, watery diarrhea that produces a relatively clear stool containing mucus flecks (rice water stool) is most closely associated with an infection caused by
A. *Escherichia coli*
B. *Shigella dysenteriae*
C. *Vibrio cholerae*
D. *Yersinia enterocolitica*

88. An example of a halophilic microorganism would be
    A. *Vibrio parahaemolyticus*
    B. *Yersinia pestis*
    C. *Escherichia coli*
    D. *Morganella morganii*

89. All the following statements about *Brucella* are true *except*
    A. Infection may occur via abrasions of the oral mucosa, conjunctiva, and genitals
    B. Thiamine, niacin, and biotin are required for growth
    C. The risk of accidental laboratory infection is no greater than with any other organism
    D. Phage and dye sensitivity test are used for identification to the species level

90. Infection of the gastric mucosa leading to gastritis or peptic ulcers is most commonly associated with
    A. *Helicobacter pylori*
    B. *Salmonella typhi*
    C. *Campylobacter jejuni*
    D. *Shigella sonnei*

91. Mycobacteria can be examined by using the
    A. Dieterle stain
    B. Gimenez stain
    C. Albert stain
    D. Kinyoun stain

92. All the following describe *Acinetobacter* sp. *except*
    A. Commonly susceptible to most antimicrobials
    B. Generally coccobacillary in morphology
    C. Oxidase negative
    D. Infections associated with use of medical devices

93. Explosive watery diarrhea with severe abdominal pain, after eating raw shellfish is most characteristic of infection caused by
    A. *Helicobacter pylori*
    B. *Vibrio parahemolyticus*
    C. *Shigella dysenteri*
    D. *Campylobacter jejuni*

94. The production of H_2S is one characteristic used to differentiate which of the aerobic gram-positive bacilli?
    A. *Corynebacterium*
    B. *Lactobacillus*
    C. *Erysipelothrix*
    D. *Nocardia*

95. Identify the motile, oxidase- and nitrate-positive, gram-negative bacillus that was isolated from a case of endocarditis following the implantation of a prosthetic heart valve. Related species have long been recognized as plant pathogens.
    A. *Erwinia carotivorum*
    B. *Agrobacterium radiobacter*
    C. *Mycobacterium terrae*
    D. *Sphingobacterium mizutaii*

96. An unheated suspension of *Salmonella typhi* typically produces agglutination of Vi antisera. After heating the same suspension, agglutination will occur in which grouping sera?
    A. A
    B. B
    C. C_1
    D. D

97. Growth in a 48-hour gelatin stab culture that shows lateral filamentous growth resembling a test tube brush is most characteristic of which organism?
    A. *Streptobacillus moniliformis*
    B. *Legionella pneumophila*
    C. *Erysipelothrix rhusiopathiae*
    D. *Plesiomonas shigelloides*

98. The species of *Campylobacter* noted to produce septicemia, septic arthritis, meningitis, jaundice with hepatomegaly, and thrombophlebitis in debilitated patients is
    A. *C. sputorum* bv. *sputorum*
    B. *C. fetus* ssp. *fetus*
    C. *C. fetus* ssp. *venerealis*
    D. *C. gracilis*

99. A clinical problem has emerged concerning infections after prosthetic heart valve insertion or other cardiac procedures with methicillin-resistant strains of
    A. *Staphylococcus epidermidis*
    B. *Serratia marcescens*
    C. *Streptococcus salivarius*
    D. *Enterococcus faecalis*

100. The former species of *Corynebacterium* that is a pathogen of swine, horses, and cattle is also known to cause disease in compromised hosts. This organism when grown on culture media produces pale pink colonies that help to presumptively identify it as
    A. *Gardnerella vaginalis*
    B. *Actinomyces naeslundii*
    C. *Aracnobacterium hemolyticum*
    D. *Rhodococcus equi*

101. *Shigella sonnei* is differentiated from the other species by
    A. Its ability to ferment lactose
    B. Its positive phenylalanine deaminase reaction
    C. Its negative oxidase reaction
    D. Its ability to demonstrate motility at 42 °C

102. A negative methyl red reaction is characteristic of
    A. *Escherichia coli*
    B. *Enterobacter aerogenes*
    C. *Proteus vulgaris*
    D. *Providencia rettgeri*

103. Which of the following is not true regarding virulent strains of *Vibrio cholerae?*
    A. Toxigenic
    B. Colonize the large intestine
    C. Adherent
    D. Motile

104. The classic toxigenic strains of which serogroup are implicated in epidemic infections of *Vibrio cholerae?*
    A. O1
    B. O2
    C. O3
    D. O4

105. Which one of the following is not appropriate when describing *Streptococcus pneumoniae?*
    A. Lancet-shaped, gram-positive diplococcus
    B. Bile-resistant
    C. Alpha hemolytic
    D. Encapsulated, with an antiphagocytic polysaccharide capsule

106. Which of the following is not characteristic of the genus *Mycobacterium?*
    A. Obligate aerobes
    B. Slow growing
    C. Transmission usually by the respiratory route
    D. High peptidoglycan content in the cell wall

107. Which of the following would be appropriate when discussing *Haemophilus influenzae?*
    A. The etiologic agent of influenza
    B. Most infections caused by capsular serotype b
    C. Always sensitive to ampicillin
    D. Common cause of bacterial pneumonia

108. *Nocardia* can be differentiated from *Actinomyces* based on

A. *Nocardia* being an obligate anaerobe

B. The partial-acid fast staining reaction of *Actinomyces*

C. The production of sulfur granules in cases of nocardiosis

D. *Nocardia* being catalase positive

109. *Enterococcus faecium* is characteristically

A. Inhibited by the presence of bile in the culture media

B. Able to grow in the presence of high concentrations of salt

C. PYR negative

D. Sensitive to penicillin G

110. *Brucella* species are

A. The etiologic agents of relapsing fever

B. Small spiral organisms

C. Primarily a cause of endogenous human infections

D. Intracellular pathogens

111. A urine specimen from a maternity patient with the complaint of cystitis was received in the laboratory. The culture of this sample grew a lactose-positive, gram-negative bacillus that was presumptively identified as *Escherichia coli*. On differential and selective media this organism would demonstrate which reaction?

A. MacConkey agar-colorless colonies

B. Hektoen enteric agar-green colonies with black centers

C. Eosin methylene blue agar-dark colonies with a metallic sheen

D. Xylose lysine desoxycholate agar-colorless colonies

112. A negative PYR (l-pyrolidonyl-B-naphthylamide) test is demonstrated by

A. *Viridans streptococci*

B. *Enterococcus faecalis*

C. *Lactococcus garviae*

D. *Streptococcus pyogenes*

113. *Yersinia pestis* is characteristically

A. Urease negative

B. Hydrogen sulfide positive

C. Motile at 20–25 °C

D. Oxidase positive

114. A sputum specimen from a suspected case of lobar pneumonia patient shows on Gram stain the presence of many WBCs and many gram-positive cocci, which are primarily in diplococci. Which of the following statements would be appropriate, given these findings on a smear?

A. A PYR test should be performed on the culture isolate

B. An ELEK test should be performed on the culture isolate

C. A CAMP test should be performed on the culture isolate

D. An optochin test should be performed on the culture isolate

115. Lack of motility is characteristic of

A. *Tatumella ptyseos*

B. *Morganella morganii*

C. *Kluyvera ascorbata*

D. *Cedacea davisae*

116. In cases of legionellosis

A. Penicillin has proven to be an effective treatment

B. Person-to-person transmission is common

C. There are two clinical forms: acute pneumonia and a self-limited, nonpneumonic febrile illness

D. Specimens may be cold enriched to enhance recovery of the organism

117. *Calymmatobacterium granulomatis* is

A. Resistant to ampicillin and tetracycline

B. Grown easily on blood agar

C. The causative agent of granuloma inguinale

D. A gram-positive organism

118. Select from the following mycobacteria the one that has as its optimal growth temperature 30–32 °C
    A. *M. ulcerans*
    B. *M. bovis*
    C. *M. xenopi*
    D. *M. avium-intracellulare*

119. A pink zone on a DNase plate containing toluidine blue would be seen in 24 hours around colonies of
    A. *Enterococcus faecalis*
    B. *Serratia marcescens*
    C. *Escherichia coli*
    D. *Staphylococcus epidermidis*

120. A child presented in August at the pediatric clinic with a superficial skin infection of the hands. The large, itchy lesions were cultured, and the diagnosis of impetigo was made. One of the etiologic agents of this clinical condition is
    A. *Erysipelothrix rhusiopathiae*
    B. *Pasteurella multocida*
    C. *Staphylococcus saprophyticus*
    D. *Streptococcus pyogenes*

121. A 36-year-old man was seen in the emergency room. He complained of fever and headache. He had returned 1 week previously from a 6-week visit to a village in India. Among the differential diagnoses was typhoid fever. The most critical laboratory test necessary to establish or eliminate that diagnosis was:
    A. Blood cultures
    B. Sputum cultures
    C. Stool cultures
    D. Urine cultures

122. A negative citrate reaction is characteristic of
    A. *Klebsiella pneumoniae*
    B. *Enterobacter aerogenes*
    C. *Serratia marcescens*
    D. *Shigella dysenteriae*

123. Isolation of *Neisseria gonorrhoeae*
    A. Is enhanced by cold enrichment
    B. Requires incubation under increased CO_2
    C. From contaminated sites is made easier by the use of a selective medium such as CIN agar
    D. For susceptibility testing is made on nutrient agar devoid of blood

124. A positive indole reaction is characteristic of
    A. *Escherichia coli*
    B. *Proteus mirabilis*
    C. *Salmonella cholerae-suis*
    D. *Serratia marcescens*

125. Which one of the following drugs is not considered as primary antimycobacteria therapy?
    A. Rifampin
    B. Streptomycin
    C. Isoniazid
    D. Kanamycin

126. On TSI agar a gram-negative bacillus produced a yellow slant and a yellow butt. Select the organism from the list below that would produce this reaction.
    A. *Shigella sonnei*
    B. *Proteus mirabilis*
    C. *Escherichia coli*
    D. *Salmonella typhimurium*

127. An identifying characteristic of *Staphylococcus aureus* is
    A. DNase negative
    B. Negative mannitol fermentation reaction
    C. Growth inhibition in presence of increased salt
    D. Positive coagulase test

128. Pyocyanin is characteristically produced by
    A. *Xanthornonas maltophillia*
    B. *Pseudomonas fluorescens*
    C. *Shewanella putrefaciens*
    D. *Pseudomonas aeruginosa*

129. Which of the following organisms is able to hydrolyze sodium hippurate to benzoic acid and glycine?
    A. *Streptococcus agalactiae*
    B. *Enterococcus faecalis*
    C. *Streptococcus pneumoniae*
    D. *Listeria monocytogenes*

130. Color Plate 28 shows the Gram stain of cerebrospinal fluid (CSF) from a 6-month-old girl who became ill with fever and lethargy and was convulsing. Which of the following organisms should be presumptively identified as the causative agent based on your observations?
    A. *Neisseria meningitidis*
    B. *Haemophilus influenzae*
    C. *Streptococcus pneumoniae*
    D. *Listeria monocytogenes*

131. A positive CAMP reaction is produced by
    A. *Legionella pneumophila*
    B. *Streptococcus equi*
    C. *Helicobacter pyloris*
    D. *Streptococcus agalactiae*

132. Which of the following is a correct statement concerning *Campylobacter jejuni*?
    A. Isolated best at 24 °C
    B. A leading cause of bacterial diarrhea worldwide
    C. Hydrogen sulfide positive
    D. Catalase negative

133. Of the following microorganisms, which will turn a dark purple or black when tetramethyl-*p*-phenylenediamine hydrochloride is applied?

    A. *Francisella tularensis*
    B. *Moraxella (Branhamella) catarrhalis*
    C. *Yersinia enterocolitica*
    D. *Listeria monocytogenes*

134. *Cardiobacterium hominis*, an inhabitant of the upper respiratory tract of humans, has been recovered as the etiologic agent from cases of endocarditis. An identifying characteristic of the organism is
    A. Motility
    B. Positive catalase
    C. Positive oxidase
    D. Gram-positive bacillus

135. *Vibrio vulnificus* is a well-established human pathogen that is known to cause
    A. Pyelonephritis
    B. Gastroenteritis
    C. Pneumonia
    D. Wound infections

136. Which of the following gram-negative fermentative bacteria require special selective procedures for isolation?
    A. *Actinobacillus actinomycetemcomitans*
    B. *Francisella tularensis*
    C. *Cardiobacterium hominis*
    D. *Chromobacterium violaceum*

137. *Kluyvera* species do not produce a positive reaction for which of the following biochemical tests?
    A. Indole
    B. Citrate
    C. Oxidase
    D. Malonate

138. Which of the following organisms produce a positive phenylalanine deaminase reaction?
    A. *Kluyvera ascorbata*
    B. *Klebsiella pneumoniae*
    C. *Tatumella ptyseos*
    D. *Yersinia enterocolitica*

139. Which of the following is a true statement about *Tatumella ptyseos?*
    A. It is more active biochemically at room temperature than at 35–37 °C
    B. It is oxidase positive
    C. It is motile by means of peritrichous flagella
    D. It is phenylalanine negative

140. Which of the following non-lactose fermenting organisms is not able to produce fluorescein?
    A. *Pseudomonas fluorescens*
    B. *Pseudomonas putida*
    C. *Burkholderia pseudomallei*
    D. *Pseudomonas aeruginosa*

141. Which of the following properties of *Staphylococcus aureus* is not associated with virulence?
    A. Coagulase production
    B. Deoxyribonuclease production
    C. Hemolysin production
    D. Catalase production

142. Which of the following is *not* a characteristic of staphylococci that would help in its isolation and identification?
    A. High salt tolerance
    B. No growth at 40 °C
    C. Resistance to drying
    D. Resistance to bacteriostatic triphenyl methane dyes

143. Which of the following organisms is unable to grow on MacConkey agar?
    A. *Kingella denitrificans*
    B. *Bordetella bronchiseptica*
    C. *Plesiomonas shigelloides*
    D. *Acinetobacter anitratus*

144. All the following statements about *Haemophilus* sp. are true *except*

A. The preferred culture medium is sheep blood agar
B. Small, pleomorphic, gram-negative coccobacilli
C. Obligate parasites
D. Many are found as normal flora in the human respiratory tract

145. *Legionella pneumophila*
    A. Infections acquired from environmental sources
    B. Are biochemically active
    C. Most species are nonmotile
    D. Stains easily by the Gram stain technique

146. Which of the following is not true about *Coxiella burnetii?*
    A. Is an obligate intracellular parasite
    B. Is transmitted from animals to man by inhalation
    C. A rash appears first on the extremities then on the trunk
    D. Is the etiologic agent of Q fever, which may be acute or chronic

147. What is the optimal clinical specimen for the recovery of *Legionella pneumophilia?*
    A. Nasopharyngeal swab
    B. Blood
    C. Stool
    D. Bronchial washings

148. The recovery of *Brucella* from blood cultures is said to be enhanced by the use of
    A. Biphasic media
    B. Anaerobic media
    C. Broth-only media
    D. Selective and differential media

149. Which of the following is not a selective media for primary isolation of *Bordetella pertussis?*

A. Modified Skirrow's medium

B. Regan-Lowe

C. Bordet-Gengou

D. Modified Jones-Kendrick charcoal

150. Production of a yellow pigment is characteristic of which species of Enterobacter?

A. *E. taylorae*

B. *E. aerogenes*

C. *E. cloacae*

D. *E. sakazakii*

151. Which of the following is not considered a zoonotic disease?

A. Leptospirosis

B. Anthrax

C. Botulism

D. Erysipeloid

152. A gram-negative bacillus was recovered from the urine of a child with a history of recurrent urinary tract infections. The organism was oxidase negative, lactose negative, urease positive, and motile. The most likely identification of this agent would be

A. *Proteus mirabilis*

B. *Escherichia coli*

C. *Pseudomonas aeruginosa*

D. *Klebsiella pneumoniae*

153. *Acinetobacter baumanii* is characteristically

A. Sensitive to penicillin

B. Motile

C. Able to grow on MacConkey agar

D. Oxidase positive

154. Which of the following species formerly classified in the genera *Moraxella* has been reclassified as *Pyschrobacterium* sp.?

A. *M. osloensis*

B. *M. lacunata*

C. *M. phenylpyruvica*

D. *M. urethralis*

155. Which of the following bacterial agents may cause human skin infections following contact with infected tissue of cattle suffering with "woody tongue"?

A. *Bacillus anthracis*

B. *Actinobacillus lignieresii*

C. *Streptobacillus moniliformis*

D. *Capnocytophaga sputigena*

156. Which of the following is not characteristic of *Eikenella corrodens?*

A. It is found in the mouth and upper respiratory tract of man

B. Colonies pit the surface of the agar medium

C. It is usually found in pure culture when recovered from uncompromised patients

D. It is a thin, gram-negative bacillus

157. Which of the species of *Pasteurella* is associated with human infections?

A. *P. aerogenes*

B. *P. haemolytica*

C. *P. pneumotropica*

D. *P. multocida*

158. *Legionella* species are all catalase and urease positive. Which of the following is positive for hippurate hydrolysis?

A. *L. micdadei*

B. *L. longbeachae*

C. *L. gormanii*

D. *L. pneumophila*

159. *Haemophilus influenzae* biogroup *aegyptius*, which is associated with cases of acute conjunctivitis, is characterized by all the following reactions *except*

A. Indole negative

B. X factor negative

C. Ornithine negative

D. V factor positive

160. According to the American Thoracic Society's "Levels of Service for Mycobacterial Laboratories," which of the following may be performed by level II laboratories?
    A. May process specimens for culture on standard agar egg-base media
    B. May perform drug susceptibility studies against secondary antituberculous drugs
    C. May identify *Mycobacterium tuberculosis*
    D. May conduct research and provide training

161. *Kingella denitrificans* can be differentiated from *Neisseria gonorrhoeae* because it is
    A. Oxidase positive
    B. Able to grow on Thayer-Martin agar
    C. Glucose positive
    D. Able to reduce nitrates

162. Which of the following is a species of *Plesiomonas?*
    A. *P. shigelloides*
    B. *P. hydrophila*
    C. *P. sobria*
    D. *P. salmonicida*

163. Of the following statements, which is true in relation to *Cardiobacterium hominis?*
    A. Motile
    B. Oxidase negative
    C. Pleomorphic gram-positive bacillus
    D. Etiologic agent of endocarditis

164. Which of the following is a true statement about mycoplasmas?
    A. Resistant to penicillin
    B. Easily stained using the Gram method
    C. Grow on routine nonselective culture media
    D. Not able to survive extracellularly

165. A commercial vendor of povidone iodine, tincture of iodine prep pads, swabsticks, and other sterile products has voluntarily recalled all products in several lots manufactured over the past three years. Microbial contamination has been confirmed in some lots representing a potential public health hazard. The most likely organism to be isolated in this case would be:
    A. *Klebsiella pneumoniae*
    B. *Pseudomonas aeruginosa*
    C. *Streptococcus pyogenes*
    D. *Staphylococcus aureus*

166. Outbreaks of brucellosis associated with contaminated food are most commonly associated with eating
    A. Improperly cooked hamburger
    B. Raw shellfish
    C. Imported cheese
    D. Contaminated potato salad

167. Which of the following species of *Bacillus* is nonmotile?
    A. *B. cereus*
    B. *B. subtilis*
    C. *B. anthracis*
    D. *B. thuringiensis*

168. *Serratia* species are unique in the family *Enterobacteriaceae* because of their ability to produce extracellular hydrolytic enzymes. Which of the following is not produced by *Serratia* species?
    A. Gelatinase
    B. Lipase
    C. Beta-galactosidase
    D. DNase

169. Which of the following is a species of group C streptococci?
    A. *S. faecium*
    B. *S. equisimilis*
    C. *S. agalactiae*
    D. *S. sanguis*

170. The mycobacterial isolate most closely associated with enteric infections in patients with acquired immune deficiency syndrome would be
    A. *M. avium* complex
    B. *M. kansasii*
    C. *M. bovis*
    D. *M. terrae*

171. The Frei test has previously been used as a diagnostic procedure for which of the following diseases?
    A. Trachoma
    B. Whooping cough
    C. Lymphogranuloma venereum
    D. Leprosy

172. Which one of the following tests would be appropriate in the diagnosis of a mycobacterial infection?
    A. Anton test
    B. Frei test
    C. Nagler test
    D. PPD test

173. Which one of the following disease processes involves erythrogenic toxin?
    A. Syphilis
    B. Leprosy
    C. Cutaneous anthrax
    D. Scarlet fever

174. Detection of antibody against cardiolipin is useful for the diagnosis of which of the following diseases?
    A. Whooping cough
    B. Syphilis
    C. Leprosy
    D. Tuberculosis

175. Corneal scrappings are collected and examined microscopically using a DFA test to detect elementary bodies for the diagnosis of infection caused by
    A. *Gardnerella vaginalis*
    B. *Brucella canis*
    C. *Haemophilus influenzae* biogroup *aegyptius*
    D. *Chlamydia trachomatis*

176. The optimal specimen for the recovery of *Bordetella pertussis* is
    A. Coughed sputum
    B. Blood
    C. Nasopharyngeal swab
    D. Anterior nares swab

177. Cultures of the posterior pharynx are most commonly submitted to the clinical laboratory for the detection of
    A. *Haemophilus influenzae*
    B. *Staphylococcus aureus*
    C. *Streptococcus pyogenes*
    D. *Corynebacterium diphtheriae*

178. Which of the following genera is the most commonly associated with bacterial vaginosis?
    A. *Gardnerella*
    B. *Listeria*
    C. *Eikenella*
    D. *Capnocytophaga*

179. Blood cultures are the optimal specimens for the recovery of which of the following microorganisms?
    A. *Yersinia enterocolitica*
    B. *Brucella canis*
    C. *Chlamydia trachomatis*
    D. *Mycobacterium leprae*

180. *Streptococcus sanguis* is most commonly associated with which of the following clinical conditions?
    A. Relapsing fever
    B. Subacute bacterial endocarditis
    C. Otitis media
    D. Pharyngitis

181. Rust-colored sputum production in cases of lobar pneumonia is characteristic of which of the following possible etiologic agents?
    A. *Klebsiella pneumoniae*
    B. *Staphylococcus aureus*
    C. *Pseudomonas aeruginosa*
    D. *Streptococcus pneumoniae*

182. *Yersinia pseudotuberculosis* is known to commonly manifest which of the following clinical conditions?
    A. Epiglottitis
    B. Pseudomembranous colitis
    C. Mesenteric lymphadenitis
    D. Peliosis hepatica

183. Epiglottitis in children is a common manifestation of an infection with which of the following?
    A. *Streptococcus pyogenes*
    B. *Haemophilus influenzae*
    C. *Stomatococcus mucilaginosus*
    D. *Streptococcus mutans*

184. A 23-year-old female is seen by her physician for symptoms of uncomplicated cystitis. A culture of her urine grew a gram-positive coccus, which would most likely be
    A. *Staphylococcus saprophyticus*
    B. *Enterococcus faecalis*
    C. *Streptococcus bovis*
    D. *Lactococcus garviae*

185. Cystine-tellurite blood agar plates are recommended for the isolation of
    A. *Yersinia enterocolitica*
    B. *Legionella pneumophila*
    C. *Corynebacterium diphtheriae*
    D. *Francisella tularensis*

186. A 45-year-old man was seen in the emergency room with fever, chills, nausea, and myalgias. He reported that 2 days earlier, he had eaten raw oysters at a popular seafood restaurant. On admission he was febrile and had hemorrhagic, fluid-filled bullous lesions on his left leg. The patient had a history of diabetes mellitus, chronic hepatitis B, and heavy alcohol consumption. The patient, who had a temperature of 102.2 °F, was admitted to the ICU for presumed sepsis and treatment was begun. A curved gram-negative rod was isolated from blood cultures drawn on admission and fluid from the bullous leg wound. On the third day, disseminated intravascular coagulation (DIC) developed and he died. The source of the oysters eaten by the deceased patient was the Gulf of Mexico. The most likely etiologic agent in this case would be
    A. *Yersinia enterocolitica*
    B. Plesiomonas *shigelloides*
    C. *Aeromonas hydrophila*
    D. *Vibrio vulnificus*

187. CIN agar is a recommended culture medium for the recovery of
    A. *Yersinia enterocolitica*
    B. *Cardiobacterium hominis*
    C. *Rhodococcus equi*
    D. *Brucella suis*

188. The appropriate culture media for the recovery of *Gardnerella vaginalis* is
    A. BCYE agar
    B. HBT agar
    C. CIN agar
    D. Middlebrook agar

189. Buffered charcoal yeast extract agar is the recommended medium for the recovery of
    A. *Erysipelothrix rhusiopathiae*
    B. *Tatumella ptyseos*
    C. *Shewanella putrefaciens*
    D. *Legionella pneumophila*

190. Which one of the following mycobacteria is known as the radish bacillus because of its association with soil and vegetables?
   A. *M. gordonae*
   B. *M. terrae*
   C. *M. xenopi*
   D. *M. gastri*

191. A primary agent of human intestinal tuberculosis in uncompromised hosts is
   A. *M. gordonae*
   B. *M. xenopi*
   C. *M. bovis*
   D. *M. fortuitum*

192. Association with patients with AIDS is most characteristic of
   A. *Mycobacterium avium* complex
   B. *M. marinum*
   C. *M. kansasii*
   D. *M. bovis*

193. Which of the following mycobacteria produces an orange pigment and is most commonly recovered from water?
   A. *M. intracellulare*
   B. *M. gordonae*
   C. *M. asiaticum*
   D. *M. kansasii*

194. Which of the following mycobacteria appears as buff-colored colonies after several weeks on culture media and is niacin positive?
   A. *M. bovis*
   B. *M. scrofulaceum*
   C. *M. ulcerans*
   D. *M. tuberculosis*

195. Swimmer's ear, a form of external otitis media, is commonly caused by
   A. *Mycobacterium marinum*
   B. *Pseudomonas aeruginosa*
   C. *Streptococcus pneumoniae*
   D. *Haemophilus influenzae*

196. The etiologic agent of "swimming pool granuloma" is
   A. *Mycobacterium marinum*
   B. *Pseudomonas aeruginosa*
   C. *Streptococcus pneumoniae*
   D. *Haemophilus influenzae*

197. Countless numbers of vacationers who have traveled outside of the United States have had their holidays interrupted by a case of "traveler's diarrhea," which is commonly associated with which etiologic agent?
   A. *Vibrio parahemolyticus*
   B. *Aeromonas hydrophila*
   C. *Escherichia coli*
   D. *Proteus mirabilis*

198. A 3-year-old was brought to the emergency room by her parents. She had been febrile with a loss of appetite for the past 24 hours. Most recently they noted that it was difficult to arouse her. She attended a day-care center and her childhood immunizations were up to date. On examination she demonstrated a positive Brudzinski sign indicative of meningeal irritation. Cultures of blood and cerebrospinal fluid were sent to the laboratory. Her CSF was cloudy and the Gram stain showed many polymorphonuclear cells with cell-associated gram-negative diplococci. The white blood cell count was 25,000/μl, with 88% PMN forms. The CSF protein was 100 mg/dL and the glucose was 15 mg/dL. Cultures of the blood and CSF grew the same gram-negative diplococcal organism. The most etiologic agent in this case was presumptively identified as
   A. *Neisseria meningitidis*
   B. *Haemophilus influenzae*
   C. *Moraxella catarrhalis*
   D. *Listeria monocytogenes*

199. The pulmonary form of anthrax is known as
  A. Valley fever
  B. Walking pneumonia
  C. Farmers' lung
  D. Woolsorters' disease

200. "Chinese letters" best describe which of the following seen on Gram stain?
  A. *Bacillus anthracis*
  B. *Yersinia pseudotuberculosis*
  C. *Campylobacter jejuni*
  D. *Corynebacterium pseudodiphtheriticum*

201. A bamboo fishing pole is the most common description of the appearance of which of the following microorganisms on Gram stain?
  A. *Bacillus anthracis*
  B. *Haemophilus ducreyi*
  C. *Campylobacter jejuni*
  D. *Neisseria gonorrhoeae*

202. Select the microorganism that on Gram stain has a characteristic arrangement that is said to resemble schools of fish
  A. *Bacillus anthracis*
  B. *Haemophilus ducreyi*
  C. *Campylobacter jejuni*
  D. *Neisseria gonorrhoeae*

203. On Gram stain a morphology that resembles seagull wings is most characteristic of
  A. *Bacillus anthracis*
  B. *Yersinia pseudotuberculosis*
  C. *Campylobacter jejuni*
  D. *Neisseria gonorrhoeae*

204. The flattened adjacent sides of the cellular appearance of which microorganism is said to resemble kidney beans?
  A. *Bacillus anthracis*
  B. *Yersinia pseudotuberculosis*
  C. *Campylobacter jejuni*
  D. *Neisseria gonorrhoeae*

205. The ability to grow on MacConkey agar is a characteristic of which species of mycobacteria?
  A. *M. marinum*
  B. *M. tuberculosis*
  C. *M. fortuitum*
  D. *M. avium* complex

206. Which of the following *Mycoplasmataceae* does not have a well-established connection with human infections?
  A. *Mycoplasma pneumoniae*
  B. *Mycoplasma hominis*
  C. *Ureaplasma urealyticum*
  D. *Mycoplasma genitalium*

207. All the following areas of the body are sites normally colonized by large numbers of normal flora organisms, *except*
  A. Trachea
  B. Colon
  C. Vagina
  D. Skin

208. During childbearing years the normal flora of the vagina is predominantly
  A. *Enterococcus* sp.
  B. *Lactobacillus* sp.
  C. *Propionibacterium* sp.
  D. Coagulase-negative *Staphylococcus* sp.

209. Susceptibility to TCH or thiophene-2-carboxylic acid hydrazide is characteristic of which of the following mycobacteria?
  A. *M. bovis*
  B. *M. kansasii*
  C. *M. avium* complex
  D. *M. tuberculosis*

210. All the following demonstrate a positive urease test *except*
  A. *Edwardsiella tarda*
  B. *Proteus mirabilis*
  C. *Corynebacterium urealyticum*
  D. *Helicobacterium pylori*

211. The most widely used target nucleic acid amplification method is
    A. Ligase chain reaction (LCR)
    B. Polymerase chain reaction (PCR)
    C. Restriction enzyme analysis (REA)
    D. Gas-liquid chromatography (GLC)

212. The aerobic gram-positive rod known to cause bacteremia in HIV-infected patients is
    A. *Corynebacterium ulcerans*
    B. *Corynebacterium jeikeium*
    C. *Corynebacterium urealyticum*
    D. *Corynebacterium auris*

213. Hansen's bacillus is another name for
    A. *Listeria monocytogenes*
    B. *Moraxella catarrhalis*
    C. *Mycobacterium leprae*
    D. *Chlamydia trachomatis*

214. *Actinomyces pyogenes* are now classified as members of the genus
    A. *Flavobacterium*
    B. *Corynebacterium*
    C. *Agrobacterium*
    D. *Arcanobacterium*

215. Identify the *Neisseria* sp. that produces the carbohydrate fermentation reaction (CTA base) of acid in glucose, negative in maltose, lactose, and sucrose.
    A. *Neisseria lactamica*
    B. *Neisseria gonorrhoeae*
    C. *Neisseria meningitidis*
    D. *Neisseria sicca*

216. Identify the *Neisseria* sp. that produces the carbohydrate fermentation reaction (CTA base) of acid in glucose, acid in maltose and negative in sucrose and lactose.
    A. *Neisseria lactamica*
    B. *Neisseria gonorrhoeae*
    C. *Neisseria meningitidis*
    D. *Neisseria sicca*

217. Which of the following is not a correct statement regarding blood cultures?
    A. Collection of 10–20 mL per culture for adults is recommended
    B. Two or 3 blood cultures recommended as optimum
    C. Volume of blood cultured more criticial than timing of culture
    D. Blood drawn for culture may be allowed to clot

218. The causative agent of the septicemic, hemolytic disease known as Oroya fever is
    A. *Mycoplasma hominus*
    B. *Abiotrophia adjacens*
    C. *Borrelia recurrentis*
    D. *Bartonella bacilliformis*

219. All the following are true about *Chlamydia pneumoniae* (formerly *Chlamydia* Twar) *except*
    A. Third most common agent of lower respiratory tract infection
    B. Intracellular pathogen
    C. Humans become infected from animal reservoirs
    D. Tetracycline and erythromycin effective treatments

220. A positive gelatin reaction is characteristic of
    A. *Serratia liquefaciens*
    B. *Proteus vulgaris*
    C. *Morganella morganii*
    D. *Salmonella enteritidis*

221. A positive phenylalanine deaminase reaction is characteristic of
    A. *Serratia liquefaciens*
    B. *Proteus vulgaris*
    C. *Moraxella (Branhamella) catarrhalis*
    D. *Salmonella arizona*

222. A positive indole reaction would be characteristic of
    A. *Serratia liquefaciens*
    B. *Morganella morganii*
    C. *Enterobacter aerogenes*
    D. *Salmonella enteritidis*

223. A positive malonate reaction is characteristic of
    A. *Serratia liquefaciens*
    B. *Salmonella arizona*
    C. *Enterobacter aerogenes*
    D. *Shigella sonnei*

224. Lack of motility is a characteristic of
    A. *Serratia liquefaciens*
    B. *Salmonella arizona*
    C. *Enterobacter aerogenes*
    D. *Klebsiella pneumoniae*

225. Violet-colored colonies are typically produced by
    A. *Chromobacterium violaceum*
    B. *Flavobacterium meningosepticum*
    C. *Pseudomonas aeruginosa*
    D. *Serratia marcscens*

226. All the following statements about *P. multocida* are true *except*
    A. Humans harbor the organism as part of their normal flora
    B. Most common human infections occur in soft tissues, bones, and joints
    C. It is the most virulent of the species
    D. There are no NCCLS guidelines for susceptibility testing

227. Pus was aspirated from an empyema. A Gram stain of the aspirated material showed many WBCs and numerous gram-negative bacilli. The culture grew many blue-green-colonies. The most likely etiologic agent in this case would be
    A. *Chromobacterium violaceum*
    B. *Legionella pneumophila*
    C. *Pseudomonas aeruginosa*
    D. *Serratia marcescens*

228. Red-colored colonies are typically produced by
    A. *Chromobacterium violaceum*
    B. *Chryseobacterium meningosepticum*
    C. *Pseudomonas aeruginosa*
    D. *Serratia marcescens*

229. A bone marrow transplant patient on immunosuppressive therapy developed a pulmonary abscess with symptoms of neurologic involvement. A brain abscess was detected by MRI and aspirated material grew an aerobic, filamentous, branching gram-positive organism, which stained weakly acid-fast. The most likely etiologic agent in this case would be
    A. *Mycobacterium tuberculosis*
    B. *Nocardia asteroides*
    C. *Actinobacillus israelii*
    D. *Propionibacterium acnes*

230. Which of the following is catalase negative?
    A. *Edwardsiella tarda*
    B. *Aeromonas hydrophila*
    C. *Campylobacter sputorum*
    D. *Listeria monocytogenes*

231. Which of the following is not a correct statement regarding *Aeromonas hydrophila?*
    A. Peritrichous flagella
    B. Beta hemolytic
    C. Catalase positive
    D. Oxidase positive

232. *Edwardsiella tarda* biochemically may be confused with *Salmonella* in that it is
    A. Lactose positive
    B. Hydrogen sulfide positive
    C. Urea positive
    D. Nonmotile

233. Colonies of *Listeria monocytogenes* on a sheep blood agar plate most closely resemble colonies of
    A. *Streptococcus agalactiae*
    B. *Corynebacterium diphtheriae*
    C. *Rhodococcus equi*
    D. *Haemophilus influenzae*

234. The porphyrin test determines an organism's requirement for
    A. Cystiene
    B. Thiol
    C. NAD
    D. X factor

235. Which of the following is commonly recovered from the oral cavity of guinea pigs and rabbits?
    A. *Escherichia coli*
    B. *Staphylococcus epidermidis*
    C. *Gardnerella vaginalis*
    D. *Bordetella bronchiseptica*

236. Which of the following is the etiologic agent of a variety of skin diseases such as strawberry foot and lumpy wool in domestic animals and has been isolated from a tongue infection in an HIV-positive patient that resembled "hairy" leukoplakia?
    A. *Prototheca wickerhamii*
    B. *Dermatophilus congolensis*
    C. *Stomatococcus mucilaginosus*
    D. *Streptobacillus moniliformis*

237. *Streptococcus sanguis* is
    A. Recovered most commonly from the female genital tract
    B. Recovered frequently from uncomplicated urinary tract infections
    C. Recovered most commonly from the oral cavity of humans
    D. Recovered most commonly from the skin surface of normal humans

238. The most common etiologic agent of infections associated with the surgical insertion of prosthetic devices such as artificial heart valves and cerebrospinal fluid shunts is
    A. *Staphylococcus aureus*
    B. *Serratia marcescens*
    C. *Streptococcus mutans*
    D. *Staphylococcus epidermidis*

239. One of the most common etiologic agents of uncomplicated cases of cystitis is
    A. *Klebsiella pneumoniae*
    B. *Escherichia coli*
    C. *Enterobacter aerogenes*
    D. *Proteus vulgaris*

240. The colonial description of Medusa head colonies on solid agar is most characteristic of
    A. *Mycoplasma pneumoniae*
    B. *Haemophilus ducreyi*
    C. *Yersinia pestis*
    D. *Bacillus anthracis*

241. What is the new gold standard for detection of *Chlamydia trachomatis* in cases of sexually transmitted disease?
    A. Nonculture EIA methods
    B. Tissue culture
    C. Culture of Thayer-Martin agar
    D. DNA-amplification techniques

242. Colonies said to have the appearance of a "fried egg" are characteristic of
    A. *Nocardia asteroides*
    B. *Bordetella pertussis*
    C. *Mycoplasma pneumoniae*
    D. *Streptobacillus moniliformis*

243. The characteristic growth pattern known as satelliting is associated with
    A. *Haemophilus influenzae*
    B. *Campylobacter jejuni*
    C. *Yersinia pestis*
    D. *Bacillus anthracis*

244. Colonies that are said to resemble "droplets of mercury" are characteristic of
    A. *Bordetella pertussis*
    B. *Campylobacter jejuni*
    C. *Yersinia pestis*
    D. *Bacillus anthracis*

245. An extracellular toxin is produced by all the following *except*
    A. *Pseudomonas aeruginosa*
    B. *Moraxella catarrhalis*
    C. *Bordetella pertussis*
    D. *Corynebacterium diphtheriae*

246. A capsular polysaccharide is a major virulence mechanism for all the following *except*
    A. *Legionella pneumophila*
    B. *Streptococcus pneumoniae*
    C. *Neisseria meningitidis*
    D. *Haemophilus influenzae*

247. Cultures from the anterior nares of health care workers often yield
    A. *Streptococcus pneumoniae*
    B. *Neisseria meningitidis*
    C. *Staphylococcus aureus*
    D. *Haemophilus influenzae*

248. Ethylhydrocupreine HCl susceptibility is a presumptive test for the identification of
    A. Viridans streptococci
    B. *Streptococcus pyogenes*
    C. *Streptococus agalactiae*
    D. *Streptococcus pneumoniae*

249. Solubility in the presence of sodium desoxycholate is characteristic of
    A. *Streptococcus pneumoniae*
    B. *Streptococus agalactiae*
    C. *Enterococcus faecalis*
    D. *Streptococcus mutans*

ANAEROBIC BACTERIA

250. An anaerobically incubated blood agar plate shows colonies surrounded by an inner zone of complete red cell lysis and an outer zone of incomplete cell lysis that gives a discolored appearance. The most likely rapid presumptive identification of this isolate would be
    A. *Clostridium perfringens*
    B. *Fusobacterium nucleatum*
    C. *Prevotella melaninogenica*
    D. *Clostridium tetani*

251. A cervical mucosal abscess specimen was sent to the laboratory for bacteriologic examination. The culture of this sample grew an anaerobic gram-negative bacillus that was inhibited by bile, pigmented brown, and was negative for indole production, positive for glucose, sucrose, and lactose fermentation. This isolate would most likely be
    A. *Bacteroides fragilis* group
    B. *Bacteroides ureolyticus*
    C. *Prevotella melaninogenica*
    D. *Porphyromonas gingivalis*

252. Which one of the following is not a true statement concerning *Clostridium tetani?*
    A. Spores in soil contaminate puncture wounds
    B. Disease caused by an exotoxin acting on the central nervous system
    C. It is a facultative anaerobe
    D. It is a gram-positive, spore-forming bacillus

253. The characteristic colonial morphology of *Actinomyces israelii* on solid agar resembles
    A. Bread crumbs
    B. A molar tooth
    C. A fried egg
    D. Ground glass

254. What is the predominant indigenous flora of the colon?
    A. Anaerobic, gram-negative, non-spore-forming bacteria
    B. Anaerobic, gram-positive, non-spore-forming bacteria
    C. Aerobic, gram-negative, non-spore-forming bacteria
    D. Aerobic, gram-positive, spore-forming bacteria

255. Obligately anaerobic, gram-negative bacilli, recovered from an abdominal wound, were found to be resistant to penicillin. Growth of this organism was not inhibited in the presence of bile. What is the most likely identification of this isolate?
    A. *Eubacterium lentum*
    B. *Fusobacterium nucleatum*
    C. *Bacteroides fragilis* group
    D. *Clostridium septicum*

256. Obligately anaerobic gram-positive cocci are called
    A. *Propionibacterium*
    B. *Peptostreptococcus*
    C. *Capnocytophaga*
    D. *Veillonella*

257. Color Plate 29 shows the filamentous gram-positive rod recovered from an aspirate of a closed chest abscess. It grew only under anaerobic conditions and was not acid-fast. What is the most likely presumptive identification of the isolate seen?
    A. *Cardiobacterium hominus*
    B. *Bacteroides fragilis* group
    C. *Actinomyces israelii*
    D. *Propionibacterium acnes*

258. The anaerobic organism that is presumptively identified by its ability to grow on kanamycin, vancomycin, laked blood agar (KVL) medium is

    A. *Clostridium perfringens*
    B. *Peptostreptococcus anaerobius*
    C. *Bifidobacterium dentium*
    D. *Bacteroides fragilis* group

259. The recommended selective agar for the detection of *Clostridium difficile* is
    A. Cycloserine cefoxitin fructose agar (CCFA)
    B. Buffered charcoal yeast extract agar (BCYE)
    C. Laked kanamycin-vancomycin blood agar (LKV)
    D. Thiosulfate citrate bile salts sucrose agar (TCBS)

260. The anaerobic, gram-negative, curved, motile bacilli associated with bacterial vaginosis is
    A. *Bifidobacterium* sp.
    B. *Mobiluncus* sp.
    C. *Atopobium* sp.
    D. *Lactobacillus* sp.

261. An infant was seen in the emergency room with symptoms of neuromuscular weakness and constipation. The diagnosis of infant botulism was confirmed by the demonstration of toxin in the child's stool. The child most likely contracted this disease by
    A. Ingestion of spores that germinated in the intestine
    B. A puncture wound with a contaminated household item
    C. A scratch wound caused by a cat
    D. Ingestion of performed toxin found in a contaminated jar of pureed vegetables

262. The majority of the gram-positive, non-spore-forming, anaerobic bacilli isolated from clinical material will be
    A. *Propionibacterium acnes*
    B. *Capnocytophagia* ochracea
    C. *Bifidobacterium dentium*
    D. *Eubacterium limosum*

263. Which of the following Clostridia has a terminal spore that swells the sporangium?
    A. *C. perfringens*
    B. *C. botulinum*
    C. *C. tetani*
    D. *C. difficile*

264. The gram-negative, non-spore-forming, anaerobic bacillus frequently implicated in such serious clinical infections as brain and lung abscesses is
    A. *Leptotrichia buccalis*
    B. *Bilophilia wadsworthia*
    C. *Fusobacterium nucleatum*
    D. *Eubacterium lentum*

265. Production of exotoxin is recognized as a major mediator of disease by all the following *except*
    A. *Clostridium ramosum*
    B. *Clostridium difficile*
    C. *Clostridium tetani*
    D. *Clostridium botulinum*

266. All the statements below describe a characteristic of *Clostridium botulinum except*
    A. It produces a positive Nagler reaction
    B. Of the seven toxicologic types, types A, B, E, and F are associated with human botulism
    C. Pathogenicity is related to a potent neurotoxin
    D. Oval spores are located either centrally or subterminally

267. A tube of semisolid medium that has resazurin incorporated in it appears pink. Which of the following organisms inoculated in this medium would be expected to be able to be recovered?
    A. *Bacteroides thetaiotaomicron*
    B. *Wolinella curva*
    C. *Fusobacterium necrophorum*
    D. *Gardnerella vaginalis*

268. Identify the *Fusobacterium* species that is considered to be the most frequent isolate recovered from clinical infections.
    A. *F. varium*
    B. *F. nucleatum*
    C. *F. mortiferum*
    D. *F. necrophorum*

269. Septicemia caused by which of the following is generally associated with an underlying malignancy?
    A. *Clostridium septicum*
    B. *Bifidobacterium dentium*
    C. *Lactobacillus catenaforme*
    D. *Eubacterium lentum*

270. Which of the following is the most potent exotoxin known?
    A. Botulinal toxin
    B. Erythrogenic toxin
    C. Tetanospasmin
    D. *C. difficile* toxin B

271. Which *Clostridium* sp. is most commonly recovered from cases of gas gangrene?
    A. *C. bifermentans*
    B. *C. perfringens*
    C. *C. sordellii*
    D. *C. difficile*

272. Which of the following organisms is not gram-positive?
    A. *Eubacterium lentum*
    B. *Bifidobacterium dentium*
    C. *Propionibacterium acnes*
    D. *Leptotrichia buccalis*

273. All the following statements about Clostridia are true *except*
    A. Botulism is caused by ingesting preformed toxin and can be prevented by boiling food prior to eating
    B. Pseudomembranous colitis is due to a toxin produced by *C. difficile*

C. *C. tetani* spores will form in the presence of oxygen; therefore, anaerobiosis in a wound is not required to cause tetanus

D. Clinically significant Clostridia are found in the normal flora of the colon and in the soil

274. Which is the correct concerning *Clostridium difficile?*

A. Produces lecithinase and lipase

B. Grows on cycloserine cefoxitin fructose agar

C. Is aerotolerant

D. All isolates are toxigenic

275. Which is the correct concerning the genus *Veillonella?*

A. Gram-positive, anaerobic cocci

B. Significant pathogens found in pure culture in infections

C. Ferment a variety of carbohydrates

D. Obligate anaerobes

276. All the following statements are correct regarding *Clostridium perfringens except*

A. There are five serologic types

B. Spores are oval and centrally located

C. Alpha toxin is produced by all strains

D. Spores are readily seen in laboratory media

277. Which is a correct statement regarding *Clostridium tetani?*

A. It is characteristically nonmotile

B. It is lecithinase positive

C. It is proteolytic

D. Pathogenicity is associated with its neurotoxin

278. Which anaerobic gram-negative rod can be presumptively identified by its Gram stain morphology, growth on in the presence of bile and inhibition by a 1 μg kanamycin disk?

A. *Fusobacterium nucleatum*

B. *Eubacterium lentum*

C. *Bacteroides fragilis* gp.

D. *Porphyromonas gingivalis*

279. Which of the following tests is most appropriate for the rapid presumptive identification of *Prevotella melaninogenica?*

A. SPS test

B. Nagler test

C. Cytotoxin assay

D. Fluorescence test

280. Which of the following tests is most appropriate for the rapid identification of *Clostridium difficile?*

A. SPS test

B. Nagler test

C. Cytotoxin assay

D. Fluorescence test

281. Which of the following tests is most appropriate for the rapid presumptive identification of *Clostridium perfringens?*

A. SPS test

B. Nagler test

C. Cytotoxin assay

D. Fluorescence test

282. Which of the following tests is most appropriate for the rapid presumptive identification of *Peptostreptococcus anaerobius?*

A. SPS test

B. Nagler test

C. Cytotoxin assay

D. Fluorescence test

283. A curved appearance on Gram stain is characteristic of which of the following?

A. *Propionibacterium acnes*

B. *Clostridium ramosum*

C. Actinomyces israelii

D. *Clostridium septicum*

284. Purulent material from a cerebral abscess was submitted to the laboratory for smear and culture. On direct Gram stain, gram-positive cocci in chains and gram-negative bacilli with pointed ends were seen. Culture results from this specimen will not be available for 48 hours. Therefore, on the basis of the organisms seen on the smear, what is the most likely presumptive identification of the etiologic anaerobic agents?
   A. *Veillonella* sp. and *Clostridium* sp.
   B. *Fusobacterium* sp. and *Peptostreptococcus* sp.
   C. *Peptostreptococcus* sp. and *Nocardia* sp.
   D. *Eubacterium* sp. and *Veillonella* sp.

285. Which of the following descriptions is most characteristic of *Bifidobacterium dentium?*
   A. Pale staining, gram-negative bacilli with tapered ends
   B. Slender, long, carved, gram-positive bacilli
   C. Bifurcated, branched, or filamentous gram-positive bacilli
   D. Gram-positive bacilli, diphtheroidal, filamentous, and branching forms

286. Which of the following is an important virulence factor of *Bacteroides fragilis* gp.?
   A. Endotoxin
   B. Protease
   C. Exotoxins
   D. Polysaccharide capsule

287. Which of the following descriptions is most characteristic of *Fusobacterium nucleatum?*
   A. Pale staining, gram-negative bacilli with tapered ends
   B. Slender, long, curved, gram-positive bacilli
   C. Bifurcated, branched, or filamentous gram-positive bacilli
   D. Gram-positive bacilli with swollen sporangia with round terminal spores

288. All the following are true about *Bacteroides fragilis* gp. *except*
   A. Anaerobic gram-negative bacilli
   B. Among the most antibiotic-sensitive anaerobic bacteria
   C. Commonly associated with intra-abdominal infections
   D. Endotoxin production is not associated with virulence

289. A 59-year-old man with a history of alcohol abuse was taken to the emergency room. He had been found unconscious laying face up on the sidewalk. There was evidence that he had vomited and it was suspected that he had aspirated his gastric or oral secretions. A pneumonia developed. Which of the following would not be a likely causative agent in this case?
   A. *Prevotella melaninogenica*
   B. *Bacteroides gracilis*
   C. *Mobiluncus* sp.
   D. *Porphpyromonas* sp.

SPIROCHETES

290. During the first week of the disease leptospirosis, the most reliable way to detect the presence of the causative agent is by the direct
   A. Culturing of urine
   B. Examination of cerebrospinal fluid
   C. Culturing of blood
   D. Examination of blood

291. The placenta is at a developmental stage that permits the maternal transmission of *Treponema pallidum* to the fetus during the _____ month of pregnancy.
   A. First
   B. Fourth
   C. Third
   D. Fifth

292. A helicoidal, flexible organism was demonstrated in a blood smear. This motile organism was approximately 12 μm long, approximately 0.1 μm wide, and had semicircular hooked ends. The description of this organism corresponds most closely to the morphology of
A. *Campylobacter*
B. *Leptospira*
C. *Borrelia*
D. *Treponema*

293. The etiologic agent of epidemic relapsing fever is *Borrelia recurrentis,* which is transmitted by
A. *Ornithodoros hermsi*
B. *Pediculus humanus*
C. *Ornithodoros erraticus*
D. *Ornithodoros parkeri*

294. All the following statements related to the VDRL test are true *except*
A. The antibody titer will decline if the patient is adequately treated
B. False-positive tests are more frequent than with the FTA-ABS test
C. Inactivated *Treponema pallidum* serves as the antigen
D. The test is usually positive in secondary syphilis

295. A research technologist was bitten on the hand by a laboratory rodent. After a week the technologist experienced regional lymphadenitis, fever, a rash spreading from the site of the bite, and liver enlargement. Wound exudate, node tissue, and blood cultures failed to grow the etiologic agent. Dark-field examination and Giemsa stain of clinical material showed short, thick, spiral cells with bipolar tufts of flagella. The etiologic agent in this case was identified as
A. *Leptospira interrogans*
B. *Treponema pertenue*

C. *Spirillum minus*
D. *Borellia recurrentis*

296. *Borrelia burgdorferi*, a spirochete transmitted by *Ixodes dammini* in the northeastern United States, is the etiologic agent of
A. Sodoku
B. Q fever
C. Lyme disease
D. Rat-bite fever

297. The axial fibrils of spirochetes most closely resemble which bacterial structure?
A. Cytoplasmic membrane
B. Flagellum
C. Pilus
D. Sporangium

298. Which of the following is not correct regarding spirochetes?
A. Motility is via axial filaments
B. Spirochetes are gram-positive
C. Those associated with human disease are 0.1–0.5 μm in diameter and 5–30 μm in length
D. They are visualized best using dark-field or phase optics

299. A positive VDRL test for syphilis was reported on a young woman known to have hepatitis. When questioned by her physician she denied sexual contact with any partner symptomatic for a venereal disease. Which of the following would be the appropriate next step for her physician?
A. Identify her sexual contacts for serologic testing
B. Test her serum using a fluorescent treponemal antibody-absorbed (FTA-ABS)
C. Treat her with penicillin
D. Reassure her that it was a biologic false-positive caused by her liver disease

SUSCEPTIBILITY TESTING

300. The concentration of calcium and magnesium ions in the susceptibility testing medium is significant when testing the susceptibility of *Pseudomonas aeruginosa* to
    A. Tetracycline
    B. Polymyxin B
    C. Cephalothin
    D. Gentamicin

301. A patient has a serious infection caused by *Staphylococcus aureus*. The patient has been diagnosed with endocarditis and is to be discharged soon. The antimicrobial agents used for therapy will be given to him in an oral form. In a discussion with the Infectious Disease Service, the Director of the Microbiology Laboratory suggests that Serum Bactericidal Test (Schlicter Test) may be helpful in managing this patient's care. The experimental specimen (analyte) in this assay is
    A. A bacteria with an unknown antimicrobial susceptibility
    B. A standardized serum sample and the patient's bacterial isolate
    C. The patient's serum containing an unknown amount of antimicrobial agent
    D. The patient's bacterial isolate with a known MIC but an unknown MBC

302. The broth culture suspension of the test organism for use in broth dilution and disk diffusion testing is adjusted to match the turbidity of a
    A. 0.5 McFarland standard
    B. 1.0 McFarland standard
    C. 2.0 McFarland standard
    D. 3.0 McFarland standard

303. When testing the antimicrobial susceptibility of *Haemophilus influenzae* strains by disk-agar diffusion, the recommended medium is

A. Charcoal-yeast extract agar
B. Mueller-Hinton agar supplemented with 1% hemoglobin and 1% IsoVitaleX
C. Trypticase soy agar supplemented with 5% defibrinated sheep blood
D. Hemophilus Test Medium

304. The chemotherapeutic agents that are structurally similar to the vitamin *p*-aminobenzoic acid and act to inhibit bacteria by the inhibition of folic acid synthesis are
    A. Aminoglycosides
    B. Penicillins
    C. Macrolides
    D. Sulfonamides

305. A new Internal Medicine Resident comes the Microbiology Laboratory to discuss the fact that some bacterial isolates do *not* have in vitro susceptibility testing performed, even when they are isolated in pure culture from clinically important body sites. Which of the following organisms would not be routinely tested?
    A. *Escherichia coli*
    B. *Proteus mirabilis*
    C. *Staphylococcus aureus*
    D. *Streptococcus pyogenes*

306. When testing the effectiveness of penicillin, its ability to inhibit _____ is evaluated on actively growing bacterial cells.
    A. Reduction of dihydrofolic acid
    B. Protein synthesis at the 30S ribosomal subunit
    C. Peptidoglycan synthesis
    D. Nucleic acid function

307. The minimum bactericidal concentration (MBC) of an antimicrobial agent is defined as the lowest concentration of that antibiotic that kills at least _____ of the original inoculum.

A. 95.5%

B. 97%

C. 99.9%

D. 100%

308. The optimal specimen for the assay of common antimicrobial agents is
    A. Urine
    B. Ascitic fluid
    C. Serum
    D. Cerebrospinal fluid

309. The term that denotes a situation in which the effect of two antimicrobial agents together is greater than the sum of the effects of either drug alone is
    A. Antagonism
    B. Sensitivity
    C. Additivism
    D. Synergism

310. β-lactamase-producing strains of *Haemophilus influenzae* are resistant to
    A. Erythromycin
    B. Chloramphenicol
    C. Trimethoprim sulfamethoxazole
    D. Penicillin

311. The agar recommended by the NCCLS for routine susceptibility testing is
    A. Mueller-Hinton agar
    B. MacConkey agar
    C. Trypticase soy agar
    D. Middlebrook 7H10 agar

312. The pH of the test agar used for the Bauer-Kirby test should be
    A. 7.0–7.2
    B. 7.2–7.4
    C. 7.4–7.6
    D. 7.6–7.8

313. Which drug known to be active against parasitic infections has importance as a therapeutic agent in cases of disease caused by anaerobic bacteria?
    A. Trimethoprim
    B. Metronidazole
    C. Isoniazid
    D. Rifampin

314. An example of a bactericidal antibiotic is
    A. Chloramphenicol
    B. Tetracycline
    C. Tobramycin
    D. Erythromycin

315. Proficiency surveys of the disk-agar diffusion method for susceptibility testing identified those variables that lead to discrepancies. Among those identified were
    A. The use of reference organisms such as *Klebsiella pneumoniae* and *Streptococcus pyogenes*
    B. The use of cotton swabs on wooden applicator sticks
    C. The selection and concentration of the antimicrobial disks
    D. The use of trypticase soy broth for the inoculum preparation

316. While reading the routine broth dilution susceptibility test panels, a Medical Technologist notices that a patient's isolate labeled as "*Streptococcus pneumoniae*" did not grow in the growth well. Remembering that *S. pneumoniae* is a fastidious organism that may not grow in routine broth medium, the technologist checks the procedure manual. Which of the following media should be used for the in vitro susceptibility testing of that *S. pneumoniae*?
    A. Charcoal-yeast extract broth
    B. Mueller-Hinton broth supplemented with 1% hemoglobin and 1% IsoVitaleX
    C. Mueller-Hinton broth supplemented with 5% lysed horse blood
    D. Walker Fastidious Medium

317. Rapid testing for β-lactamase production is recommended, prior to initiation of antimicrobial therapy, for isolates of
    A. *Staphylococcus epidermidis*
    B. *Haemophilus influenzae*
    C. *Staphylococcus aureus*
    D. *Streptococcus pyogenes*

318. The phenomenon of bacterial resistance to the bactericidal activity of penicillins and cephalosporins, with only inhibition of the organism's growth, is known as
    A. High-level resistance
    B. Intrinsic resistance
    C. Tolerance
    D. Inducible resistance

319. The supervisor of a microbiology laboratory has been asked to begin performing in vitro antimicrobial susceptibility testing of *Mycobacteria tuberculosis* due to an increase in the reported resistance in their community. Having reviewed the literature, and talked to the pharmacist and the local infectious disease specialists, he has decided that providing this service is important. Which of the following methods would be appropriate for this testing?
    A. Broth microdilution method using Mueller-Hinton broth
    B. Bauer-Kirby method
    C. BACTEC method
    D. Schlichter method

ANTIMICROBIAL AGENTS

320. β-lactam antimicrobials comprise the penicillins, cephalosporins, carbapenams, and monobactams. These antimicrobials are bactericidal to susceptible bacteria. Their therapeutic application is recommended for all the following etiologic agents *except*
    A. *Mycoplasma*
    B. *Escherichia coli*

    C. Non-penicillinase-producing strains of *Staphylococcus aureus*
    D. *Streptococcus agalactiae*

321. Which of the following antimicrobial agents acts by inhibiting cell wall synthesis?
    A. Vancomycin
    B. Clindamycin
    C. Naladixic acid
    D. Gentamicin

322. Metronidazole is most commonly recommended for treatment of infections caused by
    A. Obligate intracellular microorganisms
    B. Microaerophilic microorganisms
    C. Aerobic microorganisms
    D. Obligate anaerobic microorganisms

323. Which of the following antimicrobial agents act by inhibiting protein synthesis?
    A. Rifampin
    B. Methicillin
    C. Gentamicin
    D. Vancomycin

324. Chloramphenicol was an important antimicrobial agent for the treatment of pediatric meningitis as well as several other significant infections. Unfortunately, chloramphenicol exhibits a major complication that limit its clinical usefulness. These effects include:
    A. Allergic reactions and anaphylaxis
    B. Bone marrow suppression and aplastic anemia
    C. Significant gastrointestinal manifestations
    D. Photosensitivity

MYCOLOGY

325. A bulldozer operator became ill while working on a new highway in the San Joaquin Valley. He developed chest pain, anorexia, headache and general malaise,

and myalgia with fever. Chest X ray showed pneumonic infiltrate and a single, well-defined nodule in the left lower lobe. His leukocyte count and sedimentation rate were slightly elevated. Although no fungus was seen in direct examination of a sputum specimen, processing included a culture on Sabouraud's dextrose agar with chloramphenicol and cycloheximide. Within 3 days at 28 °C this culture produced moist, grayish growth, and a white aerial mycelium began to develop (see Color Plate 30). A lactophenol blue mount of this organism is seen in Color Plate 31. If this fungus was the cause of infection, it was most probably

A. *Asperigillus fumigatus*
B. *Blastomyces dermatitidis*
C. *Coccidioides immitis*
D. *Histoplasma capsulatum*

326. A Methodist minister from Ohio presented to his physician with a mild influenzalike illness including headache and malaise. His chest X ray showed no infiltrates. His past medical history was unremarkable. He had no history of travel but reported recently cleaning the bell tower at his church, which was littered with bird excrement. The most likely agent causing his disease is

A. *Aspergillus fumigatus*
B. *Coccidioides immitis*
C. *Candida albicans*
D. *Histoplasma capsulatum*

327. A rose gardener pricked himself with a contaminated thorn. A subcutaneous fungal infection characterized by the development of necrotic ulcers followed this direct inoculation of fungal spores into the skin. The causative fungus was cultured as a small yeast form at 36 °C (see Color Plate 32) and as a mold at room temperature with delicate hyphae and conidia. This disease is

A. Blastomycosis
B. Chromomycosis

C. Mycetoma
D. Sporotrichosis

328. A yeastlike fungus was isolated from sputum. No hyphae were produced in morphology agar. It was negative for nitrate assimilation and positive for inositol assimilation and produced urease at 37 °C. These findings are typical of

A. *Candida krusei*
B. *Cryptococcus terreus*
C. *Cryptococcus neoformans*
D. *Trichosporon beigelii*

329. A Vietnamese refugee was seen at a church-sponsored clinic in Houston. His chief complaints were weight loss and fever. A CBC confirmed he was suffering from anemia as well. Multiple skin lesions were present on his arms, some of them draining pus. Gram stain of the pus revealed what appeared to be yeastlike cells. A culture of the pus grew a green mold at 25 °C, which produced a red soluble pigment (see Color Plate 33). A lactophenol blue mount of this organism is seen in Color Plate 34. The causative agent in this case was

A. *Aspergillus fumigatus*
B. *Gliocladium* sp.
C. *Trichoderma* sp.
D. *Penicillium marneffei*

330. A section of a lymph node stained with the Gomori silver stain and hematoxylin and eosin is shown in Color Plate 35. A lactophenol blue mount of a mold that grew from this specimen is shown in Color Plate 36. Large, one-celled, smooth to tuberculate macroconidia and smooth or echinulate microconidia are typical of mycelial phase growth of

A. *Bastomyces dermatitidis*
B. *Coccidioides immitis*
C. *Histoplasma capsulatum*
D. *Paracoccidioides brasiliensis*

331. Which of the following types of *Candida albicans* infection is commonly acquired from an exogenous source?
    A. Diaper rash
    B. Neonatal thrush
    C. Perianal infection
    D. Urinary tract infection

332. In direct examination of a KOH mount of a nail specimen, *Epidermophyton floccosum* could be detected as
    A. Arthroconidia
    B. Blastoconidia
    C. Macroconidia
    D. Microconidia

333. The mold phase of the systemic fungus *Blastomyces dermatitidis* must be differentiated from which of the following fungi?
    A. *Scedosporium apiospermum*
    B. *Sporothrix schenckii*
    C. *Aspergillus* sp.
    D. *Penicillium notatum*

334. It is usually difficult or impossible to identify a fungal culture before it is mature. However, the presence of hyaline, septate hyphae, and a young conidiophore with a foot cell (see Color Plate 37) and a swollen vesicle are excellent clues to the identification of
    A. *Acremonium*
    B. *Aspergillus*
    C. *Paecilomyces*
    D. *Penicillium*

335. Zygomycetes are fast-growing, airborne saprobes. In clinical specimens they
    A. Are common as normal, human microflora
    B. Are found only as contaminants
    C. May be seen in a dimorphic tissue phase
    D. May be found as a cause of rapidly fatal infection

336. *Trichophyton rubrum* and *Trichophyton mentagrophytes* may be differentiated by the
    A. Consistently different appearance of their colonies
    B. Endothrix hair infection produced by *T. rubrum*
    C. Fluorescence of hairs infected with *T. rubrum*
    D. In vitro hair penetration by *T. mentagrophytes*

337. Broad, cenocytic hyphae found in tissue would be most typical of infection with
    A. *Aspergillus*
    B. *Blastomyces*
    C. *Microsporum*
    D. *Rhizopus*

338. A fungus infecting only skin and nails typically produces in culture
    A. Spindle-shaped, hyaline, echinulate macroconidia and microconidia
    B. Cylindrical or club-shaped, smooth, thin-walled macroconidia and microconidia
    C. Many microconidia in clusters or along the hyphae
    D. Large, thin-walled, club-shaped conidia without microconidia

339. The most useful finding for prompt, presumptive identification of *C. albicans* is its
    A. Failure to assimilate sucrose
    B. "Feathering" on EMB
    C. Production of chlamydoconidia
    D. Production of germ tubes

340. Identify the dimorphic fungus that typically has a tissue phase in which the large mother cells have one to a dozen narrow-necked buds and a slow-growing mycelial form with intercalary chlamydoconidia and coiled hyphae
    A. *Blastomyces dermatitidis*
    B. *Coccidioides immitis*

C. *Histoplasma capsulatum*

D. *Paracoccidioides brasiliensis*

341. An immunodiffusion test has been useful for diagnosis and prognostic evaluation of one important mycosis. Two precipitin lines have been recognized as significant in this test: the m line, which is found early in infection and in persons who have recovered from the disease, and the h line, which generally indicates active infection. The antigen used in this test is

A. Aspergillin

B. Coccidioidin

C. Histoplasmin

D. Sporotrichin

342. The formation of arthroconidia is a characteristic important in the identification of all the following *except*

A. *Coccidioides*

B. *Geotrichum*

C. *Trichosporon*

D. *Sporothrix*

343. Four types of fungal structures are given below. Which of these is not produced by causative agents of chromomycosis?

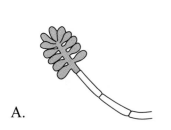

A.

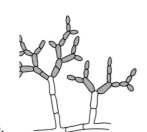

B.

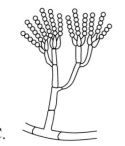

C.

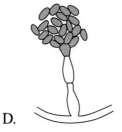

D.

344. Fungi considered to be opportunistic pathogens include all the following *except*

A. *Absidia*

B. *Aspergillus*

C. *Coccidioides*

D. *Fusarium*

345. Observation of hyaline or dematiacious hyphae is an early clue in the identification of common, airborne fungi. Which of the following genera contains species found as dematiacious contaminants?

A. *Alternaria*

B. *Penicillium*

C. *Paecilomyces*

D. *Fusarium*

346. Which of the following fungi is most likely to be found as a common saprobe and as an agent of keratitis?

A. *Exophiala*

B. *Phialophora*

C. *Fusarium*

D. *Wamgiella*

347. Host conditions that are associated with an increased incidence of *Candida albicans* infections include all the following *except*

A. Diabetes

B. Childhood viral infections

C. Prolonged antibiotic usage

D. Pregnancy

348. Chronic mucocutaneous candidiasis (CMCC) in children is associated with genetic defects in cellular immunity. Which of the following syndromes has been found to predispose to CMCC?

A. Flu

B. Hepatitis syndrome

C. DiGeorge's syndrome (with absence of thymus)

D. Bruton's hypogammaglobulinemia (humoral immunity deficiency)

349. Hyaline septate hyphae, branched or un-branched conidiophores, and multicelled banana-shaped conidia are characteristic of which of the following:
   A. *Fusarium*
   B. *Curvularia*
   C. *Acremonium*
   D. *Trichophyton violaceum*

350. All the following statements correctly de-scribe the yeast *Rhodotorula rubra except*
   A. It has been isolated from dairy products, air, soil, and water
   B. It is the most common fungal cause of diaper rash
   C. It has been identified as a nosocomial pathogen
   D. It has been found as a contaminant or commensal in specimens of urine, sputum, and feces

351. A track star from a university was in the locker room after a competition when one of his teammates noticed light brown circular lesions on his upper back. The agent most likely responsible for this condition is
   A. *Candida albicans*
   B. *Tinea versicolor*
   C. *Sporobolomyces*
   D. *Malassezia furfur*

352. Which of the following is likely to be found in clinical specimens as normal microflora and as clinically significant isolates?
   A. *Aspergillus niger*
   B. *Scopulariopsis*
   C. *Penicillium notatum*
   D. *Candida albicans*

353. A 4-year-old child's hair is falling out in patches. The hair fluoresces when subjected to the UV light from a Wood's lamp. When the hair is cultured, a white cottony mold grows at 25 °C on SDA. Microscopically, rare microconidia, septate hyphae, and ter-minal chlamydospores are seen. Macroco-nidia are absent. The mold fails to grow on polished rice grains. The causative agent is
   A. *Microsporum audouinii*
   B. *Microsporum gypseum*
   C. *Trichophyton mentagrophytes*
   D. *Trichophyton rubrum*

354. In tissues infected with *Histoplasma capsulatum*
   A. The hyphae usually invade blood vessels
   B. Encapsulated yeast cells are typical
   C. Tuberculate macroconidia are typical
   D. The fungus is usually intracellular

For each numbered mycosis below, choose the lettered environment most commonly associated with an increased incidence of that infection.

---

355. Blastomycosis

356. Coccidioidomycosis

357. Cryptococcosis
   A. Lower Sonoran Life Zone
   B. Mississippi and Ohio River basins
   C. Pigeon roosts
   D. Bat roosts

For each numbered mycosis below, choose the lettered environment most commonly associated with an increased incidence of that infection.

---

358. Histoplasmosis

359. Sporotrichosis
   A. Sphagnum moss
   B. Starling roosts
   C. Pigeon roosts
   D. Colorado River Valley

For each incomplete statement, select the most appropriate lettered species.

360. The cause of white piedra

361. The cause of black piedra

362. The cause of tinea nigra
    A. *Exophiala werneckii*
    B. *Trichosporon beigleii*
    C. *Piedraia hortae*
    D. *Fonsecaea compacta*

For each incomplete statement, select the most appropriate lettered species.

363. The cause of pityriasis (tinea) versicolor

364. A keratinophilic saprophyte

365. A cause of otittis externa (external ear)
    A. *Aspergillus niger*
    B. *Malassesia furfur*
    C. *Trichosporon ajelloi*
    D. *Geotrichum candida*

The incomplete statements below describe the appearance of growth of yeast or yeastlike fungi in morphology agar, such as rice agar or cornmeal agar with Tween 80, a finding helpful in the presumptive identification of these organisms. For each numbered description, select the most appropriate lettered species.

366. True hyphae and arthrospores only

367. True hyphae, arthrospores, and blastospores

368. Pseudohyphae, blastospores, and chlamydospores
    A. *Candida albicans*
    B. *Geotrichum*
    C. *Trichosporon*
    D. *Aspergillus fumigatus*

The incomplete statements below describe the appearance of growth of yeast or yeastlike fungi in morphology agar, such as rice agar or cornmeal agar with Tween 80, a finding helpful in the presumptive identification of these organisms. For each numbered description, select the most appropriate lettered species.

369. Pseudohyphae and blastospores only

370. Blastospores only, without hyphae or pseudohyphae
    A. *Mucor* sp.
    B. *Candida tropicalis*
    C. *Cryptococcus neoformans*
    D. *Candida albicans*

Select the most appropriate lettered specimen source for isolation of each numbered species.

371. *Cryptococcus neoformans*

372. *Histoplasma capsulatum*

373. *Pseudallescheria boydii*

374. *Trichophyton mentagrophytes*
    A. Bone marrow
    B. Cerebrospinal fluid
    C. Chronic draining sinus tract of foot
    D. Chronic interdigital lesion of foot

QUALITY ASSURANCE

375. Proper specimen handling increases the success of virus isolation. When specimens cannot be processed directly, viruses are better recovered from samples held at 2–6 °C. Specimens that must be held for longer than several days should be promptly frozen to
    A. -20 °C
    B. -40 °C
    C. -60 °C
    D. -70 °C

376. In capnophilic incubators carbon dioxide concentrations should be maintained between
    A. 1% and 5%
    B. 5% and 10%
    C. 10% and 15%
    D. 15% and 20%

377. The recommended anticoagulant for use when a body fluid or joint fluid that may clot is sent for microbiologic examination is
    A. Heparin
    B. Sodium polyethanolsulfonate
    C. Sodium EDTA
    D. Sodium citrate

378. Which of the following is not one of the standard control organisms used for the weekly testing of antimicrobial disks?
    A. *Staphylococcus epidermidis* (ATCC 25833)
    B. *Pseudomonas aeruginosa* (ATCC 27853)
    C. *Escherichia coli* (ATCC 25922)
    D. *Enterococcus fecalis* (ATCC 29212)

379. *Neisseria meningitidis* and *Neisseria gonorrhoeae* are extremely sensitive to environmental conditions. Specimens submitted for their recovery should never be held
    A. At incubator temperature
    B. At refrigerator temperature
    C. In a moist state
    D. In an increased CO_2 environment

380. Which strain of mycobacteria should not be routinely used to test each batch of prepared or purchased lot of mycobacterial culture media?
    A. *Mycobacterium leprae*
    B. *Mycobacterium tuberculosis*
    C. *Mycobacterium kansasii*
    D. *Mycobacterium avium complex*

381. To ensure that anaerobic conditions have been achieved in anaerobic jars or chambers, an oxygen-sensitive indicator is employed such as
    A. Phenol red
    B. Methylene blue
    C. Bromcreosol purple
    D. Methyl red

382. A suggested quality control organism that would demonstrate a positive reaction on Simmons citrate agar slants is
    A. *Shigella sonnei*
    B. *Klebsiella pneumoniae*
    C. *Escherichia coli*
    C. *Morganella morganii*

INFECTION CONTROL

383. Passengers on a plane that was traveling from California to Philadelphia became ill about 2 hours after eating lunch in flight. The illness was characterized by rapid onset of violent vomiting. The most likely bacterial cause of such symptoms would be
    A. Salmonella food poisoning
    B. Clostridial food poisoning
    C. Staphylococcal food poisoning
    D. Shigella food poisoning

384. When an epidemiologic survey for the detection of upper respiratory carriers of *Neisseria meningitidis* or *Bordetella pertussis* is being conducted, the optimal type of specimen to be obtained for culture is
    A. Throat
    B. Anterior nares
    C. Buccal cavity
    D. Nasopharyngeal

385. The most significant intrinsic factor of humans that affects their response to infectious disease has been shown to be
    A. Race
    B. Age

C. Economic status

D. Sex

386. Chronic carriers, persons who remain infected with an organism for long periods, are typically associated with the dissemination of

A. *Salmonella typhi*

B. *Corynebacterium diphtheriae*

C. *Streptococcus pneumoniae*

D. *Bordetella pertussis*

387. A slaughterhouse worker was seen by his physician for a febrile respiratory illness in the form of an atypical pneumonia. The laboratory studies confirmed the physician's diagnosis of the rickettsial disease, Q fever. Human infection with the causative agent of Q fever is usually acquired by

A. The bite of a mite (chigger)

B. The bite of an infected body louse

C. A blood meal taken by the arthropod *Phlebotomus*

D. Inhalation of infectious material (fomites)

388. Milk has classically been the primary food associated with disease transmission, especially for those diseases of cattle that are transmissible to man, such as

A. Meliodosis

B. Cryptococcosis

C. Diphtheria

D. Brucellosis

389. Laboratory professionals are at special risk for disease transmission. The majority of cases of laboratory-related infections are associated with

A. Infectious aerosols

B. Contamination of abraded skin

C. Puncture wounds

D. Bite of a laboratory test animal

390. Association with sink and faucet aerators and humidifiers used with ventilators in the intensive care units is most commonly a factor in outbreaks of infections with which of the following microorganisms?

A. *Serratia marcescens*

B. *Mycobacterium marinum*

C. *Pseudomonas aeruginosa*

D. *Salmonella enteritidis*

PROCEDURES, MEDIA, REAGENTS, AND STAINS

391. The ability of a microorganism to deaminate phenylalanine can be assessed by inoculating a phenylalanine agar slant with the test organism. Following incubation, if the organism is positive, a green color develops with the addition of the reagent

A. 10% ferric chloride

B. 2% sulfanilamide

C. 2 N sodium carbonate

D. 5% alpha naphthol

392. Which of the following media are both selective and differential?

A. Chocolate agar

B. Blood agar

C. Mannitol salt agar

D. Trypticase soy agar

393. The paper strip test for the demonstration of hydrogen sulfide production is impregnated with a solution of

A. Sodium desoxycholate

B. Lead acetate

C. Potassium tellurite

D. Sodium thiosulfate

394. All the following are used for the cultivation of *Neisseria gonorrheae, except*

A. Martin-Lewis

B. Thayer-Martin

C. CVA agar

D. Chocolate agar

395. The selective nature of Hektoen agar is due to the inclusion of which one of the following in the formulation?
    A. NaCl
    B. Bis-sodium metasulfate
    C. Bile salts
    D. Phenol red

396. An example of a selective enrichment broth would be
    A. Thioglycollate broth
    B. Chopped meat glucose broth
    C. Selenite broth
    D. Trypticase nitrate broth

397. Which of the following stains greatly enhances the visibility of fungi by binding to the cell walls, causing the fungi to fluoresce blue-white or apple green?
    A. Rhodamine-auramine
    B. Warthin-Starry
    C. Calcofluor white
    D. Periodic acid-Schiff

398. A technologist in the northeastern region of the United States receives a call from a physician. This physician has seen six patients in the last two days with the major complaint of diarrhea. Although she can't come up with a common source, she suspects food poisoning from a local raw oyster bar. She will contact the Health Department, but needs the technologist's help to identify the possible cause. She will be sending stool cultures on these patients to rule out *Vibrio cholera*-like disease. For the selective isolation of *Vibrio* species causing cholera, diarrhea, and food poisoning, the recommended agar is
    A. Thiosulfate citrate bile salt sucrose agar (TCBS)
    B. Charcoal yeast extract agar (BCYE)
    C. Tinsdale agar
    D. Mannitol salt agar

399. Paired, acute, and convalescent blood samples are needed for diagnostic viral serology testing. The recommended intervals for collection are

	Acute	Convalescent
A.	13–15 days	50–60 days
B.	11–13 days	40–50 days
C.	7–9 days	20–30 days
D.	5–7 days	10–20 days

400. The flagellar staining technique most commonly used in clinical laboratories is the
    A. Wayson
    B. Kinyoun
    C. Dienes
    D. Leifson

401. In the nitrate test, reduction is demonstrated by the development of a red color, following the addition of
    A. Alpha-naphthol and potassium hydroxide
    B. *p*-Dimethylaminobenzaldehyde and amyl alcohol
    C. Ninhydrin and acetone
    D. Alpha-naphthylamine and sulfanilic acid

402. The Moeller test for the detection of decarboxylase activity is dependent upon
    A. An alkaline pH shift in the medium
    B. The oxidation of gluconate
    C. An acid pH basal medium
    D. A deamination of tryptophan

403. The medium used to determine whether an organism is oxidative or fermentative with respect to its metabolic activities is
    A. CTA medium
    B. O-F medium
    C. HE medium
    D. XLD medium

404. The Voges-Proskauer broth medium is methyl red-Voges-Proskauer (MR/VP). After inoculation with the test organism and a period of incubation, two reagents must be added before the test can be read. The reagents used in this test are
    A. Creatine and 1 N HCl
    B. 10% $FeCl_3$ and alpha-naphthol
    C. Kovac's reagent and zinc dust
    D. Alpha-naphthol and 40% KOH

405. Which of the following is appropriate when discussing CTA medium?
    A. Turns a red color, indicating acid production from the metabolism of the carbohydrate present
    B. Requires incubation in increased CO_2 atmosphere
    C. Is used as a presumptive test for the identification of *Neisseria gonorrhoeae*
    D. Is inoculated with a heavy suspension of the test organism in the upper third of the column of medium

406. Which of the following would be negative using the acid-fast stain?
    A. *Cryptosporidium* sp.
    B. *Actinomyces israelii*
    C. *Mycobacterium leprae*
    D. *Isospora belli*

407. The novobiocin susceptibility test is used for the identification of
    A. *Peptostreptococcus anaerobius*
    B. *Helicobacter pylori*
    C. *Streptococcus mutans*
    D. *Staphylococcus saprophyticus*

408. Egg yolk agar showing a precipitate in the medium surrounding the colony is positive for
    A. Lecithinase production
    B. Starch hydrolysis
    C. Lipase production
    D. Protease activity

409. Which procedure is not correct for the collection and transportation of specimens for bacterial or viral isolation?
    A. Specimens be obtained before antibiotic therapy has been initiated
    B. Double-mailing containers, properly labeled, be used when shipping samples to other laboratories
    C. A holding medium be used to prevent dehydration in transit for those specimen types or organisms most susceptible to the effects of drying
    D. Glass containers used for optimal shipping of specimens

410. Which of the following is not appropriate when discussing cultures of blood for the recovery of bacteria?
    A. No more than three cultures should be drawn in one day
    B. Should be drawn before the expected fever spike
    C. Cultures incubated aerobically and anaerobically
    D. Collect 5 mL of blood for optimal recovery of pathogen

411. Which of the following systems is used to remove antibiotics from body fluids that have been sent to the laboratory for bacteriologic culture?
    A. Port-A-Cult system
    B. ARD system
    C. Roll tube system
    D. Isolator system

412. When performing the oxidase test, which of the following would not be appropriate?
    A. The reagent used is *o*-nitrophenyl-β-D-galactopyranoside
    B. The reagent must be freshly prepared or refrigerated for no longer than 1 week
    C. Do not use a Nichrome wire loop to rub a portion of the suspect colony on a paper strip
    D. A positive colony turns dark purple within 10 seconds of the application of the reagent

413. Tellurite reduction isused for the presumptive identification of
A. *Bordetella pertussis*
B. *Corynebacterium diphtheriae*
C. *Haemophilus influenzae*
D. *Vibrio parahemolyticus*

414. The SPS disk is used for the presumptive identification of
A. *Peptostreptococcus anaerobius*
B. *Helicobacter pylori*
C. *Streptococcus mutans*
D. *Moraxella catarrhalis*

415. The porphyrin test is most useful for the identification of which of the following?
A. *Streptococcus* sp.
B. *Moraxella* sp.
C. *Nocardia* sp.
D. *Haemophilus* sp.

RAPID METHODS

416. More recent BACTEC Systems (9240 and 9120) used for the rapid detection of microorganisms in clinical samples such as blood detect CO_2 produced by bacterial metabolism by
A. Fluorescence
B. ^{14}C detection
C. Colorimetry
D. Changes in headspace pressure

417. When using the rapid chromogenic cephalosporin method for the detection of beta-lactamase production by an organism, a positive test is indicated by the color
A. Yellow
B. Green
C. Red
D. Blue

418. An organism that demonstrates a positive colorimetric assay for the detection of chloramphenicol acetyltransferase (CAT) is reported as
A. Susceptible to penicillin
B. Resistant to chloramphenicol
C. Resistant to cephalosporins
D. Susceptible to beta-lactam antibiotics

419. LCR and PCR are DNA-amplification testing methods that have become the new gold standard for the direct detection of
A. *Chlamydia trachomatis*
B. Hantavirus
C. *Legionella pneumophila*
D. *Vibrio cholerae*

420. The nucleic acid probe procedure that analyzes DNA is called a
A. Western blot
B. Lectin assay
C. Northern blot
D. Southern blot

421. The initial step in the preparation of a gene probe is the isolation and removal of the desired gene by digesting DNA with
A. A nitrocellulose filter
B. Restriction endonuclease enzymes
C. Sodium hydroxide
D. DNA ligase

422. All the following are EIA tests used to detect many of the causative agents of gastrointestinal disease *except*
A. Rotovirus solid-phase EIA
B. *Cryptosporidium* EIA
C. *E. coli* 0157:H7 EIA
D. *Giardia lamblia* EIA

423. All the following are true about the laboratory diagnosis of pertussis *except*
    A. Regan-Lowe medium has replaced Bordet-Gengou medium in many labs
    B. DFA test results (positive or negative) are definitive and do not need to be confirmed by culture
    C. Calcium alginate or Dacron swabs recommended over cotton-tipped swabs for specimen collection
    D. The DFA test is currently the most rapid test available for the diagnosis of *B. pertussis*

424. The commonly used confirmatory test for HIV infection is the
    A. Enzyme immunosorbent assay
    B. Northern blot
    C. Lymulus amebiocyte lysate assay
    D. Western blot

425. Which of the following statements does not apply to the acridine orange stain?
    A. Binds to the teichoic acid of the cell wall
    B. Requires the use of a fluorescence microscope
    C. Is more sensitive than the Gram stain
    D. Is recommended for fluid and exudates with low bacterial concentrations

INFECTIOUS DISEASES

426. An infant was hospitalized with a severe, tender erythema that started on the face and then spread to the trunk and extremities. The child's epidermis was loose, and large areas of skin could be peeled off, leaving the sensitive underlying dermis exposed. The condition described is most consistent with a clinical syndrome associated with which organism?
    A. *Streptococcus pyogenes*
    B. *Staphylococcus aureus*
    C. *Bacillus anthracis*
    D. *Erysipelothrix rhusiopathiae*

427. A young woman was seen by her physician for a dermatologic problem that developed 48 hours after she used the whirlpool at her health spa. She was afebrile with a macular, pustular skin rash on her chest, abdomen, and back. A gram-negative, nonfermentative, motile organism was recovered from a culture of one of the lesions. This case is most consistent with which of the following infectious processes?
    A. Q fever
    B. Erysipelas
    C. *Acinetobacter* cellulitis
    D. *Pseudomonas* dermatitis

428. Pleomorphic gram-positive rods (slightly curved to straight) were recovered from the chest fluid drawn from a teenager with right lower lobe pneumonia who lived on a dairy farm. At 24 hours pinpoint colonies grew on sheep blood that showed faint zones of beta hemoloysis. The isolate was catalase negative and demonstrated a positive CAMP test. Which of the following is the most likely etiologic agent in this case?
    A. *Listeria monocytogenes*
    B. *Streptococcus agalactiae*
    C. *Arcanobacterium pyogenes*
    D. *Streptobacillus moniliformis*

429. Exotic pets are often associated with the transmission of
    A. *Helicobacter* sp.
    B. *Campylobacter* sp.
    C. *Salmonella* sp.
    D. *Vibrio* sp.

430. The observation of Koplik's spots along with the clinical symptoms of fever and rash strengthens the diagnosis of
    A. Measles
    B. Rocky Mountain spotted fever
    C. Varicella
    D. Scarlet fever

431. The etiologic agent of the majority of all adult joint infections is
    A. *Staphylococcus aureus*
    B. *Neisseria gonorrhoeae*
    C. *Streptococcus pneumoniae*
    D. *Haemophilus influenzae*

432. A 35-year-old man came to the gastrointestinal clinic with symptoms of fever, chills, nausea, sore throat, headache, and diarrhea of 3 days duration. Blood, stool, and urine cultures were taken, and he was told to return in 2 days. When he returned, the doctor noted that the patient had developed rose-colored spots on his trunk. The blood culture was found to be positive for a gram-negative bacillus that gave the following biochemical reactions:

TSI	Alkaline/acid, no gas, slight H_2S
Citrate	Negative
Urea	Negative
Lysine	Positive
Motility	Positive
ONPG	Negative
Indole	Negative

    Given the previous description, the most likely diagnosis would be
    A. *Salmonella typhi*
    B. *Vibrio cholerae*
    C. *Shigella dysenteriae*
    D. *Yersinia pseudotuberculosis*

433. A young street person with the complaint of fever and leg pain was seen by an emergency room physician. The patient resided in a crowded housing shelter and did not practice good hygiene. A tentative diagnosis of trench fever was made, and laboratory studies were initiated. The mode of transmission for this disease is the body louse, which carries the infectious agent

A. *Bartonella quintana*
B. *Coxiella burnetii*
C. *Bartonella bacilliformis*
D. *Rickettsia prowazekii*

434. A young woman complaining of symptons of sudden onset of fever, vomiting, diarrhea, and rash was seen by her gynecologist. She was admitted to the hospital, where a culture of vaginal discharge grew many coagulase-positive staphylococci. The most likely diagnosis in this case would be
    A. Kawasaki disease
    B. Scalded skin syndrome
    C. Pelvic inflammatory disease
    D. Toxic shock syndrome

435. A 32-year-old male was seen in the emergency room with symptoms of lower right quadrant abdominal pain and diarrhea. A CBC showed a leukocytosis with an increased number of neutrophils. He was admitted, and a stool culture was obtained. The culture showed many bipolar-staining, gram-negative bacilli, which were oxidase negative, citrate negative, and indole negative. The TSI reaction was acid over acid, but there was no evidence of gas or H_2S production. The organism was positive for urease and ONPG and negative for phenylalanine. The characteristic symptomatology and the biochemical reactions confirmed that the etiologic agent was
    A. *Campylobacter jejuni*
    B. *Yersinia enterocolitica*
    C. *Vibrio parahaemolyticus*
    D. *Tatumella ptyseos*

436. Blood cultures from a patient admitted to the hospital with fever, malaise, skin rash, and painful joints grew a pleomorphic, gram-negative coccobacillus, which showed branching and swollen, club-shaped cells in chains. It was noted by the technologist that in the culture bottle growth resembled

breadcumbs on the surface of the red cells, which settled to the bottom. The most likely identification of this isolate would be

A. *Listeria monocytogenes*
B. *Leptospira interrogans*
C. *Streptobacillus moniliformis*
D. *Erysipelothrix rhusiopathiae*

437. A patient presented in August at a community hospital in New England with symptoms of a skin rash, headache, stiff neck, muscle aches, and swollen lymph nodes. A silver-stained biopsy of a skin lesion showed spirochetes. On the basis of the clinical syndrome and laboratory detection of a causative agent the patient was diagnosed as having the tick-borne illness

A. Relapsing fever
B. Plague
C. Rabbit fever
D. Lyme disease

438. The etiologic agent implicated in cases of repeated abortion is

A. *Listeria monocytogenes*
B. *Streptobacillus moniliformis*
C. *Streptococcus agalactiae*
D. *Actinobacillus lignieresii*

439. Dozens of international participants in an Eco-Challenge adventure race in Borneo became ill with symptoms of chills, diarrhea, headaches, and eye infections. The racers hiked in the mountains and jungles, swam in rivers and slogged through flooded streams for two weeks. Contact with contaminated water and soil during the race was highly associated with illness. What is the most likely etiologic agent in this case?

A. *Borellia recurrentis*
B. *Leptospira interrogans*
C. *Franciscella tularensis*
D. *Brucella canis*

440. An anemic patient was transfused with packed red blood cells. Approximately 50 minutes after the transfusion was begun, the patient developed fever and hypotension consistent with endotoxic shock. The RBCs had been processed and stored at 4 °C for approximately 30 days prior to their use. The organism most likely to be involved in this case, based on the stated conditions would be

A. *Yersinia enterocolitica*
B. *Staphylococcus aureus*
C. *Neisseria meningiditis*
D. *Campylobacter jejuni*

441. A college student got a summer job working at a marina. While working on one of the outboard motors on a rental boat, he received several lacerations on his right forearm. No medical treatment was sought at the time of the injury but after several weeks he noted that the lesions were not healing and sought the opinion of his physician. A biopsy of one of the lesions showed it to be a cutaneous granulomatous condition. Given the history, which of the following microorganisms would most likely be the etiologic agent in this case?

A. *Vibrio vulnificus*
B. *Pseudomonas aeruginosa*
C. *Mycobacterium marinum*
D. *Nocardia asteroides*

442. A young man developed keratitis associated with the use of contact lenses that had been immersed in a contaminated cleaning solution. The most common etiologic agent in such cases is

A. *Chryseobacterium meningosepticum*
B. *Pseudomonas aeruginosa*
C. *Staphylococcus aureus*
D. *Escherichia coli*

443. The organism believed to be a cause of human peptic ulcer disease as well as the most frequent cause of gastritis is
    A. *Salmonella typhimurium*
    B. *Campylobacter jejuni*
    C. *Yersinia enterocolitica*
    D. *Helicobacter pylori*

444. *Bacillus cereus* has been implicated as the etiologic agent in cases of
    A. Impetigo
    B. Toxic shock syndrome
    C. Pelvic inflammatory disease
    D. Food poisoning

445. A woman who had recently returned from a vacation in Mexico was admitted to the hospital. She was febrile and complained of flulike symptoms. Her case history revealed that she had eaten cheese that had been made from unpasteurized milk while on vacation. The most likely etiologic agent in this case would be
    A. *Staphylococcus aureus*
    B. *Listeria monocytogenes*
    C. *Yersinia enterocolitica*
    D. *Bordetella pertussis*

446. The causative agent in cases of malignant pustule is
    A. *Yersinia pseudotuberculosis*
    B. *Brucella suis*
    C. *Bacillus anthracis*
    D. *Mycobacterium avium complex*

447. A young child became ill with an intestinal illness after visiting a petting zoo featuring baby farm animals such as calves, lambs, and chickens. She had bloody diarrhea and went on to develop hemolytic uremic syndrome, a life-threatening condition. The most likely etiologic agent in this case is
    A. *Vibrio cholerae* 01
    B. *Eschericia coli* 0157:H7

    C. *Vibrio cholerae* 0139
    D. *Shigella dysenteriae*

448. *Streptobacillus moniliformis* is the etiologic agent of
    A. Scalded skin syndrome
    B. Rat bite fever
    C. Acute gastroenteritis
    D. Human plague

449. The pathogenesis of which of the following diseases does not involve an exotoxin?
    A. Botulism
    B. Typhoid fever
    C. Scarlet fever
    D. Toxic shock syndrome

450. A middle-aged man with a history of smoking and drinking for over 40 years developed shortness of breath, fever, frontal headache, diarrhea, and cough. He worked in the produce section of a supermarket, which routinely misted the fresh greens. His medical history included a kidney transplant several years ago for which he remains on antirejection therapy. His sputum Gram stain showed polys but no organisms. An X ray of his chest showed an infiltrate in the left lower lobe and a diagnosis of atypical pneumonia was made. Which of the following is the most likely etiologic agent in this case?
    A. *Bordetella pertussis*
    B. *Moraxella catarrhalis*
    C. *Klebsiella pneumoniae*
    D. *Legionella pneumophila*

VIRUSES AND RICKETTSIAE

451. The retrovirus responsible for causing acquired immune deficiency syndrome (AIDS) is known by the name
    A. EBV
    B. HAV
    C. HIV
    D. HSV

452. The appearance of Koplik spots in the oral mucosa of patients is characteristic of infection with what viral agent?
    A. Hepatitis
    B. Measles
    C. Rabies
    D. Yellow fever

453. *Ornithodoros hermsii* is an important vector for the transmission of the etiologic agent of what disease, which is characterized by a febrile illness, with spontaneous resolution and subsequent recrudescence days later?
    A. Borreliosis
    B. Campylobacteriosis
    C. Leptospirosis
    D. Tularemia

454. For nonspecific staining of *Rickettsia* the recommended stain is
    A. Gimenez stain
    B. Gram stain
    C. Grocott-Gomori stain
    D. Kinyoun stain

455. Rotavirus is the most common etiologic agent of
    A. Acute nonbacterial encephalitis in children
    B. Acute nonbacterial gastroenteritis in infants and young children
    C. Chronic nonbacterial pharyngitis in children and young adults
    D. Chronic nonbacterial retinitis in children

456. Kaposi's sarcoma and B cell lymphomas are highly associated with infection by which group of viral agents?
    A. Bunyaviridae
    B. Parvoviridae
    C. Picornaviridae
    D. Retroviridae

457. The target of the virus causing acquired immune deficiency syndrome (AIDS) is the
    A. B lymphocyte
    B. Erythrocyte
    C. Granulocyte
    D. T lymphocyte

458. The type of cell culture that best supports the growth of human cytomegalovirus (CMV) is
    A. HeLa cells
    B. HEp-2 cells
    C. Human fibroblast cells
    D. Primary monkey kidney (PMK) cells

459. Which of the following viruses is predominantly associated with respiratory disease and the cause of epidemics of keratoconjunctivitis?
    A. Adenovirus
    B. Arenavirus
    C. Bunyavirus
    D. Rotavirus

460. A patient presented with multiple cold sores in the mouth. Material from the mucocutaneous lesions was obtained by needle aspiration and directly inoculated to human embryonic fibroblasts (MRC-5 cells). After 1 day, the cytopathic effect (CPE) included foci of ballooned and lysed cells. These data suggest infection with
    A. Adenovirus
    B. Cytomegalovirus
    C. Epstein-Barr virus
    D. Herpes simplex virus

461. The method of choice for the presumptive diagnosis of an enterovirus infection with the exception of group A Coxsackie viruses is
    A. Cell culture
    B. Electron microscopy
    C. Enzyme-linked immunoassay
    D. Serologic screening

462. The highly fatal arenavirus first described and predominantly occurring in Africa is
    A. Congo-Crimean hemorrhagic fever
    B. Lassa fever
    C. Marburg-Ebola hemorrhagic fever
    D. Yellow fever

463. Rocky Mountain spotted fever is transmitted by the bite of a tick congenitally infected with
    A. *Rickettsia akari*
    B. *Rickettsia conorii*
    C. *Rickettsia prowazekii*
    D. *Rickettsia rickettsii*

464. The viral disease shingles, which causes extreme tenderness along the dorsal nerve roots and a vesicular eruption, has the same etiologic agent as
    A. Rubeola
    B. Vaccinia
    C. Varicella
    D. Variola

465. The etiologic agents of many common colds are RNA viruses that grow better at 33 °C than at 37 °C. These viruses are
    A. Adenoviruses
    B. Orthomyxoviruses
    C. Paramyxoviruses
    D. Rhinoviruses

466. The disease of domestic fowl and wild birds that is caused by a paramyxovirus is
    A. Avian leukemia
    B. Newcastle disease
    C. Norwalk disease
    D. Psittacosis

467. Negri bodies may be found in brain tissue of humans or animals infected with
    A. Arenavirus
    B. Filovirus
    C. Measles virus
    D. Rabies virus

468. Which of the DNA viruses is the causative agent of molluscum contagiosum?
    A. Adenoviruses
    B. Herpesviruses
    C. Papovaviruses
    D. Poxviruses

469. Transmission of the sylvatic form of typhus infection caused by *Rickettsia prowazekii* is associated with
    A. Bats
    B. Flying squirrels
    C. Rabbits
    D. Raccoons

470. The mild type of typhus fever that is caused by recrudescence of an initial attack of epidemic typhus is known as
    A. Brill-Zinsser disease
    B. Q fever
    C. São Paulo typhus
    D. Tsutsugamushi disease

471. The causative agent of endemic or murine typhus is
    A. *Rickettsia akari*
    B. *Rickettsia conorii*
    C. *Rickettsia prowazekii*
    D. *Rickettsia typhi*

472. *Rickettsia akari* is the causative agent of
    A. Boutonneuse fever
    B. Rickettsial pox
    C. Rural typhus
    D. Trench fever

473. The classic European or epidemic typhus fever is caused by
    A. *Rickettsia prowazekii*
    B. *Rickettsia rickettsii*

C. *Rickettsia tsutsugamushi*

D. *Rickettsia typhi*

474. The causative agent of scrub typhus, the rickettsial disease prevalent in the Far East that is similar to spotted fever, is
    A. *Coxiella burnetti*
    B. *Rickettsia rickettsii*
    C. *Rickettsia tsutsugamushi*
    D. *Bartonella Quintana*

475. The etiologic agent of the South and Central American diseases Oroya fever and verruga peruana is the small, motile, aerobic, gram-negative bacillus
    A. *Bartonella bacilliformis*
    B. *Calymmatobacterium granulomatis*
    C. *Bartonella Quintana*
    D. *Streptobacillus moniliformis*

476. A baby was admitted to the hospital in February for dehydration due to severe diarrhea. An ova and parasite examination on a stool specimen was negative. Cultures for bacterial pathogens are pending. Which of the following additional tests would be most appropriate given the case history?
    A. Heterophile antibody test
    B. McCoy cell inoculation for Chlamydia
    C. Rotavirus antigen assay
    D. Urine microscopic analysis for presence of CMV cellular inclusion bodies

477. The chronic human degenerative viral disease of the central nervous system seen among New Guineans that was spread by ritualistic cannibalism is
    A. Guillain-Barré syndrome
    B. Kuru
    C. Progressive multifocal leukoencephalopathy
    D. Subacute sclerosing panencephalitis

478. Jaundice is a major clinical symptom of which of the following viral infections?
    A. Colorado tick fever
    B. Hepatitis A
    C. Rabies
    D. Varicella

479. One of the Herpesviridae, Epstein-Barr (EB) virus, is the causative agent of
    A. Fever blisters
    B. Infectious mononucleosis
    C. Molluscum contagiosum
    D. Shingles

480. The poliovirus, an RNA virus, is a(n)
    A. Coxsackie virus
    B. Echovirus
    C. Enterovirus
    D. Rhinovirus

481. The virus that causes hepatitis B is characterized as a
    A. Defective DNA virus requiring delta virus to complete its replication cycle
    B. DNA virus utilizing reverse transcriptase
    C. Nonenveloped DNA virus
    D. Single-stranded DNA virus

482. Hepatitis C virus infections
    A. Are commonly characterized by jaundice
    B. Are uncommon in the United States
    C. May be acquired by needle-sharing
    D. Seldom result in chronic infection

483. Paramyxoviruses such as respiratory syncytial virus (RSV), in contrast to orthomyxoviruses such as influenza virus
    A. Are not effective in syncytium formation
    B. Exhibit antigenic stability
    C. Possess a segmented genome
    D. Replicate within the nucleus of the host cell

484. The virus genus associated with warts is
    A. Bunyavirus
    B. Flavivirus
    C. Morbillivirus
    D. Papillomavirus

485. Colorado tick fever is a viral disease transmitted by the
    A. Body louse
    B. Rat flea
    C. Triatomid bug
    D. Wood tick

486. Group B Coxsackie viruses are associated with
    A. Gastrointestinal disease (i.e., severe diarrhea)
    B. Herpangina
    C. Myocarditis
    D. The common cold

487. The tubular cells of the human kidney shed which of the following viruses for prolonged periods?
    A. Adenovirus
    B. Cytomegalovirus
    C. Epstein-Barr virus
    D. Rubella virus

488. The togavirus known to produce fetal defects is
    A. Influenza
    B. Rotavirus
    C. Rubella
    D. Varicella

489. Intranuclear inclusions were found in epithelial cells from the urine of an infant who was admitted with symptoms of low birth weight, jaundice, and neurologic defects. The most likely clinical diagnosis in this case would be
    A. Cytomegalovirus infection
    B. Epstein-Barr virus infection
    C. Herpes simplex virus infection
    D. Rubella virus infection

490. Herpes simplex virus (HSV) causes rapidly fatal infections in
    A. Elderly patients
    B. Neonates
    C. Sexually active women
    D. Sickle cell patients

491. Select the statement that is correct concerning the influenza viruses.
    A. Humans are the only animal hosts for influenza viruses
    B. Pandemics are characteristically produced by influenza A
    C. The incidence of infection peaks in the summer months
    D. They are DNA viruses

492. An example of a latent viral infection occurring in humans is
    A. Influenza
    B. Rotavirus
    C. Rubella
    D. Varicella-zoster

493. The use of cell cultures has enabled microbiologists to isolate and identify many clinically important viruses. However, in some diseases the agents are best diagnosed by serologic testing. Such an agent is
    A. Adenovirus
    B. Cytomegalovirus
    C. Hepatitis C
    D. Measles virus

494. Which of the following may be associated with the rubella virus?
    A. A DNA virus
    B. A member of the same taxonomic family as measles virus
    C. Able to produce defects in fetuses during the early stages of pregnancy
    D. Transmitted by an arthropod vector

495. Steps involved in virus pathology include all the following *except*
    A. Attachment
    B. Mitosis
    C. Penetration
    D. Release

496. Opportunistic diseases that are closely associated with the acquired immune deficiency syndrome (AIDS) include all the following *except*
    A. Cryptococcosis
    B. Cryptosporidiosis
    C. Malaria
    D. Mycobacteriosis

497. Which of the following is a progressive neurologic disorder associated with the class of infectious agents termed "prions"?
    A. Creutzfeldt-Jakob disease
    B. Dengue
    C. Hepatitis C
    D. Shingles

498. The genome of a virus may consist of
    A. Amino acids
    B. Cytoplasm
    C. DNA or RNA
    D. Mitochondria

499. Viruses have been successfully detected by the use of all the following techniques *except*
    A. Cytopathic effect (CPE)
    B. Enzyme-linked immunosorbent assay (ELISA)
    C. Growth on selective agar media
    D. Immunofluorescence

500. Herpes simplex virus is associated with all the following conditions *except*
    A. Cold sores
    B. Encephalitis
    C. Genital herpes
    D. Thrush

PARASITOLOGY

501. *Enterobius vermicularis* infection is usually diagnosed by finding
    A. Eggs in perianal specimens
    B. Larvae in feces
    C. Larvae in perianal specimens
    D. Eggs in the feces

502. The best direct diagnosis of *Echinococcus granulosus* infection in humans is made by identification of
    A. Adult worms in the intestine
    B. Adult worms in tissues
    C. Eggs in feces
    D. Hydatid cysts in tissues

503. The formalin-ethyl acetate sedimentation concentration method is recommended for routine use primarily because it
    A. Preserves most parasites
    B. Recovers protozoa
    C. Is safer than formalin-ether sedimentation method
    D. All the above

504. Because of fecal contamination, a urine specimen may contain the flagellate
    A. *Balantidium coli*
    B. *Entamoeba coli*
    C. *Trichomonas hominis*
    D. *Trichomonas tenax*

505. Eggs or larvae recovered in the stool are routinely used to diagnose infections caused by all the following helminths *except*
    A. *Trichinella spiralis*
    B. *Necator americanus*
    C. *Strongyloides stercoralis*
    D. *Ascaris lumbricoides*

506. Many parasites have different stages of growth within different hosts. The host where the sexual reproductive stage of the parasites exist is called the
    A. Intermediate host
    B. Definitive host
    C. Vector
    D. Commensual

507. Species identification of an immature amebic cyst can be very difficult. This parasite stage would not, however, be found in infections caused by
    A. *Entamoeba coli*
    B. *Endolimax nana*
    C. *Dientamoeba fragilis*
    D. *Entamoeba histolytica*

508. Which of the following is typical in cysts of *Iodamoeba bütschlii?*
    A. A glycogen mass
    B. Blunt chromatoidal bars
    C. Four nuclei with large karyosomes
    D. Many ingested bacteria

509. Which of the following is the most important feature in differentiating cysts of *Entamoeba histolytica* from *E. dispar?*
    A. Number of nuclei
    B. Size of the cyst
    C. Shape of the karyosome
    D. Cysts cannot be morphologically differentiated

510. Which of the following findings in a peripheral blood smear is especially associated with tissue-invading helminths but may also be found in a variety of allergic conditions and other diseases?
    A. Eosinophilia
    B. Leukopenia
    C. Neutropenia
    D. Lymphocytosis

511. A 72-year-old man from Texas developed fever and weakness 16 days after a hunting trip in northwest Tanzania. Several days after the onset of fever, he noticed a raised, tender, erythematous nodule (6–8 cm in diameter) on the posterior aspect of his right arm. He was hospitalized in Africa and treated for 5 days with a cephalosporin for presumed cellulitis. After little improvement, he returned to Texas. On arrival, the patient had a temperature of 38.9 °C (102 °F), a morbilliform rash of the trunk, and right-sided, anterior cervical lymphadenopathy. Cerebrospinal fluid (CSF) contained 12 red cells and 18 mononuclear cells/mm^3, with a normal protein level (32 mg/dL). Laboratory tests revealed a hemoglobin level of 107 g/L (10.7 g/dL), a white cell count of 2.4×10^9/L (2.4×10^3/µL), and a platelet count of 75×10^9/L (75,000/µL). The diagnosis was made by finding the extracellular flagellate parasite in a peripheral blood smear. Which of the following is the most probable etiologic agent of this infection?
    A. *Leishmania donovani*
    B. *Trypanosoma brucei rhodesiense*
    C. *Toxoplasma gondii*
    D. *Trypanosoma cruzi*

512. Which species of malaria parasite usually has growing trophozoites with ameboid cytoplasm and produces small reddish dots in the red blood cell cytoplasm?
    A. *Plasmodium knowlesi*
    B. *Plasmodium falciparum*
    C. *Plasmodium malariae*
    D. *Plasmodium vivax*

513. With a fecal specimen, which one of the following is the most dependable procedure for the accurate, specific diagnosis of an intestinal amebic infection?
    A. Direct saline wet mount
    B. Iodine-saline wet mount
    C. Formalin-ether sedimentation technique
    D. Permanently stained smear

514. *Babesia* sp. is an organism that has been recovered in a number of human infections worldwide. In an examination of stained blood films, these organisms are likely to resemble
   A. *Leishmania donovani*
   B. *Plasmodium falciparum*
   C. *Toxoplasma gondii*
   D. *Trypanosoma cruzi*

515. Which of the following is not a fixative or preservative used for detection of parasites in stool specimens?
   A. PVA
   B. Formalin
   C. Buffered glycerol
   D. MIF

516. Examination of a fecal smear following acid-fast stain reveals round acid-fast positive structures 8–10 μm in diameter. You should suspect
   A. Microsporidia
   B. *Cryptosporidium*
   C. *Isospora*
   D. *Cyclospora*

517. Visceral leishmaniasis is caused by
   A. *Trypanosoma cruzi*
   B. *Trypanosoma brucei gambiense*
   C. *Leishmania donovani*
   D. *Loa loa*

518. *Pneumocystis carinii* is detected by obtaining specimens from the
   A. Lung
   B. Liver
   C. Brain
   D. Kidney

519. Diagnosis of pediculosis (louse infection) depends upon detection of
   A. Eggs (nits) attached to hair or clothing
   B. Larvae in domestic surroundings

C. Tunnel of insects in skin
D. Specific antibodies in patient serum

520. A patient with history of human immuno-deficiency virus infection presents with a 5-day history of diarrhea and weight loss. A series of stool specimens is collected and examined for the presence of ova and parasites. An acid-fast stain on direct smear reveals pink-stained round structures approximately 4 μm in diameter. The most likely pathogen is
   A. *Blastocystis hominis*
   B. *Cryptosporidium* sp.
   C. *Isospora* sp.
   D. Microsporidium

521. A 65-year-old female presents to her physician complaining of a fever that "comes and goes" and fatigue. A CBC reveals decreased red blood cell count and hemoglobin. History reveals the patient recently traveled through Europe and Africa. You should suspect
   A. Filariasis
   B. Cutaneous larval migrans
   C. Trichinella
   D. Malaria

522. The disease most commonly associated with *Acanthamoeba* sp. is
   A. Meningoencephalitis
   B. Diarrhea
   C. Keratitis
   D. Liver abscess

523. A modified trichrome stain of a fecal smear can be used to detect microsporidia. Which of the following would describe the appearance of this parasite in this stain?
   A. Purple circles, 10–15 μm in diameter
   B. Pink ovals, 1–3 μm in diameter
   C. Blue ovals, 4–6 μm in diameter
   D. Fluorescent circles, 8–12 μm in diameter

524. Hydatid cysts in humans are due to ingestion of a tapeworm stage normally infective for herbivores. This stage is the
   A. Embryonated egg
   B. Cercocystis
   C. Cysticercus
   D. Cercaria

525. Which of the following is a stage of *Toxoplasma gondii* infective for humans?
   A. Cercocyst
   B. Gonad
   C. Leptomonad
   D. Oocyst

526. A 15 μm pear-shaped flagellate with a visible parabasal body and "falling leaf" motility in a direct saline mount of a diarrheal stool specimen is most probably
   A. *Chilomastix mesnili*
   B. *Enteromonas hominis*
   C. *Giardia lamblia*
   D. *Trichomonas hominis*

527. Humans, especially children, are occasional hosts of this cestode parasite of dogs, cats, and wild carnivora. Transmission results from accidental swallowing of infected fleas from dogs or cats. Finding the proglottids or eggs in the feces is diagnostic. This parasite is
   A. *Dipylidium caninum*
   B. *Echinococcus granulosus*
   C. *Hymenolepsis diminuta*
   D. *Toxocara canis*

528. Knowledge of nocturnal periodicity is especially important in the diagnosis of certain infections caused by
   A. *Plasmodium*
   B. *Babesia*
   C. Microfilaria
   D. *Sarcoptes scabei*

529. For which of the following diseases is close contact with an infected human host the most important mechanism of transmission?
   A. Toxoplasmosis
   B. Schistosomiasis
   C. Trichinosis
   D. Trichomoniasis

530. Which of the following helminths produces an elongate, barrel-shaped egg (50 × 22 μm) with a colorless polar plug at each end?
   A. *Ascaris lumbricoides*
   B. *Trichuris trichiura*
   C. *Hymenolepsis nana*
   D. *Necator americanus*

531. Which species of *Plasmodium* may readily be identified when crescent-shaped gametocytes are found in stained blood films?
   A. *P. vivax*
   B. *P. falciparum*
   C. *P. malariae*
   D. *P. ovale*

532. Cysticercosis is caused by the disseminated larvae of
   A. *Echinococcus granulosus*
   B. *Hymenolepsis nana*
   C. *Necator americanus*
   D. *Taenia solium*

533. Visceral larval migrans is associated with which of the following organisms?
   A. *Ancylostoma duodenale*
   B. *Dracunculus medinensis*
   C. *Onchocerca volvulus*
   D. *Toxocara canis*

534. A free-living ameba that causes primary amebic meningoencephalitis is
   A. *Naegleria fowleri*
   B. *Entamoeba gingivalis*
   C. *Entamoeba histolytica*
   D. *Entamoeba polecki*

535. Decontamination of drinking water, fruits, and vegetables before consumption is necessary in countries without well-developed public sanitation. Which of the following diseases would probably be least affected by that kind of precaution?
    A. Amebiasis
    B. Ascariasis
    C. Filariasis
    D. Giardiasis

536. Which stage of *Taenia saginata* is usually infective for humans?
    A. Cysticercus larva
    B. Embryonated egg
    C. Filariform larva
    D. Rhabditiform larva

537. This amebic cyst has an average size of 6–8 μm and is usually spherical. When mature, it has four nuclei, but immature cysts with one or two nuclei are often seen. The nuclei have fine uniform granules of peripheral chromatin and small, discrete, usually central karyosomes. Chromatoidal bars with bluntly rounded ends are often present. Name the species.
    A. *Endolimax nana*
    B. *Entamoeba coli*
    C. *Entamoeba hartmanni*
    D. *Entamoeba histolytica*

538. Which stage of *Trichuris trichiura* is infective for humans?
    A. Rhabditiform larva
    B. Fully embryonated egg
    C. Filariform larva
    D. Proglottid

539. For which of the following diseases do reduviid bugs serve as vectors?
    A. Chagas' disease (American trypanosomiasis)
    B. African sleeping sickness
    C. Kala azar
    D. Malaria

540. Sanitary disposal of human feces is the most important factor in decreasing the incidence of most infections with intestinal parasites. Which of the following diseases would not be affected by that kind of sanitation?
    A. Ascariasis
    B. Hookworm infection
    C. Trichinosis
    D. Taeniasis

541. With which species of malarial parasite are Schüffner's dots found in the infected erythrocytes?
    A. *Plasmodium falciparum*
    B. *Plasmodium knowlesi*
    C. *Plasmodium malariae*
    D. *Plasmodium ovale*

542. The World Health Organization currently has a campaign to eliminate step wells to prevent transmission of the nematode parasite that is thought to have been the "fiery serpent" of the ancient Israelites. This parasite, which has various species of *Cyclops* (water fleas) as its intermediate host, is
    A. *Dicrocoelium dendriticum*
    B. *Dracunculus medinensis*
    C. *Diphyllobothrium latum*
    D. *Dipylidium caninum*

543. The rhabditiform larva of *Strongyloides stercoralis*
    A. Is rarely passed in the feces
    B. Has a prominent genital primordium
    C. Has a notched tip of tail
    D. Is infective for humans

544. Because of the possibility of drug resistance or the persistence of exoerythrocytic parasites, identification of the causative species can be important in the choice of treatment for malaria. Which species of *Plasmodium* may have exoerythrocytic stages capable of causing relapses up to 3 or more years after initial infection?
    A. *P. falciparum*
    B. *P. ovale*
    C. *P. malariae*
    D. *P. cynomolgi*

545. A Giemsa-stained thick blood film showed many ring forms with no older stages, and a number of the rings had double chromatin dots. These findings are characteristic of
    A. *Plasmodium falciparum*
    B. *Plasmodium vivax*
    C. *Plasmodium malariae*
    D. *Plasmodium ovale*

546. Which of the following nematode (round-worm) parasites is acquired from eating inadequately cooked, infected pork?
    A. *Strongyloides stercoralis*
    B. *Taenia solium*
    C. *Taenia saginata*
    D. *Trichinella spiralis*

547. Which of the following pairs of helminths *cannot* be reliably differentiated by the appearance of their eggs?
    A. *Ascaris lumbricoides* and *N. americanus*
    B. *Hymenolepsis nana* and *H. diminuta*
    C. *Necator americanus* and *Ancylostoma duodenale*
    D. *Diphyllobothrium latum* and *Dipylidium caninum*

548. Which of the following forms of *Toxoplasma gondii* are produced in infected humans?
    A. Bradyzoites
    B. Macrogametes
    C. Sporoblasts
    D. Oocysts

549. Hematuria is one typical sign of human infection caused by
    A. *Trypanosoma cruzi*
    B. *Trichinella spiralis*
    C. *Trichomonas vaginalis*
    D. *Schistosoma haematobium*

550. Which of the following is the most important vector for *Babesia* sp.?
    A. Fleas
    B. Ticks
    C. Lice
    D. Mosquitoes

551. Chagas' disease (American trypanosomiasis) is caused by
    A. *Trypanosoma brucei rhodesiense*
    B. *Trypanosoma cruzi*
    C. *Leishmania braziliensis*
    D. *Mansonella perstans*

552. A 40-year-old resident of Virginia presented to his physician with fever, muscle pain, periorbital edema, and eosinophilia. The case history revealed the patient had consumed locally produced pork sausage about 10 days previously. From what disease is this patient most likely suffering?
    A. Chagas' disease
    B. Cryptosporidiosis
    C. Trichinosis
    D. Giardiasis

553. Refer to Color Plate 38. This is a photomicrograph of a trichrome stain of a fecal smear, magnification 400×. The parasite measures 65 × 45 μm. What is the identification of this parasite?
    A. *Balantidium coli*
    B. *Diphyllobothrium latum*
    C. *Giardia lamblia*
    D. *Schistosoma japonicum*

554. Refer to Color Plate 39. This is a photomicrograph of an iodine wet prep made from a stool sample; magnification is 400×. The ovum is about 70 × 50 μm. What is the identification of the parasite?
    A. Hookworm
    B. *Enterobius vermicularis*
    C. *Trichuris trichiura*
    D. *Ascaris lumbricoides*

555. Refer to Color Plate 40. This is a photomicrograph of an iron hematoxylin stain from a fecal smear. The magnification is 1,000×. The parasite is approximately 20 μm long and 15 μm wide. What is the identification of this parasite?
    A. *Chilomastix mesnili* trophozoite
    B. *Giardia lamblia* trophozoite
    C. *Trichomonas hominis* trophozoite
    D. *Trichomonas tenax* trophozoite

556. Refer to Color Plate 41. This is a photomicrograph of an iron hematoxylin stain from a fecal smear. The magnification is 1,000×. The parasite is approximately 12 μm in diameter. What is the identification of this parasite?
    A. *Entamoeba histolytica* trophozoite
    B. *Entamoeba hartmanni* trophozoite
    C. *Dientamoeba fragilis* trophozoite
    D. *Entamoeba coli* trophozoite

557. Refer to Color Plate 42. This is a photomicrograph of an iodine wet-mount from a fecal sample. The magnification is 1,000×. The parasite is approximately 25 μm in diameter. What is the identification of this parasite?
    A. *Entamoeba histolytica* cyst
    B. *Entamoeba histolytica* trophozoite
    C. *Entamoeba coli* cyst
    D. *Entamoeba coli* trophozoite

558. Refer to Color Plate 43. This is a photomicrograph of an iodine wet-mount from a fecal sample. The magnification is 400×. The ovum is approximately 70 × 38 μm. What is the identification of this parasite?
    A. Hookworm
    B. *Ascaris lumbricoides*
    C. *Diphyllobothrium latum*
    D. *Taenia solium*

559. Refer to Color Plate 44. This is a photomicrograph of a trichrome stain from a fecal smear. The magnification is 1,000×. The parasite is approximately 15 μm in diameter. What is the identification of this parasite?
    A. *Entamoeba hartmanni*
    B. *Dientamoeba fragilis*
    C. *Iodamoeba bütschlii*
    D. *Blastocystis hominis*

560. Refer to Color Plate 45. This is a photomicrograph of a blood smear stained with Wright's stain. Identify the parasite.
    A. *Babesia* sp.
    B. *Plasmodium malariae*
    C. *Plasmodium falciparum*
    D. *Trypanosoma cruzi*

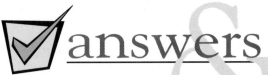
answers & rationales

AEROBIC BACTERIA

1.

A. The etiologic agents of brucellosis are the *Brucellae*, which are small, nonmotile, gram-negative coccobacilli that are intracellular parasites. Isolation of these organisms is difficult. In suspected cases, which are generally job related, multiple blood cultures are recommended for optimal recovery of the agent. Bone marrow cultures have been found to be positive when cultures of blood failed to recover the organism.

2.

B. Members of the genus *Klebsiella* have a capsule and appear mucoid on cultures. *Klebsiella pneumoniae* is the species most frequently recovered from the vast majority of clinical cases. This highly encapsulated organism can cause severe pneumonia, nosocomial infections of several types, infantile enteritis, and other extraintestinal infections.

3.

B. Mycobacteria characteristically possess a high lipid content, unlike gram-positive cocci, and gram-negative bacteria. The high lipid content acts to protect these organisms from dehydration and the lethal effects of alkali, various germicides, alcohol, and acids. Thus an acid-fast staining technique can be used for the demonstration of these organisms.

4.

A. Enterotoxins are produced in the intestinal tract and cause diarrhea or vomiting in the patient. The heat-la-bile enterotoxin of *Escherichia coli,* which resembles cholera toxin, acts to stimulate the enzyme adenylate cyclase. Diarrhea results following stimulation of the net output of chloride ions by the cells lining the small intestine. The stimulation of the enzyme adenylate cyclase by the toxin increases the output of cyclic AMP, causing rapid gastrointestinal fluid loss.

5.

A. *Chlamydia trachomatis,* one of the four species of *Chlamydia,* is the causative agent of trachoma, STD, inclusion conjunctivitis and lymphogranuloma venereum. Trachoma is a primary cause of blindness in the world. The disease is preventable, but when it is not treated, the organism produces hypertrophy of the lymphoid follicles on the inner surface of the upper eyelid. This process causes the upper eyelid to evert (entropion), which ultimately leads to blindness. Smears and culture of scrapings from the conjunctiva will demonstrate the organism.

6.

C. The genus *Neisseria* contains organisms that possess cytochrome oxidase activity. Colonies can be identified by the development of a dark purple color following the application of tetramethyl-*p*-phenylenediamine dihydrochloride. The reaction relies on the property of the dye to substitute for oxygen as an electron acceptor. In the presence of the enzyme and atmospheric oxygen the dye is oxidized to form indophenol blue.

7.

B. *Enterococcus* or group D streptococci in particular are able to be presumptively identified based on their ability to hydrolyze esculin in the presence of 1–4% bile salts. The medium is made selective for streptococci either by the addition of sodium azide or bile salts in the concentration of 4%. Organisms able to grow in this medium produce esculetin, which reacts with an iron salt to form a black color in the agar.

8.

A. The optimal growth temperature of *Mycobacterium xenopi* is 42 °C, which enables its survival and replication as an environmental contaminant in hot water systems. Human infections caused by *M. xenopi* are rare. The majority of clinically significant species, those not known to cause cutaneous infections, have an optimal growth temperature of 37 °C.

9.

A. *Shigella* has a low infecting dose and has been reported to cause outbreaks in day-care centers and can be spread to family members. These organisms are found in humans only at the time of infection; they are not part of the normal flora. Transmission is by the fecal-oral route. Infection is by ingestion of contaminated foods or water.

10.

A. *Chryseobacterium* species are ubiquitous in the environment and are especially associated with moist soil and water. *Chryseobacterium* (previously identified as *Flavobacterium meningosepticum*), a known nosocomial pathogen, has been implicated in outbreaks of meningitis in hospitals associated with the use of contaminated respiratory therapy equipment. Adult human infections are rare, with these opportunistic microorganisms occurring primarily in immunocompromised patients.

11.

D. *Mycobacterium leprae* cannot be cultivated on artificial media to date. The growth of *Mycobacterium leprae* can be supported in experimental animals: the armadillo and the foot pads of mice. All the other organisms can be cultivated on artificial media.

12.

A. Growth on MacConkey agar is a test used for the differentiation of rapid-growing mycobacteria. For the test a MacConkey agar plate is inoculated with a 7-day broth culture of the test organism. The in-

oculated plate is then incubated at 37 °C for at least 5 days. Plates are checked for growth at 5 days, and if no growth is detected, they are checked daily until day 11, at which time they are discarded as negative. *M. fortuitum* and *M. chelonei* are the only mycobacteria able to grow on MacConkey agar in 5 days. *Mycobacterium phlei* is recommended as a negative growth control for this test.

13.

D. *Shigella dysenteriae*, the type species of the genus, is a causative agent of bacillary dysentery. Differential and selective media for the recovery of enteric pathogens from stool samples would demonstrate *Shigella* species as non-H_2S-producing, non-lactose-fermenting, gram-negative bacilli. Further biochemical testing would generally show these organisms to be unable to use citrate as their sole carbon source, unable to decarboxylate the amino acid lysine, and unable to degrade urea. On triple sugar iron (TSI) agar, *Shigella* species generally produce acid in the butt, an alkaline reaction on the slant, and no gas or H_2S.

14.

D. Strains of *Corynebacterium diphtheriae* infected by a lysogenic bacteriophage produce an extremely potent acidic globular protein toxin. Absorption of the toxin may cause a rapidly fatal hypertoxic disease characterized by myocarditis and neuritis. This disease most commonly affects children ages 1 to 10 years. Transmission is by contact with a human carrier or contact with contaminated fomites.

15.

B. Staphylococcal enterocolitis food poisoning cases result from the ingestion of contaminated foods containing preformed thermostable enterotoxin. This form of intoxication causes a perfuse and watery diarrhea due to the loss of electrolytes and fluids into the lumen. In many cases, the causative agent may never be recovered from patient specimens.

16.

A. *Aeromonas hydrophila* have a water source as their habitat and have been implicated in human infections. Growth on MacConkey agar and a positive oxidase reaction are key tests for the presumptive identification of this organism. A positive oxidase reaction eliminates this organism from the Enterobacteriaceae. On blood agar many strains of *Aeromonas* produce zones of beta hemolysis, which aids in their differentiation.

17.

B. A highly selective media, TCBS is used for the isolation of *Vibrio* species. Vibrios that are able to ferment sucrose, such as *V. cholerae,* produce yellow colonies. Non–sucrose fermenting organisms produce green colonies.

18.

B. The K antigen (envelope) surrounds the bacterial cell and acts to mask the somatic antigens of the cell wall, which are used to group members of the *Enterobacteriaceae.* These heat-labile antigens are able to be removed by heating a suspension of the unagglutinable culture at 100 °C for 10 to 30 minutes. Antisera that contain K antibody (Vi antiserum) can be used to demonstrate the presence of the envelope antigens. *Salmonella typhi* and certain strains of *Escherichia coli* possess the K antigen.

19.

D. *Mycoplasma pneumoniae*, part of the normal flora of humans, causes primary atypical pneumonia. The convalescent serum of infected patients shows an increase in cold agglutination titers. The typical clinical syndrome has a 2- to 3-week incubation period leading to fever, headache, and a characteristic nonproductive paroxysmal cough. Chest films of such patients may show bilateral infiltrates, although physical examination reveals few chest findings.

20.

B. Nutritionally variant streptococci (NVS) are now termed *Abiotrophia*. These clinically significant microorganisms, which account for 5 to 6% of the cases of endocarditis, are frequently not able to be recovered because of insufficient quantities of vitamin B_6 in the culture medium selected. The routine use of a pyridoxal disk, a streak of *Staphylococcus,* or vitamin B_6 supplemented culture media is required for isolation.

21.

C. Scalded skin syndrome is a form of dermatitis produced by strains of *Staphylococcus aureus* that elaborate exfoliative toxin. Two types of this toxin have been identified, exfoliation A and exfoliation B. This potent toxin acts by disturbing the adhesive forces between cells of the stratum granulosum, which causes the appearance of the clear, large, flaccid bullae and the skin to actually peel away. Infants and children are most commonly affected with this form of dermatitis, beginning about the face and trunk with subsequent spread to the extremities.

22.

C. *Mycobacterium scrofulaceum* is defined as a scotochromogen because of its characteristic of pigmenting in the dark. This slow-growing *Mycobacterium* is a cause of cervical adenitis and other types of infections predominantly in children. Therapy may require susceptibility studies that include the secondary drugs, since the organism is known in some cases to be resistant to isoniazid and streptomycin.

23.

A. Cold hemagglutinins were first noted in the serum of patients with primary atypical pneumonia in 1943. When incubated at 0–10 °C, these macroglobulins in serum cause human erythrocytes to clump. Although this is not a specific test, for *Mycoplasma pneumoniae* infections, a single titer of greater than 1:128 is considered significant. Approximately half of patients with atypical pneumonia demonstrate a positive result. The most widely used tests today are complement fixation (CF) and the enzyme-linked immunosorbent assay (ELISA).

24.

C. Presumptive identification of group A streptococci can be achieved through the PYR (L-pyrrolidonyl-β-naphthlylamide) disk test. The use of a 0.04-u bacitracin disk is no longer recommended because groups C and G streptococci are also susceptible to this agent. A positive test result is interpreted as a bright red color change within 5 minutes.

25.

B. *Burkholderia pseudomallei* can survive in macrophages. It is found in soil and water in subtropical areas of Southeast Asia and Australia. Melioidosis has several forms from skin abscesses to abscess formation in internal organs.

26.

D. *Francisella tularensis* requires the presence of these amino acids for growth. Glucose-cysteine with thiamine and cystine heart agar are commercially available for suspected cases of tularemia. They both require the addition of 5% sheep or rabbbit blood.

27.

A. The family *Micrococcaceae* contains both *Staphylococcus*, which is an important human pathogen, and the genus *Micrococcus*. In the clinical laboratory the differentiation of *Micrococcus* from *Staphylococcus* assumes importance. A series of tests for the identification of *Micrococcus* are used.

28.

C. A recent development for the definitive identification of *Mycobacterium malmoense* and *Mycobacterium szulgai* has been the use of gas-liquid chromatography. Differences in lipid content of the mycobacterial cell walls can be determined. Previously unrecognized species such as *Mycobacterium szulgai* demonstrate unique lipid patterns, which have enabled their characterization.

29.

B. Decubitus ulcers frequently contain normal intestinal flora. In the case presented the microorganism isolated was *Escherichia coli*, which is characteristically indole positive and citrate negative and ferments lactose. *Escherichia coli* is associated with a variety of diseases, being the predominant organism associated with cases of neonatal meningitis, specticemia, cystitis, appendicitis, and endocarditis.

30.

D. *Pseudomonasa aeruignosa* is the most commonly encountered gram-negative species that is not a member of the family *Enterobacteriaceae*. It is ubiquitous in nature and is found in environments in homes and hospitals. It is an opportunistic pathogen that is responsible for nosocomial infections.

31.

A. *Capnocytophaga* are fermentative gram-negative bacteria that are inhabitants of the human oral cavity. These organisms have been identified as a cause of disease in the oral cavity, and in compro-

mised hosts they have been implicated in systemic disease being isolated from CSF, pleural fluid, and pulmonary secretions. The gliding motility is best observed during the log phase of growth and can be demonstrated by dark-field microscopy and on blood agar medium by the production of concentrically spreading growth around primary colonies.

32.

C. *Vibrio vulnificus* is implicated in wound infections and septicemia. The organism is found in brackish or salt water. Ingestion of contaminated water or seafood is the mode of transmission; wound infections are associated with contamination at the site with organisms in water.

33.

D. The Waterhouse-Friderichsen syndrome of disseminated intravascular clotting occurs in cases of fulminant meningococcemia. Invasion of the circulatory system by *Neisseria meningitidis* may produce only a transient bacteremia or meningitis or may go on to cause a rapidly fatal infection. In cases of meningococcemia with intravascular coagulation, acute adrenal insufficiency due to hemorrhage into the adrenal gland may result.

34.

A. *Chlamydia* are obligate intracellular parasites. In chlamydial infections the recovery of the organism is often required for a definitive diagnosis. Tissue culture techniques are therefore required, and McCoy cells are the recommended host cell type. The monolayer of inoculated cells is stained and examined microscopically for the presence of intracellular inclusions.

35.

D. Human infections with *Chlamydia psittaci* (psittacosis) occur after exposure to infected birds and their droppings. A true zoonosis, psittacosis is a disease of birds that may be contracted by humans. The disease produced by this organism may be mild or fulminant, with a high mortality rate. Clinical manifestations of the disease include severe headache, weakness, and mild pulmonary symptoms.

36.

A. Nocardiosis, a bacterial disease, is characterized by mycetoma or chronic suppurative infection. Draining sinus tracts in the subcutaneous tissue are a common manifestation of the disease. *Nocardia* are soil saprophytes that may produce disease in humans either by the inhalation of contaminated material or through skin abrasions. Microscopic examination of pus from suspected cases will demonstrate this partially acid-fast, gram-positive, branching filamentous or coccoid organism.

37.

B. The strain of *Haemophilus influenzae* found to be implicated in the majority of cases of bacterial meningitis is surrounded by a polyribitol phosphate capsule and identified as the specific antigenic type b. Meningeal infections with this agent were most common in children 1 to 6 years of age. The widespread use of Hib vaccine beginning in 1985 has significantly reduced the incidence of invasive *H. influenzae* type b disease.

38.

A. Infection caused by *Erysipelothrix rhusiopathiae* in humans is primarily erysipeloid. Erysipeloid is usually the result of contact with an infected animal or contaminated animal product. The characteristic appearance is one of cutaneous spreading lesions of the fingers or hand that are raised and erythematous. Although disease is generally confined to the skin, it has been implicated in rare cases of endocarditis.

39.

B. Improperly home-canned foods, especially low-acid-content vegetables, cause the majority of the cases of food-borne botulism. The ubiquitous nature of *Clostridium botulinum* enables the spores to contaminate a variety of foods. Contamination and subsequent germination under anaerobic conditions stimulate toxin formation. The patient becomes ill following the ingestion of food that contains nanograms of preformed toxin.

40.

C. The *N*-acetyl-L-cysteine-sodium hydroxide (NALC-NaOH) method is recommended since the addition of NALC reduced the concentration of NaOH to only 2%. The NALC is a mucolytic agent which frees trapped organisms in the sample and the NaOH acts to decontaminate the sample. The optimal treatment reduces the numbers of indigenous microorganisms present in the sample without significantly reducing the number of tubercle bacilli.

41.

A. Unlike typical *Salmonellae*, *Salmonella typhi* produces only a small amount of hydrogen sulfide, produces no gas in glucose, is not able to utilize citrate, and possesses the K antigen. Identification of *Salmonella typhi*, the etiologic agent of typhoid fever, may be delayed if laboratory professionals do not have a good appreciation of its atypical characteristics. Also important to note is that the presence of the bacilli in the patient's circulatory system several days before culture of stool will be positive for this agent.

42.

B. *Streptococcus agalactiae* isolates can be presumptively identified by the demonstration of a positive CAMP reaction. Group B streptococci elaborate the CAMP factor, which acts to enhance the zone of hemolysis produced by beta-lysin-producing strains of *Staphylococcus aureus*. Incubation of test plates should be carried out in normal air, since increased CO_2 and anaerobic incubation increase the rate of false-positive CAMP reactions by group A streptococci.

43.

D. DNA probes are widely used for the detection of clinically significant organisms, which are difficult to grow or grow slowly such as *M. tuberculosis*. Gen-Probe (San Diego, CA), as an example, has developed probes targeted to bacterial ribosomal RNA. There are hybridization and amplification methods available, both of which are based on the specificity of a nucleotide sequence for a particular organism.

44.

B. The recovery rate of coagulase-negative *Staphylococcus saprophyticus* from urinary tract infections in young females is second only to that of *Escherichia coli*. The organism has a predilection for the epithelial cells of the urogenital tract and is often seen in large numbers adhering to these cells on Gram stain. Key to the identification of this coagulase-negative *Staphylococcus* is its resistance to novobiocin.

45.

A. Chancroid or soft chancre is caused by *Haemophilus ducreyi*, a small, gram-negative coccobacillus. Painful genital lesions and painful swelling of the inguinal lymph nodes characterize the disease chancroid. The incubation period following contact with an infected person ranges from 1 to 5 days, after which the patient notes the painful, round, nonindurated primary lesion on the external genitalia. Signs of regional lymphadenitis appear in about one-half of the cases a few days after the appearance of the primary lesion. Isolation of the agent is the only definitive diagnostic method.

46.

B. The organism seen in Color Plate 26 is *Listeria monocytogenes. Listeria* is a significant human and animal pathogen, which is known to cause abortion, meningitis, and septicemia in humans. This gram-positive rod is actively motile at room temperature, hydrolyzes esculin, produces catalase, and is oxidase negative. When recovered on sheep blood agar plates from clinical samples, it is often initially confused with group A or group B streptococci because of its beta hemolysis.

47.

C. Disseminated gonococcal infection (DGI) produces symptoms of arthritis, especially in the major joints of the body. Samples of joint fluid from these patients should be inoculated to a selective medium for the isolation of *Neisseria gonorrhoeae* in addition to nonselective media. Thayer-Martin agar is basically a chocolate agar with the addition of antibiotic inhibitors that has been formulated to support the growth of fastidious species of *Neisseria* while suppressing the growth of normal or indigenous flora.

48.

C. Leprosy (Hansen's disease) is caused by the acid-fast bacterium *Mycobacterium leprae*. Chronic skin lesions and sensory loss characterize this disease. Skin or biopsy specimens taken from within the margin of a lesion will demonstrate the causative agent. Cultures of this agent on artificial media, unlike other mycobacteria, have not been successful to date. Cultivation can be accomplished by injecting bacilli into the foot pads of mice or systemically into armadillos.

49.

B. *Campylobacter jejuni* rivals *Salmonella* as the most common bacterial cause of diarrheal disease in humans. *Campylobacter* enterocolitis is characterized by fever, bloody diarrhea, and abdominal pain. Special selective culture media and incubation under a microaerophilic atmosphere at 42 °C are required for the recovery of this organism from clinical samples.

50.

C. *Streptococcus agalactiae* (group B streptococci) is a principal cause of bacterial meningitis and septicemia in neonates. The organism, which is a part of the indigenous microbial flora of the vagina, is transmitted by the mother of the child before birth, usually as it passes through the birth canal. Neonatal infection with group B streptococci may occur either as an early onset disease (at birth) or as a delayed-onset syndrome that manifests itself weeks after birth.

51.

A. Screening procedures for the recovery of the enteric pathogen *Salmonella* rely heavily on differential media, which indicate lactose fermentation and the production of H_2S. Isolates of *Shewanella putrefaciens* recovered from stool samples on a medium such as Hektoen enteric agar would resemble *Salmonella* in that the organism is not able to ferment lactose and does produce a significant amount of H_2S. Diagnostic serotyping of such suspect isolates from TSI using polyvalent salmonella antisera would be negative.

52.

C. Molecular relationship studies among the *Salmonellae* have shown that the "Arizona group" of organisms, once considered to be a separate genus, should be reclassified as members of the genus *Salmonella*. The former *Arizona hinshawii* is now reported by reference laboratories as *Salmonella* serotype 47:r:z. Reclassification of *Enterobacteriaceae* is based on several types of testing: DNA-DNA hybridization, phenotypic characteristics, biochemical features, and susceptibility patterns.

53.

C. The vegetative cells and spores of *Bacillus cereus* are widely distributed in the environment. The virulence mechanisms of *B. cereus* are an enterotoxin and a pyogenic toxin. Traumatic introduction into a normally sterile site through the use of contaminated medical equipment, an accident in nature, intravenous drug abuse, or ingestion of contaminated foods are associated with infection.

54.

D. Whooping cough or pertussis is caused by *Bordetella pertussis,* a minute, encapsulated, non-motile, gram-negative, pleomorphic bacillus. The best identification method is PCR. For isolation of this agent the recommendation is Regan-Lowe medium. The disease is characterized by a peculiar paroxysmal cough, ending in a whooping inspiration; culture usually negative after paroxysmal coughing begins.

55.

D. The formation of the characteristic *Corynebacterium diphtheriae* granules and cellular morphology seen in methylene blue stains is enhanced when the organism is grown on Loeffler's serum medium. Although this medium is primarily designed for the recovery of *Corynebacterium diphtheriae* from clinical samples, the beef serum in it makes Loeffler's medium generally useful for the demonstration of an organism's proteolytic activity. The grayish white agar slant, when inoculated, may demonstrate growth of corynebacteria within 8 to 24 hours. Since this is not a differential medium, colonies present are smeared to observe their morphology, and suspect growth removed to be streaked on tellurite agar.

56.

C. *Francisella tularensis,* a small, nonmotile, aerobic, gram-negative bacillus requires enriched culture media such as blood-cysteine-glucose agar for isolation from clinical specimens. Clinical material for culture of this highly infectious agent should be handled with care. Ordinary microbiology labs should not attempt isolation but send instead to a reference lab for handling. The amount of inoculum per plate should not exceed 0.2–0.3 mL. Culture plates should be kept free of surface moisture, which is inhibitory, and should be incubated at 35–37 °C in an air or CO_2 incubator. On enriched media, smooth, gray colonies should appear after 18 to 24 hours.

57.

D. *Neisseria gonorrhoeae* is a primary pathogen of the urogenital tract. It is a leading cause of sexually transmitted disease. Surface structures such as pili aid in attachment to mucosal epithelial cells and invasion of submucosa to produce infection.

58.

C. Tinsdale medium, for the primary isolation of *Corynebacterium diphtheriae*, not only inhibits indigenous respiratory flora but differentiates colonies of *Corynebacterium diphtheriae*. The potassium tellurite in the medium is taken up by colonies of *Corynebacterium*, causing them to appear black. Colonies of *Corynebacterium diphtheriae* are presumptively identified when black colonies surrounded by a brown halo are seen on this agar medium.

59.

A. *Salmonella enteritidis* characteristically produces hydrogen sulfide in triple sugar iron (TSI) agar. As seen in Color Plate 27 they demonstrate a positive lysine and a negative urease reaction, which differentiates them from *Proteus* species, which also produce H_2S. It is important to be able to quickly differentiate those organisms that resemble *Salmonella* from other H_2S producing organisms such as *Citrobacter* and *Edwardsiella.*

60.

A. *Neisseria* and *Moraxella (Branhamella)* are most commonly described as having a "kidney bean" cellular morphology. These gram-negative coccal organisms appear characteristically as diplococci with the paired cells having adjacent walls, which are flattened. *Neisseria* are an important human pathogen, causing the venereal disease gonorrhea and meningitis most notably. In males suspected of having *Neisseria gonorrhoeae* a clinical diagnosis can be made based on the presence of characteristic symptoms and the observation of gram-negative diplococci in a smear of urethral discharge.

61.

D. The Elek immunodiffusion test is recommended for the detection of toxigenic strains of *Corynebacterium diphtheriae*. In the test, diphtheria antitoxin is impregnated on a sterile filter paper strip, which is pressed onto the surface of an Elek agar plate. Test strains and control strains are then inoculated perpendicular to the strip on both sides and without contacting the strip. A positive reaction, given by toxigenic strains, demonstrates the formation of a precipitin line at a 45-degree angle to the inoculum streak.

62.

C. Erysipelas results from person-to-person transmission of group A streptococci. Symptoms occur when nasopharyngeal infection spreads to the face. The rare complication of an upper respiratory infection with *Streptococcus pyogenes* is characterized by sensations of burning and tightness at the site of invasion. Erythema associated with this superficial cellulitis rapidly spreads with an advancing elevated margin. The causative agent may be recovered from these lesions from either the center of the erysipeloid or the advancing margin.

63.

A. Phenylethyl alcohol agar (PEA) is a selective culture medium for the isolation of gram-positive cocci. Blood agar medium is supplemented with 0.15% phenylethyl alcohol to create a medium that will be inhibitory to most gram-negative aerobic bacilli. This medium is particularly helpful when a specimen containing gram-positive cocci is contaminated with a *Proteus* species due to the inhibition of swarming by PEA.

64.

C. The Center for Disease Control has adopted the diagnostic standards recommended by the American Thoracic Society as published in 1981. This is a method of reporting the number of acid-fast bacilli observed in fuchsin stained smears of clinical material. A count of up to nine acid-fast bacilli per field should be reported as a positive at 3+.

65.

C. *B. cepacia* is the most common *Burkolderia* spp. in clinical specimens. *P. aeruginosa* is the most common gram-negative bacillus that is not in the *Enterobacteriaceae* family and *Stenotrophomonas maltophilia* the second most common. *B. pseudomallei* is not commonly isolated in the United States

66.

D. Viridans or greening streptococci are the most common normal flora in upper respiratory cultures. They are opportunistic pathogens with low virulence. Subacute endocarditis is seen in patients with previously damaged heart valves.

67.

A. Ophthalmia neonatorum, a specific form of conjunctivitis, is the most common manifestation of neonatal infection with *Neisseria gonorrhoeae*. The infection is transmitted to the child by the mother as it passes through the birth canal. The use of an ophthalmic solution of silver nitrate is recommended for the prevention of this form of conjunctivitis.

68.

B. *Neisseria lactamica* is a component of the normal nasopharyngeal flora of humans. In the laboratory this agent may be mistakenly identified as *Neisseria meningitidis*, an organism of significant pathogenicity. Differentiation of these two species is easily accomplished by demonstrating the fermentation of lactose or an ONPG (*o*-nitrophenyl-beta-galactopyranoside) positive test.

69.

A. Previously known as *Haemophilus aegyptius*, the causative agent of "pinkeye" is now known to be a biotype III of *Haemophilus influenzae*. This form of conjunctivitis is highly contagious and is frequently seen in children attending day-care centers. The agent is an aerobic gram-negative bacillus that is nonmotile and requires both hemin (X factor) and nicotine adenine dinucleotide (NAD, V factor) for growth.

70.

D. *Hafnia* is a member of the *Enterobacteriaceae* family. It was previously known as *Enterobacter hafnia* and thought to be a cause of extraintestinal infections of humans. This organism has been reclassified as the genus *Hafnia,* which contains the single species *alvei*. The characteristics of this organism are positive motility and lysine, ornithine, ONPG, and KCN reactions.

71.

C. *Acinetobacter* sp. are opportunistic pathogens for humans. They are similar to *Neisseriaceae* with the exception of being oxidase negative. Their gram-negative coccoid appearance frequently leads to a microscopic reporting of the presence of *Neisseria* in a clinical specimen.

72.

A. Pontiac fever is caused by *Legionella pneumophila*, as is Legionnaires' disease, but it is not as serious an infection. This febrile illness is characteristically self-limited and does not demonstrate significant pulmonary symptoms. The incubation period, unlike that for Legionnaires' disease, is short, followed by symptoms of malaise, muscle aches, chills, fever, and headache.

73.

D. *Brucella* species are fastidious, gram-negative, coccobacillary organisms. They are predominantly animal pathogens but occasionally produce disease in humans. The differentiation of the species is made by noting the differences in their physiologic and biochemical properties. *Brucella melitensis* does not require increased carbon dioxide for growth, is able to produce hydrogen sulfide, and can grow in the presence of both basic fuchsin and thionine.

74.

A. *E. coli* O157:H7 produces a toxin similar to Shiga toxin produced by *Shigella dysenteriae*. It is transmitted by ingestion of undercooked ground beef or raw milk most commonly. Hemorrhagic colitis is characteristic of infection but it can also lead to hemolytic uremic syndrome resulting from toxin-mediated kidney damage.

75.

B. *Aeromonas* species are found in bodies of fresh water and salt water that can be flowing or stagnant and contaminated with sewage. These organisms are known as one of the animal pathogens that cause "red leg disease" in frogs. The largest number of cases of human infection occur between May and November and seem to be highly associated with exposure to water or soil.

76.

B. *Campylobacter jejuni* are small, curved, motile gram-negative rods. They are found in the gastrointestinal tract of a variety of animals. Campy agar is used for insolation from stool and must be incubated at 42 °C under microaerophilic conditions (10% CO_2, 5% O_2 with balance N_2) for 72 hours.

77.

C. Whether growing aerobically or anaerobically, streptococci obtain all their energy requirements from the fermentation of sugars to lactic acid. Streptococci are all catalase negative and grow on coventional media such as sheep blood agar. Most are part of the normal flora of human skin, throats, and intestines but produce a wide variety of infections when introduced in tissues or blood.

78.

D. Organisms that synthesize the enzyme catalase are able to protect themselves from the killing effects of H_2O_2 by converting it to H_2O and O_2. Streptococci are unable to synthesize the heme prosthetic group for this enzyme and are therefore catalase negative.

79.

C. Streptolysin S is primarily responsible for the beta hemolysis seen on the surface of a blood agar plate inoculated with a betahemolytic *Streptococcus*. Of the two hemolysins secreted by beta-hemolytic streptococci, streptolysin S is stable in the presence of atmospheric oxygen. Streptolysin O is reversible, is inactivated in the presence of oxygen, and is best demonstrated when the agar has been stabbed and shows subsurface hemolysis.

80.

B. *Hafnia alvei*, the only species in the genus, is a member of the family *Enterobacteriaceae* and is therefore characteristically oxidase negative and has been isolated from a variety of clinical specimens but is not considered pathogenic. *Aeromonas, Plesiomonas*, and *Vibrio* are all characteristically oxidase positive. *Pseudomonas* is a nonfermentative bacillus that produces a positive oxidase reaction.

81.

D. *Streptococcus mutans* produces a dextransucrase that forms an insoluble polymer of glucose known as glucan. It is the glucan that by adhering to the surface of the teeth keeps these streptococci in contact with the enamel surface of the teeth. Decay is caused when the streptococci ferment fructose cleaved from sucrose and form lactic acid.

82.

B. *Neisseria gonorrhoeae* is the causative agent of gonorrhoea and is very sensitive to drying and temperature variations. Incubation under CO_2 is required for recovery and selective media like Thayer-Martin are recommended. The organism appears in smears as an encapsulated gram-negative diplococcus.

83.

D. Resistance to penicillin by production of beta-lactamase has become widespread among *N. gonorrhoeae*. Resistance to ceftriaxone has not been described. In males it commonly produces purulent urethritis. In females the infection is often asymptomatic, with the primary site being the cervix.

84.

B. *Nocardia asteroides* causes a variety of disease states but is most associated with cavitary, pulmonary infections. These gram-positive organisms may appear filamentous, bacillary, or coccoid and usually stain irregularly. *Nocardia asteroides* in a clinical sample can be separated from indigenous bacterial flora by incubating the culture at greater than 37 °C. *Nocardia asteroides* are able to grow well at temperatures up to 45 °C.

85.

C. The anatomy of the female urethra allows bacteria from the perirectal region to easily reach the bladder. *E. coli* is the most common pathogen in uncomplicated community-acquired UTIs. Other organisms are more prevalent in nosocomial or recurrent infections.

86.

D. The most commonly used method for typing *Klebsiella* is based on the K or capsular antigens. Routine grouping based on the O antigens is not practiced because the heat-stable capsules interfere with O agglutination. The Quellung procedure can be performed for the identification of *Klebsiella* types much the same as for the identification of *Streptococcus pneumoniae*.

87.

C. *Vibrio cholerae* is a virulent organism that causes those infected to lose massive amounts of fluids. Severe dehydration is usually the cause of death in untreated patients. Proper therapy begins with intravenous fluid replacement to restore the patient's electrolyte balance and water volume.

88.

A. *Vibrio parahaemolyticus* is associated with gastroenteritis following ingestion of contaminated seafood. This organism is classified as a halophilic *Vibrio* species, which makes routine biochemical test media less than optimal because of its low NaCl content. Growth in the presence of 1% NaCl but no growth in media without the added Na+ is the test for the differentiation of halophilic microorganisms.

89.

C. *Brucella* spp. are class III pathogens and appropriate biohazard facilities must be used. It is important for the laboratory to be notified whenever brucellosis is suspected. Most laboratories send isolates to a reference laboratory for confirmation or definitive identification because they lack the specialized media and containment facilities.

90.

A. *Helicobacter pylori* are found in the human gastric mucosa colonizing mucous layer of the antrum and fundus but do not invade the epithelium. Approximately 50% of adults over age 60 are infected, with the incidence of gastritis increasing with age. *H. pylori* have been cultured from feces and dental plaque, supporting the theory of a fecal-oral or oral-oral route of transmission.

91.

D. Acid-fast bacilli can be demonstrated in stained smears of clinical material using Ziehl-Neelsen or Kinyoun acid-fast stains. The Kinyoun carbolfuchsin method adds a detergent or wetting agent such as Tergitol No. 7 to accelerate the staining process. If a fluorescent method is used as the primary staining method, it is recommended that all positive slides be confirmed with either the Kinyoun or Ziehl-Neelsen stains.

92.

A. *Acinetobacter* is widely distributed in nature and commonly colonizes patients in the hospital environment. Infection occurs mainly in compromised hosts. Their resistance to many of the commonly used antimicrobial agents limits the selection of optimal therapeutic agents.

93.

B. *Vibrio parahemolyticus* is found in brackish or salt water. The mode of transmission is the ingestion of contaminated water or seafood. *V. parahemolyticus* is know as a halophilic vibrio and the case history illustrates a common association with infection.

94.

C. *Erysipelothrix* is a nonmotile, catalase-negative, gram-positive bacillus that often appears as long filaments. Unlike other aerobic gram-positive bacilli, this organism produces H_2S, which can be demonstrated in triple sugar iron agar. Erysipeloid, a skin disease of the hands usually associated with the handling of infected animals, is the human infection produced most commonly by this agent.

95.

B. *Agrobacterium*, the causative agent of crown gall and hairy root in plants, has been shown to cause human disease. These gram-negative, oxidase-positive, motile organisms must be differentiated from *Pseudomonas* and *Achromobacter* species. This highly antimicrobial-resistant organism has been recovered in a case of endocarditis but can be effectively treated with a combined therapy of trimethoprim-sulfamethoxazole and polymyxin.

96.

D. Organisms biochemically resembling *Salmonella* are typically tested using a polyvalent antiserum composed of antibodies against all the commonly isolated strains including antisera against the Vi antigen. The Vi antigen is a heat-labile capsular antigen associated with *Salmonella typhi*. After heating of a *Salmonella typhi* suspension the Vi antigen has been removed and the organism can now react with the somatic grouping antisera. *Salmonella typhi* demonstrates a positive agglutination reaction in D-grouping sera.

97.

C. Primarily an animal pathogen, *Erysipelothrix rhusiopathiae* is a pleomorphic, gram-positive bacillus transmitted to humans by contact with an infected animal or animal product. This organism when grown in the laboratory produces alpha hemolysis and is nonmotile, hydrogen sulfide-positive, and catalase and oxidase-negative. Its unique reaction in a gelatin stab culture is helpful for identification.

98.

B. *Campylobacter fetus* ssp. *fetus* is occasionally implicated in human disease. These organisms, unlike *C. jejuni*, are characterized as producing extraintestinal symptoms. Those persons most at risk of infection are those with preexisting disease who are in a debilitated condition.

99.

A. Methicillin-resistant *Staphylococcus epidermidis* strains are becoming a problem for clinicians treating infected patients. *Staphylococcus epidermidis* has long been associated with infections following the surgical insertion of prosthetic devices such as heart valves and cerebrospinal fluid shunts. Methicillin resistance makes treatment difficult because it is heterogenic, and clinical cases may require combination antibiotic therapy.

100.

D. *Rhodococcus equi* is found in soil and commonly produces disease among livestock. These gram-positive bacilli can demonstrate primary mycelia and were formerly in the genus *Nocardia*. This species is characterized by its pigmentation on culture media and its inability to ferment carbohydrates.

101.

A. *Shigella sonnei* is identified as a group D *Shigella* and is characterized by its ability to ferment lactose. This species of *Shigella* is the most common cause of bacillary dysentery in the United States. The genus *Shigella* is characterized biochemically by being negative for citrate, urease, motility, and lysine decarboxylation, and it does not produce gas from glucose.

102.

B. The methyl red test is a broth test that detects the presence of acidity from the breakdown of glucose in the medium. Red indicates a positive reaction, and yellow a negative reaction. The genera *Providencia, Escherichia, Salmonella*, and *Proteus* all produce a positive methyl red test.

103.

B. *V. cholerae* has as its pathogenic mechanisms adherence, motility, enzymes such as protease and mucinase, and the production of an enterotoxin. Epidemic strains colonize the small intestine where they elaborate choleragen. Disease is produced when the enterotoxin stimulates the secretion of large volumes of fluids into the intestinal lumen.

104.

A. Classic epidemic strains of *Vibrio cholerae* are included in the antigenic O group 1. The Ogawa and Inaba strains are considered the predominant epidemic strains. More recently the O139 strain has also been associate with outbreaks of cholera.

105.

B. *Streptococcus pneumoniae*, a primary etiologic agent of lobar pneumonia, is an encapsulated, gram-positive, lanceolate diplococcus. Fastidious in its growth requirements, the organism on blood agar produces characteristic alpha-hemolytic colonies, which are convex and often mucoid in appearance and bile soluble. Upon aging, colonies of *Streptococcus pneumoniae* undergo autolytic changes. The polysaccharide capsule provides the most useful means of identification: the Neufeld Quellung reaction. There are 82 types of pneumococci based on specific capsular antigens.

106.

D. Members of the genus *Mycobacterium* are characterized as slow-growing, obligately aerobic bacilli that because of the high lipid content of their cell wall exhibit acid fastness when stained. *Mycobacterium tuberculosis* is the primary etiologic agent of tuberculosis in humans. These microorganisms are resistant to adverse environmental conditions and can remain viable in respiratory secretions for weeks or months. The most common route of infection is the respiratory tract through inhalation of droplet nuclei or infected fomites.

107.

B. *Haemophilus influenzae* is a well-established human pathogen known to produce highly fatal meningeal infections. Children in daycare between 1 to 5 years of age are most commonly infected. The number of infections has been reduced due to Hib vaccination. This organism's association with the disease influenza is merely as a secondary bacterial infection and not as the primary agent. *Haemophilus* spp. are part of the indigenous oral flora of humans. Most infections are produced by

serotype b, which have been found to be resistant to the bactericidal effect of complement.

108.

D. Species of the genus *Nocardia* are ubiquitous in the soil and thus characteristically produce exogenous forms of infection as a result of inhalation of contaminated fomites or a traumatic incident with soil contamination. A diagnostic characteristic, depending on the species, is the acid fastness of the filamentous bacilli or coccoid forms. Unlike *Actinomyces* species, which are catalase-negative, gram-positive, non-spore-forming anaerobic bacilli, *Nocardia* species are catalase-positive aerobic organisms. "Sulfur granules" are characteristic of actinomycotic pus and upon examination would reveal non-acid-fast branching filaments.

109.

B. *Enterococcus faecium* is an important agent of human infection. Their differentiation from other enterococcal strains is of importance because of their resistance to most clinically useful antibiotics including vancomycin. The ability to tolerate a high concentration of salt is characteristic of the clinically significant species of *Enterococcus.*

110.

D. *Brucella* species are small gram-negative intracellular parasites that are implicated in zoonotic infection of humans. The disease brucellosis produces a characteristic undulant febrile illness. In the United States, disease caused by *Brucella* species is mainly job related or involves food or animal associations such as in hunters or those who drink raw milk. Primarily an agent of disease in animals, the species reflects in its name the animal for which it is primarily pathogenic (*Brucella canis*, a pathogen of dogs).

111.

C. *Escherichia coli* is a lactose-fermenting member of the family *Enterobacteriaceae*. Various selective and differential agars are available for the differentiation of lactose fermenters from those that do not degrade lactose. In some media H_2S production may be demonstrated. Isolates of *Escherichia coli*, it is true, would produce yellow colonies at 24 hours on xylose-lysine-desoxycholate agar (XLD). Non-lactose-fermenters such as *Shigella* species would produce red colonies on XLD agar. On MacConkey agar, lactose fermenters produce pink colonies; on Hektoen enteric agar, colonies would be orange; and on eosin methylene blue agar (EMB) *Escherichia coli* would be blue-purple and produce a green metallic sheen at 24 hours.

112.

A. Viridans streptococci do not produce the enzyme pyroglutamyl aminopeptidase and therefore do not produce a positive or red color when tested on PYR agar. The PYR test is used predominantly for the presumptive identification of group A streptococci and *Enterococcus*. *Micrococceae* and *Lactococcus* are known to produce a positive reaction as well, although the reaction may be delayed.

113.

A. *Yersinia pestis* is causative agent of human plague. The organism is endemic in rodents and transmitted to man by the rat flea. This oxidase-negative organism is nonmotile at 20–25 °C and is negative for H$_2$S and urea; it is coccobacillary in shape and is said to resemble a safety pin.

114.

D. *Streptococcus pneumoniae* is a leading cause of lobar pneumonia as well as other serious bacterial infections. The Gram stain smear of clinical specimens can provide a rapid presumptive diagnosis when the characteristic morphology and Gram reaction is observed. The optochin disk test can be performed to presumptively identify this organism. Optochin lyses pneumococci producing a zone of inhibition around the disk.

115.

A. Motility is an important consideration in an identification procedure for microorganisms. Of the *Enterobacteriaceae*, the genera *Klebsiella* and *Shigella* are characteristically nonmotile as is *Tatumella*. Motility of the *Enterobacteriaceae* can normally be detected by the use of a semisolid motility medium, which is grossly observed for the determination of motility. The hanging-drop method is perhaps the most accurate means of detecting motility of nonfermentative microorganisms.

116.

C. Pneumonic legionellosis and the nonpneumonic illness, known as Pontiac fever, are the two clinical forms of the disease caused by *Legionella pneumophila*. The optimal temperature for cultivation

is 35 °C and cold enrichment is not appropriate. Direct fluorescent antibody is often used diagnostically, and erythromycin is the drug of choice for therapy.

117.

C. The etiologic agent of granuloma inguinale is *Calymmatobacterium granulomatis*, a pleomorphic, gram-negative, encapsulated bacillus. First described as Donovan bodies or inclusions seen in mononuclear cells from genital ulcers, these organisms are extremely difficult to recover. Following a gradual onset, lesions develop and go on to erode and indurate, resulting in a red, hypertrophic granulation of the tissue. Buboes and pseudobubo formation occur occasionally in the inguinal area much the same as in chancroid.

118.

A. *Mycobacterium ulcerans* and *Mycobacterium marinum* have both been implicated in skin infections. Their predilection for surface areas of the body is related to their optimal growth temperature range of 30–32 °C. At body temperature (37 °C) or higher these organisms grow poorly, if at all.

119.

B. When streaked on DNase test medium, colonies of *Staphylococcus aureus* and *Serratia marcescens* will demonstrate a positive reaction for DNase activity. Inoculated plates are incubated for 18 to 24 hours after which the growth plates are flooded with a 0.1% solution of toluidine blue. DNase-producing organisms are differentiated by the development of pink in the agar around the colonies.

120.

D. Bacteriologic cultures of a typical impetigo lesion may yield either a pure culture of *Streptococcus pyogenes* or a mixed culture of *Streptococcus pyogenes* and *Staphylococcus aureus*. The thick crust form of impetigo, which is most commonly seen, is primarily caused by group A streptococci. It is the bullous form of impetigo for which *Staphylococcus aureus* is the etiologic agent. The route of infection is direct inoculation of the causative agents into abraded or otherwise compromised areas of the skin.

121.

A. *S. typhi*, the causative agent of typhoid fever, is commonly associated with invasion of the bloodstream. The presence of organisms is the result of an extravascular site of infection. The extravascular sites in the case of typhoid fever are the small intestine, regional lymph nodes of the intestine, and the reticuloendothelial system. The bacteremic phase is seen before the organism can be recovered in stool.

122.

D. Citrate utilization is one of the common tests used for the differentiation of members of the family *Enterobacteriaceae*. Both *Escherichia coli* and *Shigella dysenteriae* are incapable of using citrate as the sole source of carbon as an energy source. Organisms such as *Klebsiella pneumoniae* and *Enterobacter aerogenes* when tested on citrate agar are able to grow, and a color change occurs from green to blue in the medium.

123.

B. *N. gonorrhoeae* is a fastidious organism requiring the addition of serum or blood to the culture media in order to grow. A selective medium such as Thayer-Martin should be used for primary isolation, especially from sites that may be contaminated. Collection and processing of specimens must be done under optimal conditions, since this organism is sensitive to drying and low temperatures.

124.

A. The indole reaction is one of the most widely used methods for differentiating lactose-positive *Escherichia coli* from other members of the family *Enterobacteriaceae*. Organisms such as *Escherichia coli,* which possess the enzyme tryptophanase, are able to metabolize the amino acid tryptophan with the production of indole, pyruvic acid, and ammonia. Indole represents the I in the IMViC reactions, an early battery of tests used for the identification of *Enterobacteriaceae*.

125.

D. Rapid development of drug resistance is a concern in the treatment of tuberculosis. Patients are treated generally with a combination of at least two of the primary drugs such as isoniazid and streptomycin. Those drugs such as kanamycin or ethionamide, which are considered secondary treatment modalities, are used only when primary drug resistance is detected.

126.

C. *E. coli* produces an acid over acid (A/A) reaction on TSI agar that indicates that glucose and either lactose or sucrose or both have been fermented. Bacteria that ferment lactose or sucrose produce large amounts of acid in the medium because of the greater concentration of these carbohydrates as compared to that of glucose (10:1) in the medium. The enteric pathogens *Salmonella* and *Shigella* can be ruled out when such a reaction is observed, since they are generally not able to utilize either lactose or sucrose.

127.

D. Identifying characteristics of *Staphylococcus aureus* include the production of the extracellular enzyme coagulase and DNase and its ability to grow in the presence of high salt concentrations. Differential and selective media such as mannitol salt agar have been developed for the recovery of this organism. Selective media and rapid identification tests are important for this known etiologic agent of food poisoning.

128.

D. Pyocyanin is the blue-green, diffusable pigment that is nonfluorescent. *Pseudomonas aeruginosa* is the only gram-negative rod able to produce this pigment. Most *Pseudomonas aeruginosa* strains can be identified presumptively by their characteristic grapelike odor, colonial morphology, and blue pigment.

129.

A. Group B streptococci, unlike other streptococci, can hydrolyze sodium hippurate to benzoic acid and glycine. If glycine is produced by the action of the test organism, the addition of ninhydrin to the medium will reduce the glycine to produce a purple color. The use of ninhydrin to detect glycine is a more sensitive and rapid test of hippurate hydrolysis.

130.

B. Color Plate 28 shows the Gram stain of a CSF specimen from an 8-month-old. The slide showed many WBCs and short gram-negative rods and "coccobacillary" forms characteristic of *Haemophilus influenzae*. Bacterial meningitis is a true medical emergency. A Gram stain of CSF often provides rapid presumptive identification of the causative agent for emperical therapy. *H. influen-*

zae, *Streptococcus pneumoniae* and *Neisseria meningitidis* are all frequent causes of meningitis in children.

131.

D. *S. agalactiae* produces an extracellular factor known as the CAMP factor. The test is performed by making a streak of the test isolate perpendicular to a streak of *Staphylococcus aureus*. A positive CAMP reaction is indicated by a zone of enhanced beta hemolysis at the point where the zone of hemolysis produced by a *Staphylococcus aureus* joins with that produced by the beta-hemolytic test isolate.

132.

B. *Campylobacter jejuni* is an important human pathogen that is associated most commonly with cases of bloody diarrhea, fever, and abdominal pain in humans. Special handling of cultures suspected to contain this organism is required for optimal recovery. Cultures should be incubated at 42 °C in a microaerophilic atmosphere and examined at 24 and 48 hours for spreading nonhemolytic colonies, which may be slightly pigmented. Wet mounts demonstrate the typical "darting" motility of this isolate. Erythromycin is an effective agent for treatment.

133.

B. *Moraxella catarrhalis* possess the enzyme indophenol oxidase. When a 1% solution of tetramethyl-*p*-phenylenediamine is applied to colonies of these organisms, the colonies turn a purple color, which rapidly darkens. *Neisseria gonorrhoeae* growing on selective media inoculated with a urogenital specimen can be presumptively identified by a positive oxidase test and a smear showing the characteristic gram-negative diplococcal morphology.

134.

C. *Cardiobacterium hominis* is a rare pathogen, which is recovered predominantly from cases of endocarditis. It is characterized as a fermentative, gram-negative bacillus that is nonmotile, catalase negative, and oxidase positive. Growth of this microorganism on laboratory media is enhanced by the addition of yeast extract.

135.

D. *Vibrio vulnificus* is a halophilic lactose-fermenting organism. The isolate has an association with two distinct clinical conditions, primary septicemia and wound infection. Septicemia with this organism appears to be correlated in most cases with preexisting hepatic disease. Infection of the blood with *Vibrio vulnificus* characteristically produces a fulminant disease with a high mortality rate. Wound infection with this organism is usually associated with trauma and contact with a marine environment.

136.

B. Only *Francisella tularensis* requires special selective procedures for cultivation; all others listed will grow on media such as blood and chocolate agar plates. Tularemia is a zoonotic disease transmitted to man through the handling of infected animals, ingestion of contaminated food or water, or by the bite of an insect. The disease produced is a febrile illness characterized by lymphadenopathy, malaise, chills, severe headache, myalagia, and local erythematous lesions. Isolation of this agent requires the use of glucose-cysteine agar media enriched with defibrinated rabbit blood.

137.

C. There are two species in the genus *Kluyvera*: *K. ascorbata* and *K. cryocrescens*. All species are positive for ornithine decarboxylase, indole, citrate, malonate, esculin, ONPG, and ferment lactose. *Kluyvera ascorbata* is considered more clinically significant and is differentiated from cryocrescens by its positive ascorbate test and resistance to cephalothin and carbenicillin.

138.

C. *Proteus vulgaris, Tatumella ptyseos*, and *Morganella morganii* are all phenylalanine-positive. *Proteus* species are characteristically positive in this test, and *Morganella* was formerly classified in the genus *Proteus*. *Tatumella*, which has several unusual characteristics, is in the family *Enterobacteriaceae* and is able to deaminate phenylalanine, although it is not positive for urease as are the other organisms.

139.

A. *Tatumella* is a genus of *Enterobacteriaceae* was formerly classified as CDC group EF–1. This organism has been isolated from a variety of clinical specimens including blood and is classified as a rare but potentially important human pathogen. In the laboratory these isolates demonstrate a rather inert pattern of biochemical activity, being more active at room temperature than at 35–37 °C.

140.

C. The water-diffusible greenish yellow pigment fluorescein is produced by *Pseudomonas aeruginosa*, *P. fluorescens*, and *P. putida*. The production of pyoverdins can be detected when a culture of the organism is exposed to a short-wavelength, ultraviolet light source. It is necessary, when checking for fluorescence, that special media such as Sellers medium be used, since the production of fluorescent pigments is dependent upon nutritional factors. Cationic salts such as magnesium sulfate, when present in the medium, act to intensify luminescence.

141.

D. The production of hemolysins and the enzymes coagulase and deoxyribonuclease are associated with the virulence of staphylococci. The coagulase-producing staphylococci are most commonly producers of staphylolysins, which create beta hemolysis when the isolate is grown on blood agar. There are many factors that act to create staphylococcal virulence by overcoming the host's natural defenses.

142.

B. The physiology of staphylococci enables them to remain infectious in the environment longer than many other pathogenic bacteria. Staphylococci are heat resistant and have a high maximum growth temperature. Their high salt tolerance enables strains to grow in salt-preserved foods and causes cases of food poisoning through enterotoxin production. *Staphylococci* are more like other gram-positive cocci in their sensitivity to trephenyl methane dyes, many broad-spectrum antibiotics, and penicillin.

143.

A. *Kingella* species are gram-negative bacilli or coccobacilli that may appear in short chains. *Kingella denitrificans* can be isolated from the human upper respiratory tract, will grow on Thayer-Martin agar, and is oxidase-positive. The growth of this organism is inhibited by MacConkey agar, and growth is poor on TSI agar.

144.

A. Chocolate agar is the preferred culture medium. Unlike 5% sheep blood agar it provides both the hemin and NAD factors required for growth. *H. ducreyi* requires a special media such as Mueller-Hinton based chocolate agar, supplemented with 1% IsoVitaleX and 3 μg/mL of vancomycin for growth.

145.

A. *L. pneumophila* requires the use of special laboratory media for cultivation and does not stain well by the conventional Gram stain. The primary mode of transmission is by the airborne route, usually in association with an environmental source of bacteria. Most species are motile and biochemically inert.

146.

C. Unlike rickettsial diseases there is no rash involved in *C. burnetti* infections. The organism is an obligate intracellular parasite that is able to survive for long periods in the environment and is transmitted most often by fomites. Tetracycline is the drug of choice for uncomplicated infections.

147.

D. Tissue samples from the respiratory tract and associated fluids such as pleural fluid are optimal for the laboratory isolation of *Legionella pneumophila*. This agent of severe pneumonic disease is seldom recovered from blood specimens. The diagnosis of this disease can be facilitated by the direct staining of tissue using the immunofluorescence technique with specific antibody conjugates.

148.

A. Blood cultures are positive in greater than 70% of patients with brucellosis. The organisms are slow growing, fastidious, intracellular parasites and require special techniques for optimal recovery. Biphasic media or the use of the Isolator system may release the intracellular organisms enhancing growth and speeding up recovery time. Similarly the use of lysis-centifugation or an automated system optimize recovery and reduce incubation time; cultures must be held for 3 weeks before reporting as negative.

149.

A. Modified Skirrow's media is a primary plating media for *Campylobacter* spp. The diagnosis of pertussis or whooping cough is confirmed by culture. Isolation of the etiologic agent is best done within the first week of the illness. Selective media have been developed for optimal recovery. Plates are held for 12 days before discarding as negative; most positive cultures are detected in 3 to 5 days.

150.

D. Both *Enterobacter sakazakii* and *E. agglomerans* produce a yellow pigment that aids in their presumptive identification. Speciation of *Enterobacter agglomerans* relies on biochemical tests that demonstrate its failure to decarboxylate lysine, arginine, and ornithine. *Enterobacter sakazakii* can be definitively identified by its production of DNase and an acid reaction from d-sorbitol.

151.

C. Zoonotic diseases are diseases of lower animals that are transmissible to humans. Leptospirosis is primarily a disease of small animals such as rabbits. It is contracted by humans through contact with infected carcasses or contaminated water. *Bacillus anthracis* is found in the environment. Anthrax is transmitted to humans by exposure to contaminated animal products such as cattle hides, goat hair, or wool. Erysipeloid considered an occupational disease is caused by *Erysipelotyrix rhusiopapthiae,* a cause of disease in animals.

152.

A. *P. mirabilis* is commonly associated with urinary tract infections as well as infections in other parts of the body. It is a motile organism that characteristically swarms across the surface of sheep blood agar plate. Members of the genus Proteus are characteristically rapidly urea positive, lactose negative, and phenylalanine deaminase positive.

153.

C. *Acinetobacter baumanii* is not able to reduce nitrate either to nitrites or to gas. This species is positive in O-F glucose media and in 10% lactose. *Acinetobacter* species are able to grow on MacConkey agar, and they are oxidase negative, nonmotile, and characteristically resistant to penicillin.

154.

C. *Moraxella phenylpyruvica* has been reclassified as *Pyschrobacter* spp. They are small, MacConkey-positive, gram-negative diplobacillary, oxidase-positive, nonglucose utilizing organisms. Because of their morphology and reaction on Gram stain and oxidase reaction, these organisms may be presumptively misidentified as *Neisseria gonorrhoeae* when found in clinical samples. The former *M. urethralis* has also been reclassified and is now named *Oligella urethralis*.

155.

B. Both *Actinobacillus lignieresii* and *A. equuli* are etiologic agents of "woody tongue" in cattle. These agents, in addition to producing granulomatous lesions in the upper gastrointestinal tract of cattle, are also associated with suppurative skin and lung lesions in sheep. *Actinobacillus lignieresii* and *A. equuli* are small gram-negative bacilli that are urease, catalase, and oxidase positive, able to reduce nitrates, and nonmotile.

156.

C. *Eikenella corrodens* is a facultatively anaerobic gram-negative bacillus that requires hemin in the culture medium to grow aerobically. This organism, which is a part of the normal indigenous flora of man, is seldom found in pure culture. They are commonly found in infections following bite or clenched-fist wounds. Infections of the face and neck may also involve this organism, which produces pitting of the agar on which it is isolated.

157.

D. In the genus *Pasteurella, P. multocida* is the species commonly recovered in clinical specimens. This gram-negative coccobacillus is a normal inhabitant of the oral cavity of domestic animals. Humans most often become infected from a bite or scratch of a cat or dog, which produces a rapidly progressing, painful, suppurative wound infection. Penicillin is an effective drug for the treatment of *Pasteurella* infections.

158.

D. *Legionella pneumophila* is able to hydrolyze hippurate. Although most of the studies done on legionellosis are based on this species, *L. pneumophila* is not the only one associated with human disease. *Legionella micdadei* is called the Pittsburgh pneumonia agent and is the causative agent of Fort Bragg fever.

159.

B. *Haemophilus influenzae* biogroup *aegyptius* was previously known as *Haemophilus aegyptius*. It is a causative agent of the purulent conjunctivitis known as pinkeye. The factors X and V are both positive. On culture colonies of this biogroup resemble those of *H. influenzae* but are smaller at 48 hours.

160.

C. The extent of laboratory services offered in various hospitals varies according to the level of need for the isolation and identification of mycobacteria. The American Thoracic Society has published suggested levels of service, with larger facilities being designated reference laboratories or level III and equipped for identification and susceptibility testing of mycobacteria isolates. Smaller, lower level laboratories send cultures to reference laboratories instead of attempting isolation and identification at their own institutions.

161.

D. *Kingella denitrificans* is found as normal flora in the upper respiratory and genitourinary tracts. It is morphologically similar to *Neisseria gonorrhoeae* both on Gram stain and colonies on culture media. Confusion is further compounded by its ability to grow on Thayer-Martin medium and its positive oxidase and glucose reaction. The ability of *Kingella denitrificans* to reduce nitrates and its resistance to amylase are key tests for its differentiation from *N. gonorrhoeae*.

162.

A. *Plesiomonas* belongs to the family *Vibrionaceae* and is found in water sources. Infection in humans has been mainly diarrheal diseases, and it is most likely that a waterborne mode of transmission was involved. *P. shigelloides* is the only species in this genus of gram-negative bacilli, which have polar flagella, are oxidase and catalase positive, and have been isolated from freshwater fish as well as a variety of animals.

163.

D. *Cardiobacterium hominis* is a pleomorphic, gram-negative bacillus that is oxidase positive, catalase and urea negative, and nonmotile. This normal inhabitant of the human upper respiratory tract is known to be one cause of endocarditis. On culture these organisms grow slowly, and colonies are shiny, circular, and opaque and may pit the agar.

164.

A. Mycoplasmas are small, pleomorphic organisms that lack a cell wall and are best visualized by dark-field or phase microscopy. Species of the genus *Mycoplasma* are well-known human pathogens that cause a variety of disease processes. Penicillin is not an effective treatment because of their lack of a cell wall, and isolation requires media supplemented with peptone, yeast extract, and serum.

165.

B. The recall described illustrates the ubiquitous nature of *P. aeruginosa* in the environment. Their minimal nutritional requirements and ability to tolerate a wide range of temperatures (4°–42 °C) make them ideal opportunistic organisms. They are resistant to many disinfectants such as povidone iodine and thus able to contaminate a variety of sterile products.

166.

C. Ingestion of unpasteurized and contaminated milk or cheese is one of the four primary routes of infection. Brucellosis is found worldwide and symptoms vary from asymptomatic to a debilitating systemic infection. Only four of the six species are pathogenic for humans; *B. abortus*, *B. melitensis*, *B. suis*, and *B. canis*.

167.

C. Motility is a key test for the differentiation of *Bacillus anthracis* from other species of *Bacillus*. Suspect *Bacillus* colonies are inoculated in a broth media and allowed to grow to a visible turbidity. A sample of this actively growing culture should be examined using the hanging-drop technique for motility. *Bacillus anthracis* is nonmotile and can therefore be easily differentiated from commonly encountered motile species.

168.

C. The production of DNase, lipase, and gelatinase differentiates the genus *Serratia* from other *Enterobacteriaceae*. *Serratia* species, especially *S. marcescens*, have a close association with nosocomial infections. *Serratia* species can produce severe infections such as septicemia and meningitis and are frequently difficult to eradicate because of their characteristic antibiotic-resistant strains found in the hospital environment.

169.

B. Group C streptococcal species include *S. equi, S. equisimilis, S. dysgalactiae*, and *S. zooepidemicus*. These organisms are primarily pathogenic for animals and only rarely are isolated in the clinical laboratory. The human infections with group C organisms closely resemble those caused by group A streptococci, and therefore their identification is of clinical importance.

170.

A. *M. avium* complex (MAC) are the species of mycobacteria most frequently implicated in enteric infections among patients with AIDS. In suspected cases, several stool cultures should be collected and submitted to the laboratory for smear and culture for acid-fast organisms. These organisms are resistant to many of the antituberculosis drugs and are generally treated with multiple drugs in combination.

171.

C. A delayed hypersensitivity reaction following an intradermal injection of *Chlamydia trachomatis* extract has been used as a diagnostic procedure for lymphogranuloma venereum (LGV). The procedure, which is known as the Frei test, has many limitations such as lack of sensitivity and specificity, and it is no longer relied upon in the United States. The hypersensitivity in LGV patients develops between weeks 1 and 6 following infection and is lifelong. Diagnosis is now established by isolation of an LGV strain from a bubo or other infected site.

172.

D. A positive tuberculin skin test reaction is an example of a hypersensitivity reaction. Tuberculin preparations are prepared from culture filtrates, which are precipitated with trichloroacetic acid and are known as PPD or purified protein derivative. A positive test demonstrates an area of induration following an intradermal injection of PPD.

173.

D. The Schultz-Charlton phenomenon demonstrates immunity to erythrogenic toxin. The classic rash of scarlet fever is a result of the action of the erythrogenic toxin. Patients who are exhibiting the characteristic bright red rash, when injected with convalescent serum, will demonstrate a blanching or fading of the rash within 6 hours.

174.

B. Cardiolipin is a tissue lipid produced as a byproduct of treponemal infection. Nontreponemal tests for syphilis take advantage of antibodies made to cardiolipin. The most commonly used tests are the RPR for blood and the VDRL for CSF.

175.

D. *Chlamydia trachomatis*, a leading cause of blindness, can be recovered from corneal scrapings in suspected cases of trachoma. Clinical material can be cultured on McCoy cells and examined directly using fluorescent antibody techniques. Trachoma is a chronic inflammatory process of the conjunctiva which, as reinfections occur, results in corneal involvement.

176.

C. Nasopharyngeal cultures are recommended over cough plates for the recovery of *Bordetella pertussis* in suspected cases of whooping cough. Swabs of the nasopharynx are inoculated on the selective agar Bordet-Gengou. Penicillin may be added to the culture medium to inhibit the growth of contaminating indigenous flora.

177.

C. Cultures of the tonsillar fossae and posterior pharynx are most commonly obtained in suspected cases of streptococcal pharyngitis. *Streptococcus pyogenes* is most often associated with cases of pharyngitis but is also the agent of scarlet fever and erysipelas in addition to wound infections. Rapid identification of this organism and prompt antimicrobial therapy are required to prevent the diseases that are related to sequelae.

178.

A. *Gardnerella vaginalis* is associated with cases of bacterial vaginosis formerly called "nonspecific vaginitis." Vaginal cultures for the recovery of this microorganism should be inoculated on HBT (human blood Tween) agar. These small, gram-negative bacilli are frequently seen in great numbers on the surface of epithelial cells from an infected area (clue cells).

179.

B. Cultures of blood are the recommended specimens for the isolation of *Brucella* species. A biphasic culture bottle is recommended as the culture system to be used for the recovery of these intracellular parasites. If cultures of the blood are negative, bone marrow cultures have proven useful.

180.

B. Subacute bacterial endocarditis is an inflammation of the lining membrane of the heart, which most often is caused by a member of the viridans group of streptococci. *Streptococcus sanguis* is one of several species that may lodge in an abnormal heart or on valves damaged by rheumatic fever. Viridans streptococci are normal inhabitants of the human upper respiratory tract.

181.

D. *Streptococcus pneumoniae* is most commonly associated with cases of lobar pneumonia. Patients characteristically produce blood-tinged, rust-colored sputum in which the characteristic gram-positive lanceolate diplococci can be found. A diagnosis can be made directly from the clinical material using Omniserum and observing a positive capsular swelling reaction. Coagglutination and latex agglutination tests are used for serologic identification of culture isolates.

182.

C. Mesenteric lymphadenitis is one of the common manifestations of human *Yersinia pseudotuberculosis* infections. Symptoms produced by this agent closely resemble those of acute appendicitis. This gram-negative coccobacillus grows well on routine culture media and has an optimal growth temperature of 25–30 °C.

183.

B. Epiglottitis is a severe inflammation of the epiglottis, which most often occurs in children. The most frequent cause of this condition is *Haemophilus influenzae*. Symptoms of epiglottitis include sore throat, fever, and cough and may progress to airway obstruction and cyanosis.

184.

A. *Staphylococcus saprophyticus* is recognized as an etiologic agent of uncomplicated cystitis cases oc-

curring in young females. These nonhemolytic, coagulase-negative staphylococci closely resemble *Staphylococcus epidermidis* on blood agar medium. Identification of these microorganisms is facilitated by demonstrating their resistance to novobiocin using the disk diffusion test.

185.

C. Clinical material sent to the laboratory for the recovery of *Corynebacterium diphtheriae* should be inoculated on cystine-tellurite agar plates or Tinsdale medium. On these tellurite-containing media, colonies of this pathogen will appear dark-brown to black, which aids in their differentiation. Suspicious colonies should be further tested for their biochemical activity and toxin production.

186.

D. *Vibrio vulnificus* is responsible for septicemia after consumption of contaminated raw oysters. Infections are most severe in patients with hepatic disease, hematopoietic disease, or chronic renal failure and those receiving immunosuppressive drugs. Mortality in patients with septicemia can be as high as 50% unless antimicrobial therapy is started rapidly.

187.

A. Cefsulodin-irgasan-novobiocin (CIN) agar is recommended for the primary isolation of *Yersinia* spp. and *Aeromonas* spp. *Y. enterocolitic* produces "bull's-eye" colonies at 48 hours; colonies show a dark red center surrounded by a translucent border. This is a selective and differential agar that supresses the growth of normal fecal flora and differentiates colonies of *Y. enterocolitica*.

188.

B. *Gardnerella vaginalis* is a causative agent of bacterial vaginosis and may be overlooked on routine cultures unless a selective medium is used. HBT (human blood Tween) agar is the selective agar recommended for the recovery of this small, pleomorphic, gram-negative bacillus. Isolates resembling this agent can be definitively identified by fermentation studies.

189.

D. *Legionella pneumophila*, the causative agent of Legionnaires' disease, can be recovered from respiratory tract secretions. The culture medium recommended most commonly is buffered charcoal yeast extract (BCYE) agar, which is incubated in a moist chamber at 35 °C. Growth on this medium may not be visible for 3 to 4 days, after which further identification procedures may be carried out.

190.

B. The "radish bacillus" is the name given to *Mycobacterium terrae*. This slow-growing organism has been isolated from soil and agricultural products. It is not believed to be pathogenic for humans, although it is occasionally recovered in the clinical laboratory.

191.

C. The bovine bacillus is the name given to *Mycobacterium bovis*. This agent is known to be an etiologic agent of tuberculosis in humans, and it must be differentiated from *Mycobacterium tuberculosis* when recovered from clinical material. Unlike *M. tuberculosis*, *M. bovis* is negative for niacin production and nitrate reduction.

192.

A. The *M. avium* complex is sometimes referred to as *Mycobacterium avium-intracellulare* complex. These slow-growing bacilli are members of the Runyon group III. The organisms in this complex that cause human disease are *M. avium*, *M. iintracellulare*, and *M. paratuberculosis*.

193.

B. *Mycobacterium gordonae* has been recovered from water stills, faucets, and bodies of water in nature, which is why it has been called the tap water scotochromogen. These organisms are not considered to be pathogenic for humans, but since they may be recovered because of sample contamination, their identification is recommended. Members of Runyon group II, they are slow growing and form yellow-orange colonies that do not depend on exposure to light.

194.

D. The human tubercle bacillus is *Mycobacterium tuberculosis*. Growth of this well-known human pathogen appears in 2 to 3 weeks when incubated at 35 °C. These niacin-positive mycobacteria produce good, eugonic growth on culture media, and colonies are buff colored.

195.

B. Swimmer's ear is a form of external otitis common to persons who swim as a hobby and fail to completely dry their ear canals when they get out of the water. The organism most commonly associated with this condition is *Pseudomonas aeruginosa*. It is an organism known to be an opportunistic pathogen and one that favors a watery environment.

196.

A. *Mycobacterium marinum* is the causative agent of "swimming pool granuloma." Most typically, patients with abraded skin that has come in contact with water containing this agent develop granulomatous skin lesions, from which this agent may be cultured. Lesions generally occur on the extremities, since the skin temperature is at its lowest there, which is in keeping with the organism's optimal growth temperature of 25–32 °C.

197.

C. Traveler's diarrhea is caused by strains of toxin producing invasive or enteropathogenic *Escherichia coli*. It has been discovered that there are two distinct types of *E. coli* enterotoxins, one that is heat stable and one that is heat labile. Contaminated food products in foreign countries seem to be the major vehicle for human infection with these agents.

198.

A. *N. meningitidis* is a leading cause of bacterial meningitis. Disease is transmitted by respiratory droplets among people in prolonged close contact such as in a day-care center. Chemoprophylaxis with rifampin is appropriate for those in close contact with the patient: household, day-care staff, and classmates.

199.

D. *Bacillus anthracis* is the causative agent of woolsorters' disease or the pulmonary form of anthrax. The mode of infection is the inhalation of spores by the patient, usually during the performance of his/her occupation (sheep shearing or processing of animal hair). Prompt diagnosis and treatment of this disease is needed, since it is known to progress rapidly to a fatal form of septicemia.

200.

D. *Corynebacterium pseudodiphtheriticum* is morphologically similar to all other members of the genus *Corynebacterium*. They are all gram-positive, non-spore-forming bacilli that characteristically resemble Chinese characters or palisades. These bacteria often stain irregularly and have a pleomorphic club-shaped appearance.

201.

A. Because of the characteristic arrangement of the bacilli of *Bacillus anthracis*, they are said to resemble a bamboo pole when seen on Gram stain. The large, square-ended, gram-positive, spore-forming bacilli are arranged in long chains when grown in primary culture. The virulent forms of this organism typically demonstrate chains of encapsulated bacilli.

202.

B. *Haemophilus ducreyi*, the causative agent of chancroid, is a small, gram-negative, coccobacillary organism. On Gram stain, a culture of this organism shows a characteristic arrangement of cells in long parallel strands that are said to resemble schools of fish. Material aspirated from the soft chancre lesion is used to inoculate an enriched culture medium for the isolation of this agent.

203.

C. Isolates of *Campylobacter jejuni* can be presumptively identified on Gram stain by their characteristic gull-wing appearance. These gram-negative bacilli are motile with a typical darting pattern. They stain poorly using the Gram stain method, and it is recommended that 0.06% carbolfuchin be substituted for the safranin counterstain.

204.

D. *Neisseria gonorrhoeae* is said to resemble a kidney bean on Gram stain because of its characteristic gram-negative diplococcal morphology in which the adjacent sides are flattened. Typically these organisms are found intracellularly when direct smears of clinical material are examined. Smears from the female genital tract must be interpreted with caution, since other normal flora microorganisms are morphologically similar.

205.

C. *Mycobacterium fortuitum* complex species are differentiated from other species by their ability to grow on MacConkey agar without crystal violet. Growth of species in this complex appears within 5 days. The MacConkey agar used in this test

is not the same formulation as the agar used for the recovery of gram-negative bacteria. The crystal violet inhibits the growth of mycobacteria species. These mycobacteria are also able to reduce tellurite.

206.

D. *M. pneumoniae, U. urealyticum,* and *M. hominis* commonly colonize and infect humans. They are part of of the normal flora of humans colonizing the oropharynx, upper respiratory tract, and genitourinary tract. These organisms are one of the leading causes of sexually transmitted disease (STDs) worldwide.

207.

A. The host has several mechanisms that protect the respiratory tract from infection. The trachea, unlike other body sites listed, is not typically colonized with bacterial flora. When diagnosing lower respiratory track infections, procedures such as bronchoscopy or percutaneous transtracheal aspitate are used to obtain a specimen that is not contaminated by upper tract flora.

208.

B. The flora of the female genital tract changes with age and the associated effects of pH and estrogen concentration in the mucosa. *Lactobacillus* spp. are the predominant flora during childbearing years. Earlier and late in life staphylococci and corynebacteria predominate.

209.

A. *Mycobacterium bovis* is susceptible to 5 µg/mL of thiophene-2-carboxylic acid hydrazide (T2H). This *Mycobacterium* is associated with cattle and is rarely isolated from humans in the United States. Growth occurs only at 35 °C and is differentiated from other mycobacteria by its susceptibility to TCH.

210.

A. *E. tarda* is urease negative and H_2S positive. The negative urease reaction would help to differentiate it from an H_2S positive *Proteus* spp. Urease production is a key test for the identification of *H. pylori*. *C. urealyticum* is a component of the normal skin flora but has been recovered in urinary tract and wound infections in compromised hosts.

211.

B. It is a powerful amplification tool that enhances the sensitivity of molecular diagnostic techniques by increasing the target nucleic acid. The polymerase chain reaction combines the principles of complementary nucleic acid hybridization with nucleic acid replication. PCR can multiply a single copy of target nucleic acid up to 10^7 or more in 30–50 replication cycles.

212.

B. *Corynebacterium jeikeium* is a low virulence organism that is resistant to multiple antimicrobials. Its multiple drug resistance allows it to remain in hospital environments and is often cultured from the skin of hospitalized patients. In compromised patients it has been implicated in cases of septicemia, wound infections, and endocarditis in association with intravenous catheters used.

213.

C. Hansen's bacillus or *Mycobacterium leprae* is the etiologic agent of leprosy. The *Mycobacterium* has never been grown in an artificial medium but can be replicated in foot pads of mice and in the armadillo. There are two distinct types of disease caused by this agent; one is called tuberculoid, which is the more benign, and the other is the lepromatous form.

214.

D. *Arcanobacterium* spp. are catalase-negative, gram-positive, non-spore-forming rods. They may demonstrate delicate curves, pointed ends, and rudimentary branching. On culture they may have a narrow zone of beta-hemolysis and may be confused with beta-hemolytic streptococci on respiratory cultures. They are ubiquitous in the nature and some species are part of the normal skin and pharyngeal flora of humans.

215.

B. *Neisseria gonorrhoeae* is identified in the clinical laboratory by its ability to degrade only glucose when fermentation studies are done using tubes of glucose, sucrose, maltose, and lactose. The diagnosis of the venereal disease caused by this agent can be definitively made only by the isolation and identification of *Neisseria gonorrhoeae* in the clinical laboratory. Morphologically all members of the genus are alike, and all are oxidase positive,

which makes definitive identification procedures a necessity.

216.

C. *Neisseria meningitidis* is a well-known human pathogen that is most commonly associated with cases of meningitis. These oxidase-positive, gram-negative diplococci are identified either by fermentation tests or serologic methods that use specific antiserum. Positive fermentation reactions are demonstrated by *Neisseria meningitidis* in both glucose and maltose.

217.

D. Most commercially available blood culture media contain the anticoagulant sodium polyanetholsulfonate (SPS). Anticoagulation is important because certain bacteria do not survive well within clotted blood. Within the clot neutrophils and macrophages remain active and phagocytosis can occur.

218.

D. *Bartonella bacilliformis* is the causative agent of Oroya fever and verruga peruana. It is a pleomorphic gram-negative rod that can destroy RBC's and can be cultured from blood in the critical stage of the disease. The disease is rare occuring only in certain areas of the Andes mountains.

219.

C. *Chlamydia* are obligate intracellular pathogens. The lower respiratory disease caused by this agent is sporadic and epidemic and is characterized as atypical pneumonia. The organism has been associated epidemiologically to coronary heart disease. Most infections are diagnosed serologically. PCR for direct detection and diagnosis is effective and overcomes difficulties of culture and serologic methods.

220.

A. *Serratia liquefaciens*, as its name implies, is able to liquefy gelatin. This member of the genus is not thought to be a primary pathogen, being only rarely isolated from clinical specimens. The positive arabinose test reaction is one way of differentiating this isolate from Serratia marcescens. A positive KCN test reaction is also characteristic of this microorganism.

221.

B. *Proteus vulgaris* is able to deaminate phenylalanine. The test is performed by inoculating the test isolate on a slant of test medium containing phenylalanine and after incubation adding a 10% solution of ferric chloride. If the test is positive, a dark green color will develop on the slant after the addition of the reagent.

222.

B. *Morganella morganii*, previously classified as a member of the genus *Proteus*, has many of the same biochemical characteristics as *Proteus vulgaris* and *Proteus mirabilis*. This microorganism is positive for phenylalanine deaminase, indole production, and KCN. Its negative reaction for hydrogen sulfide production and negative gelatin reaction aids in its differentiation from the genus *Proteus*.

223.

B. Malonate broth has been used commonly for the differentiation of *Arizona* from the genus *Salmonella*. *Arizona* isolates are positive in malonate and turn the medium blue after incubation. They also are able to liquefy gelatin, although slowly, which is not a characteristic of *Salmonella* species. Recently the genus *Arizona*, which has always been known to be similar to *Salmonella*, has been classified as a type of *Salmonella*.

224.

D. *Klebsiella pneumoniae* produces positive reactions in malonate and KCN. *Klebsiella* species are all nonmotile, which aids in their identification. *Klebsiella pneumoniae* produces a capsule that can be used as a definitive means of identification by application of the Quellung procedure using specific antisera.

225.

A. *Chromobacterium violaceum* is a motile, gram-negative bacillus that is found in soil and water and that can be pathogenic for humans. The production of a non-water-soluble violet pigment by these organisms aids in their identification. *Chromobacterium* is catalase and oxidase positive and generally attacks carbohydrates fermentatively.

226.

A. *P. multocida* is the species most encountered in the clinical laboratory. They are normal flora in animals, not man, and are opportunistic in that the mode of transmission generally involves traumatic inoculation of the organism through human skin. Penicillin is the drug of choice for infections although a validated testing method is unavailable.

227.

C. *Pseudomonas aeruginosa* has not only a characteristic grapelike odor but also a blue-green color. These oxidative, motile organisms are oxidase positive and are able to grow at 42 °C. In humans these opportunistic organisms cause many types of infections, but they are primarily associated with burn wound infections.

228.

D. *Serratia marcescens* is a chromogenic member of the family *Enterobacteriaceae*. *S. marcescens* is the most clinically significant of the genus and is frequently involved in nosocomial infection. The red pigment produced is not water soluble and is demonstrated more readily at room temperature rather than at 35 °C.

229.

B. In immunocompromised patients *Nocardia asteroides* can cause invasive pulmonary infection and can often spread hematogenously throughout the body. Lesions in the brain are commonly associated with dissemination and have a poor prognosis. The organism is ubiquitous in nature and infection is acquired by traumatic inoculation or inhalation.

230.

C. *Campylobacter* species of clinical importance are characteristically oxidase positive and catalase positive. *Campylobacter sputorum* is differentiated from the other species because it does not produce the enzyme catalase. *C. sputorum* is not considered to be one of the clinically significant species of the genus.

231.

A. *Aeromonas* can be differentiated from other fermentative gram-negative bacilli such as the *Enterobacteriaceae* in that they are oxidase positive. Motility is made possible by a single polar and not peritrichous flagella. *Aeromonas hydrophila* is found in soil and water and has been isolated from a variety of human infections. On blood agar medium, colonies of this agent are beta hemolytic.

232.

B. *Edwardsiella tarda* is classified as a motile member of the family *Enterobacteriaceae* and as such is characteristically peritrichously flagellated. These organisms are infrequently isolated in the clinical laboratory. Biochemically they may initially resemble *Salmonella* in many ways such as hydrogen sulfide production and the inability to ferment lactose.

233.

A. *Listeria monocytogenes* is a small, gram-positive, motile bacillus that is actively motile. When grown on blood agar medium, this organism produces small translucent beta-hemolytic colonies, which may be visually mistaken for beta-hemolytic streptococci. Biochemically *L. monocytogenes* organisms differ from streptococci because they possess the enzyme catalase.

234.

D. The porphyrin test is most commonly used to test for the X factor requirement of *Haemophilus* isolates. A positive test result indicates that the organism posessed the enzymes to convert delta-aminolevulinic acid (ALA) into porphyrins and therefore would not require hemin or X factor. This rapid test will show a red fluorescence under UV light after a 4-hour incubation if porphyrins were produced.

235.

D. *Bordetella bronchiseptica* in humans produces either a respiratory illness or wound infections. The organism is a part of the normal respiratory flora of laboratory animals such as rabbits and guinea pigs. *Bordetella bronchiseptica* may cause problems for researchers, since it can cause outbreaks of bronchopneumonia in the experimental animals.

236.

B. *Dermatophilus congolensis* is a gram-positive organism with hyphal-like forms that is the etiologic agent of dermatophilosis, a skin disease of domestic animals. The organism is best visualized by making a touch preparation from the scabbing dermatitis, which is then stained with methenamine silver or Giemsa stain. Reports of human infections are rare and involve immunocompromised hosts.

237.

C. *Streptococcus sanguis* is a member of the viridans group of streptococci. These organisms produce a characteristic alpha hemolysis on blood agar media. A part of the normal indigenous flora of the oral cavity, they are pathogenic most commonly for humans who have damaged heart valves. In such patients this group of microorganisms is a major cause of subacute endocarditis.

238.

D. *Staphylococcus epidermidis* is a saprophytic microorganism found on the skin and mucous membranes of humans. This coagulase-negative *Staphylococcus* is seen frequently as a contaminant in blood cultures when proper venipuncture technique has not been used. *Staphylococcus epidermidis* has been implicated in serious human infections associated with the surgical insertion of prosthetic devices.

239.

B. *Escherichia coli* is frequently the etiologic agent of cystitis. This agent can be easily recognized by its fermentation of lactose, negative citrate reaction, and positive indole test. On EBM agar *Escherichia coli* produces the characteristic dark colonies with a metallic sheen.

240.

D. *Bacillus anthracis* is the etiologic agent of human anthrax that occurs in any of three forms: cutaneous, pulmonary, gastrointestinal. On Gram stain this organism appears as a large, spore-forming, gram-positive bacillus that characteristically grows in long chains. Colonies on agar plates are large and opaque with fingerlike projections that are typically referred to as "Medusa head" forms.

241.

D. PCR and LCR DNA amplification techniques have been shown to be more sensitive than cell culture and nearly 100% specific for the detection of *C. trachomatis*. Suitable specimens for detection are vaginal or cervical secretions or urine. When confirmation of *C. trachomatis* is needed, tissue culture remains the test of choice.

242.

C. *Mycoplasmas* are implicated in a variety of human infections. *Mycoplasma pneumoniae*, in particular, is a clinically important respiratory tract pathogen. When grown on culture media, colonies are said to have a "fried egg" appearance because the central portion of the colony has grown into the agar and thus appears more dense.

243.

A. "Satellitism" is the name given to the appearance of colonies of *Haemophilus influenzae* on blood agar media around colonies of organisms that provide the needed growth factor. *Haemophilus influenzae* requires both hemin and coenzyme I, nicotinamide adenine dinucleotide (NAD). Colonies of some organisms such as *Staphylococcus* and *Neisseria* produce coenzyme I, which diffuses into the surrounding agar enabling *Haemophilus influenzae* to grow.

244.

A. *Bordetella pertussis* is the etiologic agent of whooping cough. On Bordet-Gengou agar the organism forms small, round colonies, which appear pearlike, as if they were mercury droplets. A nasopharyngeal swab is now recommended as the optimal specimen type for the recovery of this agent.

245.

B. Organisms use toxins to establish infection and multiply in the host; a virulence mechanism. Activities of toxins range from enzymes that assist in tissue invasion to highly specific activities—for example, diptheria toxin inhibits protein synthesis. The toxin of *P. aeruginosa* is similar to diphtheria toxin but the role of the toxin produced by *B. pertussis* is not clear.

246.

A. The capsule a gelatinous layer covering an entire bacterium is a determinant of virulence of many bacteria. It limits the ability of phagocytes to engulf the bacteria. Capsular polysaccharides are used as the antigens in certain vaccines, since they are capable of eliciting protective antibodies. *Legionella pneumophila* do not possess a capsule.

247.

C. Staphylococci colonize various skin and mucosal surfaces in humans. The carrier state is common and infections are frequently acquired when a colonizing strain is introduced in a normally sterile site during an invasive procedure. Hospital personnel may harbor resistant strains, and person-to-person contact is a substantial infection control concern. Cultures of the anterior nares are recommended when screening for carriers in the hospital environment.

248.

D. The susceptibility of alpha-hemolytic streptococcal isolates to optochin or ethylhydrocupreine HCl is a presumptive test for the differentiation of *Streptococcus pneumoniae* from viridans species. Viridans streptococci are typically resistant to this agent and show no zone of inhibition or a zone of less than 10 mm when tested. *S. pneumoniae* characteristically is susceptible and produces a zone of inhibition equal to 10–12 mm.

249.

A. Solubility of *Streptococcus pneumoniae* colonies by surface-active agents, such as sodium desoxycholate, is a widely used presumptive identification procedure. When a 10% solution of this reagent is applied to test colonies, *S. pneumoniae* will be totally dissolved. Colonies of viridans streptococci typically remain intact when bile is applied.

ANAEROBIC BACTERIA

250.

A. Isolates of the anaerobic, spore-forming, bacillus *Clostridium perfringens* characteristically produce a pattern of double-zone hemolysis on blood agar plates. A smear of such colonies should demonstrate a medium-sized gram-positive bacillus that does not contain spores. For further identification the isolate should be inoculated on an egg yolk agar plate to look for lecithinase production (opalescence).

251.

C. *Prevotella melaninogenica* was isolated from this cervical abscess. This anaerobic organism is part of the indigenous microflora of the respiratory, gastrointestinal, and genitourinary tracts and is considered a significant human pathogen. The black pigment appears after several days when growing on laked blood agar plates. Prior to pigmentation this isolate can be presumptively identified by its brick-red fluorescence under UV light. Pigmented *Porphpyromonas* sp. are asaccharolytic.

252.

C. *Clostridium tetani* is an obligate anaerobe. Spores are widespread in nature and cause disease by contaminating puncture wounds. The exotoxin, tetanospasmin, produced by this organism is one of the most powerful toxins known.

253.

B. The gram-positive, non-spore-forming, anaerobic bacillus *Actinomyces israelii* is a slow-growing organism that is considered to be an opportunistic pathogen. Colonies may not be visible before 5 to 7 days or longer. When colonies are seen, they appear white, opaque, lobate, irregular, and shiny and are described as resembling a molar tooth. *Actinomyces israelii* is part of the indigenous flora of the human mouth, and a few species of *Actinomyces* have been found to inhabit the vagina. Pathogenesis generally involves trauma to tissues of a mucous membrane and the introduction of this endogenous organism.

254.

A. The predominant indigenous flora of the human intestinal tract are anaerobic, gram-negative, non-spore-forming bacilli. The *Bacteroides fragilis* group, in particular, predominate in the fecal flora. Trauma involving the intestinal area or bowel surgery predisposes patients to an endogenous anaerobic infection. Although these organisms are present in large numbers, their routine identification in fecal cultures is of no diagnostic value.

255.

C. *Bacteroides fragilis* group, the most commonly isolated anaerobes and a predominant part of the indigenous fecal flora in humans, are not inhibited by the presence of bile. Bile-esculin agar plates are used for the selection and presumptive identification of *Bacteroides fragilis* group. Although not used as a component of selection media for the *Bacteroides* group, it is important to note that in general gram-negative, non-spore-forming, anaerobic bacilli are susceptible to penicillin. The *Bacteroides fragilis* group is an exception in that it is known to be resistant to penicillin.

256.

B. The second most commonly encountered group of anaerobes in human infections are the anaerobic, gram-positive cocci *Peptostreptococcus*. The species most commonly encountered in infection is *Peptostreptococci anaerobius*, which is easily identified by SPS disk test; growth is inhibited by sodium polyanethol sulfonate.

257.

C. The close chest abscess described is characteristic of human actinomycosis, which is caused by *Actinomyces israelii* an anaerobic, gram-positive, non-spore-forming bacilli. The organism is not acid-fast, which helps to differentiate it from a *Nocardia* sp. Actinomycotic pus characteristically shows "sulfur granules" or solid yellow particles made up of masses of the filamentous bacilli seen on the Gram stain in Color Plate 29.

258.

D. KVL agar is selective for the *Prevotella* and *Bacteroides* spp. Presumptive identification of *Bacteroides fragilis* group can be accomplished utilizing its antimicrobial resistance pattern. *Bacteroides* are resistant to vancomycin and kanamycin, unlike *Fusobacterium* species, which are resistant to vancomycin but susceptible to kanamycin. A kanamycin-vancomycin laked sheep blood agar plate should be part of the primary plating media for anaerobic cultures. After incubation, organisms present on this selective medium can be removed for more definitive testing.

259.

A. Cycloserine cefoxitin fructose agar (CCFA) is the recommended selective agar for *C. difficile*. *C. difficile* is spread from person to person in the hospital environment. Hospitalized patients treated with broad spectrum antibiotics become colonized when their normal intestinal flora is diminished.

260.

B. *Mobiluncus* stains gram-variable to gram-negative although it has a gram-positive cell wall. This curved and motile bacillus seems to contribute to the pathology of bacterial vaginosis. A Gram stain of the discharge that is produced in this condition can be used for the detection of these distinctively curved organisms.

261.

A. Infant botulism or "floppy infant" syndrome is seen in children up to 6 months of age. This infective process begins with the ingestion of food contaminated with spores of *Clostridium botulinum*.

Following ingestion viable spores are carried to the lower bowel, where they germinate and elaborate the powerful neurotoxin that produces the characteristic flaccid paralysis.

262.

A. *Propionibacterium acnes* is the most frequently isolated of all the gram-positive, non-spore-forming, anaerobic bacilli. It is a part of the normal human bacterial flora and predominates on the surface of the body but may also be recovered from the upper respiratory tract, intestines, and urogenital tract. This organism is a common contaminant of blood culture specimens because of its presence on the skin. Care in the preparation of the skin before venipuncture and interpretation of serial blood cultures helps to eliminate confusion caused by the recovery of this anaerobic isolate.

263.

C. The spore of *Clostridium tetani* is located terminally and is larger than the sporangium. Characteristically, when seen on Gram stain, the cells of *Clostridium tetani* resemble a drumstick or tennis racket. Spores can be readily seen in late growth phase cultures at 37 °C.

264.

C. *Fusobacterium nucleatum*, a gram-negative, anaerobic bacillus, is part of the indigenous microbial flora of the respiratory, gastrointestinal, and genitourinary tracts. It is frequently implicated as the causative agent in metastatic suppurative infections such as brain abscesses. These pale-staining bacilli characteristically appear as long, thin bacilli with pointed ends (spearlike morphology).

265.

A. *Clostridium tetani* produces two primary toxins, one of which is responsible for the characteristic symptoms of tetanus. The toxin produced by *C. botulinum* is the most powerful toxin known. The pathogenicity of *C. difficile* is produced by a toxin.

266.

A. *Clostridium botulinum* is the causative agent of botulism, a disease produced by an exotoxin that acts on the central nervous system. Types A, B, E, and F are all causes of human botulism; types C and D and less commonly types A and B are associated with disease in animals and birds. Type G has not been associated with disease in humans or animals. This anaerobic organism produces oval central or subterminal spores that germinate in food products or less commonly in wounds. Following germination they release a potent neurotoxin, which can be fatal in very small quantities.

267.

D. Resazurin is an Eh indicator used in anaerobic culture media. When the oxygen concentration is reduced, the resazurin indicator is colorless. A pink color in the medium as described would therefore indicate aeration and an unsuitable environment for the preservation of obligate anaerobic organisms.

268.

B. *Fusobacterium nucleatum* is the most frequent clinical isolate of the species of *Fusobacterium*. These anaerobes are part of the indigenous flora of human mucous membranes, oral cavity, intestine, and urogenital tract. *F. necrophorum* is, however, much more virulent.

269.

A. *Clostridium septicum* is isolated in the clinical laboratory in cases of serious or often fatal infections. Bacteremia seen in association with an underlying maglignancy. The most common types of cancer are colon or cecum, breast, or leukemia-lymphoma.

270.

A. Botulinal toxin is the most potent exotoxin known. When absorbed this exotoxin produces the paralyzing disease botulism. Toxin acts in the body by blocking the release of acetylcholine transmitters in the neuromuscular junction of the peripheral nervous system, causing muscle paralysis.

271.

B. *Clostridium perfringens* is the species most commonly associated with clostridial myonecrosis or gas gangrene. These soil and water saprophytes gain entrance to the human body through traumatic wounds most frequently. Once they have been introduced into injured tissue, the characteristic syndrome of gas gangrene due to the elaboration of exotoxins may occur. Following *C. perfringens*, *C. novyi* is the second most common cause of this clinical syndrome.

272.

D. *Eubacterium*, *Bifidobacterium*, and *Propionibacterium* are all anaerobic, gram-positive, non-spore-forming bacilli. This group of anaerobic micro-organisms is difficult to identify in the clinical laboratory and often requires the use of gas chromatography. These organisms are rarely isolated, and of those listed, only *Bifidobacterium dentium* is considered to be a major pathogen. Morphologic identification cannot be relied upon, since these organisms frequently appear coccoid and decolorize easily, making them at times appear gram-negative.

273.

C. *Clostridium tetani* is an obligate anaerobe. Spores are widespread in the soil. When introduced into a puncture wound the spores require the reduced oxygen environment produced by the necrotic tissue and poor blood supply in the wound. Cleaning and debridement of the wound is important as is the administration of a tetanus toxoid booster.

274.

B. *Clostridium difficile* is an obligate anaerobe that may be difficult to recover using the GasPak anaerobic procedure because of its oxygen sensitivity. Use of the selective and differential medium CCFA enables the microbiologist to make a rapid presumptive identification in suspected cases of pseudomembranous colitis. *Clostridium difficile* has oval subterminal spores and is negative for lipase, lecithinase, indole production, and lactose fermentation.

275.

D. *Veillonella* are obligate anaerobic, gram-negative cocci. They characteristically do not ferment carbohydrates but can reduce nitrates to nitrites and are esculin negative. These organisms, which are part of the normal flora of humans, are considered opportunistic and are commonly found in mixed infections.

276.

D. *Clostridium perfringens* produces spores that are oval and central in location but that are rarely seen in cooked foods or on laboratory cultures. This organism has five antigenic types, A to E, which can be used for the identification of strains. Type A is responsible for human cases of gas gangrene and food poisoning. Alpha toxin or lecithinase is produced by all strains of *C. perfringens*.

277.

D. *Clostridium tetani* is a strict anaerobe that is motile and produces terminal round spores. Biochemically it does not attack carbohydrates, with the rare exception of glucose. *C. tetani* is gelatinase and indole positive but is nonproteolytic and H_2S negative. The clinical manifestations of tetanus are the result of the release of a neurotoxic exotoxin.

278.

A. *Fusobacterium nucleatum* characteristically appears on Gram stain as a gram-negative rod with pointed ends. Their growth is inhibited by a 1 μg kanamycin disk and the presence of bile. The *Bacteroides fragilis* gp. and the pigmented species *Prevotella* and *Porphyromonas* are not inhibited by kanamycin.

279.

D. *Prevotella melaninogenica* can be rapidly presumptively identified on media containing laked blood with the use of an ultraviolet light source. This important anaerobic pathogen can be differentiated after 5 to 7 days' incubation by its black pigmentation. The use of ultraviolet enables a more rapid differentiation because of the appearance of a brick red fluorescence before the pigment is demonstrated.

280.

C. The pathogenic mechanism of *Clostridium difficile* is toxin mediated. This organism is known to cause pseudomembranous colitis associated with the use of antimicrobial therapy. The cytotoxin assay is performed in a cell culture monolayer, which is examined after incubation for evidence of cytotoxicity.

281.

B. The Nagler reaction aids in the identification of *Clostridium perfringens*. This test is appropriate because it identifies alpha-toxin producers, which include perfringens. Performed on egg yolk agar, this test is done by applying *C. perfringens* type A antitoxin on one half and then streaking the test isolate at a right angle in a line across the plate. After incubation a positive test is indicated by inhibition of lecithinase production on the side containing antitoxin.

282.

A. The identification of *Peptostreptococcus anaerobius* is made easier by the use of the SPS disk. The test is performed by growing the organism in the presence of a disk impregnated with sodium polyethanol sulfonate (SPS). A zone of inhibition of 12–18 mm around the disk is considered a positive test for the presumptive identification of this organism.

283.

B. *Clostridium ramosum* produces oval subterminal spores, but they are seldom seen in the laboratory. This organism decolorizes easily and is curved in appearance on Gram stain. *C. ramosum* produces positive carbohydrate fermentation reactions in glucose, lactose, maltose, sucrose, and salicin.

284.

B. Anaerobes are a major cause of brain abscess. *Peptostreptococcus* sp. are most often associated with human disease and are easily seen on a Gram stain of clinical material. The characteristic Gram stain morphology of *Fusobacterium* would enable a physician to make a presumptive identification of the presence of anaerobic flora in this clinical case.

285.

C. *Bifidobacterium dentium* is a normal inhabitant of the human body that is most commonly recovered from pulmonary infections. A Gram stain reveals the characteristic gram-positive, bifurcated, diphthcroid-to-filamentous bacillus. Gas chromatographic analysis of metabolic end products and carbohydrate fermentation reactions are characteristics used for identification.

286.

D. *Bacteroides fragilis* gp. predisposes to abscess formation. The capsule may be a contributing factor to the pathology produced by this anaerobe. The polysaccharide capsule is an important virulence mechanism for *Bacteroides fragilis* gp.

287.

A. The morphology of *Fusobacterium nucleatum* helps to distinguish these organisms from other anaerobic, gram-negative, non-spore-forming bacilli such as bacteroides. They appear as long, thin rods that have pointed or spearlike ends. Most commonly they are recovered from brain and lung abscesses.

288.

B. The *Bacteroides fragilis* gp. is among the most antibiotic-resistant anaerobes. Beta-lactamase production is responsible for their resistance to penicillin. They are also resistant to first-generation cephalosporins, and aminoglycosides.

289.

C. The common agents in cases of aspiration pneumonia are oral anaerobes such as the black-pigmented *Prevotella* sp. and *Porphpyromonas* sp., species of *Bacteroides*, fusobacteria and anaerobic streptococci. These endogenous organisms, when in an abnormal site, possess virulence factors that enable them to produce disease. Often these are polymicrobic infections mixing anaerobes with aerobic or facultative organisms such as *Enterobactericeae* or *Staphylococcus aureus*.

SPIROCHETES

290.

C. *Leptospira* species are most reliably detected during the first week of illness by the direct culturing of a blood sample. The media of choice are Fletcher semisolid and Stuart liquid media, both of which are supplemented with rabbit serum. One or two drops of the patient's blood are added to 5 mL of culture medium, which is incubated in the dark at 30 °C or room temperature for up to 6 weeks. After the first week of disease and lasting for several months, the urine becomes the specimen of choice for isolation of the organism. Direct microscopic examination is not reliable for detection because of the low numbers of organisms normally present in body fluids.

291.

D. Congenital syphilis may result in termination of fetal development, premature birth, or fetal death, or the pregnancy may go to term. Not until the fifth month is the placental development such that spirochetes can be transmitted to the fetus. Following in utero infection, the infant is most often born with lesions characteristic of secondary syphilis; perinatal death is not an uncommon consequence of infection.

292.

B. The description given is characteristic of members of the genus *Leptospira*. Blood and other fluids such as cerebrospinal fluid and urine are examined by direct dark-field microscopy and stained preparations for the presence of these organisms in suspected cases of leptospirosis. The number of organisms present in clinical samples is low, and detection is difficult even when concentration methods are used. Cultural and serologic tests are available for the diagnosis of disease produced by these organisms.

293.

B. The body louse, *Pediculus humanus*, is the vector for the transmission of *Borrelia recurrentis*. Pathogenic species not only have specific vectors but also well-defined geographical distributions. Epidemic relapsing fever is found in Ethiopia, Sudan, and parts of South America.

294.

C. The antigen in the VDRL test is cardiolipin. In this flocculation test reagin, an antibody-like protein, is produced by infected patients. The reagin binds to cardiolipin-lecithin-coated cholesterol particles causing the particles to flocculate indicating a positive test result.

295.

C. *Spirillum minus* is the etiologic agent of sodoku or rat-bite fever. There are two types of rat-bite fever, each with a different causative agent. The disease, first described in Japan as sodoku, was not described in the United States until 1920. In the United States the disease is known as Haverhill fever and was first associated with the ingestion of contaminated milk. The etiologic agent of Haverhill fever is *Streptobacillus moniliformis,* whereas sodoku is caused by a spiral microorganism. *Spirillum minus* cannot be cultured on artificial media but can be visualized by dark-field microscopy or Gimenez stain. Treatment with a combination of penicillin and tetracycline is recommended.

296.

C. Lyme disease was first described in 1975 following an outbreak in Lyme, Connecticut. The etiologic agent, *Borrelia burgdorferi*, is transmitted to humans by the tick vector *Ixodes dammini*. Clinically the disease peaks in the summer and pro-

duces an epidemic inflammatory condition characterized by skin lesions, erythema, headache, myalgias, malaise, and lymphadenitis. A second clinical picture may present weeks later in some patients with symptoms of meningoencephalitis, myocarditis, or chronic arthritis.

297.

B. The basic structure of spirochetes is an outer membrane, cytoplasmic membrane-peptidoglycan complex, cytoplasm, and axial fibrils. The fibrils are attached to the cytoplasmic membranes close to the ends of the cell extending along the body under the outer membrane. The axial fibrils most closely resemble bacterial flagella and are associated with motility of the organism.

298.

B. Spirochetes are gram-negative but most do not stain with Gram stain. Silver impregnation can be used to visualize them in smears. The direct observation using dark-field or phase optics is recommended to view these delicate, coiled cells in body fluids or tissue sections.

299.

B. Infections other than syphilis can cause a positive VDRL result. The VDRL test detects an antibody that is not directed against *T. pallidum* antigens. It is a good screening test for syphilis but it is not highly specific. Confirmation with a specific treponemal test is required.

SUSCEPTIBILITY TESTING

300.

D. The concentration of the divalent cations Ca^{++} and Mg^{++} in the Mueller-Hinton agar test medium may affect the test results for aminoglycosides. The performance of each new lot of cation-supplement Mueller-Hinton should be tested with the control strain of *Pseudomonas aeruginosa* (ATCC 27853) before use. Increased concentrations of these cations, especially when testing *P. aeruginosa* to aminoglycosides such as gentamicin, may produce smaller zones of inhibition and result in the reporting of false resistance.

301.

C. In addition to determining the in vitro susceptibility of a bacterial isolate, a laboratory can measure the activity of the patient's own serum (containing the antimicrobial agent with which she/he is being treated) against his/her specific pathogen. A serum sample is obtained from the patient at a specific time after the antimicrobial dose, serially diluted and the antimicrobial activity against the infecting bacteria is determined. The lowest dilution of the patient's serum that kills a standardized inoculum is call the serum bactericidal titer or level.

302.

A. Standardization of the susceptibility testing procedure is essential for the determination of the susceptibility of an organism to antimicrobial agents. A 0.5 McFarland standard is used when adjusting the turbidity of the suspension of test organism. An 0.5 McFarland standard has a turbidity consistent with approximately $1–2 \times 10^8$ organisms per mL of broth or saline.

303.

D. Hemophilus Test Medium was developed by Dr. James Jorgenson and is recommended for use in the disk-agar diffusion susceptibility testing procedure. This medium will support the growth of most bacterial pathogens. The testing of Haemophilus isolates requires that this medium be supplemented to support the growth of this fastidious organism. In vitro growth of *Haemophilus influenzae* requires the presence of accessory growth factors: X factor (hemin) and V factor (nicotinamide-adenine dinucleotide).

304.

D. Sulfonamides act to interfere with the ability of bacterial cells to use *p*-aminobenzoic acid, which is a part of the folic acid molecule, by competitive inhibition. These chemotherapeutic agents are bacteriostatic and not bactericidal. The drug sulfisoxazole is a member of this group and is widely used in the treatment of urinary tract infections, especially those caused by *Escherichia coli*, which must synthesize folic acid for growth.

305.

D. Antimicrobial susceptibility testing is not routinely performed on all types of bacteria. Certain organisms are predictably susceptible to a variety of antimicrobial agents. Therefore, testing is not usually performed even when these organisms are the etiological agents of infection. Bacteria for which susceptibility tests are usually not performed include: *Streptococcus pyogenes* (Group A strep), *Streptococcus agalactiae* (Group B strep), and *Neisseria meningitidis*.

306.

C. Inhibitors of peptidoglycan synthesis such as penicillin act to inhibit cell wall development. Bacteria unable to produce the peptidoglycan for their cell walls are subject to the effects of varying osmotic pressures. The peptidoglycan component of the cell wall protects the bacterium from lysis.

307.

C. The requirement of 99.9% killing defines the minimum bactericidal concentration (MBC) of an antimicrobial agent. The MBC test is an additional quantitative assessment of the killing effect of a drug on a specific patient isolate. This test, done to evaluate a drug's activity, is one of the most commonly requested procedures in cases of life-threatening clinical conditions.

308.

C. Serum is the most appropriate clinical specimen for the assay of antimicrobial agents. Antibiotics such as aminoglycosides, vancomycin, and chloramphenicol demonstrate a narrow range between efficacy and excess. The trough level concentration (minimum concentration), which occurs between doses, is thought to be the more sensitive indicator of defective clearance. Blood for trough levels should be collected just before the next dose of antimicrobial agent is to be given.

309.

D. The therapeutic effect of antimicrobial therapy is often increased by the use of a combination of drugs. A combination of antimicrobials is said to be synergistic when the sum of their effects is greater than that derived from either drug when tested independently. A tenfold decrease in the number of viable cells from that obtained by the most effective drug in the combination is the definition of synergism. Synergistic combinations of antimicrobials are used primarily in the treatment of tuberculosis, enterococcal endocarditis, and certain gram-negative bacillus infections.

310.

D. β-lactamase production by strains of *Haemophilus influenzae* renders them resistant to the antibacterial effect of penicillin and ampicillin. It is recommended that rapid beta-lactamase testing be performed on isolates in life-threatening clinical infections such as meningitis. The rapid tests all rely on this enzyme's ability to act on a beta-lactamase ring and in turn produce a color change, which denotes a positive acidic condition as a result of the production of penicilloic acid.

311.

A. The recommended plating medium for use in both the disk diffusion and tube dilution susceptibility test procedures is Mueller-Hinton agar. Low in tetracycline and sulfonamide inhibitors, this medium has been found to show only slight batch-to-batch variability. For the susceptibility testing of fastidious organisms, 5% defibrinated sheep blood may be added or chocolatized for testing *Haemophilus* species.

312.

B. The Bauer-Kirby or disk-agar diffusion susceptibility test requires that the pH of the test agar be tested at room temperature to ensure an optimal range of 7.2–7.4 before use in the procedure. A sample of the Mueller-Hinton medium can be tested by macerating it in distilled water and testing with a pH meter electrode; a surface electrode is acceptable if available for direct testing. Another acceptable method is to allow the agar to solidify around the electrode of a pH meter and then obtain a reading.

313.

B. Metronidazole, a drug recommended for the treatment of amoebic dysentery and trichomoniasis, is a synthetic compound that acts by effecting DNA synthesis. The use of this drug for treating anaerobic infections has gained emphasis in light of resistance patterns of many of the commonly recovered anaerobes. Metronidazole is consistently active against all gram-negative, anaerobic bacilli, is able to cross the blood-brain barrier, and is the only agent consistently bactericidal against susceptible isolates.

314.

C. Tobramycin, an aminoglycoside aminocyclitol, is the only antibiotic, of those listed, that is bactericidal. Bactericidal antibiotics actually destroy the bacteria, whereas bacteriostatic drugs only arrest the growth of the microorganism. All aminoglycosides, with the exception of spectinomycin, are bactericidal in their activity.

315.

C. The selection and concentration of the antimicrobial disks and the storage and handling of the disks have been identified as two of five variables that account for discrepancies in the disk-diffusion procedure. Other variables were noted to be the selection of the plating medium, age of the agar, depth of the agar, methodology of testing, and criteria for the interpretation of results. The standardization of the procedure for disk-diffusion susceptibility testing must be followed to obtain reproducible and clinically useful information.

316.

C. Most fastidious bacteria do not grow satisfactorily in standard in vitro susceptibility test systems that use unsupplemented media. For certain species such as *Haemophilus influenzae, Neisseria gonorrheae, Streptococcus pneumoniae,* and other *Streptococcus* species, modifications have been made to the standard National Committee for Clinical Laboratory Standards (NCCLS) methods. In the case of *S. pneumoniae,* current NCCLS broth dilution test conditions include cation supplemented Mueller-Hinton broth with 5% lysed horse blood. Other fastidious organism may require different supplements, different incubation times and/or incubation in an atmosphere with increased CO_2.

317.

B. Detection of β-lactamase production can be performed directly, and the methods are reliable for the detection of penicillin and ampicillin resistance. Rapid test methods, in general, rely on a color change to detect the presence of this enzyme. A pH indicator may be used to detect the penicilloic acid produced when the beta-lactam ring of penicillin is cleaved; the penicillic acid may be detected by its ability to reduce iodine in a starch-iodine mixture, or a color change can be observed when the beta-lactam ring of a chromogenic cephalosporin is hydrolyzed by the enzyme.

318.

C. Tolerance is described as the ability of certain strains of organisms to resist lethal concentrations of antimicrobial agents like penicillin. The growth of these organisms is only inhibited by these cidal drugs. This new mechanism of bacterial resistance is attributed to a deficiency of cell wall autolysins.

319.

C. The rise in antimicrobial resistant isolates of *Mycobacteria tuberculosis* has been a major public health crisis. Currently, the accepted methods for determining the in vitro antimicrobial susceptibility of mycobacteria are based on the growth of the microorganisms on or in a solid or liquid medium containing a specified concentration of a single drug. Two such methods that have been described and are in common use in the United States are the agar proportion method and the BACTEC method.

ANTIMICROBIAL AGENTS

320.

A. The mode of action of these drugs is to inhibit cell wall synthesis. Both gram-positive and gram-negative organisms have cell walls composed of peptidoglycan. Organisms that do not have a cell wall, such as *Mycoplasma*, are not susceptible to these antimicrobial agents.

321.

A. Vancomycin is produced by an actinomycete, which acts to inhibit cell wall synthesis of susceptible bacteria. The main activity of this drug is to inhibit peptidoglycan synthesis, but it also has an effect on other aspects of bacterial metabolism. Vancomycin is a bactericidal antibiotic.

322.

D. Metronidazole, a nitroimidazole derivative, is active against most of the clinically significant anaerobes. Only some of the non-spore-forming gram-positive anaerobic bacilli and gram-positive anaerobic cocci are not susceptible to this agent. This drug acts to disrupt bacterial DNA through the production of cytotoxic intermediates.

323.

C. Gentamicin is a member of the aminoglycoside aminocyclitol group of antibiotics. These drugs act on the 30S ribosomal subunit site to inhibit protein synthesis. Gentamicin is particularly effective against a wide variety of gram-negative bacilli.

324.

B. Bone marrow toxicity is the major complication of chloramphenicol use. Reversible bone marrow suppression with anemia, leukopenia, and thrombocytopenia occurs as a direct result of the agent on hematopoiesis. The second form of bone marrow toxicity is a rare but usually fatal aplastic anemia. The mechanism of this response is not known.

MYCOLOGY

325.

C. Areas of the San Joaquin Valley are highly endemic for *C. immitis*, and infectious arthroconidia of this fungus can be distributed in dust aerosols produced by construction and other disturbances. Symptomatic pulmonary disease patterns vary, but the signs and symptoms given are found in many cases. The fungus grows more rapidly than do other systemic fungal pathogens, and the aerial mycelium will typically produce the characteristic barrel-shaped arthrospores.

326.

D. The distribution of *Histoplasma capsulatum* is probably worldwide but most clinical disease occurs in the western hemisphere. Most cases in the United States occur in the Ohio and Mississippi River valleys. This organism is found in areas contaminated by large amounts of bird excrement, such as starling and blackbird roosts. Inhalation of the spores results in a respiratory illness usually with clinical symptoms within two weeks of exposure. Disease ranges from a mild influenzaelike illness to acute fulminant lung infection resembling tuberculosis.

327.

D. *Sporothrix schenckii* is the agent of sporotrichosis. It usually enters the skin by traumatic implantation. This fungus grows in vitro as a small yeast at 36 °C and as a mold at room temperature (25–30 °C) with delicate hyphae and conidia.

328.

C. All species listed may be urease positive, but *C. terreus* does not grow at 37 °C and may assimilate nitrate. *C. krusei* is inositol negative, and these species of *Candida* and *Trichosporon* produce hyphae on morphology agar. *C. neoformans* typically does not produce hyphae and is nitrate negative, inositol and urease positive, and grows at 37 °C.

329.

D. Infections due to *Penicillium marneffei* seem to originate in eastern and southeastern Asia. This fungi was first isolated in 1959 from a hepatic lesion from a bamboo rat, a rodent found throughout Southeast Asia. Clinical disease includes fever, weight loss, anemia, and death if untreated. Skin lesions may be present and may drain pus. Diagnosis is made via culture or histopathologic exam of lesions of skin, bone, or liver. The yeastlike cells of *P. marneffei* are oval (3–8 μm) and scattered throughout tissue. Elongated, sausage-shaped cells often contain crosswalls. At 25–30 °C structures typical of the genus *Penicillium* develop. At 35–37 °C round or oval yeastlike cells are seen.

330.

C. Diagnostic features of *H. capsulatum* include large, 8–14 μm macroconidia with tuberculate projections. Tuberculate and smooth macroconidia may be seen in the same colony. Microconidia are also produced.

331.

B. Neonatal thrush is the oral candidiasis most commonly associated with mothers having vaginal *Candida*, and the newborn acquires the organism from the mother. Antepartum treatment with clotrimazole has been shown to decrease markedly vaginal Candida infestation and thrush of newborn infants. Diaper rash due to *C. albicans* usually follows oral and perianal candidiasis of the infant. The other three infections are associated with physiologic changes in the host, which permit proliferation of *C. albicans* already present in the host's microflora.

332.

A. KOH wet mounts should be used routinely for direct examination of nail, skin, or hair for fungal elements. KOH digests the keratinous tissue and facilitates observation of any fungi present. *Epidermophyton floccosum* and *Trichophyton* species invade nails, and the former typically is found as chains of arthroconidia in nail tissue.

333.

A. At 25–30 °C *Blastomyces dermatitidis* forms septate hyphae with delicate conidiophores of various lengths that bear round or oval conidia. It is important not to confuse the mold phase of *B. dermati-*

tidis with either *Scedosporium apiospermum* or *Chrysosporium* species. *S. apiospermum* appears as septate hyphae with simple conidiophores of various lengths that bear oval conidia singly or in groups. *Scedosporium apiospermum* is the causative agent of mycetoma and can infect brain, bones, eyes, lungs, etc. *Chrysosporium* sp. appears as septate hyphae with simple to branched conidiophores that bear oval conidia. *Chrysosporium* sp. is commonly considered a contaminant.

334.

B. Conidiophores of *Aspergillus* arise from a foot cell and terminate in a vesicle. The vesicle produces phialides; the phialides then produce the conidia. Before the culture is mature, the presence of a young conidiophore with a foot cell and vesicle is a good clue to the identity of the fungus.

335.

D. Zygomycosis caused by members of the Mucorales is an acute disease that often results in death within a few days in acidotic patients. Fungal agents of mucormycosis include *Rhizopus, Mucor*, and *Absidia*, which are common fungi found free in the environment.

336.

D. When speciation of *T. mentagrophytes* or *T. rubrum* is not certain on morphology alone, the in vitro hair test is useful; *T. mentagrophytes* is positive; *T. rubrum* is negative. Urease production by *T. mentagrophytes* is less reliable. Neither species produces endothrix infection, and *T. rubrum* rarely infects hair.

337.

D. *Rhizopus* and other fungal agents of mucormycosis are characterized by having cenocytic (nonseptate) hyphae. The finding of broad, nonseptate hyphal elements in sterile body fluids or tissue can provide rapid confirmation of a clinical diagnosis of mucormycosis.

338.

D. *Epidermophyton floccosum* infects skin and nails. This dermatophyte produces thin-walled macroconidia, usually in clusters, but no microconidia. *Microsporum* species produce infections in hair and skin; *Trichophyton* species may produce infection of the nails, hair, and skin.

339.

D. Essentially all strains of *Candida albicans* typically produce germ tubes within 2 hours incubation at 37 °C in serum or a similar proteinaceous substrate. Chlamydoconidia are produced by most strains of *C. albicans* after 24 to 48 hours at 22–26 °C in cornmeal Tween 80 agar or a similar substrate. *C. albicans* is sucrose positive, thus differing from *Candidia stellatoidea*. Use of eosin methylene blue (EMB) medium to screen for *C. albicans* may require 24 to 48 hours incubation.

340.

D. The dimorphic pathogenic fungi include the species named. The parasitic or tissue phase of *P. brasiliensis* produces large, multiple-budding yeasts, 20–60 μm long. The saprophytic or mycelial phase colonies resemble *B. dermatitidis*, but all cultures produce intercalary chlamydoconidia and coiled hyphae, and production of conidia is delayed or absent. Clinical types of paracoccidioidomycosis include relatively benign, primary pulmonary infection, progressive pulmonary disease, disseminated disease, or an acute, fulminant, juvenile infection. The disease is endemic in certain areas of Central and South America.

341.

C. Histoplasmin is an extract of the mycelial phase of *Histoplasma capsulatum*, and the immunodiffusion test for histoplasmosis, using histoplasmin as the antigen, appears to become positive within the first month of infection. The h line of antigen-antibody precipitation has been shown to correspond to the presence of active infection, but it may be present up to 2 years following cure. Some variations and cross reactions have been found in this test, but it is still an important serologic procedure for histoplasmosis.

342.

D. Barrel-shaped arthroconidia, alternating with empty cells, are typical of the mature mycelial phase of *Coccidioides immitis*. Species of *Geotrichum* produce chains of hyaline arthroconidia, and *Trichosporon* is characterized by production of hyaline arthroconidia, blastoconidia, hyphae, and pseudohyphae. *Aureobasidium* produces dematiacious arthroconidia. Sporothrix is the sole member of the list that does not produce arthroconidia.

343.

C. Several species of dematiacious fungi are causative agents of chromoblastomycosis. Among the most common are *Fonsecaea pedrosoi, Fonsecaea compacta, Cladosporium carrionii,* and *Phialophora verrucosa*. In tissue these fungi produce brown, spherical cells called Medlar bodies or sclerotic bodies. In cultures Phialophora verrucosa usually produces Phialophora-type conidiophores and conidia and sometimes *Cladosporium* type. *Fonsecaea* isolates may produce any of the three types of conidia.

344.

C. *Absidia* and *Mucor* are genera in the order Mucorales that can cause mucormycosis in debilitated patients. Rhino-facial-cranial syndrome is the form of this infection most often seen in the United States. Species of *Aspergillus* are ubiquitous and opportunistic, causing a variety of human infections. *Fusarium* is one of the saprobic fungi most often found in external mycotic keratitis following corneal trauma. *Coccidioides* is considered a true pathogen that can attack normal healthy people.

345.

A. Observation of pigmented hyphae in a culture is evidence that the fungus is in one of the dematiacious genera. Typically, the reverse of a plate will be black. *Alternaria* is a common dematiacious contaminant.

346.

C. Mycotic keratitis due to *Fusarium* has been reported following injury or cortisone treatment. An ulcerative lesion develops on the cornea. Corneal scrapings may be received for direct exam and culture.

347.

B. Five general conditions may disrupt the normal equilibrium between the host and *C. albicans*. These are extreme youth, physiologic change, prolonged administration of antibacterial antibiotics, general debility and the constitutionally inadequate patient, and iatrogenic and barrier-break conditions. Pregnancy and diabetes are physiologic conditions that increase colonization with *C. albicans* and concurrent opportunities for infection. Childhood viral infections are not associated with an increase in fungal infection.

348.

C. DiGeorge's syndrome includes absence of the thymus. It is associated with an increase in CMCC due to genetic defects in cellular immunity. Patients with Bruton's hypogammaglobulinemia are deficient in humoral immunity only and have no increased incidence of candidiasis. None of the other syndromes results in defects in cellular immunity.

349.

A. Diagnostic features of *Fusarium* sp. include hyaline septate hyphae, sickle- or banana-shaped macroconidia. Macroconidia are multiseptate with long or short branched or unbranched conidiophores. Microconidia (one or two celled) are also produced.

350.

B. *R. rubra* has been isolated from air, soil, and water and a number of food sources, especially dairy products, and as a contaminant of skin, lung, urine, or feces. *Rhodotorula* fungemia has been caused by contaminated catheters, intravenous solutions, and dialysis machines. These infections can be marked by endotoxic shock. *C. albicans* is a more common cause of diaper rash.

351.

D. *Malassezia furfur* is the causative agent of tinea or pityriasis versicolor—a superficial skin infection that occurs commonly on the upper back, chest, shoulders, upper arms, and abdomen. Initially lesions are discrete but in time may coalesce. Lesions may be hyper- or hypopigmented. *M. furfur* is part of the normal skin flora of over 90% of adults. There may be an association between the disease and excessive sweating. Disease is more common in tropical and subtropical areas. Diagnosis is made by KOH preparation of skin scrapings from the lesions that demonstrate the characteristic yeastlike cells and hyphae (spaghetti and meatballs). Most lesions will fluoresce yellow under a Wood's lamp.

352.

D. *C. albicans* is an endogenous species causing a variety of opportunistic infections. Infection is usually

secondary to a predisposing debility. The other fungi are common saprophytic contaminants.

353.

A. *Microsporum audouinii* most commonly effects children. Only rarely are adults infected. Colonies are flat, downy to silky, and gray to white in color. Colony reverse is salmon to brown with a reddish brown center. Microscopic exam reveals septate hyphae, terminal chlamydoconidia, occasional microconidia (borne singly). Macroconidia are very rare or absent. Infected hair fluoresces. Growth on polished rice grains aids in differentiating *M. audouinii* from other *Microsporum* species that grow well on rice grains.

354.

D. *H. capsulatum* is found primarily within histiocytes and in macrophages or monocytes in specimens from sternal punctures, biopsies, or the buffy coat of centrifuged blood. Unstained cell wall of the tissue (yeast) form of *H. capsulatum* may be mistaken for a capsular halo in stained preparations.

355.

B. Although *Blastomyces dermatitidis* is rarely found in the environment and there is no reliable skin test for screening for past or subclinical blastomycosis, the incidence of clinical cases in the United States is highest in the Mississippi and Ohio River basins and part of the Missouri River drainage. In 1970, Furcolow reported the highest number of infections in Kentucky and other states south of the Ohio River and east of the Mississippi.

356.

A. The most highly endemic regions of coccidioidomycosis are semiarid, with dry, hot seasons and wetter, cooler seasons still above freezing. The areas of southwestern United States and northern Mexico with this typical Lower Sonoran Life Zone climate have the highest incidence of coccidioidomycosis. The peak endemic period is fall when the fungus becomes airborne from the desert surface.

357.

C. Although *Cryptococcus neoformans* does not appear to infect pigeons, it apparently passes unharmed through the gut. It has been found in large numbers, even as the predominant microorganism, from the debris of old pigeon roosts. Viable, virulent, desiccated cells, small enough to be inhaled into the alveoli, can be present in the dust of these roosts.

358.
B. The most highly endemic areas of histoplasmosis (Missouri, Kentucky, southern Illinois, Indiana, and Ohio) also have the most starlings, whose flocks produce large accumulations of guano. *Histoplasma capsulatum* has been found growing in almost pure culture in accumulated starling guano. Exposure to aerosols containing many spores of this fungus has been associated with a number of "common source" outbreaks of histoplasmosis.

359.
A. In temperate countries including the United States, sporotrichosis is an occupational hazard of gardeners and nursery workers and is frequently associated with contact with sphagnum moss. In Mexico, it has been associated with working with grass, and a well-known epidemic in South Africa involved gold mine workers in contact with untreated mine poles.

360.
B. White piedra is caused by *T. beigelii*, which produces soft, white to light brown granules around and in the hair shaft. These are composed of hyphae, yeastlike arthroconidia, and sometimes blastoconidia. There may also be bacteria present within the granules. The beard and body hair are more often affected than scalp hair.

361.
C. Black piedra is caused by *P. hortae*, which produces brown to black, gritty nodules on the outside and under the cuticle of the hair shaft. Direct microscopic examination of portions of these nodules in KOH wet mounts can show septate dematiacious hyphae and ascospores.

362.
A. Tinea nigra is a superficial skin infection caused by *E. werneckii*, which has also been known as *Cladosporium werneckii*. The pigmented, painless lesion, which usually occurs on the palms or fingers, may be mistaken for melanoma, and accurate laboratory findings in a KOH preparation of a skin scraping are important in preventing surgical mutilation of the patient. Microscopic examination of skin scrapings from tinea nigra shows dematiacious, septate hyphae, and budding cells.

363.
B. Pityriasis versicolor is a chronic, mild, superficial skin infection caused by *M. furfur*, which may also be found on normal skin. These fungi have also been placed in the genus *Pityrosporum*. Tinea versicolor has been used as one of several synonyms for this infection, but the causative fungus is not a dermatophyte.

364.
C. *T. ajelloi* is a keratinophilic fungus easily isolated from the soil by hair baiting. It has been isolated rarely from human infections and from some animal infections, but it is more often found as a geophilic saprophyte. It is a rapid grower, producing numerous thick-walled smooth macroconidia and pyriform microconidia.

365.
A. *A. niger* causes approximately 90% of the external ear infections due to fungi. *Aspergillus fumigatus* also causes otomycosis. Other fungi, far less often involved, include *Scopulariopsis, Penicillium, Rhizomucor, Candida* species, and other species of *Aspergillus*.

366.
B. *Geotrichum* species typically produce numerous hyphae and arthrospores. Germinating arthrospores of *Geotrichum*, however, may be mistaken for blastospore production. This may cause confusion between *Geotrichum* and *Trichosporon*.

367.
C. *Trichosporon* species produce hyphae and arthrospores. They may also produce blastospores, although these may be rare. If present, blastospores can differentiate *Trichosporon* from *Geotrichum*.

368.
A. *C. albicans* and *Candida stellatoidea* both produce pseudohyphae and usually blastospores. Both are capable of producing chlamydospores, although these are uncommon with *C. stellatoidea*. It has been suggested that *C. stellatoidea* should be reclassified as a variety of *C. albicans*.

369.

B. In morphology agar, *C. tropicalis* typically produces long-branched pseudohyphae. Blastospores are produced singly or in short chains. This species does not produce chlamydospores. The carbon assimilation pattern of *C. tropicalis* is very like that of *C. albicans*, and some strains of *C. tropicalis* may produce a positive germ tube test if incubated more than 3 hours.

370.

C. *C. neoformans* produces only blastospores when growing in morphology agar. This species is usually identified by its encapsulated cells, production of urease, failure to assimilate nitrate, and its production of brown pigment on Niger seed agar.

371.

B. The most frequently diagnosed form of cryptococcosis is central nervous system infection. There may be few or many organisms in the cerebrospinal fluid, but a clinical diagnosis of meningitis can often be confirmed by cryptococcal antigen test. In the past the use of a microscopic examination of a spun specimen with India ink has been used. The encapsulated yeast cells are outlined by contrast with the dark background. The cryptococcal antigen test is much more sensitive and is the recommended test.

372.

A. *H. capsulatum* is a parasite of the reticuloendothelial system and is seldom extracellular. Specimens such as sternal marrow, lymph nodes, liver and spleen biopsies, or buffy coat of blood should be stained with Giemsa or Wright's stain and examined for intracellular yeast cells.

373.

C. *P. boydii* is the most common cause of eumycotic mycetoma in the United States. Mycetoma is a clinical syndrome of localized abscesses, granulomas, and draining sinuses that develops over months or years. It usually occurs on the foot or hand after traumatic implantation of soil organisms.

374.

D. *Trichophyton mentagrophytes* is a common cause of intertriginous tinea pedis or athlete's foot. This is a chronic dermatitis most often affecting the areas between the fourth and fifth and third and fourth toes. The acute inflammation often subsides, but recurrences are common.

QUALITY ASSURANCE

375.

D. Specimens for virus isolation that must be held for prolonged periods before processing should be frozen to -70 °C or below. In general, if there is only a delay of 1 or 2 days before processing, specimens should be held at refrigerator temperatures (2–6 °C). Freezing to -20 °C is not recommended because of the rapid loss of the infectivity of viruses at that temperature.

376.

B. Incubation of inoculated bacteriologic culture media requires that attention be given to optimal temperature ranges, adequate moisture, and proper atmospheric conditions for growth. The optimal atmosphere for many clinically significant isolates is one that contains 5–10% carbon dioxide. Capnophilic environments may be obtained through the use of incubators equipped with a tank of carbon dioxide and a regulator or GasPak carbon dioxide generators. Candle jars, although widely used, produce only about a 3% concentration of carbon dioxide. The portable Fyrite carbon dioxide gas analyzer may be used for the daily monitoring of capnophilic incubators.

377.

B. Microbiologic examination of body fluids is less effective when bacteria become trapped in clotted specimens. The most effective anticoagulant for use in the microbiology laboratory is sodium polyanetholsulfonate (SPS) in a concentration of 0.025–0.05%. Fluids known to clot on standing should be transported to the laboratory in a sterile tube containing SPS. This polyanionic anticoagulant is also anticomplementary and antiphagocytic.

378.

A. Standard quality control strains maintained by the American Type Culture Collection (ATCC) should be tested routinely as recommended by the National Committee for Clinical Laboratory Standards (NCCLS). Guidelines developed for the quality assurance of the disk-diffusion antimicrobial susceptibility test procedure recommended that the following organisms be used for this purpose: *Pseudomonas aeruginosa* (ATCC 27853), *Staphylococcus aureus* (ATCC 25923), *Escherichia coli* (ATCC 25922), and *Enterococcus fecalis* (ATCC 29212). Cultures of these organisms should be frozen or lyophilized to maintain their antimicrobial susceptibility pattern. Testing should not be done from stored cultures but rather from freshly grown 18- to 24-hour cultures.

379.

B. Pathogenic species of *Neisseria* sp. are extremely sensitive to adverse environmental conditions. Careful attention to specimen transport is needed to ensure the viability of the organism. Clinical samples frequently contain small numbers of the agent. Chilling and dehydration of a specimen before processing will substantially reduce, if not preclude, the isolation of *Neisseria gonorrhoeae* and *Neisseria meningitidis*. Nonnutritive transport media were originally created as appropriate transit systems for gonococci.

380.

A. Control organisms, as for other organisms, are also available for quality assurance programs in mycobacteriology laboratories. Culture media for the recovery of mycobacteria from clinical samples should routinely be performance tested by using isolates of *M. tuberculosis*, *M. kansasii*, *M. avium* complex, and *M. fortuitum*. Characteristics such as rate of growth, pigmentation, colonial characteristics, and temperature range can be assessed by the use of these isolates, which represent various Runyan groups.

381.

B. Methylene blue strips are the most commonly used oxidation-reduction (E_h) indicators. When anaerobic conditions are achieved, the methylene blue indicator will turn from blue (oxidized state) to white, indicating reduction. Resazurin, another E_h indicator, is used in anaerobic transport systems and anaerobic culture media such as the prereduced anaerobically sterilized (PRAS) system. Resazurin when oxidized is pink; when reduced, the color fades, indicating anaerobiosis.

382.

B. One of the metabolites in the tricarboxylic acid cycle, sodium citrate can serve as an energy source for some bacteria. The assessment of the ability of an organism to utilize citrate as its sole

source of carbon aids in the identification of the Enterobacteriaceae. *Klebsiella pneumoniae* is able to utilize citrate with the production of alkaline by-products. A blue color and/or growth of the isolate on the streak line or both are indicative of a positive reaction.

INFECTION CONTROL

383.

C. The ingestion of food contaminated with enterotoxin produced by *Staphylococcus aureus* is the most likely cause of the disease in the case described. *Staphylococcus aureus* multiplies rapidly. Within a few hours levels of 10^5 organisms per gram of food can be found. Enterotoxin is elaborated when the organism reaches stationary growth phase. Food contaminated with enterotoxin usually does not taste or smell unusual. Ingestion of small amounts of toxin results in a rapid onset (1–6 hours) of vomiting and diarrhea as a result of a neural response. Staphylococcal food poisoning is a self-limiting condition, which lasts no longer than 24 hours.

384.

D. *Neisseria meningitidis* is the etiologic agent of one form of inflammation of the meninges, which is known as epidemic cerebrospinal meningitis. Infection with *Bordetella pertussis* produces the highly contagious upper respiratory infection whooping cough. Both diseases are spread by droplet infection or fomites contaminated with respiratory secretions. The microorganisms are present in greatest numbers in the upper respiratory tract, and specimens for isolation and identification should be collected on nasopharyngeal swabs.

385.

B. Factors that influence how humans react to epidemic disease are both intrinsic and extrinsic. Intrinsic factors relate to the human body, with age being the most important response determinant. Specific infectious diseases are associated with age groups, and therefore specific populations are at greatest risk, and the incidence of disease is increased.

386.

A. *Salmonella typhi* is spread most commonly by chronic carriers. This enteric bacillus may be carried throughout a person's life, being sequestered most often in the gallbladder. Carriers are usually symptomless, and the presence of the organism can be confirmed only by isolation and identification in the clinical laboratory.

387.

D. Q fever is caused by infection with *Coxiella burnetii*, which has unique characteristics. Unlike other rickettsiae, this organism is able to resist heat and drying for long periods and does not rely on an arthropod vector for transmission. Infectious fomites such as dust from contaminated cattle hides are considered to be the primary mode of infection.

388.

D. *Brucella* sp. infect cattle and may be transmitted to man by the ingestion of contaminated milk or other dairy products. Milk is able to support the growth of many clinically significant microorganisms and may often be ingested in the unpasteurized state. Humans generally consume large quantities of milk, and in diseases such as brucellosis the infective dose is relatively small.

389.

A. Infectious aerosols put laboratory professionals at risk for acquiring many diseases. The handling of clinical specimens that require pipetting, centrifugation, or decanting may produce infectious aerosols. Bacteria frequently are present in greater numbers in aerosol droplets than in the liquid medium.

390.

C. *Pseudomonas aeruginosa* is a major cause of hospital-acquired infections. These opportunistic organisms are able to survive in moist environments for prolonged periods and may be transferred to compromised patients. Pseudomonas infections in recent years have accounted for as much as 10% of the nosocomial infections.

PROCEDURES, MEDIA, REAGENTS, AND STAINS

391.

A. The deamination of the amino acid phenylalanine by a microorganism results in the formation of phenylpyruvic acid. Detection of the activity of

this deaminase enzyme is accomplished by adding a 10% solution of ferric chloride to the growth on an overnight agar culture. Visualization of a green color in the liquid on the agar slant indicates the presence of phenylpyruvic acid.

392.

C. Mannitol salt agar is highly selective and differential. It is used for the isolation and identification staphylococcal species. The 7.5% concentration of sodium chloride results in the inhibition of most bacteria other than staphylococci. Mannitol fermentation, as indicated by a change in the phenol red indicator, aids in the differentiation of staphylococcal species since most *S. aureus* ferment mannitol (changing the color of the medium to yellow) and most coagulase-negative staphylococci are unable to ferment mannitol.

393.

B. When inoculated on a sulfur-containing medium, organisms that produce hydrogen sulfide will demonstrate a partial blackening of a strip impregnated with a 5% solution of lead acetate. The strip is inserted above the medium in the tube and is secured under the closure, which seals the tube. The presence of liberated, dissolved sulfide reacts with the lead on the strip, and a black (lead sulfide) color develops. This test is useful for the detection of weak hydrogen sulfide-producing organisms, since the TSI agar is not a sensitive indicator.

394.

C. A variety of media has been developed to aid in the isolation of *Neisseria gonorrhoeae* from specimens containing mixed flora. Examples include: Martin-Lewis, Thayer-Martin media. The common base medium for the isolation of *N. gonorrhoeae* is Chocolate agar. In 1964, Thayer and Martin formulated a Chocolate agar–based medium, which included polymixin B and vistocetin, with added hemoglobin and yeast extract. All specimens collected for the possible isolation of *N. gonorrhoeae* must be plated to selective media.

395.

C. Hektoen enteric agar was developed in 1967 by King and Metzger of the Hektoen Institute to improve the isolation of *Shigella* and *Salmonella*. The selective nature of this agar is due to the bile salts. The medium also contains three carbohydrates, lactose, sucrose, and salicin, along with a pH indicator to detect carbohydrate fermentation. Fermentative organisms turn the medium yellow. Ferric ammonium citrate and sodium thiosulfate are included in the medium to detect H_2S production. H_2S producing organisms appear as black-centered colonies.

396.

C. Selective enrichment media such as selenite broth are designed to reduce the numbers of normal bacterial flora in order to isolate enteric pathogens from clinical specimens. The broth, through the addition of chemicals and nutrients, is able to eliminate gram-positive cocci and to retard the growth of enteric gram-negative bacilli for 12 to 24 hours. At 24 hours, the broth is subcultured to differential and selective plating media.

397.

C. The calcofluor white stain requires the use of a fluorescence microscope. It is a rapid staining method, requiring only one minute to complete. Stain binds to cellulose in the cell wall of certain prokaryotic and eukaryotic fungi.

398.

A. TCBS agar is recommended for use in the selective isolation of *Vibrio* species associated with cholera, diarrhea, or food poisoning. The selective agent in this medium to inhibit gram-positive organisms is oxgall, a naturally occurring substance containing bile salts and sodium cholate. Sucrose is the carbohydrate utilized by vibrio. *Vibrio cholera* and *Vibrio alginolyticus* appear as large yellow colonies, and *Vibrio parahemolyticus* exhibits colonies with blue to green centers. Routine screening of stool specimens for *Vibrio* species is not cost effective in the United States; however, it is recommended that TCBS be used as a primary isolation media when patients present with a compatible illness and a history of eating raw seafood.

399.

D. Blood samples for the serologic diagnosis of viral diseases should be collected during the acute phase of the disease (shortly after onset) and during the convalescent stage, which is generally 1 or 2 weeks later. The separated serum should be stored at refrigerator temperatures or frozen until testing can be accomplished. Serologic confirmation of a viral illness generally requires a fourfold rise in a specific antibody titer. In other cases a significant ratio of antibody levels between the acute and convalescent sera has been defined as diagnostic.

400.

D. The Leifson flagellar staining technique is most commonly used in clinical laboratories. The morphology and location of flagella are observable by light microscopy after staining with the tannic acid-base fuchsin technique of Leifson. Although not a difficult technique, the test procedures must be strictly adhered to for accurate results. Proper pH of the stain, clean glass slides, the optimal growth phase of the organism, and the timing of the staining procedure itself are all critical factors.

401.

D. Nitrate reduction is a general characteristic of members of the Enterobacteriaceae. An organism with this ability removes oxygen from nitrates, and nitrites are produced in the medium. After incubation alpha-naphthylamine and sulfanilic acid are added to the medium. The presence of nitrites is indicated by the production of a red color within 30 seconds. If the reduction has gone all the way to nitrogen gas, the color change will not occur. The addition of zinc dust with no resulting color change confirms the reduction of nitrate.

402.

A. The decarboxylase activities of members of the *Enterobacteriaceae* are important tests for their identification. When a decarboxylase broth is inoculated with a test organism, the organism first ferments the glucose present, which produces a color change from purple to yellow. The yellow color indicates acid production. An organism that possesses decarboxylase activity will then be able to attack the amino acid present, producing alkaline amines. The amines in turn raise the pH, and a color change from yellow back to purple results. The lowered pH activates the decarboxylase enzyme.

403.

B. Oxidative-fermentative (O-F) medium was first devised by Hugh and Leifson in an attempt to detect weak acid production from nonfermentative bacilli. By decreasing the amount of peptone (0.2%) used in conventional media, the formation of oxidative products from amino acids, which may neutralize the weak acids produced by the organism, is reduced, and the metabolic reaction can be demonstrated. Demonstration is further facilitated by an increase in the concentration of carbohydrate (1.0%) in the medium, along with a semisolid consistency and the use of bromthymol blue as the indicator.

404.

D. Glucose metabolism by certain organisms produces acetyl methyl carbinol (acetoin) as the chief end product. To demonstrate this reaction 40% potassium hydroxide is added, which oxidizes the acetoin to diacetyl. The prior addition of alpha-naphthol, which acts as a catalyst, produces a red color complex if acetoin is oxidized. Members of the *Klebsiella, Enterobacter, Hafnia*, and *Serratia* groups of organisms produce a positive reaction in this test.

405.

D. Carbohydrate degradation tests using cystine trypticase agar (CTA) medium are particularly useful for the definitive identification of *Neisseria* species. An organism's acid production from specific carbohydrates is indicated by the production of a yellow color in the phenol red indicator used in the medium. Satisfactory test results can be achieved if inoculation and incubation procedures are adhered to. A dense suspension of a pure culture of an isolate is inoculated heavily just below the surface of the medium. Incubation of this medium is at 35–37 °C in an air incubator, not under increased CO_2.

406.

B. The acid-fast stain would be positive for all the organisms listed with the exception of *Actinomyces israelii*. Not only is the stain used to identify bacterial microorganisms, it is also positive for oocysts of *Cryptosporidium* sp. and *Cyclospora* sp. These coccidian parasites have been associated with outbreaks of diarrheal diseases associated with consumption of contaminated food and water.

407.

D. Most strains of *Staphylococcus saprophyticus* are resistant to novobiocin. This organism is frequently found in urine culture of young women and may be misidentified as *S. epidermidis*. A 5 μg disk is used in the test and a zone of 16 mm or less determines resistance.

408.

A. An area of precipitate in the agar around the colonies of *Clostridium perfringens* indicates that the organism produces lecithinase. Organisms that produce a pearly sheen on their surface are producing lipase. Lecithinase is identified as alpha toxin.

409.

D. Faulty collection or transportation procedures frequently result in failure to isolate the etiologic agent of an infectious disease. Samples should always be collected before therapy has been initiated and sent to the laboratory in appropriate collection systems to prevent loss of viability due to adverse environmental conditions. When samples must be sent through the mail, the use of special double containers is mandated by the Code of Federal Regulations. In the laboratory, refrigeration is not always an acceptable alternative when processing is delayed.

410.

D. Blood cultures are one of the most important specimen types sent for bacteriologic examination. A knowledge of the various clinical conditions that produce bacteremia is essential for optimal recovery of the causative agent. Not all conditions produce continuous bacteremia, and organisms may be present in low numbers. Cultures should always be drawn before antimicrobial therapy is initiated and optimally before a fever spike. There is a period of 1 to 2 hours from the time of the release of bacteria into the bloodstream and the subsequent physiologic chill response. It is recommended that cultures of blood be held in the laboratory for at least 1 week before being discarded as negative.

411.

B. ARD is the system that contains synthetic antibiotic-removing resins. Blood culture bottles incorporating this system are reported to yield significantly higher numbers of bacterial isolates. Bottles containing these resins should be used when the patient has already received antibiotic therapy.

412.

A. The oxidase test detects those organisms that produce the enzyme cytochrome oxidase. A freshly prepared 1% solution of dimethyl or tetra-methyl-*p*-phenylenediamine dihydrochloride is applied to filter paper, and the test organism is then rubbed into the impregnated area. A platinum loop on wire or wooden applicator stick should be used to pick the colony, since Nichrome wire may cause a false-positive reading. A positive oxidase test will demonstrate the rapid development of a dark purple color in the area where the organism was inoculated. *Pseudomonas aeruginosa* and *Aeromonas hydrophila* both produce cytochrome oxidase and would produce a positive test reaction. A negative oxidase test would be demonstrated by *Acinetobacter lwoffi*, which does not possess the enzyme.

413.
B. On serum-cystine-sodium thiohiosulfate-tellurite medium (Tinsdale medium), *Corynebacterium diphtheriae* is differentiated from other cornybacterium species and other bacteria of the respiratory tract by its ability to produce black colonies surrounded by a brown-black halo after 48 hours of incubation. Growth factors needed by *C. diphtheriae* are provided by the addition of the serum. Potassium tellurite is inhibitory to many gram-positive and gram-negative bacteria, but corynebacterium species are resistant. An interaction between tellurite and hydrogen sulfide produced from cystine causes the halo production by colonies *C. diphtheriae*.

414.
A. The SPS disk test is used for the presumptive identification of *Peptostreptococcus anaerobius*. A 12-mm or greater zone of inhibition identifies the anaerobic gram-positive coccus tested as susceptible and therefore identified as *P. anaerobius*. Anaerobic cocci are frequently recovered in the laboratory from wounds and body fluids in association with other microorganisms.

415.
D. Strains of *Haemophilus* that are able to synthesize heme are identified by the porphyrin test. Species such as *H. influenzae*, which require heme, would give a negative test reaction, while *H. parainfluenzae* would be positive. A red color is indicative of a positive reaction in this test.

RAPID METHODS

416.
A. Bacterial metabolism of carbohydrates in the culture media produces the by-product carbon diox-

ide, which is captured as head gas in sealed culture vials. Within only a few hours of inoculation it is possible using BACTEC 9240 or BACTEC 9120 to detect a bacterial infection by fluorescence. There is continuous monitoring of the sample with detection external to the bottle.

417.
C. The chromogenic cephalosporin method is the most sensitive test for the detection of the production of beta-lactamase enzymes. This yellow compound will become red in color if the organism tested produces the enzyme that is able to break the beta-lactam ring. Nitrocefin, the commonly used compound, has a high affinity for most bacterial beta-lactamases.

418.
B. Rapid tests can detect the chloramphenicol-modifying enzyme chloramphenicol acetyotransferase. If the enzyme is detected the organism is reported as resistant. A negative test result, however, does not rule out resistance mediated by another mechanism.

419.
A. *Chlamydia trachomatis* and *Neisseria gonorrhoeae* can be directly detected in suitable samples such as vaginal or cervical secretions or urine using the PCR and LCR DNA-amplification techniques. Amplification techniques have been shown to be more sensitive than culture and 100% specific for the identification of *N. gonorrhoeae* and much the same for *C. trachomatis*. Abbot Diagnostic's Ligase Chain Reaction assay for these two common sexually transmitted organisms is an example of a commercial molecular system for direct detection of infections.

420.
D. DNA sequences are detected by the southern blot test. DNA fragments are separated by electrophoresis on an agarose gel. The separated fragments then are overlaid with a nitrocellulose membrane and reacted with a labeled probe; hence specific DNA fragments are detected.

421.
B. Digestion of DNA with restriction endonucleases is the preparatory step in the construction of a DNA probe for use as a diagnostic reagent for the identification of specific microorganisms. Restric-

tion endonucleases reduce the DNA to linear fragments that contain the desired sequence. Once the specific gene has been isolated, it can be inserted into a carrier, which will enable the insertion of this DNA into another cell from which many copies of the probe will be made (cloning).

422.

C. Enzyme immunoassays (EIAs) or latex agglutination tests are used in clinical laboratories for the rapid identification of many agents of gastrointestinal diseases. EIA methods have proven accurate and sensitive for the diagnosis of rotovirus, cryptosporidiosis, and giardiasis. There is a simple screening procedure for *E. coli* 0157:H7, which uses a DFA stain.

423.

B. Direct fluorescent antibody (DFA) test results for *Bordetella pertussis* are presumptive. Both positive and negative test results must be confirmed by culture. The quality of the test result depends greatly on the experience of the microscopist, the quality of the antibody, and the microscope.

424.

D. The western blot assay is used for confirmation of HIV infection. In this assay peptide components of the agent are seperated on a gel. The separated fragments are then tested with patient serum suspected of containing antibodies against the agent and binding can be detected using visual methods.

425.

A. The acridine orange (AO) stain is used for the detection of low numbers of microorganisms in fluid and exudate samples. The application of this fluorescent dye enables the microbiologist to screen samples at low-power magnification. This technique is recommended for the routine screening of blood cultures and on cerebrospinal fluid sediment smears because of its superior sensitivity as compared to the Gram stain.

INFECTIOUS DISEASES

426.

B. Scalded skin syndrome is the dermatitis associated with the effects of the exfoliative toxin produced by strains of *Staphylococcus aureus*. The exfoli-

atin produced acts in humans to disrupt the adhesive forces between cells of the stratum granulosum, creating large flaccid bullae. This syndrome occurs primarily in infants and children, with the primary infection usually unrelated to the areas where lesions appear.

427.

D. Pseudomonads are ubiquitous microorganisms generally associated with moist environments. Cases such as the one described have been occurring more frequently as the popularity of health spas increases. In some cases the pattern of dermatitis caused by these organisms matches the areas covered by the host's swimsuit. When not properly maintained, whirlpools create a favorable environment for the growth of these organisms.

428.

C. *Arcanobacterium pyogenes* has been reclassified several times. It was formerly a member of the genera *Corynebacterium* and *Actinomyces*. *A. pyogenes* is a well-known animal pathogen causing soft tissue infections in a wide variety of farm animals. Mode of transmission to humans is unknown but most cases occur in a rural environment and include a history of abrasion or undetected wounds with animal exposure. The organism can be successfully identified in the lab using the API 20 Strep System, the API Coryne system, or the automatic Vitek system.

429.

C. Exotic pets such as iguanas, snakes, and turtles are known to transmit *Salmonella* sp. Young children who do not practice good handwashing after touching family pets are particularly at risk for infection. Natural medicinal products made from snakes or other animals known to carry *Salmonella* have been implicated in cases of salmonellosis.

430.

A. Koplik's spots are small, bluish-white spots on a red areolar base that appear in the mouth just before the onset of the characteristic measles rash. These spots are actually inflamed submucosal glands that appear white because of necrosis. It is relatively difficult to isolate this viral agent in the laboratory, so a serologic diagnosis is optimal. Uncomplicated cases of measles last only 7 to 10 days.

431.

A. *Staphylococcus aureus* is the predominant pathogen involved in joint infections of adults. Bacterial arthritis can occur following infection in other parts of the body or bacteremia. *Streptococcus pyogenes* and *Neisseria gonorrhoeae* each account for a significant number of adult infections, whereas *Streptococcus pneumoniae* and *Haemophilus influenzae* predominate in childhood infections.

432.

A. Blood cultures are appropriate in cases of fever of unknown etiology. In this case, which was diagnosed as typhoid fever, the blood is usually positive during the first or second week of illness. In the laboratory diagnosis of suspected cases of typhoid fever it is important to note that the etiologic agent can be isolated in blood before the stool becomes positive. Urine may also yield *Salmonella typhi* in many cases, although an enrichment procedure may be needed.

433.

A. Seen among soldiers in Europe during World War I and World War II, trench fever was a major cause of illness. The disease is caused by *Bartonella quintana,* which is transmitted by the body louse or inoculation with infected louse excreta. The disease has a long incubation period; infection may persist for long periods, and relapse may occur years later. The most common symptom is leg pain with intermittent fever. *B. quintana* can be cultivated on artificial media containing erythrocytes and serum.

434.

D. *Staphylococcus aureus* has been isolated from a majority of the reported cases of the clinical syndrome described, which has been termed toxic shock syndrome. First reported in the late 1970s, the disease was associated with the use of a specific brand of tampons. Symptoms are thought to be associated with the production of a pyrogenic exotoxin by the coagulase-positive staphylococcus.

435.

B. The etiologic agent in this case was *Yersinia enterocolitica*. Disease caused by this organism frequently mimics the symptoms of appendicitis, although it has been implicated in a variety of clinical illnesses such as bacteremia, cholecystitis, and mesenteric lymphadenitis. *Yersinia enterocolitica* grows slowly at 35 °C and, unless in large numbers or pure culture, may be overlooked in the laboratory.

436.

C. The disease described is known as Haverhill or rat bite fever and is caused by *Streptobacillus moniliformis.* This organism is a part of the normal oral flora of mice and rats. The most common form of transmission to humans is the bite of a rodent, but infection may also occur following ingestion of contaminated milk and other foods. For the cultivation of this agent artificial media must be supplemented with ascitic fluid, blood, or serum.

437.

D. Lyme disease is an epidemic inflammatory disease seen predominantly in the northeast United States during the summer months. The etiologic agent of this tick-borne disease is *Borrelia burgdorferi.* The spirochetes causing Lyme disease have not been able to be demonstrated in peripheral blood films. An indirect immunofluorescence test and an ELISA test are available for the detection of specific antibody in the patient's serum. The initial symptoms of this disease may be followed months later by more serious complications, such as meningoencephalitis, myocarditis, and arthritis of the large joints.

438.

A. *Listeria monocytogenes* is a cause of human and bovine abortion. The mother's symptoms are usually mild, resembling the flu and causing a low-grade fever generally late in the pregnancy. The organism can be isolated from aborted fetuses as well as from the maternal placenta. When infection with this etiologic agent is detected early, appropriate therapy can be initiated, which may prevent the death of the fetus.

439.

B. Human infections caused by *Leptospira* characteristically produce the clinical symptoms of fever, anemia, and jaundice. Weil's disease or infectious jaundice are other names for the disease leptospirosis. Infections result from contact with the urine or tissue of infected animals like rats and mice or from water contaminated with urine of these animals. Most infections resolve in about a week but they can go on for much longer and can cause fatal kidney and liver damage.

440.

A. *Yersinia enterocolitica* causes a variety of infections. This organism is able to grow at refrigerator temperatures. Contamination of banked blood is not visually detected because the organism is able to reproduce in RBCs without causing lysis or a color change.

441.

C. *Mycobacterium marinum* produces lesions on the skin or the extremities of humans. This species of *Mycobacterium* is a free-living organism found in salt or brackish water. Human infection characteristically follows trauma to the body in or around water.

442.

B. Keratitis is a serious clinical condition that is characterized by an inflammation of the cornea, which, if not appropriately treated, may lead to loss of the eye. *Pseudomonas aeruginosa* is the most common agent of keratitis associated with lens-cleaning solution. Pseudomonads are opportunistic pathogens that are commonly associated with contaminated fluids, requiring minimal nutrients for growth.

443.

D. *Helicobacter pylori* is implicated as an etiologic agent of gastritis and peptic ulcer disease. This organism can be demonstrated in gastric biopsy specimens. *H. pylori* produces a strong positive urease test result.

444.

D. Bacillus species are gram-positive, spore-forming bacilli found widely in the environment. *Bacillus cereus* is of particular interest as an etiologic agent of human cases of food poisoning. This enterotoxin-producing microorganism is most commonly associated with cases of food poisoning following ingestion of reheated rice served at oriental restaurants.

445.

B. *Listeria monocytogenes* has been associated with human disease following the ingestion of unpasteurized dairy products. The organism is capable of replicating at refrigerator temperatures and is commonly found in low numbers in animal products. Listeriosis associated with contaminated food, in uncompromised patients, usually produces a self-limiting, nonspecific febrile illness.

446.

C. *Bacillus anthracis* infects humans by three routes, each of which produces a characteristic form of disease: respiratory, gastrointestinal, and cutaneous. Malignant pustule is the name given to cutaneous anthrax in humans. The disease is transmitted by contact with infected animal products and produces a localized abscess on the skin, which forms a characteristic black eschar.

447.

B. *Escherichia coli* 0157:H7 is associated with HUS. These strains produce verotoxin and are associated with outbreaks of diarrheal disease following ingestion of undercooked hamburger at fast-food restaurants and contact with calves at petting zoos. Cattle infected with this strain serve as the reservoir and humans become infected by eating products made from their meat or contaminated with their excretions.

448.

B. One form of rat bite fever is caused by *Streptobacillus moniliformis*. Haverhill fever is another name for disease caused by the microorganism. The bite of an infected rodent and the ingestion of contaminated food products such as milk are the modes of transmission. *Streptobacillus* is a gram-negative bacillus, whereas the other agent of rat bite fever or sodoku is the spiral organism *Spirillum minor*.

449.

B. Typhoid fever does not involve an exotoxin. The organisms enter, multiply in the mononuclear phagocytes of Peyer's patches, then spread to the liver, gallbladder, and spleen. Bacteremia follows with the onset of fever and other symptoms such as constipation. Gastrointestinal symptoms are seen later in the disease.

450.

D. The clinical presentation suggests that the etiologic agent is *Legionella pneumophila*. The Gram stain was not helpful in making the diagnosis due to the poor staining quality of its gram-negative cell wall. Examination of the sputum using fluorescent antibody to *Legionella pneumophila* would provide a rapid positive identification.

VIRUSES AND RICKETTSIAE

451.

C. Retroviruses are RNA viruses that replicate by means of DNA intermediates produced by the viral enzyme reverse transcriptase. In human infections with retroviruses, T cells are major targets. The viruses associated with acquired immune deficiency syndrome are human immunodeficiency viruses (HIV). Two subtypes are known: HIV-1 and HIV-2.

452.

B. Measles (rubeola) is a highly infectious childhood disease. Infection with this virus is followed by a prodromal syndrome characterized by cough, coryza, conjunctivitis, and fever. The most characteristic lesions, Koplik spots, are seen on the buccal mucosa. Koplik spots are diagnostic for measles infection and represent necrotic vesicles with a white center surrounded by erythema.

453.

A. The soft-shelled tick *Ornithodoros hermsii* is the arthropod vector for *Borrelia hermsii,* one of the etiologic agents of relapsing fever (borreliosis) in North America. *Borrelia* bacteria are species-specific in that they are perpetuated and transmitted exclusively by their specific tick vector. The transmission of tick-borne spirochetes to humans occurs when infected ticks feed on humans.

454.

A. Direct microscopic examination for *Rickettsia* organisms is possible using such stains as Giemsa, Machiavello, or Gimenez. The recommended procedure is the nonspecific Gimenez stain, which colors the organisms a brilliant red against a green background. The staining technique calls for flooding a thin smear, which has been air-dried, with a solution of carbol-fuchsin for 1 to 2 minutes. Washing with tap water is followed by the application of a malachite green solution for 6 to 9 seconds before the final washing with tap water.

455.

B. One of the major viral agents associated with cases of acute gastroenteritis is the rotavirus. In particular this agent is the cause of epidemic non-bacterial gastroenteritis in infants and young children that occurs most commonly during the winter months. Rotavirus belongs to the family of RNA viruses known as Reoviridae. Rotavirus has a fecal-oral route of transmission and has been documented as a nosocomial pathogen in pediatric areas of hospitals.

456.

D. The family of viruses known as the Retroviridae contains the subfamily Lentiviridae. This subfamily contains the human immunodeficiency viruses (HIV), the causes of acquired immune deficiency syndrome (AIDS). Kaposi's sarcoma and B-cell lymphomas are associated with a loss of T-helper cell function, predisposing the patient to assault by a variety of infectious agents.

457.

D. HIV is a member of the group known as retroviruses. The major target of the virus in this syndrome is the T-helper cell, which would normally function to control disease. As the disease progresses, the T-cell population is depleted, leaving the patient vulnerable to a variety of infectious agents as well as specific cancers.

458.

C. Commercially available cell cultures of human fibroblasts are optimal for the cultivation of CMV. The human cytomegalovirus will not replicate in other cell culture systems such as HeLa, HEp-2, or PMK. CMV can be identified with a high level of confidence solely on the basis of its characteristic cytopathology. Infected cells in the monolayer appear enlarged, rounded, and refractile.

459.

A. Adenoviruses are well known as respiratory pathogens, having been the cause of acute respiratory disease among military recruit populations. Also associated with adenoviral infection is the severe ocular disease known as keratoconjunctivitis that typically occurs in epidemic form. Adenoviruses may remain in tissues, lymphoid structures, and adenoids and become reactivated.

460.

D. Cell cultures recommended for the isolation of herpes simplex virus (HSV) are human embryonic fibroblasts. The usual period needed to detect

HSV destruction of the cell monolayer is 1 to 2 days. The most common of the two recognized types of HSV CPE begins with a granulation of the cytoplasm followed by cell enlargement and a ballooned appearance. Monoclonal antibodies and immunofluorescence are commonly used to differentiate between HSV-1 and HSV-2.

461.

A. The diagnosis of enterovirus infection from clinical specimens is best accomplished by the cell culture technique. A dual cell culture system of primary monkey kidney and human diploid fibroblast cells is recommended for optimal sensitivity and rapid recovery. The clinical history, including the season of onset, the type of specimen cultured, and growth in a specific cell culture line all contribute to the presumptive identification of an enterovirus infection. The sensitivity and specificity of the other methods of identification listed have not been defined as compared to those of the cell culture technique.

462.

B. The first case of Lassa fever occurred in Nigeria and was described in 1969. It is believed that primary infection results from contact with infected rodent urine. Secondary cases have resulted from contact with an index case or contact with infectious material such as blood. Lassa fever is characterized by a high fever, respiratory symptoms, abdominal pain, myalgia, vomiting, and diarrhea, which may last from 1 to 3 weeks.

463.

D. Transovarian passage from generation to generation in the ticks perpetuates *Rickettsia rickettsii* for several generations outside an animal host. A blood meal serves to reactivate the rickettsiae carried by the arthropod vector. Rodents and small mammals are the natural reservoir hosts for the rickettsiae causing this form of spotted fever.

464.

C. Zoster or shingles occurs predominantly in adults, whereas varicella occurs more commonly in children. The varicella virus, following the primary infection known as chicken pox, remains latent in the sensory ganglia. Reactivation of this virus, which may occur years later, is usually associated with an immunocompromised state.

465.

D. Rhinoviruses, members of the picornavirus group, are a common cause of the respiratory disease known as the common cold. Hand transmission, not aerosols, appears to be the primary means of transmission. In contrast to other picornaviruses, the optimum temperature for rhinoviruses is 33 °C.

466.

B. Newcastle disease is an avian disease that may be transmitted to humans. Outbreaks of this disease in domestic poultry flocks can produce heavy economic losses. Disease in humans has a short incubation period and is characterized by conjunctivitis, malaise, and chills but not fever.

467.

D. Rabies is a neurotropic virus causing extensive destruction in the brain. Negri bodies are seen in the cytoplasm of large ganglion cells and are demonstrated by Seller's stain and the fluorescent antibody staining technique. Rabies in humans or lower animals can be diagnosed by demonstration of these characteristic inclusions, but the more common test is the direct fluorescent antibody (DFA) test.

468.

D. Molluscum contagiosum is an infectious disease with worldwide distribution caused by a poxvirus. Nodules develop in the epidermis of the face, arms, back, and buttocks, which undergo necrosis. Examination of epithelioid cells from affected areas will show characteristic eosinophilic cytoplasmic inclusions (molluscum bodies).

469.

B. Flying squirrels, *Glaucomys volans*, are associated with cases of the sylvatic form of typhus in the United States. The squirrel louse transmits the organism among the squirrel population. Humans contract the disease through association with infected squirrels. The disease is more common in the winter months when squirrels seeking shelter enter dwellings.

470.

A. Humans who have had the classic form of typhus may remain infected with the causative agent *Rickettsia prowazekii*. Relapses or recrudescence of disease may occur in these persons years or decades after the initial attack. The latent form of infection is known as Brill-Zinsser disease and may serve as an interepidemic reservoir for epidemic typhus.

471.

D. Murine typhus is transmitted to humans by fleas infected with *Rickettsia typhi*. Prevalent in the southern United States, it is primarily a disease of rodents sometimes transmitted to humans. Control of disease outbreaks is related to rodent (rat) control and the related rat flea *(Xenopsylla cheopis)* population. The symptoms of murine or endemic typhus are similar to those of the classic epidemic form seen in Europe.

472.

B. *Rickettsia akari*, transmitted by mites, is the only rickettsia of the spotted fever group not transmitted by ixodid ticks. Rickettsial pox is a mild febrile disease with a rash and an eschar at the bite site. This rickettsial disease is most closely associated with urban areas due to its transmission by mites from the infected house mouse.

473.

A. Epidemic typhus fever is caused by *Rickettsia prowazekii*, which is transmitted by the human body louse *Pediculus humanus*. A severe headache, chills, fever, and a rash are characteristic symptoms of typhus fever. Associated with overcrowding, this disease has caused epidemics in both civilian and military populations. Examination of infected cells will demonstrate the organism only in the cytoplasm and not in the nucleus.

474.

C. *Rickettsia tsutsugamushi* is the causative agent of this disease, which is characterized by headache, orbital pain, rash, and fever. The organism is carried by infected rodents and transmitted to humans by the bite of infected mites. The name of the disease describes the geographic localities in the Asian Pacific region in which the mites are most prevalent—low, swampy areas of scrub underbrush along riverbanks.

475.

A. *Bartonella bacilliformis* is a hematotropic bacterium included in the order Rickettsiales. These Gram-negative coccobacillary organisms are transmitted to humans by an arthropod vector. The disease bartonellosis is seen in two forms: an infectious anemia and a cutaneous form characterized by nodular skin eruptions. The disease has a strict geographic limitation, being confined to South America in the Andes Mountains at elevations between 500 and 3000 feet. Oroya fever is the most severe form and frequently causes a fatal, febrile anemia due to the presence of large numbers of organisms in the erythrocytes, causing hemolysis.

476.

C. Rotavirus is the cause of diarrheal disease in at least half of all infants and young children admitted to the hospital with dehydration requiring fluid replacement therapy. Since rotaviruses are difficult to propagate in cell culture, the method of choice for the detection of rotavirus infection is the direct examination of stool for the presence of viral antigen. Rotavirus antigen assay tests, such as latex agglutination and EIA tests, employ a solid phase previously coated with antibody to which the stool sample is applied. Detection of the bound antigen identifies the causative agent.

477.

B. Kuru, the first spongiform encephalopathy proven to be of infectious origin, has an incubation period of from 4 to 20 years. The ritualistic practice of cannibalism among highland natives of New Guinea maintained the incidence of disease. Control of kuru can be accomplished by curtailment of the practice of cannibalism. The agent, found in brain tissue, can be inoculated into monkeys, producing disease; however, the agent cannot be grown on cell cultures.

478.

B. Hepatitis A is one of several infectious diseases that damage the liver and produces icterus (jaundice). The appearance of jaundice, in the icteric phase, is correlated by liver biopsy with extensive parenchymal destruction. Convalescence is usually accompanied by subsequent complete regeneration of the diseased organ.

479.

B. The double-stranded DNA enveloped, icosahedral viruses known as the family Herpesviridae contain the Epstein-Barr virus, which is associated with Burkitt's lymphoma, nasopharyngeal carcinoma, and is the etiologic agent of infectious mononucleosis. Infectious mononucleosis is an acute disease most commonly affecting children and young adults. The virus is thought to be transmitted by intimate contact and has been called the "kissing disease." The patient's blood demonstrates a leukocytosis with a marked increase in T lymphocytes and serologically is characterized by a positive heterophile antibody and antibodies to various viral antigens.

480.

C. All the viruses listed are members of the family of small RNA viruses known as Picornaviridae. Poliovirus, an enterovirus, is shed by both respiratory and fecal routes. Laboratory identification relies on isolation (especially from feces) and subsequent virus neutralization in tissue culture. Spread of the disease is associated with poor sanitary conditions and crowding.

481.

B. The hepatitis B virus is an enveloped, partially double-stranded DNA virus. During viral replication, full-length RNA transcripts of the viral genome are inserted into maturing virus particles. The viral enzyme reverse transcriptase then transcribes these RNA transcripts to a full-length DNA strand but only partially completes synthesis of the complementary DNA strand—hence a partially double-stranded DNA genome.

482.

C. Hepatitis C virus infections, unlike hepatitis A or hepatitis B infections, do not commonly produce jaundice. At one time, hepatitis C was the leading cause of transfusion-related hepatitis. Effective testing of donor units has minimized that risk. There are tens of thousands of individuals in the United States chronically infected with hepatitis C; chronic infection appears to be the rule rather than the exception. Transmission of the virus at the present time occurs mainly through needle sharing. Cases involving contact with infected blood by health care workers also occur.

483.

B. Paramyxoviruses such as RSV are noted for syncytium formation (the fusing of cell membranes to create multinucleated cells) in culture. Orthomyxoviruses such as influenza virus have segmented genomes; paramyxoviruses do not. Influenza virus is unusual among RNA viruses in that genome replication takes place in the nucleus. In contrast

to the marked antigenic instability of influenza virus (antigenic drift, antigenic shift), paramyxoviruses exhibit antigenic stability.

484.

D. The etiologic agents for the numerous benign cutaneous and mucosal lesions known as warts are the human papillomaviruses (HPVs). The diagnosis of lesions caused by these agents is based on the clinical appearance and histopathology, since there are no *in vitro* systems available for isolation. Some HPV types are strongly associated with squamous cell carcinoma of the cervix and anus.

485.

D. The wood tick *Dermacentor andersoni*, which becomes naturally infected with the virus, is apparently the sole vector of the infection. Colorado tick fever is a seasonal problem, with the majority of cases being reported between March and July in the western mountainous regions of the United States. The disease is characterized by a short febrile phase with fevers, chills, headache, and severe muscle aches. A remission period follows, but true to its diphasic nature, recrudescence of the febrile phase occurs in a few days. Antibody against the virus can be detected by a direct immunofluorescence test performed on the patient's serum.

486.

C. The Coxsackie viruses are enteroviruses named after the town of Coxsackie, New York, where they were first isolated. The viruses are divided into Groups A and B on the basis of virologic and antigenic differences. The Group B Coxsackie viruses are strongly associated with myocarditis that may cause sufficient damage to require heart transplantation. The Group A Coxsackie viruses are associated with various diseases, characterized by vesicular lesions, such as herpangina. Neither group of Coxsackie viruses is associated with gastrointestinal disease.

487.

B. Cytomegalovirus infections in humans may be asymptomatic for normal healthy hosts. Infections tend to be more severe in patients who are immunosuppressed or in neonates infected perinatally. Cytomegalovirus is readily isolated from urine, since it is shed by the tubular cells of infected hosts.

488.

C. The rubella virus is an RNA virus and a member of the Togaviridae. In adults and children rubella infections are generally a mild contagious rash disease. When a pregnant woman becomes infected, the consequences become more serious. If the fetus becomes infected during the first trimester of pregnancy, a variety of congenital defects may result. Anatomic abnormalities produced by this agent include cataracts, deafness, and cardiac problems.

489.

A. Infants usually acquire cytomegalovirus infections before birth or at the time of delivery. These infections may lead to death during the first months of life or may result in residual neurologic impairment. The virus can be isolated from several different body fluids with urine being the most commonly examined. It is recommended that several fresh urine samples be examined with exfoliative cytologic techniques for the presumptive diagnosis of this disease.

490.

B. There are two types of herpes simplex viruses (HSV-1, HSV-2), both of which are associated with latent infections. Viral lesions may develop in any part of the body, and primary infections may be subclinical or severe. In neonates, in those with immune deficiencies, or in individuals undergoing immunosuppressive therapy with anticancer drugs or steroids, HSV infections are often life-threatening.

491.

B. Influenza viruses are RNA viruses that enter the human body through the respiratory tract. These important pathogens are associated with epidemic and pandemic disease. There are two main types of influenza viruses (A and B), which differ antigenically and in epidemic periodicity. All recorded pandemics have been caused by influenza A viruses. The incidence of respiratory disease caused by these agents peaks during the winter months.

492.

D. Herpes simplex viruses (HSV), cytomegalovirus (CMV), and varicella-zoster viruses (VZV) produce latent infections. The genomes of these viruses can remain dormant in host cells for decades. Shingles (zoster) represents reactivation of latent VZV.

493.

C. Hepatitis C virus has never been grown in culture. All knowledge of the virus and diagnostic reagents have been attained through molecular techniques applied to the RNA genome. Hepatitis C virus infection can be diagnosed by detecting antibody to the virus or by amplification of viral RNA from plasma. Adenovirus, cytomegalovirus, and measles virus are readily grown in culture.

494.

C. The rubella virus (German measles) causes an exanthematous disease resembling a milder form of measles in children. This single-stranded RNA virus, transmitted from person to person, is of medical importance to females in the childbearing years due to the teratogenic effects it has on the fetus. Congenital rubella resulting from an intrauterine fetal infection is most severe when contracted during the first trimester of gestation.

495.

B. Lacking essential components for the synthesis of macromolecules, viruses are not able to reproduce by binary fission. Host cells are required to provide the synthesis of viral components. The replicative cycle has four stages: absorption, penetration (uncoating), eclipse (biosynthesis), and release (maturation). Viral replication in the host cell may result in cell death (as demonstrated by cytopathic effect—CPE), chronic infection with no observable changes, or transformation of the infected cell.

496.

C. The immunologic abnormalities demonstrated by AIDS patients predispose them to a variety of opportunistic pathogens. The absence of a cellular immune response enables opportunistic organisms to cause extensive infection. The retrovirus HIV is the causative agent of this syndrome. Malaria is not an opportunistic infection.

497.

A. Creutzfeldt-Jakob disease (CJD) has a wide geographic distribution and is one of the diseases associated with the infectious agents called "prions." These infections characteristically have a long period of latency between infection and the development of illness. The clinical syndrome produced includes progressive cerebellar ataxia and tremors.

Prions are composed of proteins and produce non-inflammatory subacute degenerative diseases of the central nervous system. Recently, a variant form of CJD (vCJD) has appeared in England and is thought to be related to consumption of nerve tissue from cattle affected with bovine spongiform encephalopathy (BSE), or "mad cow" disease.

498.

C. Viruses are obligate intracellular parasites consisting of either an RNA or a DNA genome. The nucleic acid may be single- or double-stranded and in many possible forms (circular, linear, or segmented). Viruses are divided into families based on the type of nucleic acid in the virion. There are RNA viruses and DNA viruses.

499.

C. Due to their nature as obligate intracellular parasites, successful cultivation of viruses requires living cells. Cell cultures provide homogeneous host cell systems, which are easily handled, stable for long periods, and not susceptible to host factors such as stress or physiologic changes. Viruses are not like bacteria. They will not grow on any cell-free medium.

500.

D. Cold sores and fever blisters are caused by herpes simplex virus, most often HSV-1. This recurrent infection is characterized by initial sensations of burning, pain, and irritation at the site with the rapid appearance of a cluster of erythematous papules. The papules quickly develop into thin-walled fluid-filled vesicles that burst or dry and then heal (without scarring) within 6 to 10 days.

PARASITOLOGY

501.

A. Because the eggs of *E. vermicularis* are usually deposited on the perianal area, cellulose tape slides are recommended to collect the eggs. Recovery is best if specimens are collected late in the evening or before bathing or defecating in the morning. The gravid female worms usually migrate at night to the perianal region to deposit eggs. Because their migration is sporadic, several consecutive collections may be necessary to detect the infection.

502.

D. When *E. granulosus* eggs are ingested by an intermediate herbivorous host, including humans, they usually develop into hydatid cysts in which invaginated larval scolices are produced. These cysts are most often in the liver or lung. Although clinical findings can provide a presumptive diagnosis, this is best confirmed by the finding, at surgery, of encysted larval scolices. Each scolex is capable of developing into an adult worm after ingestion by a dog or related animal, the definitive host.

503.

D. The formalin-ether concentration method preserves most parasites, including operculated and schistosome eggs, which may not be recovered by zinc sulfate flotation. Formalin-ethyl acetate sedimentation concentrates most parasites and is more effective than flotation with formalinized specimens. Ether is hazardous because it is highly flammable; ethyl acetate is used as a less volatile substitute. A newer chemical, Hemo-De, is safer to use than ethyl acetate.

504.

C. *T. hominis* is a flagellate parasite of the intestine that may be found in fecally contaminated urine and should not be mistaken for *T. vaginalis*. It has been suggested that a heavy infection with *T. hominis* may cause diarrhea, but it is generally considered to be a commensal organism. *T. tenax* is found in the mouth. *B. coli* and *E. coli* are not flagellates.

505.

A. Although the *T. spiralis* adults live in the intestinal mucosa, they are rarely seen. The female deposits living larvae into the mucosa or lymphatic vessels, from which they normally enter the bloodstream and are disseminated throughout the body. They then burrow into muscle fibers. Although larvae may occasionally be liberated into the intestinal lumen, the definitive diagnostic procedure is the demonstration of larvae in skeletal muscle, not in feces.

506.

B. In parasites with a sexual and asexual stage of development, the definitive host is the host where the sexual stage of the parasite occurs. The intermediate host is the host where the asexual stage of the parasite is found. Vectors are arthropods, like mosquitoes and ticks, that transmit infectious agents. A commensal is an organism that benefits from an existence with a host but does not damage the host.

507.

C. No cyst stage is known for *D. fragilis*. The majority of the trophozoites are binucleated, and they often appear to have rounded up in stained preparations. This species has recently been reclassified, being placed among the trichomonads on the basis of its immunologic features and ultrastructure, although movement is by pseudopodia.

508.

A. Mature cysts of *I. bütschlii* are usually ovoid, with a single nucleus with a large eccentric karyosome. The cytoplasm contains a compact mass of glycogen, which appears as a clear area in unstained or permanently stained preparations but stains dark brown with iodine. Chromatoid bodies are not present.

509.

D. *E. histolytica* and *E. dispar* cannot be morphologically differentiated. The cyst stage of both organisms has four nuclei with a centrally located karyosome. *E. histolytica* is a well recognized intestinal parasite, while *E. dispar* is considered nonpathogenic. Molecular biology assays are necessary to differentiate these two species.

510.

A. Although the condition may vary from patient to patient, eosinophilia is often found in association with infections with tissue-invading nematodes. Eosinophilia of 40–80% is not unusual in trichinosis and in visceral larva migrans. It may also be present in strongyloidiasis, early in *Ascaris* and hookworm infections, and in filariasis, which may also cause pulmonary eosinophilia.

511.

B. The symptoms and history for this patient are compatible with trypanosomiasis (African sleeping sickness). The trypomastigote form of the parasite was found in peripheral blood smears from this patient. Another key clinical sign is the presence of swollen lymph nodes at the posterior base of the neck; this is called Winterbottom's sign.

512.

D. The trophozoites of *P. vivax* often develop fine pseudopodia and large vacuoles and are described as ameboid; infected red blood cells (RBCs) contain clumps of malarial pigment called Shüffner's dots. *P. malariae* cytoplasm is much more compact, and infected RBCs lack Shüffner's dots. *P. ovale* resembles *P. vivax*. Shüffner's dots are generally found in *P. vivax* and *P. ovale* infected red blood cells; however, *P. ovale* infected RBCs have fimbriated edges. Growing trophozoites of *P. falciparum* seen in the peripheral blood remain in the ring form, and infected RBCs lack malarial pigment. *P. knowlesi* is not typically a human pathogen.

513.

D. The permanently stained smear is especially recommended for identification of trophozoites, for confirmation of species, and for keeping a permanent record of the organisms found. Species identification of amebic trophozoites can rarely be made from a single feature; permanent stains enable one to observe the cytoplasm and cytoplasmic inclusions and the nuclear morphologic features. Iron hematoxylin and trichrome are commonly used stains. Quensel's vital stain, buffered methylene blue, and chlorazol black E also give good results with fresh feces but cannot be used with preserved specimens.

514.

B. *Babesia* spp. are sporozoan parasites of erythrocytes that have been recognized as causing febrile illness in humans. *B. microti* has caused a number of tick-borne infections in the New England area. The parasites often appear as small rings within infected red blood cells, resembling *P. falciparum* trophozoites. The pathognomic form of *Babesia* is the "Maltese Cross," four ring forms inside a single red blood cell.

515.

C. Polyvinyl alcohol (PVA) is a commonly used fixative for stool specimens. This chemical is used to fix fecal samples for making permanently stained smears. Formalin is commonly used to preserve stool samples in preparation for concentration procedures. Merthiolate iodine formalin (MIF) is also used to preserve stool samples for concentration procedures. Buffered glycerol is sometimes used as a transport medium for stool samples when performing a bacterial culture.

516.

D. While all the organisms listed have some degree of acid-fast positivity, only *Cyclospora* forms oocysts in the size range of 8–10 μm. The oocysts of *Cryptosporidium* are generally 4–6 μm in diameter and are generally strongly acid-fast positive. Oocysts of *Isospora* are much larger, approximately 25 × 18 μm. Microsporidium are acid-fast variable, and this stain is not recommended for detecting microsporidium. The spores of microsporidium are generally 1–4 μm in diameter.

517.

C. Visceral leishmaniasis is the most severe form of leishmaniasis; it is characterized by fever, hepatosplenomegaly, and lymphadenopathy. Members of the *L. donovani* complex cause visceral leishmaniasis. The disease is also known as Kala azar (black poison).

518.

A. *Pneumocystis carinii* has become an important cause of pneumonia in immunocompromised patients, and as such, is most generally found in lung samples. This organism received a lot of notoriety in the early 1980s when it was associated with acquired immunodeficiency syndrome patients. *P. carinii* was originally classified as a protozoan, but DNA sequencing has determined this organism is more closely related to fungi.

519.

A. Lice, caused by *Pediculosis* sp., are generally diagnosed by detecting the adults or eggs in hair. The eggs measure about 0.8–1 mm in length and are found fastened to hair shafts. The adult forms of head and body lice are about 3–4 mm long, while crab lice are about 2 mm long. Scabies, another arthropod infestation of humans, can be diagnosed by seeing the adult forms burrowing in the outer layers of the skin.

520.

B. While all these organisms are potential pathogens of immunocompromised patients, only *Cryptosporidium* produces acid-fast positive oocysts about 4–6 μm in diameter. The oocysts of *Isospora* measure approximately 25 × 18 μm. The spores of microsporidium are generally 1–4 μm in diam-

eter. *B. hominis* is generally considered to be pathogenic in high numbers. The diagnostic form of this intestinal parasite measures 6–40 μm in diameter and is not acid-fast positive.

521.

D. One of the classical signs of malaria is a fever that occurs in cycles. As the infection is developing, all the parasites are in about the same stage of development. The fever spikes correspond to the release of the merozoites from infected red blood cells (RBCs). *Plasmodium* is an obligate intracellular parasite of RBCs; therefore, infections can result in decreased RBC counts and hemoglobin.

522.

C. *Acanthamoeba* is a free-living ameba rarely causing human infections. This organism has been associated with granulomatous infections of the skin and lung, as well as causing meningoencephalitis. However, the most common presentation is keratitis, infection of the cornea. Most keratitis cases have been associated with contact lenses.

523.

B. The small size and variable staining of the microsporidium make their detection difficult. Tissue examination by electron microscopy seems to be the most specific diagnostic method. In the modified trichrome stain, one of the stains (chromotrope 2R) is used at 10 times the normal concentration. In addition, the staining time is increased to 90 minutes. Under these staining conditions, the spores of microsporidium stain as pinkish ovals, 1–3 μm.

524.

A. *Echinococcus granulosus* is a tapeworm that lives as an adult in the small intestines of carnivores, primarily dogs and wolves, and other canines. When the embryonated egg from the feces of a carnivore is ingested by the intermediate host, usually a herbivore but sometimes a human, the liberated embryo can develop into a hydatid cyst. These cysts are most often hepatic or pulmonary, and the resulting symptoms are comparable to those of a slow-growing tumor.

525.

D. *T. gondii* is a protozoan parasite of humans and a variety of lower animals. Human infections can be congenital or can result from ingestion of material containing oocysts from cat feces or from eating undercooked beef, lamb, or pork containing toxoplasma cysts. Its life cycle includes asexual multiplication in a number of hosts and sexual multiplication only in domestic cats and some closely related species, which then excrete potentially infectious oocysts. Pregnant women should take precautions to avoid infection.

526.
C. All these flagellates except *E. hominis* are pear-shaped, but only *C. mesnili* and *G. lamblia* are usually as large as 15 μm. The typical motion of *G. lamblia* is described as "falling leaf"; *C. mesnili* has a stiff rotary motion, and the others move jerkily. *G. lamblia* is known to cause diarrheal disease and malabsorption, and the trophozoites may be found in diarrheal feces. The other intestinal flagellates of humans are nonpathogenic commensals.

527.
A. *D. caninum* infects a high percentage of dogs. The gravid proglottids are often found on the dog's fur. After the liberated eggs are ingested by larval fleas, the parasite develops into an infective cysticercoid in the adult flea. These organisms may be ingested by humans kissing the dog or by hand-to-mouth transfer. Human infections are usually single and asymptomatic, but the proglottids are passed in the host's feces.

528.
C. Transmission of filariasis depends on the presence of microfilariae in the bloodstream at the time the vector bites, and the periodicity of microfilariae in the peripheral blood varies with the species and sometimes with the geographic area. Nocturnal periodicity is marked in *W. bancrofti* in Africa, Asia, and the western hemisphere, and thick blood films for detection of these microfilariae should be made between 10 P.M. and 2 A.M. The other choices do not exhibit nocturnal periodicity.

529.
D. Sexual intercourse with infected men is thought to be the most important mode of transmission of *Trichomonas vaginalis* to women. Other routes of infection are direct contact with infected females or contact with infected toilet articles or toilet seats; these are considered rare modes of transmission. Infants may become infected while passing through the birth canal. Toxoplasmosis occurs as a

congenital infection, but it is more commonly acquired by the ingestion of infected, undercooked meat or by swallowing oocysts excreted by infected cats. Schistosomiasis and trichinosis are not passed from person to person.

530.
B. Typical eggs of *T. trichiura* are normally yellow to brown, with colorless polar plugs. They are shaped like a football or a barrel, and they are in the cell, or unsegmented, stage when passed in the feces. The usual egg range is 49–65 × 35–45 μm.

531.
B. The gametocytes of *P. vivax*, *P. malariae*, and *P. ovale* are round and somewhat similar in appearance. Those of *P. falciparum* have a typical sausage or crescent shape. The gametocytes of *P. falciparum* may remain in the peripheral blood a month or more and are often found with the ring stages.

532.
D. The larva of *T. solium* in pork or *T. saginata* in beef has been referred to as *Cysticercus cellulosae*. Human cysticercosis, or infection with *T. solium* larvae, can occur after ingestion of *T. solium* eggs passed by the same or another human host or after regurgitation of the eggs by a human harboring the adult *T. solium* in the intestine. Cysticercosis is a chronic disease whose clinical manifestations depend on the number and location of the cysticerci in the host tissues.

533.
D. When eggs of *Toxocara canis*, a tapeworm of dogs, are ingested by humans, they may hatch in the small intestine and liberate larvae, which can migrate within the hosts. This type of infection is visceral larval migrans. It occurs most often in children, who are more likely to have hand-to-mouth transfer of infected fecal material. One serious complication is retinal damage resulting in blindness caused by *T. canis* larvae in the eye.

534.
A. *Naegleria fowleri* is found in freshwater ponds and lakes, especially those with disturbed or suspended soil. It has caused a number of cases of meningoencephalitis in people who have swum in these bodies of water. Essentially, all these infec-

tions have been fulminating and fatal, and they are often not diagnosed until autopsy.

535.

C. Infectious cysts of amebas and *Giardia lamblia* and eggs of *Ascaris lumbricoides* may all be ingested in fecally contaminated water and/or on fecally contaminated plants. These infections are most prevalent in areas lacking good public sanitation, that is, sanitary disposal of human waste and adequately treated and protected drinking water. Filiariasis is transmitted by blood-feeding insects (vectors).

536.

A. Humans are infected with *T. saginata* by eating beef containing living cysticerci, the infectious larval stage of this parasite. Cattle become infected by ingesting viable eggs from human feces. Unlike *Taenia solium*, if humans ingest *T. saginata* ova, infection does not develop.

537.

C. Cysts of *E. hartmanni* are differentiated from cysts of *E. histolytica* by their small size; they are otherwise morphologically identical. *E. hartmanni*, which was formerly called "small race ameba," is considered to be nonpathogenic. The size range for *E. hartmanni* cysts is 5–10 μm, and for *E. histolytica*, the range is 10–20 μm.

538.

B. The fertilized eggs of *T. trichiura* are unsegmented when laid, and embryonic development occurs outside of the host. In moist, warm, shaded soil, the first-stage larva develops within the egg in about 2 weeks. This fully embryonated egg is infective when ingested by a susceptible host, and it hatches in the small intestine. During development from larva to adult, the worm usually passes to the cecum, where it embeds its slender anterior portion in the intestinal mucosa.

539.

A. The principal vectors for the trypanosome causing Chagas' disease (American trypanosomiasis) in humans are reduviid bugs, especially *Triatoma infestans* and *Rhodnius prolixus*, which adapt to living and breeding in human habitations. These bugs feed at night, and the bite wound is readily contaminated with the infected feces deposited by the vector. Other routes of transmission for Chagas' disease are transplacental or by blood transfusion.

540.

C. Excretion in human feces of the eggs of the hookworms, *Taenia solium*, *T. saginata*, and *Ascaris lumbricoides,* is an essential or important factor in perpetuating the cycle of infection with these parasites. Trichinosis is caused by ingestion of the living larvae of *Trichinella spiralis* encysted in the muscles of a flesh-eating host. The adults live in the host's intestine, and the viviparous females, after fertilization, produce larvae that migrate into the same host's muscle tissue.

541.

D. Typically, red blood cells (RBCs) infected with *P. ovale* are larger than normal, pale and often misshapen, and frequently contain Schüffner's dots or stippling in any stage from the fairly young ring forms onward. RBCs infected with *P. vivax* are also larger than normal, oval, and contain Schüffner's dots. Ovale malaria, however, is a comparatively rare disease.

542.

B. Historically, millions of persons in India, Africa, Asia, northeastern South America, and the West Indies have been infected with *D. medinensis*. The female adult inhabits cutaneous and subcutaneous tissues; a gravid female discharges her motile, rhabditiform larvae through a cutaneous ulcer into water. When ingested by *Cyclops*, the larvae metamorphose into infective forms that are ingested in drinking water from the contaminated wells. The World Health Organization has initiated an education program along with water filters to remove the water flea, and chemoprophylaxis to control the incidence of this infection.

543.

B. The rhabditiform larva of *S. stercoralis* is the diagnostic stage typically passed in the feces of infected persons. This larva measures up to 380 μm long × 20 μm wide, with a short buccal cavity and a prominent, ovoid, genital primordium midway along the ventral wall of the body. The infective stage is the filariform larva, which differs from the hookworm filariform larva by having a notched tail tip and a long esophagus.

544.

B. A malaria relapse is parasitemia developing from exoerythrocytic stages in the liver. These persistent stages are found in *P. ovale* and *P. vivax*, and they may cause relapses up to 4 or 5 years after the primary infection. For infections caused by these species, treatment with primaquine is used to prevent relapses after clinical cure with chloroquine or an alternate drug.

545.

A. *P. falciparum* infections tend to produce a large number of rings that frequently have double chromatin, which is only occasionally found in other species. *P. falciparum* differs from other plasmodia of humans in that only early trophozoites (ring forms) and gametocytes are found in peripheral blood except in severe cases. Sex differentiation of the gametes, when present, is difficult.

546.

D. *T. spiralis* is a nematode parasite whose infectious larvae may be found encysted in the muscles of flesh-eating mammals. Humans are infected most often by eating infected, undercooked pork. *Taenia* are cestodes (tapeworms). *S. stercoralis* and *N. americanus* are roundworms whose infectious larvae usually hatch in the environment and infect by penetration of human skin, although internal autoinfection may also occur.

547.

C. *N. americanus* and *A. duodenale* are two species of hookworms infecting humans. Their eggs are so similar when found in stool specimens, that they are reported as hookworm. The two hookworms can be differentiated by the morphologic characteristics of the adult worms, which are intestinal parasites of humans.

548.

A. The life cycle of *T. gondii* includes five forms or stages, but only bradyzoites and tachyzoites appear in the tissue phase, which is the only phase known to exist in humans. The crescent-shaped tachyzoites are characteristic of acute infection. The slowly multiplying bradyzoites develop within cysts and are typical of chronic infections. Oocysts, merozoites, and gametes have been found only in the cat, where the enteric cycle of development of *T. gondii* occurs.

549.

D. A common sign of *S. haematobium* infection is the presence of blood in the urine. This is due to the damage caused when the eggs break out of the blood vessels of the vesicular plexus into the bladder. Falciparum malaria may also cause severe hematuria or "blackwater fever."

550.

B. *B. microti* is a sporozoan parasite commonly found in voles and field mice. The vector is the tick *Ixodes* sp., normally a parasite of deer. Humans are accidental hosts when bitten by an infected tick. The majority of *B. microti* infections within the United States have been reported in the northeast. It is important to differentiate this parasite from *Plasmodium* in a stained blood film. Antimalarial drugs have not appeared to be effective in babesiosis.

551.

B. Chagas' disease is found throughout the American continents. The infectious agent, *T. cruzi*, is transmitted to humans by reduviid bugs, primarily the triatomids. Chagas' disease can be acute or chronic.

552.

C. The initial symptoms of trichinosis may include nonspecific gastroenteritis, fever, eosinophilia, myositis, and circumorbital edema. Confirmatory diagnosis is made by demonstration of the encapsulated larvae in skeletal muscle. Infections in humans originate by ingestion of improperly cooked pork and bear meat that contain encysted larvae.

553.

A. *B. coli* is the only ciliate that is pathogenic for humans. It is relatively easy to detect in stool samples due to its large size. The trophozoite is generally oval and measures 50–100 × 40–70 µm. A cytosome is present on the anterior end.

554.

D. Color Plate 39 demonstrates a fertilized egg of *A. lumbricoides*. Eggs measure 45–75 × 35–50 µm. Unfertilized *Ascaris* eggs typically do not float in the zinc sulfate concentration technique.

555.

B. Color Plate 40 demonstrates a *G. lamblia* trophozoite; notice the two prominent nuclei. Trophozoites of *C. mesnili* are approximately 6–24 µm in length but have a single nucleus, while *G. lamblia* trophozoites have two nuclei. Trophozoites of

---

answers & rationale

Trichomonas are about the same size as *G. lamblia*, but they are more round than the pear-shaped trophozoites of *B. lamblia* and *C. mesnili*. *Trichomonas* sp. have a single nucleus, and *T. tenax* is found in the oral cavity.

556.

C. Color Plate 41 demonstrates a *D. fragilis* trophozoite. Although this organism lacks a flagella and morphologically resembles the ameba, based on its ultrastructure and molecular biology studies, it is classified as a flagellate. Like the trichomonads, *D. fragilis* does not have a cyst stage. Most trophozoites of *D. fragilis* have two nuclei, like the one in this slide.

557.

C. Color Plate 42 demonstrates an *Entamoeba coli* cyst. These cysts most closely resemble *E. histolytica* and *E. dispar*. The key distinguishing feature is that *E. coli* cysts contain up to eight nuclei, while *E. histolytica* and *E. dispar* have up to four nuclei. It is often necessary to use the fine adjustment to see all the nuclei. In this slide, six nuclei can be seen. Trophozoites of all three species only contain one nucleus.

558.

A. Color Plate 43 demonstrates a hookworm ovum. Besides the size, key characteristics are the thin ovum shell and nearly symmetrical shape. *Enterobius vermicularis*, pin worm, ovum appear similar, except *E. vermicularis* has a flattened side and thicker shell; in addition, the ovum are slightly smaller. Ova of *D. latum* are unembryonated, operculated, and slightly larger than hookworm ova.

559.

D. Color Plate 44 demonstrates the "classical form" of *B. hominis*. After years of taxonomic uncertainty, this organism is now classified as a protozoan. The classic form usually seen in human feces varies in size from 6 to 40 μm in diameter. It contains a large central body, resembling a vacuole, that pushes several nuclei to the periphery of the cell.

560.

B. Color Plate 45 demonstrates a *P. malariae* trophozoite. A trophozoite stretching across the infected red blood cell (RBC) is a key characteristic of *P. malariae*. Other important characteristics include a lack of malarial pigment, and infected RBCs are about the same size as uninfected RBCs. During *Babesia* infections, only ring forms are seen.

REFERENCES

Forbes, B. A., Sahm, D. F., and Weissfeld, A. S. (1998). *Bailey and Scott's Diagnostic Microbiology,* 10th ed. Philadelphia: Mosby.

Garcia, L.S., and Bruckner, D. A. (1997). *Diagnostic Medical Parasitology,* 3rd ed. Washington, DC: American Society for Microbiology Press.

Koneman, E. W., Allen, S. D., Janda, W. M., Schreckenberger P.C., and Winn, Jr. W. C. (1997). *Color Atlas and Textbook of Diagnostic Microbiology,* 5th ed. Philadelphia: Lippincott.

Murray, P. R., Baron, E. J., Pfaller, M. A., Tenover, F. C., and Yolken, R. H. (1999). *Manual of Clinical Microbiology,* 7th ed. Washington, DC: American Society for Microbiology Press.

Murray, P. R., Rosenthal, K. S., Kibayashi, F. S., and Pfaller, M. A. (1998). *Medical Microbiology,* 3rd ed. Philadelphia: Mosby.

7 Urinalysis and Body Fluids

contents

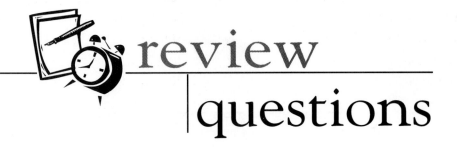
review questions

INSTRUCTIONS Each of the questions or incomplete statements that follow comprises four suggested responses. Select the *best* answer or completion statement in each case.

1. Why is the first-voided morning urine specimen the most desirable specimen for routine urinalysis?
   A. Most dilute specimen of the day and therefore any chemical compounds present will not exceed the detectability limits of the reagent strips
   B. Least likely to be contaminated with microorganisms
   C. Most likely to contain protein because the patient has been in the orthostatic position during the night
   D. Most concentrated specimen of the day and therefore it is more likely that abnormalities will be detected

2. The physical characteristic of color is assessed when a routine urinalysis is performed. What substance is normally found in urine that is principally responsible for its yellow coloration?
   A. Bilirubin
   B. Melanin
   C. Carotene
   D. Urochrome

3. In certain malignant disorders, a substance is found in the urine that turns the urine dark brown or black on exposure of the urine to air. What is this substance?

   A. Urobilinogen
   B. Indican
   C. Melanin
   D. Porphyrin

4. What is the expected pH range of a freshly voided urine specimen?
   A. 3.5 and 8.0
   B. 3.5 and 9.0
   C. 4.0 and 8.5
   D. 4.5 and 8.0

5. Urine specimens should be analyzed as soon as possible after collection. If urine specimens are allowed to stand at room temperature for an excessive amount of time, the urine pH will become alkaline because of bacterial decomposition of
   A. Protein
   B. Urea
   C. Creatinine
   D. Ketones

6. Which term is defined as a urine volume in excess of 2000 mL excreted over a 24-hour period?
   A. Anuria
   B. Oliguria
   C. Polyuria
   D. Hypersthenuria

7. Isosthenuria is a term applied to a series of urine specimens that exhibit a
   A. Specific gravity of exactly 1.000
   B. Specific gravity less than 1.007
   C. Specific gravity greater than 1.020
   D. Fixed specific gravity of approximately 1.010

8. A urine specimen that exhibits yellow foam on being shaken should be suspected of having an increased concentration of
   A. Protein
   B. Hemoglobin
   C. Bilirubin
   D. Nitrite

9. How should controls be run to ensure the precision and accuracy of the reagent test strips used for the chemical analysis of urine?
   A. Positive controls should be run on a daily basis and negative controls when opening a new bottle of test strips
   B. Positive and negative controls should be run when the test strips' expiration date is passed
   C. Positive and negative controls should be run on a daily basis
   D. Positive controls should be run on a daily basis and negative controls on a weekly basis

10. The colorimetric reagent strip test for protein is able to detect as little as 5 to 20 mg of protein per deciliter. What may cause a false-positive urine protein reading?
    A. Ammonia concentration is greater than 0.5 g/day
    B. Uric acid concentration is greater than 0.5 g/day
    C. Glucose concentration is greater than 130 mg/day
    D. pH is greater than 8.0

11. The reagent test strips used for the detection of protein in urine are most reactive to
    A. Albumin
    B. Hemoglobin
    C. Alpha-globulins
    D. Beta-globulins

12. A urine specimen is tested by a reagent strip test and the sulfosalicylic acid test to determine whether protein is present. The former yields a negative protein, whereas the latter results in a reading of 2+ protein. This difference is best explained by which of the following statements?
    A. The urine contained an excessive amount of amorphous urates or phosphates that caused the turbidity seen with the sulfosalicylic acid test
    B. The urine pH was greater than 8, exceeding the buffering capacity of the reagent strip, thus causing a false-negative reaction
    C. A protein other than albumin must be present in the urine
    D. The reading time of the reagent strip test was exceeded (the reading being taken at 2 minutes), causing a false-negative reaction to be detected

13. Two different methods are used to assess the presence of glucose in a urine specimen. A reagent test strip impregnated with glucose oxidase–peroxidase reagent yields a negative result, but a positive result is obtained with Benedict's test. What is the best explanation for these results?
    A. Benedict's test is more sensitive than the strip method
    B. A non-glucose, reducing substance is present in the urine sample
    C. The urine sample has been contaminated by hypochlorite
    D. The urine sample has been contaminated by peroxide

14. Each of the following is included in the quality assurance program for a urinalysis laboratory. Which one represents a preanalytical component of testing?
    A. Setting collection guidelines for 24-hour urines
    B. Maintenance schedule for microscopes
    C. Reporting units to be used for crystals
    D. Requiring acceptable results for control specimens before any patient results are reported out

15. The presence of ketone bodies in urine specimens may be detected by use of a reagent strip impregnated with sodium nitroprusside. This strip test is sensitive to the presence of
    A. Acetoacetic acid and beta-hydroxybutyric acid
    B. Acetoacetic acid and acetone
    C. Diacetic acid and beta-hydroxybutyric acid
    D. Beta-hydroxybutyric acid and acetone

16. A routine urinalysis is performed on a young child suffering from diarrhea. The reagent test strip is negative for glucose but positive for ketones. These results may be explained by which of the following statements?
    A. The child has Type 1 diabetes mellitus
    B. The child is suffering from lactic acidosis, and the lactic acid has falsely reacted with the impregnated reagent area for ketones
    C. The child is suffering from increased catabolism of fat because of decreased intestinal absorption
    D. The reagent area for ketones was read after the maximum reading time allowed

17. The principle of the colorimetric reagent strip test for hemoglobin is based on the peroxidase activity of hemoglobin in catalyzing the oxidation of a dye with peroxide to form a colored compound. This method may yield false-positive results for the presence of hemoglobin when the urine specimen contains
    A. Ascorbic acid
    B. Tetracycline
    C. Myoglobin
    D. Nitrite

18. A reagent test strip impregnated with a diazonium salt such as diazotized 2,4-dichloroaniline may be used to determine which analyte?
    A. Glucose
    B. Ketone
    C. Hemoglobin
    D. Bilirubin

19. Which of the following can affect a specimen's specific gravity if it is found in a patient's urine?
    A. 50–100 rbc/hpf
    B. 5 mmol/L glucose
    C. 3+ amorphous phosphates
    D. Moderate bacteria

20. With infections of the urinary system, white blood cells are frequently seen in the urine sediment. What type of white blood cell is seen the most frequently in urine sediment?
    A. Eosinophil
    B. Lymphocyte
    C. Monocyte
    D. Neutrophil

21. Which of the following when present in urine can be an early predictor of renal damage associated with Type 1 diabetes mellitus?
    A. Macroglobulinuria
    B. Paucialbuminuria
    C. Hypersthenuria
    D. Myoglobinuria

22. The identification of unstained cellular components and casts in urine sediments provides a practical method for the detec-

tion and differentiation of formed elements in urinary sediment. Which microscopic technique is used for this procedure?

- A. Fluorescent microscopy
- B. Phase-contrast microscopy
- C. Polarized microscopy
- D. Bright-field microscopy

23. Which substance found in urinary sediment is more easily distinguished by use of polarized microscopy?

- A. Lipids
- B. Casts
- C. Crystals
- D. Ketone bodies

24. Glitter cell is a term used to describe a specific type of

- A. Ketone body
- B. Oval fat body
- C. Fatty droplet
- D. Neutrophil

25. The final phase of degeneration that granular casts undergo is represented by which of the following casts?

- A. Fine
- B. Coarse
- C. Cellular
- D. Waxy

26. What condition is characterized by increased urinary excretion of protein during the day while at night there is a normal excretion of protein?

- A. Pathological proteinuria
- B. Bence Jones proteinuria
- C. Orthostatic proteinuria
- D. Functional nocturia

27. A freshly collected and processed urine specimen is examined microscopically. Which of the following statements about the major formed element in Color Plate 46 is *true?*

- A. These will lyse in the presence of 10% acetic acid
- B. The number shown in this high power field does not indicate pathology
- C. They can be found in male and female urine specimens
- D. They can be confused microscopically with white blood cells

28. Alkaptonuria, a rare hereditary disease, is characterized by the urinary excretion of

- A. Alkaptone
- B. Phenylalanine
- C. 5-Hydroxyindole acetic acid
- D. Homogentisic acid

29. Excessive lipid metabolism, as is seen in diabetes mellitus, is indicated by the presence in the urine of

- A. Hemoglobin
- B. Ketone bodies
- C. Glucose
- D. Protein

30. Metastatic carcinoid tumors arising from the enterochromaffin cells of the gastrointestinal tract are characterized by increased excretion of urinary

- A. Serotonin
- B. 5-Hydroxytryptophan
- C. Homogentisic acid
- D. 5-Hydroxyindole acetic acid

31. Some clinical conditions are characterized by unique urinalysis result patterns. Which of the following shows such a relationship?

- A. Nephrotic syndrome: positive protein on reagent strip, negative protein with sulfosalicylic acid
- B. Intensive dieting: increased ketones, negative glucose
- C. Multiple myeloma: positive protein by both reagent strip and sulfosalicylic acid
- D. Cystitis: positive nitrite and protein

32. Nitrite in a urine specimen suggests the presence of
   A. White blood cells
   B. Red blood cells
   C. Bacteria
   D. Yeasts

33. If a fasting plasma glucose level of 100 mg/dL is obtained on an individual, what is the expected fasting cerebrospinal fluid (CSF) glucose level in mg/dL?
   A. 25
   B. 50
   C. 65
   D. 100

34. A patient with diabetes mellitus complicated with kidney malfunction is admitted to the hospital. His chemical urinalysis results show a glucose level of 1000 mg/dL, a protein level of 2000 mg/dL, a protein determination of 2.04 g/dL by sulfosalicylic acid, and a ketone level of 40 mg/dL. The specific gravity is 1.018 with the use of a reagent strip. What is this patient's correct specific gravity?
   A. 1.007
   B. 1.008
   C. 1.011
   D. 1.018

35. To preserve the sensitivity of the reagent test strips used for the chemical evaluation of urine, how should the strips be handled?
   A. Used within one year after opening
   B. Kept in a loosely capped container
   C. Protected from excessive heat
   D. Stored in a refrigerator

36. Which is true about the formed element found in Color Plate 47?
   A. May be found in normal alkaline urine
   B. Always associated with renal pathology
   C. Never found at urine pH 7.0
   D. Always associated with lung pathology

37. Which formed element is *not* found in the high-power field shown in Color Plate 48?
   A. White blood cell
   B. Mucus
   C. Squamous epithelium
   D. Sperm

38. Which of the following is true about the final concentrating of urine in the kidney?
   A. The distal convoluted tubule, through active transport, reabsorbs water
   B. Water is reabsorbed under the direct influence of angiotensin II
   C. Vasopressin controls the collecting duct reabsorption of water
   D. Water reabsorption is influenced by urine filtrate levels of potassium

39. If a urine specimen is left standing at room temperature for several hours, which of the following changes may occur?
   A. Multiplication of bacteria
   B. An increase in the glucose concentration
   C. Production of an acid urine
   D. Deterioration of any albumin present

40. The diluting and concentrating ability of the kidneys may be measured by performing which of the following urine tests?
   A. Sodium
   B. Creatinine
   C. Volume
   D. Specific gravity

41. Positive results on Benedict's test would be obtained if the urine sample contained which of the following?
   A. Urea
   B. Potassium
   C. Sucrose
   D. Ascorbic acid

42. Phenylketonuria may be characterized by which of the following statements?

A. It may cause brain damage if untreated

B. It is caused by the absence of the enzyme, phenylalanine oxidase

C. Phenylpyruvic acid excess appears in the blood

D. Excess tyrosine accumulates in the blood

43. What condition is suggested by the number of the formed element that predominates in the low-power field of Color Plate 49?

A. Glomerulonephritis

B. Improperly collected specimen

C. Pyelonephritis

D. Nephrotic syndrome

44. Xanthochromia of cerebrospinal fluid (CSF) samples may be due to increased levels of which of the following?

A. Chloride

B. Protein

C. Glucose

D. Magnesium

45. All the following would be characterized by an increased number of the urinary component in Color Plate 50 *except*

A. Acute glomerulonephritis

B. Renal calculi

C. Menstrual contamination

D. Nephrotic syndrome

46. To determine amniotic fluid contamination with maternal urine, which of the following measurements could be used?

A. Creatinine concentration

B. Lecithin/sphingomyelin ratio

C. Albumin/globulin ratio

D. Lactate dehydrogenase

47. With the development of fetal lung maturity, which of the following phospholipid concentrations in amniotic fluid significantly and consistently increases?

A. Sphingomyelin

B. Phosphatidyl ethanolamine

C. Phosphatidyl inositol

D. Phosphatidyl choline

48. Which of the following amniotic fluid measurements is used as an indicator of fetal maturity?

A. Phosphatidyl glycerol

B. Phosphatidyl inositol

C. Alpha$_1$-fetoprotein

D. Delta absorbance at 450 nm

49. Contamination of amniotic fluid with even small amounts of maternal or fetal blood could significantly interfere in the measurement of which of the following?

A. Net absorbance at 450 nm

B. Creatinine

C. Alpha$_1$-fetoprotein

D. Urea nitrogen

50. Patients with diabetes insipidus tend to produce urine in _____ volume with _____ specific gravity.

A. Increased, decreased

B. Increased, increased

C. Decreased, decreased

D. Decreased, increased

51. The estimation of hyaluronic acid concentration by measurement of viscosity is useful in evaluating which type of fluid?

A. Cerebrospinal

B. Peritoneal

C. Pleural

D. Synovial

52. Which of the following is characteristic of an exudate effusion?

A. Leukocyte count greater than 1000/μL

B. Clear appearance

C. Protein concentration less than 3.0 g/dL

D. Absence of fibrinogen

53. All the following systems may be used to determine the specific gravity of urine *except*
   A. Refractometer
   B. Osmometer
   C. TS meter
   D. Polyelectrolytes

54. Which methods may be used to quantify protein in both cerebrospinal fluid and urine specimens?
   A. Sulfosalicylic acid and bromcresol green
   B. Ponceau S and Coomassie brilliant blue
   C. Bromcresol green and Coomassie brilliant blue
   D. Coomassie brilliant blue and sulfosalicylic acid

55. Which of the following characteristics is true of the urinary components in Color Plate 51?
   A. Consist entirely of Tamm-Horsfall protein
   B. Presence always indicates a disease process
   C. Can be observed with polarized microscopy
   D. Appear yellowish in brightfield microscopy

56. A characteristic of substances normally found dissolved in the urine is that they are all
   A. Water soluble
   B. Inorganic
   C. Organic
   D. Waste products

57. Which of the following statements applies to the proper collection and handling of CSF?
   A. The second tube collected should be used for chemistry analyses
   B. The third tube collected should be used for bacteriologic studies

C. CSF collected in the evening should be refrigerated and assays performed only by day-shift personnel
   D. With low-volume specimens, a culture is performed first, before cell counts are done

58. All the following characteristics are true for the urinary components in Color Plate 52 *except*
   A. Appear morphologically as octahedrals resembling envelopes
   B. Appear as dumbbell or oval forms
   C. Appear only in an acid urine
   D. Occur in a normal urine

59. Which assay is commonly performed on pleural, pericardial, and peritoneal fluids?
   A. Total protein
   B. Specific gravity
   C. Osmolality
   D. Calcium

60. Which urinalysis reagent strip test will never be reported out as "negative"?
   A. Protein
   B. Urobilinogen
   C. Bilirubin
   D. Nitrite

61. The following urinalysis results were obtained on a 40-year-old white male whose skin appeared yellowish during the clinical examination. Color and clarity—dark brown, clear; protein—negative; glucose—negative; blood—negative; ketones—negative; bilirubin—moderate; urobilinogen—0.2 mg/dL. These results are clinically significant in which of the following conditions?
   A. Bile duct obstruction
   B. Cirrhosis
   C. Hepatitis
   D. Hemolytic anemia

62. Which of the following pertains to the performance of a sperm count?
    A. Performed by means of a direct observation on a glass slide
    B. Requires dilution of the seminal fluid specimen
    C. Performed on a sample prior to complete liquefaction
    D. Manual sperm counts yield precise data

63. Which of the following may be associated with morphologic examination of spermatozoa?
    A. Evaluation should include assessment of 1000 spermatozoa
    B. A small number of sperm should have normal morphologic characteristics
    C. Papanicolaou stain may be used
    D. Presence of red or white cells and epithelial cells need not be noted

64. Which condition is characterized by increased levels of immunoglobulins in the cerebrospinal fluid, originating from within the central nervous system and not from the general blood circulation?
    A. Gout
    B. Erythroblastosis fetalis
    C. Multiple myeloma
    D. Multiple sclerosis

65. Which of the following statements pertains to screening methods used to determine pregnancy?
    A. Immunoassays will use reagent anti-CG to react with patient CG
    B. One-step pregnancy tests require the use of both anti-α-CG and anti-β-CG as reagents
    C. Internal controls provided within the kit will assess if the patient's specimen was collected correctly
    D. External quality control is not needed with these methods

66. The following urinalysis biochemical results were obtained from a 4-month-old infant who experienced vomiting and diarrhea after milk ingestion and failed to gain weight. pH—6; protein—negative; glucose—negative; ketone—negative; bilirubin—negative; Clinitest—2+ These results are clinically significant in which of the following disorders?
    A. Diabetes mellitus
    B. Ketosis
    C. Starvation
    D. Galactosemia

67. Which of the following is a *true* statement?
    A. Renal tubular cells originate from the renal pelvis
    B. Red blood cells in acid urine (pH 4.5) will usually be crenated because of the acidity
    C. Bacteria introduced into a urine specimen at the time of the collection will have no immediate effect on the level of nitrite in the specimen
    D. Pilocarpine iontophoresis is the method of choice for the collection of pericardial fluid

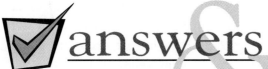
answers & rationales

1.

D. The first-voided morning urine specimen is the most desirable for chemical and microscopic analysis because it is the most concentrated specimen of the day. Protein and nitrite testing are better performed on a concentrated specimen, as are the specific gravity determination and the examination of urinary sediment. However, because of the lack of food and fluid intake during the night, glucose metabolism may be better assessed on the basis of a postprandial specimen.

2.

D. Urochrome, a yellow-brown pigment derived from urobilin, is principally responsible for the yellow coloration of normal urine. Urochrome is excreted at a constant rate, showing no diurnal variation. Therefore the color of normal urine, which may range from straw to deep amber, is dependent on the concentrating ability of the kidney and the volume of urine excreted.

3.

C. Melanin, a substance derived from tyrosine, is responsible for the pigmentation of the eyes, skin, and hair. In some malignancies, known as melanomas, the tumor or mole takes on a darkly pigmented appearance because of the melanin present. In cases of metastatic melanoma, melanogen, which is a colorless precursor of melanin, is excreted in the urine. If the urine is allowed to stand at room temperature for 24 hours, the melanogen is oxidized to melanin, imparting a dark brown or black coloration to the specimen. Qualitative screening tests for the detection of melanin in

urine utilize ferric chloride or sodium nitroprusside as the oxidation reagent systems.

4.

D. pH is a representative symbol for the hydrogen ion concentration. The kidney plays an important role in the maintenance of the acid-base balance of body fluids by either excreting or retaining hydrogen ions. A normally functioning kidney will excrete urine with a pH between 4.5 and 8.0, depending on the overall acid-base needs of the body.

5.

B. At room temperature the amount of bacteria present in a urine sample will increase. The bacteria are capable of metabolizing the urinary urea to ammonia. The ammonia formed through this process will cause an alkalinization of the urine.

6.

C. On the average, a normal adult excretes 1200–1500 mL of urine daily. Polyuria is a term used to describe the excretion of a urine volume in excess of 2000 mL/day. In oliguria, the daily urine excretion is less than 500 mL, and in anuria the urine formation is completely suppressed. Hypersthenuria refers to urines of any volume containing increased levels of dissolved solute.

7.

D. Isosthenuria is a term applied to a series of urine specimens that exhibit a fixed specific gravity of approximately 1.010. In isosthenuria there is little, if any, variation of the specific gravity between urine specimens. This condition is abnormal and denotes the presence of severe renal damage in which both the diluting ability and the concentrating ability of the kidneys have been severely affected.

8.

C. Normal urine does not foam on being shaken. However, urine containing bilirubin will exhibit yellow foaming when the specimen is shaken. In fact, the foam test was actually the first test for bilirubin, prior to the development of the chemical tests. If the shaken specimen shows a white foam, increased urine protein can be suspected.

9.

C. For quality control of reagent test strips, it is recommended that both positive and negative controls be used daily. It is necessary that any deterioration of the strips be detected in order to avoid false-positive or false-negative results. The use of positive and negative controls will act as a check on the reagents, on the technique employed, and on the interpretive ability of the person or instrument performing the test.

10.

D. The principle of the reagent strip method for the detection of protein in urine is based on a color change in an indicator system, such as tetrabromophenol blue, that is buffered to pH 3. The buffering capacity of the strip is sufficient provided that the urine pH does not exceed 8.0. Within the normal urine pH range of 4.5–8.0, a change in color in the reagent strip is an indication of the presence of protein in the urine. With a urine pH greater than 8, the buffering capacity of the strip may be exceeded, and a false-positive color change in the impregnated area will reflect the pH of the urine rather than the presence of protein.

11.

A. In healthy individuals the amount of protein excreted in the urine should not exceed 150 mg/24 hr. When protein is present in the urine, the colorimetric reagent test strips change color, indicating a semiquantification of the amount of protein present. Serum proteins are classified as being albumin or globulin in nature, and the type of protein excreted in the urine is dependent on the disorder present. Although the strip test is a rapid screening method for the detection of urinary protein, it must be noted that this method is more sensitive to the presence of albumin in the specimen than to

the presence of globulin, Bence Jones protein, or mucoprotein.

12.

C. When globulin, mucoprotein, or Bence Jones protein is present in a urine specimen, the reagent strip test may give a negative result because the strip is more sensitive to the presence of albumin than to the presence of other proteins in urine. However, the sulfosalicylic acid (SSA) test is able to detect not only albumin but also globulin, mucoprotein, and Bence Jones protein in a specimen. Therefore, it can be seen that a negative reagent strip test result for protein but a positive sulfosalicylic acid test result is possible when the protein present is some protein other than albumin. For this reason the sulfosalicylic acid test is frequently run as a confirmatory procedure in testing for urinary protein.

13.

B. The test strip impregnated with glucose oxidase–peroxidase reagent is specific for glucose. Benedict's test, however, is responsive to both glucose and a variety of non-glucose, reducing substances. Therefore a negative strip test result with a positive Benedict's test result is possible when a non-glucose, reducing substance is present in the urine specimen. It should be noted that contamination of a urine specimen with hypochlorite or peroxide would actually cause a positive reaction with the glucose oxidase–peroxidase method, and a negative/decreased result with Benedict's test.

14.

A. Preanalytical components of laboratory testing include all variables that can affect the integrity or acceptability of the patient specimen prior to analysis, such as correct collection technique. Analytical factors affect the actual analysis of the specimen (temperature, condition of equipment, timing, presence of interfering substances). Postanalytical factors affect the final handling of the results generated (reporting units, critical values, acceptability of quality control).

15.

B. Under normal metabolic conditions, the body metabolizes fat to carbon dioxide and water. With inadequate carbohydrate intake, as with dieting and starvation, or with inadequate carbohydrate metabolism, as with diabetes mellitus, there is an increased utilization of fat. Because of this increased fat metabolism, the body is unable to completely degrade the fat, resulting in a buildup of intermediary products known as ketone bodies. Ketone bodies is a collective term used to denote the presence of acetoacetic acid, beta-hydroxybutyric acid, and acetone. Reagent test strips impregnated with sodium nitroprusside are able to detect the presence of acetoacetic acid and acetone in urine specimens. Although beta-hydroxybutyric acid accounts for approximately 78% of the total ketones, it is not detected by the sodium nitroprusside test.

16.

C. Although a positive result on a urine test for ketones is most commonly associated with increased urinary glucose levels, as in diabetes mellitus, other conditions may cause the urine ketone test to show positive results while the urine glucose test shows negative results. In young children, a negative glucose reaction accompanied by a positive ketone reaction is sometimes seen. Ketones in the urine may be seen when a child is suffering from an acute febrile disease or toxic condition that is accompanied by vomiting or diarrhea. In these cases, because of either decreased food intake or decreased intestinal absorption, fat catabolism is increased to such an extent that the intermediary products, known as ketone bodies, are formed and excreted in the urine.

17.

C. The colorimetric reagent strip test for the detection of hemoglobin in urine utilizes a buffered test zone impregnated with a dye and organic peroxide. The peroxidase activity of hemoglobin catalyzes the oxidation of the dye with peroxide to form a colored compound. Like hemoglobin, myoglobin also has a peroxidase activity and when present in a urine specimen, myoglobin will react, yielding false-positive results. In the presence of large amounts of ascorbic acid, antibiotics containing ascorbic acid as a preservative, formaldehyde, or nitrite, the urine reaction may be inhibited, causing false-negative results.

18.

D. Bilirubin is a compound that is formed as a result of hemoglobin breakdown. The majority of bilirubin in the blood is bound to albumin and is known as unconjugated bilirubin. Since unconjugated bilirubin is not water soluble, it may not be ex-

creted in the urine. The remainder of the bilirubin in the blood has been processed by the liver. In the liver, the bilirubin is conjugated with glucuronic acid or sulfuric acid. This conjugated bilirubin is water soluble, and it is this portion that is excreted in increased amounts in the urine in some hepatic and obstructive biliary tract diseases. The presence of conjugated bilirubin in a urine specimen may be detected by use of the reagent test strips. The test strips are impregnated with a diazonium salt, such as diazotized 2,4-dichloroaniline, which forms a purplish azobilirubin compound with bilirubin.

19.

B. Only dissolved solutes affect specific gravity. Cells, mucus, crystals, or any other formed elements will have no effect, regardless of concentration. If the reagent strip method is used, it should be noted that only dissolved ions will affect specific gravity results. In such instances as diabetes mellitus, with urine glucose levels over 2 g/dL, there may be a discrepancy between specific gravity readings taken with a reagent strip method versus that using a refractometer.

20.

D. The majority of renal and urinary tract diseases are characterized by an increased number of neutrophilic leukocytes in the urine. To identify correctly any white blood cells present in a urine specimen, it is necessary to examine the specimen as soon as possible after collection. This is necessary since leukocytes tend to lyse easily when exposed to either hypotonic or alkaline urine.

21.

B. The ability of the glomerulus to prevent filtration of protein is one of the first renal properties affected in the renal complications of Type 1 diabetes mellitus. As microcirculation in the nephron is compromised, increasing amounts of albumin will be found in the urine. These levels will initially be less than the sensitivity level of the reagent strips usually used for urinalysis (5–10 mg/dL). Special strips with a protein sensitivity of 2 mg/dL or less must be used to detect and follow these urine protein changes in at-risk patient populations.

22.

B. To better diagnose renal and urinary tract diseases, it is necessary to examine urinary sediment carefully by the most appropriate microscopic method available. Formed elements in the urine, such as cells and casts, are more easily differentiated by the use of phase-contrast microscopy. This is especially true for the identification of the more translucent elements such as the hyaline casts. Phase microscopy tends to enhance the outline of the formed elements, allowing them to stand out and be more easily distinguished.

23.

A. Fatty materials in urinary sediment may be identified by means of staining techniques using Sudan III and oil red O or by means of polarized microscopy. Polarized microscopy is especially useful when the composition of fatty casts, fatty droplets, or oval fat bodies is primarily cholesterol. When cholesterol molecules are exposed to polarized microscopy, the effect is such that a Maltese cross formation becomes visible, simplifying the identification process.

24.

D. When neutrophils are exposed to hypotonic urine, their physical appearance becomes altered. Under hypotonic conditions, the neutrophils tend to swell and the cytoplasmic granules contained within the cells exhibit Brownian movement. This Brownian movement of the granules causes the neutrophilic contents to refract in such a way that the cells appear to glitter—thus, the name glitter cells.

25.

D. Waxy casts represent the final phase of granular cast degeneration. As the fine granules of the granular casts lyse, highly refractive, smooth, blunt-ended waxy casts are formed. When waxy casts are found in the urine sediment, the implication is that there is nephron obstruction caused by tubular inflammation and degeneration.

26.

C. Orthostatic proteinuria, also referred to as postural proteinuria, is characterized by an increased excretion of protein during the day when a patient is in an erect position. When the patient lies down, the proteinuria disappears; urine tested for protein during this time period will show a negative reaction. This condition, in which urinary protein is found during the day but not at night as a function of the patient's body position, occurs in 3–5% of young adults. These young adults appear to be

healthy, and except for the excessive protein excretion, they show no other signs of renal disease.

27.

C. The yeasts, as seen in Color Plate 46, can resemble red blood cells. They can be differentiated by introducing a drop of 10% acetic acid under the cover slip: red cells will lyse and yeasts will not. They can be found in urine from either sex as evidence of a nonbacterial type of urinary tract infection. In a fresh urine, the number of yeasts shown would suggest pathology rather than contamination.

28.

D. Alkaptonuria is a rare hereditary disease that is characterized by excessive urinary excretion of homogentisic acid. This acid, the product of phenylalanine and tyrosine metabolism, accumulates in urine because of a deficiency in the enzyme homogentisic acid oxidase, which normally catalyzes the oxidation of homogentisic acid to maleyl acetoacetic acid. Urine containing homogentisic acid turns black on standing because of an oxidative process; thus the screening test for alkaptonuria consists of the detection of a black coloration in urine that is left standing at room temperature for 24 hours.

29.

B. Diabetes mellitus is marked by an underutilization of blood glucose by the cells of the body as a result of inadequate glucose uptake by the cells. Since glucose metabolism is depressed, the cells must revert to lipid catabolism for energy production. Such an increased use of lipid results in incomplete lipid metabolism, so that intermediary products are formed. These intermediary products, known as ketone bodies, accumulate in the blood and are excreted in the urine.

30.

D. The intestinal enterochromaffin cells, sometimes called the argentaffin cells, produce a substance known as serotonin from the amino acid tryptophan. In cases of metastatic carcinoid tumors, excessive amounts of serotonin are produced. Serotonin may then undergo oxidative deamination to form the metabolite 5-hydroxyindole acetic acid (5-HIAA), which is excreted in the urine. It is the quantification of 5-HIAA that is diagnostically significant as it reflects serotonin production.

31.

B. Because of increased lipid metabolism in long-term, intensive dieting, ketone body formation will increase. Blood glucose levels in such patients will be normal or decreased. In nephrotic syndrome, the large amounts of albumin excreted will be detectable by both reagent strip and SSA methods. In multiple myeloma, however, the increased globulin light chains (Bence Jones proteins) excreted will only be detectable by SSA since the reagent strip is more sensitive to albumin. Cystitis is a lower urinary tract infection affecting the bladder but not the kidney itself. This will not have increased protein, while an upper urinary tract infection will.

32.

C. Bacteria of the *Enterobacter, Citrobacter, Escherichia, Proteus, Klebsiella,* and *Pseudomonas* species produce enzymes that catalyze the reduction of nitrate, a substance normally found in urine, to nitrite. Reagent test strips have been developed that are able to detect nitrite in urine. Therefore, a positive nitrite test result is an indirect indication of the presence of bacteria in the urine specimen.

33.

C. Cerebrospinal fluid (CSF) is a clear, colorless liquid that may be described as a modified ultrafiltrate of blood. Both active transport and passive diffusion are involved in the passage of glucose from the blood into the CSF. Normally, fasting CSF glucose levels range between 50 and 80 mg/dL, representing approximately 60–70% of the blood glucose level. In hyperglycemia with plasma glucose levels of 300 mg/dL, the active transport mechanism reaches a point of maximum response, so that CSF glucose levels reflect approximately 30% of the plasma glucose level. Decreased CSF glucose levels are associated with hypoglycemia, a faulty active transport mechanism, and excess utilization of glucose by microorganisms, red or white blood cells, or the central nervous system.

34.

D. Reagent strip methods for specific gravity are sensitive to the presence of ions in the specimen. As such, they will not be affected by unionized solutes such as glucose and protein. Measurement of the ionized components of urine represents a truer estimate of the concentrating ability of the kidneys.

35.

C. To avoid loss of sensitivity, it is necessary that the reagent test strips for chemical analysis of urine be stored in a cool, dry place and protected from both moisture and excessive heat. Because of moisture buildup, the strips should not be stored in a refrigerator. Impregnated reagent areas should be checked for discoloration and the strip not used if any discoloration is observed. To protect the strips, it is necessary that the cap be kept on the container tightly at all times and removed only long enough to remove the needed strips. To prevent contamination, the impregnated reagent areas should not be touched with the fingers or placed on a countertop.

36.

A. Normal alkaline (or neutral) urine may contain triple phosphate crystals, as seen in Color Plate 47. These crystals can be identified by the characteristic "coffin lid" appearance. They usually do not indicate any pathology.

37.

D. Refer to Color Plate 48. White blood cells are 12–15 microns in diameter with a granular cytoplasm. Mucus strands can be seen here as translucent, long, thin filaments. Squamous epithelial cells are 40–50 microns in diameter, with a large cytoplasm/nucleus ratio. They can at times have their cell membrane folded over. Not present in this field are sperm, which have a 4–6-micron-diameter head attached to a long flagellum.

38.

C. The distal convoluted tubule and collecting duct provide water reabsorption through the action of antidiuretic hormone (vasopressin). The renin-angiotensin-aldosterone system is responsible for sodium reabsorption by the distal and collecting tubules. Decreased plasma volume leads to pressure alterations detected by receptors located in the kidney's juxtaglomerular apparatus and the right atrium of the heart. These changes trigger the production of renin and antidiuretic hormone, respectively.

39.

A. Only freshly voided urine specimens should be used for urinalysis testing. If the specimen cannot be examined within 1 hour after collection, it should be refrigerated to help preserve the integrity of the specimen. When urine is left standing at room temperature for an excessive period, multiplication of bacteria will occur. The bacteria are capable of converting urea in the urine to ammonia, causing the urine to become more alkaline. Loss of carbon dioxide from the specimen will also contribute to the alkalinization of the urine. Constituents such as glucose, bilirubin, and urobilinogen will also be lost from the specimen.

40.

D. Both the specific gravity and the osmolality determinations have been used as a measure of the diluting and concentrating ability of the kidneys. Both tests are based on the measurement of the proportion of dissolved solids to total volume of urine. The specific gravity, although a somewhat easier procedure to perform, is not as exact a measurement as the osmolality. The specific gravity is dependent not only on the quantity of solute present but also on the type of solute present. Therefore, if large molecules such as protein or glucose are present in excess, a disproportionate specific gravity reading may be obtained. With an osmolality determination, such interference would be avoided because the osmolality is dependent only on the number of dissolved particles present in the urine specimen.

41.

D. Benedict's test is a copper reduction method for the detection of glucose and other reducing substances in urine. In this test, alkaline copper sulfate is reduced to cuprous oxide by any reducing substance present in urine. The drawback of this procedure is that it is nonspecific for glucose. Nonglucose reducing substances such as ascorbic acid, creatinine, and uric acid or other reducing sugars, such as galactose and lactose, can also cause a positive reaction. Therefore, when used alone, Benedict's test can only detect the presence of reducing substances in urine but cannot itself identify the exact reducing substance present.

42.

A. Phenylketonuria is inherited as an autosomal recessive trait that manifests itself in the homozygous form. The basis for the disease lies in the fact that the enzyme phenylalanine hydroxylase, which is needed for the conversion of phenylalanine to tyrosine, is absent. Because of this enzyme deficiency, phenylalanine levels rise in the blood with increased amounts of phenylpyruvic acid and other derivatives being excreted in the urine. If the disease is detected at an early stage, mental retardation may be avoided by restricting the dietary intake of phenylalanine.

43.

B. Color Plate 49 demonstrates significantly increased numbers of squamous epithelial cells in the field. This usually suggests the sample has not been collected by the preferred method of "clean midstream catch." Such proper collection would have flushed out these cells, found at the external meatus and final one-third of the urethra. Cells characteristically found in cases of glomerulonephritis are red blood cells. In pyelonephritis, white blood cells would predominate, while cases of nephrotic syndrome will show oval fat bodies and red blood cells.

44.

B. A variety of substances in CSF specimens have been associated with a xanthochromic appearance. Among those substances are oxyhemoglobin, carotenoids, bilirubin, and protein. The appearance of the specimen by itself is not usually specific for a particular disease state, but it may provide useful information in comparison with other findings. Glucose, magnesium, and chloride do not contribute to the color of the specimen.

45.

D. Refer to Color Plate 50. Erythrocytes or red blood cells (RBCs) occur in small numbers (0–2/HPF) in a normal urine. Using bright-field microscopy, unstained RBCs appear as colorless discs with an average size of 7 μm in diameter. Increased or large numbers of RBCs are commonly seen with acute glomerulonephritis, renal calculi, acute infections, and menstrual contamination. The nephrotic syndrome is characterized by heavy proteinuria, oval fat bodies, renal tubular epithelial cells, casts, and waxy and fatty casts.

46.

A. Because there may be technical problems associated with amniocentesis, contamination with maternal urine should be considered in evaluating specimens submitted for amniotic fluid analysis. Urinary concentrations of creatinine and urea nitrogen are anywhere from 10 to 50 times the amniotic fluid concentrations, and an increased concentration of either in the amniotic fluid would be sensitive indicators of urinary contamination. Measurements of albumin, total protein, or lactate dehydrogenase would be of little use for this purpose because their relative concentrations in urine and amniotic fluid are not predictably different.

47.

D. The alveolar concentrations of the various phospholipids (surfactants) change during fetal lung development, and because these changes are reflected directly in the amniotic fluid, a number of investigations have shown that analysis of the fluid can provide good predictive information for the development of respiratory distress syndrome in the newborn. The concentrations of sphingomyelin and phosphatidyl inositol increase until about 32 to 34 weeks of gestation and then decline. Conversely, lecithin (phosphatidyl choline) and phosphatidyl glycerol concentrations increase rapidly after 32 to 34 weeks of gestation, and their concentrations relative to those of the other phospholipids are useful in assessing the development of fetal lung maturity.

48.

A. Measurements on amniotic fluid that are used for determining fetal maturity can usually be related to the maturity of a particular organ. For example, the level of creatinine appears to be related to the maturity of the fetal kidney. The lecithin/sphingomyelin ratio, phosphatidyl glycerol levels, and the foam stability index have been shown to correlate well with the development of fetal lung maturity. Only those tests that measure fetal lung development will be useful in predicting the respiratory distress syndrome. The net absorbance at 450 nm measurement is not a measure of fetal maturity but is useful in monitoring the course of the isoimmunization syndrome.

49.

A. The spectrophotometric method for detection of the isoimmunization syndrome, applied to amniotic fluid, is based on the determination of bilirubin concentration by measuring the net change in absorbance at 450 nm. Hemoglobin absorbs strongly at approximately 410 nm and therefore can interfere in the net absorbance at 450 nm measurement. The presence of meconium in amniotic fluid is in itself an indication of fetal distress, and it can interfere in the spectrophotometric measurement because of its absorbance at approximately 410 nm. Creatinine and protein do not have strong absorbance bands in this spectral region and are generally not a problem.

50.

A. Diabetes insipidus is caused by a deficiency in antidiuretic hormone. Such deficiencies will result in the kidney's inability to reabsorb water at the distal and collecting tubules. This affects only water reabsorption and not the reabsorption of other urinary solutes. Excreted solute amounts will be the same, but the water volume into which they are excreted will be larger. This results in high urine volumes and low final solute concentrations. The low solute will lead to low specific gravities in these patients' specimens.

51.

D. Synovial fluid is a form of plasma ultrafiltrate with added hyaluronic acid. Decreased viscosity and poor mucin clot formation are indications of the decreased hyaluronate concentration of synovial fluid. Either of these findings is usually an indication of inflammation. Since the viscosity of synovial fluid is normally very high, it can be estimated by the length of string formed when the fluid drops from a syringe. The term mucin in the mucin clot test is a misnomer, since mucin is not present in synovial fluid.

52.

A. Effusions result from an imbalance of the flow of body fluids. Effusions are classified as exudates or transudates on the basis of certain characteristics. Exudates are generally formed in response to inflammation or infection with concomitant capillary wall damage. Exudates are characterized by protein levels greater than 3.0 g/dL, leukocyte counts greater than 1000/μL, and the presence of a sufficient amount of fibrinogen to cause clotting. In contrast, transudates are characterized by protein levels less than 3.0 g/dL, leukocyte counts less than 300/μL, and the absence of fibrinogen. Transudates are generally formed as the result of noninflammatory processes, including alterations in plasma oncotic pressure, pleural capillary hydrostatic pressure, or intrapleural pressure.

53.

B. A clinically useful test for assessing the concentrating and diluting ability of the kidneys is the determination of urine specific gravity. The specific gravity is a measure of the proportion of dissolved solids in a given volume of solvent. The TS meter is a specific type of refractometer that utilizes the close correlation of a solution's refractive index with its solute concentration to determine the specific gravity of urine. The refractive index is the ratio of the velocity of light in air to the velocity of light in a solution, this being comparable to the number of dissolved particles in that solution. Polyelectrolytes are incorporated into urinalysis reagent strips. A dye also present in the strips will change color because of a pKa change in the polyelectrolytes. The pKa varies with the ionic concentration of the urine. The color obtained is compared with a set of standard colors, each color correlating with a different specific gravity concentration.

54.

D. Trichloroacetic acid and sulfosalicylic acid are turbidimetric methods used to quantify small amounts of protein, less than 100 mg/dL, in cerebrospinal fluid (CSF) and urine specimens. Coomassie brilliant blue is a colorimetric dye binding method in which protein complexes with the dye, forming a soluble blue complex. This method also exhibits the necessary sensitivity for detecting small quantities of protein.

55.

A. As seen in Color Plate 51, hyaline casts are the most commonly observed cast, and they consist completely of Tamm-Horsfall protein. A reference urine may contain 0–2 hyaline casts per low-power field. Hyaline casts appear translucent using bright-field microscopy because they have a refractive index similar to urine. Phase contrast microscopy may be used to visualize the casts better.

56.

A. To be found in urine, a solute must be water soluble. Solutes can be inorganic (e.g., sodium) or organic (e.g., urea). Excreted waste products, meaning end products of metabolism, are creatinine, urea, and uric acid. Some excreted solutes, however, are not present as waste but as overload, such as glucose or sodium.

57.

D. Cerebrospinal fluid (CSF) must be collected in sterile tubes. The first tube is generally used for chemistry and serology studies, the second tube is employed for bacteriologic examination, and the third tube is used for cell counts. Tubes used for chemistry and bacteriologic studies should be centrifuged before use. CSF should remain uncentrifuged for cell counts. Low-volume specimens need to be cultured first (to ensure sterility) before any other test is performed. Since the analyses of CSF should be performed immediately, it is critical that personnel on all shifts be able to perform the necessary testing.

58.

C. Calcium oxalate crystals, as seen in Color Plate 52, are commonly encountered in normal acidic urine but may be observed in neutral urine and rarely in an alkaline urine. Using bright-field microscopy, calcium oxalate crystals appear as small, colorless octahedrals or envelopelike forms, and they may also be observed in dumbbell or ovoid forms. These crystals are soluble in dilute hydrochloric acid.

59.

A. When pleural, pericardial, and peritoneal fluids with unknown abnormalities are examined, the following assays are generally performed: total protein, red and white blood cell counts, differential count, Gram stain, culture, and cytologic evaluation. In addition to these tests, determination of values for any of the following may also be warranted, depending on the particular case involved: glucose, amylase, lactate dehydrogenase, pH, ammonia, creatinine, and alkaline phosphatase. The general appearance of the specimen should always be noted.

60.

B. The sensitivity of a method is the lowest concentration of the analyte that will result in a detectable reaction signal. The protein, bilirubin, and nitrite readout color scales each have a color associated with analyte concentrations less than the method's sensitivity, called "negative." Urobilinogen's readout color scale begins with its lowest reportable value, but there is no pad associated with concentrations less than this.

61.

A. In the hepatic phase of bilirubin metabolism, bilirubin is conjugated with glucuronic acid to form water-soluble conjugated bilirubin. The conjugated bilirubin passes into the bile duct and on to the intestinal tract. In the intestine, it is reduced by intestinal bacteria to form urobilinogen. Bile duct obstruction is characterized by an obstruction of the flow of conjugated bilirubin into the intestinal tract to complete its metabolism. The conjugated bilirubin, which is water soluble, will be excreted by the kidney. Since bilirubin is not entering the intestines, the normal production of urobilinogen is decreased. Therefore, the urine biochemical test will indicate a positive reagent strip test for bilirubin, positive Ictotest, and "normal" (0.2 mg/dL) urobilinogen (since there is no reagent strip pad for "negative" urobilinogen).

62.

B. Sperm counts are performed after complete liquefaction with the use of a diluted sample to charge the hemacytometer. The seminal fluid is diluted 1:20 by means of a calibrated micropipet. The diluent may be isotonic saline. The number of sperm counted in 2 mm² multiplied by 100,000 represents the quantity of sperm per milliliter. Since these counts tend to be imprecise, it is recommended that both the dilution and the count be performed in duplicate and the results averaged.

63.

C. The morphologic characteristics of spermatozoa are best evaluated by means of smears stained with Papanicolaou stain. Other stains used include Kernechtrot, Giemsa, basic fuchsin, crystal violet, and hematoxylin. When oil immersion is used, a minimum of 200 spermatozoa should be evaluated for morphologic characteristics. Although sources differ as to the exact number, it is generally established that at least 60% of the sperm should have normal morphologic features. When this microscopic analysis is performed, the presence of eryth-

rocytes, leukocytes, epithelial cells, and microorganisms should be indicated.

64.

D. Immunoglobulins (IgG) are normally present at less than 1 mg/dL in the CSF. Increased CSF IgG can result from increased CSF production (e.g., multiple sclerosis) or from increased transport from the blood plasma (compromised blood-brain barrier). Neither gout, erythoblastosis fetalis (isoimmunization syndrome), nor multiple myeloma produces increased CSF IgG levels.

65.

A. Many simplified yet immunologically sophisticated methods exist currently for determining pregnancy. All are based on the reaction between patient chorionic gonadotropin (CG) and anti-CG. Most kits will use an antibody recognizing one subunit of CG (alpha or beta), while other kits may use both anti-α-CG and anti-β-CG. Internal controls in these kits will only check if the procedural steps were performed correctly. They cannot detect problems with any pre-analytical variables, like specimen handling or appropriateness. In addition, internal quality control cannot be used to assess the kit's accuracy in distinguishing "positive" from "negative" specimens. Only the use of external quality control specimens can accomplish this.

66.

D. Galactosemia, an inborn error of metabolism, is characterized by the inability to metabolize galactose, a monosaccharide that is contained in milk as a constituent of the disaccharide, lactose. Thus galactose appears in elevated levels in the blood and urine. The condition may result in liver disease, mental retardation, and cataract formation if not treated or controlled. In the biochemical analysis of the urine, the conflicting results for the two glucose tests may be explained as follows. The glucose oxidase reagent strip test is specific for glucose, therefore, the glucose will be negative. The clinitest, a modification of the Benedict's test procedure, detects most reducing substances. Since galactose is present in the urine and is a reducing substance, the clinitest is positive.

67.

C. Renal tubular cells originate from the renal medulla or cortex. Red blood cell crenation is a phenomenon reflecting increased solute concentration (hyperosmolality), and is not caused by urine pH. Red cells will, however, lyse at high alkaline pH. The nitrite reaction requires (a) a sufficient dietary source of nitrate, (b) sufficient numbers of bacteria present in the urine, (c) sufficient incubation time (> 4 hours). Bacteria introduced at collection, even in sufficient number, will not have had sufficient incubation time to convert urine nitrate to nitrite. Pilocarpine iontophoresis is the collection method for sweat.

REFERENCES

Brunzel, N. A. (1994). *Fundamentals of Urine and Body Fluid Analysis.* Philadelphia: W. B. Saunders.

Lehman, C. A. (1998). *Saunders Manual of Clinical Laboratory Science.* Philadelphia: W. B. Saunders.

Ringsrud, K. M., and Linné, J. J. (1995). *Urinalysis and Body Fluids—A Color Text and Atlas.* St. Louis: Mosby-Year Book.

Strasinger, S. K., and DiLorenzo, M. S. (2001). *Urinalysis and Body Fluids,* 4th ed. Philadelphia: F. A. Davis Co.

Wallach, J. (1996). *Interpretation of Diagnostic Tests,* 6th ed. New York: Little, Brown and Co.

CHAPTER

8 Molecular Diagnostics

contents

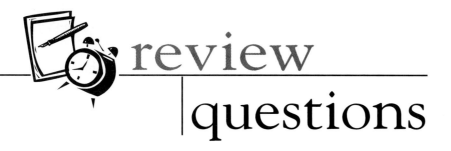

review questions

INSTRUCTIONS Each of the questions or incomplete statements that follow comprises four suggested responses. Select the *best* answer or completion statement in each case.*

1. If 20% of the nucleotides in an organism are adenine, predict the percentage of nucleotides that are guanine.
   A. 20%
   B. 30%
   C. 40%
   D. 60%

2. All the following are required for DNA replication as used in the polymerase chain reaction (PCR) *except*
   A. Oligonucleotide primers
   B. DNA polymerase
   C. DNA ligase
   D. Deoxyribonucleotides

3. In naming restriction endonucleases, the first letter of the name comes from the
   A. Bacterial genus
   B. Bacterial species
   C. Scientist who discovered it
   D. Geographic location of its discovery

4. A restriction enzyme recognizes the sequence, 5′ CT^ATAG 3′, and cuts as indicated. Predict the sticky ends that would result on the *complementary* DNA strand.
   A. 3′ G 5′   3′ ATATC 5′
   B. 3′ GA 5′   3′ TATC 5′
   C. 3′ GATA 5′   3′ TC 5′
   D. 3′ GATAT 5′   3′ C 5′

5. The absorbance of a 1:100 dilution of isolated double-stranded DNA (dsDNA) solution, measured at 260 nm, is 0.062. What is a reasonable estimate for the dsDNA concentration of the sample, expressed in μg/mL?
   A. 3.1
   B. 6.2
   C. 310
   D. 5000

*Abbreviations used frequently: **DNA**, deoxyribonucleic acid; **RNA**, ribonucleic acid; **PCR**, polymerase chain reaction; **LCR**, ligase chain reaction; **bDNA**, branched chain DNA reaction; **NaCl**, sodium chloride; **PFGE**, pulsed field gel electrophoresis; **A**, adenine; **T**, thymine; **U**, uracil; **G**, guanine; **C**, cytosine; **dNTP**, deoxyribonucleotide triphosphate; **RT-PCR**, reverse transcriptase-polymerase chain reaction; **DNases**, deoxyribonucleases; **RNAses**, ribonucleases; **HIV**, human immunodeficiency virus; **HCV**, hepatitis C virus; **CMV**, cytomegalovirus; **ss**, single-stranded; **ds**, double-stranded; **TMA**, transcription mediated amplification; **SDA**, strand displacement amplification; **NASBA**, nucleic acid sequence-based amplification.

6. In the isolation of RNA, diethyl pyrocarbonate (DEPC) is used to
   A. Inhibit RNase
   B. Lyse the cells
   C. Precipitate the DNA
   D. Remove buffer salts

7. Purification resins used to isolate DNA take advantage of the fact that DNA is
   A. Double-stranded
   B. Negatively charged
   C. Higher molecular weight than RNA
   D. Higher in concentration than RNA

8. After performance of DNA electrophoresis, the isolated bands in the kilobase size range appear too close together. Which of the following can be done with the next run to improve the appearance/separation of the bands in the samples?
   A. Increase the percent agarose concentration of the matrix
   B. Increase the running time of the electrophoresis
   C. Increase the sample volume applied to the gel
   D. Decrease the sample volume applied to the gel

9. Which of the following may be used as a label in molecular tests?
   A. ^{32}P
   B. Enzymes, such as alkaline phosphatase
   C. Biotin
   D. All the above

10. Which of the following is *not* an example of target amplification?
    A. Reverse transcription-PCR (RT-PCR)
    B. Transcription mediated amplification (TMA)
    C. Branched chain DNA amplification (bDNA)
    D. Polymerase chain reaction (PCR)

11. In forensic testing, DNA fingerprinting can identify individuals with high accuracy because
    A. Human genes are highly conserved
    B. Only a small amount of sample is needed
    C. Human gene loci are polymorphic
    D. DNA is stable and not easily contaminated

12. The technique that makes single-stranded DNA from RNA is called
    A. Strand displacement amplification
    B. Polymerase chain reaction
    C. Ligase chain reaction
    D. Reverse transcription

13. A 5850-base plasmid possesses EcoRI restriction enzyme cleavage sites at the following base pair locations: 36, 1652, and 2702. Following plasmid digestion, the sample is electrophoresed in a 2% agarose gel. A DNA ladder marker, labeled M in Color Plate 56, is included in the first lane, with base pair sizes indicated in lanes A through D. Which lane represents the sample pattern that is most likely the digested plasmid?
    A. A
    B. B
    C. C
    D. D

14. Which of the following is *not* a possible explanation for poor DNA transfer onto a Southern blot?
    A. Transfer time was too short
    B. Weight at the top of the stack was too light
    C. Presence of air bubbles in the "sandwich"
    D. Power conditions (amps) used were too high

15. The most useful feature of the molecules streptavidin and biotin is that they bind
    A. To each other with very high affinity
    B. Directly to DNA immobilized on nitrocellulose
    C. Specifically to nucleic acids
    D. Only in neutral pH conditions

16. What is the theoretical estimation of the number of DNA target sequences present (per original double-stranded DNA in solution) following 15 cycles of PCR?
    A. 30
    B. 1024
    C. 32,768
    D. 1,048,576

17. "Star activity" for a restriction enzyme refers to
    A. An ability to cleave DNA at sequences different from their defined recognition sites
    B. The enzyme's specificity for sites of methylation within the nucleotide sequence
    C. The percent increased accuracy of the enzyme when placed in ideal conditions of pH
    D. The temperature and pH conditions at which the enzyme will function optimally

18. A major difference between the transfer of DNA versus RNA onto nitrocellulose is that
    A. High temperature must be used for the RNA transfer
    B. Less time is usually needed for DNA transfer
    C. The gel is pretreated with alkaline buffer before DNA transfer
    D. RNA transfer is affected by the presence of RNA secondary structure

19. If a DNA probe is added to nitrocellulose after the transfer step but before the blocking step, which of the following will occur?
    A. The probe will nonspecifically bind to its DNA target
    B. Unoccupied spaces on the nitrocellulose will bind the probe
    C. The DNA target on the nitrocellulose will be unable to bind the probe
    D. Bound probe will be washed away in the next wash step

20. Preparation of a DNA probe for Southern blotting using random hexamer primers includes all the following *except*
    A. Template DNA
    B. Three unlabeled deoxynucleotides
    C. Dideoxynucleotides, with one of them radiolabeled
    D. DNA polymerase

21. Which of the following is considered a "high stringency" condition for DNA probe protocols?
    A. Washing the matrix with high-salt buffer
    B. Radiolabeling the probe with ^{35}S rather than ^{32}P
    C. Washing the transfer membrane (e.g., nitrocellulose or nylon) at high temperature
    D. Using wash buffer with highly acidic pH

22. When compared to Southern blot hybridization testing, polymerase chain reaction (PCR)
    A. Is less sensitive to DNA degradation than Southern blot
    B. Requires no specialized equipment
    C. Is more labor intensive
    D. Includes transfer of DNA onto a nylon membrane

23. Specimens used routinely as source material for molecular genetic tests include all the following *except*
    A. Whole blood
    B. Buccal scrapings
    C. Amniocytes
    D. Rectal swabs

24. In the presence of salt, DNA is precipitated from solution by
    A. 10 mM Tris, 1 mM EDTA
    B. Alkaline buffers, such as 0.2 N NaOH
    C. Alcohols, such as 95% ethanol or isopropanol
    D. 0.1% sodium dodecyl sulfate (0.1% SDS)

25. DNA sequencing methods include
    A. Random oligonucleotide sequencing and chemical sequencing
    B. Dideoxy sequencing and chemical sequencing
    C. Nick translation and random oligonucleotide sequencing
    D. Dideoxy sequencing and nick translation

26. For the purpose of diagnosing genetic diseases, what component of whole blood is used for the extraction of DNA?
    A. Red blood cells
    B. Platelets
    C. Plasma
    D. Leukocytes

27. Total RNA was isolated from a tissue sample in the presence of guanidine isothiocyanate and stored at −70 °C. Two weeks later, the RNA was run on a 1% agarose gel in Tris-Borate-EDTA buffer. No distinct bands were seen in the ethidium bromide stained gel. What does this indicate?

    A. RNA was degraded during the isolation procedure
    B. RNA was degraded, probably due to improper storage
    C. RNA was degraded while running the gel
    D. This is an expected result

28. Which of the following is the *least* likely inhibitor of the polymerase chain reaction?
    A. Heme
    B. Sodium heparin
    C. EDTA (ethylenediaminetetraacetic acid)
    D. DEPC (diethyl pyrocarbonate)

29. Frequently, DNA probes are used to detect target sequences in Northern or Southern blots. Hybridization occurs between DNA probe and RNA or DNA on the blot, respectively. To ensure that only exactly matched complementary sequences have bound together, the blot is washed under stringent conditions. Stringency of the wash steps to remove unbound and mismatched probe can be increased by
    A. High temperature, high NaCl concentration, and high detergent (i.e., SDS) solution
    B. High temperature, low NaCl concentration, and high detergent (i.e., SDS) solution
    C. High temperature, high NaCl concentration, and low detergent (i.e., SDS) solution
    D. Low temperature, high NaCl concentration, and high detergent (i.e., SDS) solution

30. In RNA, which nucleotide base replaces thymine of DNA?
    A. Adenine
    B. Cytosine
    C. Guanine
    D. Uracil

31. The component parts of a dNTP include a purine or pyrimidine base, a
    A. Ribose sugar, and one phosphate group
    B. Deoxyribose sugar, and three phosphate groups
    C. Ribose sugar, and two phosphate groups
    D. Deoxyribose sugar, and two phosphate groups

32. When comparing two double-stranded DNA sequences of equal length, the strand that has a higher
    A. G+C content has a higher melting temperature (T_m)
    B. A+T content has a higher T_m
    C. A+T content has more purines than pyrimidines along its length
    D. G+C content has more purines than pyrimidines along its length

33. Molecular typing of bacterial strains is based on restriction fragment length polymorphisms (RFLP) found by digesting bacterial chromosomal DNA with restriction endonucleases. The resulting large DNA fragments are separated by using which of the following techniques?
    A. DNA sequencing
    B. Pulsed field gel electrophoresis
    C. Ribotyping
    D. Reverse transcriptase–polymerase chain reaction

34. Isothermal methods for target amplification include all the following *except*
    A. Nucleic acid sequence-based amplification (NASBA)
    B. Polymerase chain reaction (PCR)
    C. Strand displacement amplification (SDA)
    D. Transcription mediated amplification (TMA)

35. Applications of molecular biological techniques in the clinical laboratory include
    A. Diagnosis and classification of B and T cell lymphomas
    B. Identification of inherited diseases, such as Fragile X and Factor V Leiden
    C. Viral load testing to determine viral burden and monitor antiviral therapy
    D. All the above

36. The central dogma is that DNA is used to make RNA, which is then used to make protein. In this scheme the two processes that are involved (i.e., DNA to RNA and RNA to protein) are termed
    A. Replication and transcription
    B. Synthesis and encryption
    C. Transcription and translation
    D. Initiation and elongation

37. How many chromosomes are contained in a normal human somatic cell?
    A. 22
    B. 23
    C. 44
    D. 46

38. An ordered sequence of events makes up the cell cycle. Which of the following describes the correct sequence of events starting at G1?
    A. G1, G2, S, M
    B. G1, S, G2, M
    C. G1, M, G2, S
    D. G1, S, M, G2

39. Purified DNA remains stable indefinitely when stored as
    A. Small aliquots at 4 °C (refrigerator)
    B. A single aliquot at 25 °C (room temperature)
    C. Small aliquots at −70 °C (ultralow freezer)
    D. A single sample at −20 °C (refrigerator freezer)

40. In Color Plate 57 the procedure of Southern blotting is diagrammed. In the upper panel, restricted genomic DNA fragments have been separated by electrophoresis in an agarose gel. In lane 1 is a molecular weight marker, in lanes 2–4 are three patient samples, and in lane 5 is a positive control DNA sequence for the probe used. After electrophoresis, DNA was transferred from the gel onto a nylon membrane and then hybridized with a radiolabeled probe that recognizes CGG trinucleotide repeat. Fragile X (FRAXA) syndrome is the most frequently inherited form of mental retardation in males (1:1,000–1:1,500 individuals). In affected individuals, expansion of the trinucleotide repeat within the Fragile X gene (FRAXA) increases to greater than 200 repeats. The bottom panel shows the resultant autoradiogram after a series of high stringency washes. The three patient samples (lanes 2–4) are DNA from individuals of a single family, one of them suffering from Fragile X (FRAXA) syndrome. In which lane is the mentally retarded patient's sample?
    A. Lane 2
    B. Lane 3
    C. Lane 4
    D. Cannot be determined by the results given

41. An advantage of amplification technologies for clinical laboratories is
    A. They lend themselves to automated methods
    B. Each target molecule sought requires a unique set of primers
    C. They require inexpensive test reagents
    D. Contamination is not a concern when performing these assays

42. The method to look for the expression of a gene rather than the mere presence or structure of a gene is termed
    A. RT-PCR
    B. TMA
    C. Multiplex PCR
    D. Ribotyping

43. RT-PCR is used for
    A. Diagnosis of *Chlamydia trachomatis* and *Neisseria gonorrhoeae* infection
    B. Detection of gene mutations for cystic fibrosis
    C. Presence of minimal residual disease in certain malignancies
    D. Viral load testing for HIV and HCV

44. One method to prevent "false-positive" PCR results includes the use of dUTP in the reaction mix resulting in PCR products containing U in place of T. The enzyme used to decrease contamination is
    A. Uracil-*N*-glycosylase
    B. *Taq* polymerase
    C. S1 nuclease
    D. DNAse

For questions 45–47, refer to Color Plate 58.

45. What temperature is used in Step 1?
    A. 35 °C
    B. 55 °C
    C. 75 °C
    D. 95 °C

46. What process occurs in Step 2?
    A. Denaturation
    B. Hybridization
    C. Elongation
    D. Ligation

47. What enzyme is used in Step 3?
    A. *Taq* polymerase
    B. T7 RNA polymerase
    C. DNA ligase
    D. RNAse H

48. The following question refers to Color Plate 59. Factor V Leiden mutation causes increased risk of thrombosis. It is caused by a single base mutation in which guanine (G) is substituted for adenine (A) with a subsequent loss of a restriction site for the enzyme *MnlI*. Primers used in this example generate a 223 bp PCR product from patient DNA. After resulting PCR products are digested with *MnlI*, normal patients produce the following DNA fragments (104 bp, 82 bp, 37 bp). In Color Plate 59, the 37 bp fragment is not seen in all lanes because it is sometimes below detectable levels. Lane identities are as follows: M (molecular weight marker), 1–5 (Patient 1–Patient 5, respectively), + (positive control showing 104, 82, and 37 bp fragments), Neg (sterile water used in place of sample DNA). Which patient is heterozygous for the Factor V Leiden mutation?

    A. Patient 1
    B. Patient 2
    C. Patient 3
    D. Patient 4

49. The translocation resulting in the Philadelphia chromosome is detected by

    A. Southern blot analysis only
    B. Cytogenetic analysis (e.g., karyotyping) only
    C. PCR, Southern blot, and cytogenetic analysis
    D. RT-PCR, Southern blot, and cytogenetic analysis

50. Which of the following is characteristic of DNA chips (i.e., DNA microarrays)?

    A. Allow detection and discrimination of multiple genetic sequences at the same time
    B. Thousands of oligonucleotide probes are labeled and placed on glass or silicon surfaces
    C. Unlabeled target sequences within the patient sample are detected by hybridization to labeled probes
    D. All the above

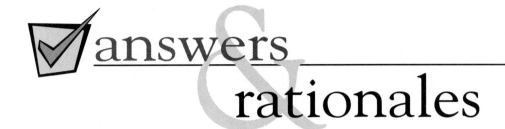

answers & rationales

1.

B. Due to the base pairing property within DNA, the presence of 20% adenine (A) means there must also be 20% thymine (T) in the organism. This means 40% of the DNA is A or T, leaving 60% of the DNA to be cytosine (C) or guanine (G). Since there must be an equal amount of each base type within the base pair, 60% divided by 2 gives 30% each of cytosine and guanine.

2.

C. DNA ligase is an enzyme that catalyzes the reaction between the 5′-phosphate end of one DNA fragment and the 3′-hydroxyl end of the next. This "nick sealing" requires energy from ATP hydrolysis, thus remaking the broken phosphodiester bond between the adjacent nucleotides. It is a very important enzyme in DNA repair, but is not used in polymerase chain reactions (PCR). PCR does require a DNA template, two primers to anneal to nucleotide sequences flanking the desired amplification sequence, deoxyribonucleotide triphosphates (dNTPs) to be used as building blocks for the growing DNA chain, DNA polymerase, and magnesium chloride as an essential cofactor for DNA polymerase activity.

3.

A. The first letter of a restriction endonuclease's name comes from the bacterial genus from which it originated. The second and third letters derive from the bacterial species. The last letter indicates the subspecies or strain from which the enzyme was obtained. The last Roman numeral represents the numerical place the enzyme has among those which have been isolated from that bacterial genus/species/strain. For example, EcoRI is the first restriction endonuclease isolated from the bacteria *Escherichia coli*, strain R, while EcoRV is the fifth such enzyme to be discovered.

4.

C. The complementary strand for this DNA sequence would be, read left to right, 3′ GATATC 5′. Restriction endonucleases require double-stranded DNA, since they take for their substrate palindromic molecules, meaning a molecule that will "read" the same left to right or right to left. In this instance, the complementary strand, read 5′ to 3′ (right to left), reads the same as the sense strand, read 5′ to 3′. If the enzyme cuts the sense strand as indicated, between the thymine and adenine, it will cut the complementary strand identically. This will leave, on the sense strand, the two sequences 5′ CT 3′ and 5′ ATAG 3′. The complementary strand will show 3′ GATA 5′ and 3′ TC 5′. Check again to see that these new sequences actually are identical, read 5′ to 3′, on both strands.

5.

C. The concentration of double-stranded DNA (dsDNA) can be estimated by taking its absorbance reading at 260 nm and multiplying that absorbance by a factor of 50, since one absorbance unit at 260 nm equals approximately 50 μg/mL. To solve this problem: 100 (dilution factor) × 0.062 (sample Abs. at 260 nm) × 50 μg/mL (conversion factor for double-stranded DNA) = 310 μg/mL. Note that for single-stranded DNA (ssDNA), the factor would be 33. For single-stranded RNA, the factor is 40.

6.

A. In the isolation of RNA, it is very important to remove all RNase activity. Such enzymes are considered ubiquitous, so precautions must always be taken. Diethyl pyrocarbonate, also known as DEPC or diethyl oxydiformate, will inactivate RNase, thus protecting RNA from degradation. It is used in solution at 0.1–0.2%$^{w/v}$ concentration.

7.

B. Resin-based purification of DNA takes advantage of the fact that DNA, at alkaline pH, possesses a net negative charge. Cells are incubated with detergent, which causes their lysis. RNA is digested with RNase, and the solution is neutralized with potassium acetate. This salt solution will precipitate the detergent and all proteins. Lysate is added to the exchange resin, and both DNA and residual RNA will bind. RNA and ssDNA are removed with a wash buffer, and the desired dsDNA will be eluted from the resin with either water or pH 8.0–8.5 buffer.

8.

B. The rate of electrophoretic separation when using polyacrylamide or agarose gels is affected by time, current, and the percent matrix used. Sample volume will not affect rate of separation, but only make the resulting bands more visible when stained. Achieving increased separation can be accomplished by increasing the time or current used. It can also be achieved by decreasing the percent matrix, since the "pores" present in a 1% agarose gel will be larger than those in a 5% gel. This larger-size pore will allow easier molecular passage of DNA molecules during the time of electrophoresis. Conversely, achieving a tighter band pattern (i.e., higher resolution of smaller DNA molecules) can be accomplished by decreasing time or current, or increasing percent matrix used.

9.

D. There are three essential parts to any molecular test performed: (1) a target, (2) a probe, and (3) a signal that can be detected. There are many ways a probe can be labeled in order for a signal to be produced and an analyte measured. Radioactive isotopes, such as ^{32}P, ^{33}P, ^{35}S, and ^{125}I are traditionally used to label probes. Positive signals are measured using X-ray exposure or scintillation counting. However, due to environmental, costs, and safety concerns, nonradioactive labels are being used with increased frequency. Nonradioactive probes are often labeled with haptens (e.g., digoxigenin), biotin, fluorescein, rhodamine, or a chemical such as acrididium esters. Detection of the hybridization (i.e., a positive test) is dependent on the type of label used, but it is generally either colorimetric, fluorescent, or chemiluminescent. Hapten-labeled and biotin-labeled probes are detected by enzyme-conjugated antihapten antibodies and enzyme-conjugated streptavidin. Enzyme conjugates used are horseradish peroxidase and alkaline phosphatase.

10.

C. Target amplification refers to a process that increases the number of copies of the target DNA or RNA nucleotide sequence. Examples include the polymerase chain reaction (PCR), reverse transcription-PCR, strand displacement amplification, transcription mediated amplification, and nucleic acid sequence-based amplification. Signal amplification will cause increased signal strength without increasing the number of target molecules. One example of signal amplification is the branched chain DNA reaction. Probe amplification will increase the number of copies of the probe that is complementary to the target. One example of probe amplification is the ligase chain reaction.

11.

C. While human genes are highly conserved in gene coding regions, human gene loci are polymorphic, which means many forms of the gene exist at a given locus, making each person "unique." Only identical twins are not "unique." Short tandem repeats (STRs) account for the many polymorphisms used in DNA fingerprinting. STRs are short, repetitive sequences of 3–7 base pairs and are abundant in the human genome. There are STR kits commercially available from several manufacturers. The common loci used in forensics to obtain DNA fingerprints are the CTT triplex and the FFv triplex. These contain the following loci: CSF1PO (proto-oncogene CSF-1), TPOX (thyroid peroxidase gene), TH01 (tyrosine hydroxylase gene), F13A01 (coagulation factor XIII gene), FES/FPS (proto-oncogene c-fes/fps), and v-WA (von Willebrand gene). This testing does not require large quantities or high-quality DNA for successful results. It uses PCR, which is highly sensitive; however, this characteristic also makes it prone to contamination.

12.

D. The process whereby a strand of RNA is synthesized from template DNA is called transcription. The enzyme involved is RNA polymerase. It is possible, however, as retroviruses have shown us, to produce DNA using template RNA. This reversal of the central nucleic acid dogma is called "reverse transcription," and the enzyme that carries this out is called reverse transcriptase. After synthesizing a single-stranded DNA molecule from RNA, a different enzyme DNA polymerase then synthesizes a complementary strand to produce a DNA double helix. The human immunodeficiency virus (HIV) is an example of a retrovirus. The other 3 answers describe amplification methods designed to increase the sensitivity of molelular diagnostic tests. They accomplish this by making copies of either the target nucleic acids, (e.g., [SDA] strand displacement amplification and [PCR] polymerase chain reaction), or the probe molecules (e.g., [LCR] ligase chain reaction), or the signal produced (e.g., [bDNA] branched chain DNA reaction).

13.

C. To solve this problem, it is necessary to recognize that plasmid DNA exists as a closed circle. This means that base pair #1 is adjacent to base pair #5850. If the enzyme cleaves the plasmid at positions 36, 1652, 2702, this will result in three pieces of DNA. One piece will contain base pairs (bp) 37 through 1652 (with a size of 1616 bp), a second will contain bp 1653 through 2702 (with a size of 1050 bp), and the third will span the sequence from bp 2703 through 5850 **AND** from 1 to 36 (with a size of 3184 bp). Note that to determine the size of each piece, subtract the numbers corresponding to each adjacent cut site. (For example, 1652–36 = 1616 and 2702–1652 = 1050.) For the third piece, subtract the highest numbered cut site (i.e., 2702) from the total size of the plasmid (i.e., 5850), and add the size of the piece beginning at bp #1 through bp #36. Then use the DNA ladder marker (lane M) in Color Plate 56 to predict the placement of these pieces (3184 bp, 1616 bp, and 1050 bp) of DNA on the final electrophoresis pattern.

14.

D. Transfer of any molecule from an electrophoresis gel to a solid matrix such as nitrocellulose is dependent on a number of physical factors: size of the molecule being transferred, size of the matrix pores (both gel and solid), amount of time used for the transfer, and presence of a clear path for the molecules being transferred. Factors that could decrease the transfer would include short transfer time, presence of air bubbles between the gel and the nitrocellulose, and inadequate weight placed on top of the transfer "stack." Routine methods for transferring DNA use capillary action. Vacuum, pressure, and electric current can be used to speed the transfer of molecules from the gel matrix onto a solid support. Increased power conditions would enhance transfer; however, too much current could cause membrane damage by generation of excessive heat.

15.

A. Biotin is a vitamin involved physiologically in single carbon transfers. Streptavidin is a protein derived from *Streptomyces avidinii,* consisting of four subunits, each of which can bind one biotin molecule. This bond formation is rapid and essentially irreversible. The interaction between streptavidin and biotin is the strongest known noncovalent biological interaction between a protein and its ligand. *In vitro* assays take advantage of this tight and specific binding by covalently attaching streptavidin to a reporter molecule (e.g., a primary antibody), then incubating this with a secondary fluorescent-labeled antibody conjugated to biotin. Each streptavidin molecule will bind four biotin-conjugated molecules, thereby increasing fourfold the signal generated.

16.

C. Assuming 100% efficiency, each cycle of the polymerase chain reaction doubles the number of DNA molecules present in the solution. Starting with one DNA template molecule, there would be $2^2 = 4$ DNA molecules present after two cycles. After 5 cycles, this would result in $2^5 = 32$. Based on a starting single molecule of double-stranded DNA, after 15 cycles there would theoretically 2^{15} molecules (32,768). *Note:* Actual yield is somewhat less than theoretical yield because PCR products, created in the first 2 PCR cycles, are slightly longer than the target amplicon. Thus, yield may be better calculated as $2^{(n-2)}$. Actual yield may be decreased by a plateau effect that may occur in later PCR cycles.

17.

A. Restriction enzymes will show specificity for a target nucleotide sequence when used under optimal conditions of temperature, glycerol content, salt concentration, and substrate concentration. If these conditions are not optimal, some enzymes will lose their specificity and begin to cleave more randomly. This undesirable, nonoptimal digestion is called "star activity." Such activity is evident when the following parameters are altered in the reaction environment: more than 100 units of enzyme per microgram of DNA, more than $5\%^{(v/v)}$ glycerol content, less than 25 mM salt concentrations, pH > 8.0, presence of dimethyl sulfoxide (DMSO), ethanol, or other organic solvents.

18.

C. The ultimate purpose of transferring DNA or RNA from a gel onto a solid matrix like nitrocellulose is to probe the bound molecule with a labeled oligonucleotide. This step requires that the bound molecule be single-stranded. Since DNA will be double-stranded in the gel, it needs to be denatured before its transfer to the nitrocellulose. This requires pretreatment of the gel with an alkaline buffer (to disrupt the hydrogen bonds holding the DNA strands together) before doing the DNA transfer. Although RNA is single-stranded, most RNAs can form secondary structures. Therefore, RNA must be electrophoresed under denaturing conditions to ensure that all RNA molecules have an unfolded, linear conformation. Denaturation is achieved by adding formaldehyde to the gel and loading buffers or by treating the RNA samples with glyoxal/dimethyl sulfoxide. Migration of RNA molecules and probe binding are affected by secondary structures; however, the presence of secondary structures does not inhibit transfer of RNA onto the membrane.

19.

B. After DNA is transferred to nitrocellulose or nylon membrane, there will be many sites on the membrane that will not be occupied. Adding a probe at this point will not only allow for specific binding of the probe to the target DNA sequence, but also the nonspecific binding of the probe to the available binding sites on the membrane. This will

cause nonspecific signal generation throughout the matrix. To prevent this, the membrane must first be treated with blocking agents. Denhardt solution and denatured nonhomologous DNA (e.g., salmon sperm DNA) are often used to bind up all the available sites on the matrix and allow for specific binding of the probe in the next step.

20.

C. Preparation of a DNA probe using random hexamer primers requires a DNA template containing the desired target sequence, four deoxynucleotides, at least one of which must be labeled (e.g., radionuclide, fluorescent, biotin, etc.), and DNA polymerase. The double-stranded DNA template (25–50 ng) is denatured and a mixture of random oligonucleotides of 6 bases in length anneal to the template DNA. The primers are extended by the action of a DNA polymerase (e.g., T7 DNA polymerase) in the presence of one or two labeled deoxynucleotide triphosphates. Random primed probes are generally 500 nucleotides in length. Solutions containing the labeled probes are incubated with the blot. Hybridization of the labeled probe will occur if the gene being sought is present in the DNA on the blot to give a positive signal. Dideoxynucleotides are used in preparing samples for DNA sequencing by the Sanger method and cause DNA polymerization to cease.

21.

C. In Southern blots, hybrids can form between molecules with similar but not necessarily identical sequences. The washing conditions used after adding the labeled probe can be varied so that hybrids with differing mismatch frequencies are controlled. The higher the wash temperature or the lower the salt concentration in the wash buffer, the higher the stringency. Increasing the stringency will decrease the number of mismatches that form between the probe and the target DNA.

22.

A. Standard Southern blot techniques recommend the use of 10 μg of high-quality genomic DNA when studying single copy genes. In a subsequent step the genomic DNA is restricted (i.e., cut into small fragments of predictable size). The resulting fragments of the gene of interest generally range in size from 1.0 to 10.0 kilobases. In contrast, the gene sequence of interest to be amplified in a routine PCR targets a smaller portion of the gene (generally 150–500 bases in length). Because the target is a smaller size, partially degraded DNA (i.e., genomic DNA samples of lesser quality) can be amplified successfully. (*Note:* Long-range PCR methods are available that extend the range of PCR products synthesized from 5 to 35 kilobases.) Because PCR targets are usually a few hundred bases in length, high-molecular-weight DNA is not necessary for successful PCR. It requires a piece of equipment, a thermocycler, to take the reaction through the cycles of 3 temperatures needed for denaturation, hybridization, and elongation steps. Turn-around time is also an advantage of PCR reactions because results can be completed in less than 4 hours, whereas Southern blotting takes up to 1 week to complete due to multiple steps required for this procedure.

23.

D. Most frequently used protocols in molecular biology involve PCR. Several substances can inhibit this reaction. For example, due to the nature of fecal material it is not routinely used, and materials in swabs have also been reported to inhibit PCR. Therefore, a more appropriate specimen that could be used for PCR would be a stool filtrate. Nucleated cells are necessary for isolation of DNA. Whole blood is an acceptable specimen. White blood cells are the source of DNA in this type of specimen and must be separated from red blood cells as soon as possible because hemoglobin will inhibit PCR. For diagnosis of blood parasites, such as *Babesia* and *Plasmodium* species, a hemolyzed and washed red blood cell sample is preferred for recovery of the DNA from the parasites. Amniocytes are used for molecular cytogenetic testing to prenatally screen for genetic diseases. Noninvasive collection of cells for genetic and forensic testing can be obtained from the buccal (mouth) mucosa.

24.

C. Alcohol precipitation of nucleic acids is a standard method in molecular biology. Sterile water, 10 mM Tris, 1 mM EDTA, or 0.1% SDS can be used to rehydrate DNA; 1 mM EDTA and 0.1% SDS are included in these mixes to inhibit DNAses. Alkaline solutions, such as 0.2 N NaOH, are used to denature nucleic acids.

25.

B. Two general methods exist for DNA sequencing: (1) dideoxy (Sanger) sequencing and (2) chemical

(Maxam-Gilbert) sequencing. In the Sanger method, four separate reaction tubes are set up with special nucleotides called 2′,3′dideoxyribonucleotides (ddNTPs). Chain growth terminates when ddNTPs are used as substrates and incorporated into oligonucleotide chains synthesized according to the template DNA being sequenced. Biochemical manipulation of the reaction results in chain termination at each occurrence of the dideoxynucleotide base. The resultant chains have variable ends specifying the sequence of the DNA. In the Maxam-Gilbert method, radioactive labeled DNA is subjected to four specific chemical reactions causing cleavages at given bases. If radioisotopes are used as labels in the reaction, resultant products are separated by electrophoresis in polyacrylamide gels and followed by autoradiography. The DNA sequence can be read from the X-ray film. However, technological advances have allowed sequencing methods to become more automated. Fluorescent labeled nucleotides are used in the reaction mix that emit light of characteristic colors when stimulated by a laser. The resultant products of each termination reaction (Sanger method) can be distinctly labeled. Upon electrophoresis, as product bands reach a designated position they are illuminated by a laser and identified by a fluorescence detector. Thus, the DNA sequence is determined by temporal order of nucleotides passing the detector and is recorded by a computer. Random oligonucleotide priming and nick translation are methods used to label nucleic acid probes.

26.

D. Leukocytes are routinely used for extraction of DNA from human blood. Mature red blood cells and platelets have no nucleus. Plasma or serum can be used for detection of viremia in the blood, but it is not used for analysis of genetic diseases.

27.

C. RNAses are ubiquitous and can act at temperatures below freezing (-20 °C). Experiments utilizing RNA are plagued at every step by them. Isolation of RNA was done in the presence of guanidine isothiocyanate, a chaotropic agent that inhibits RNAses, as recommended. When analyzing RNA in a gel, formaldehyde or other agents that denature RNAses must be included in the gel. If RNAse inhibitors are absent, RNA will be degraded and either be absent or appear as a smear at the bottom of the gel. On the other hand, high-quality (i.e., undegraded) RNA will appear as a long smear with 2 or 3 distinct areas of RNA that correspond to the ribosomal RNA subunits: 28S (~4800 bases), 18S (~1800 bases), and 5.8S (~160 bases), as seen in Color Plate 60. After isolation, purified RNA should be stored at −70 °C.

28.

C. EDTA and ACD (acid citrate dextrose) are the preferred anticoagulants for specimens that will undergo PCR. Polymerase chain reaction (PCR) can be inhibited by a variety of substances. These inhibitors are concentration dependent; inhibition can often be overcome by simply diluting the DNA sample. Heme and sodium heparin can inhibit PCR. However, there are laboratory methods that can be used to remove these inhibitors, if necessary. Diethyl pyrocarbonate (DEPC) is a substance used to inhibit RNAses; it can also inhibit PCR.

29.

B. Stringency of hybridization is accomplished at two steps in the blotting technique. The first step is hybridization conditions of the labeled probe in solution with the transferred RNA or DNA targets on the membrane. The second step occurs when the membrane is washed to remove unbound probe. In the hybridization reaction, formamide and temperature can be used to increase stringency. During wash steps, increasing temperature and increasing detergent concentration (e.g., 1% SDS) will increase stringency; while lowering NaCl concentration also increases stringency. At the end of the highest stringency wash, only specific hybrids of interest should remain on the blot.

30.

D. The four nucleotide bases found in RNA are adenine (A), guanine (G), cytosine (C), and uracil (U). The purines A and G are the same as in a DNA strand. C is present in both DNA and RNA; however, in RNA thymine (T), the DNA nucleotide base, is replaced by uracil (U). RNA is usually single-stranded, although double-stranded areas can occur. A pairs with U and C pairs with G.

31.

B. dNTP stands for <u>d</u>eoxyribo<u>n</u>ucleotide <u>t</u>riphosphate. Nucleotides are the building blocks of nucleic acids. They are composed of phosphate groups, a 5-sided sugar molecule, and a nitrogenous base. Nitrogenous bases are either purines (A, G) or pyrimidines (C, T, or U, an RNA specific base). The sugar molecules are either ribose (in RNA) or deoxyribose (in DNA), with the only difference in structure being the lack of a hydroxyl group at position 2′ in the deoxyribose molecule. Without the phosphate groups, a nucleotide is a nucleoside. A nucleotide can have 1, 2, or 3 phosphate groups, which are termed monophosphate, diphosphate, and triphosphate, respectively.

32.

A. DNA is composed of two strands of polynucleotides coiled in a double helix. The outside backbone is composed of sugar-phosphate moieties, whereas the purine and pyrimidine bases are stacked inside the helix. The size and stability of the DNA molecule is such that only specific bases can hydrogen bond to each other to hold the two strands together (A-T, C-G, and vice versa). This is referred to as complementary base pairing. An A-T base pair is less stable than a C-G base pair because 3 hydrogen bonds form between C-G, and only 2 hydrogen bonds form between A-T. The increased stability between C-G causes the melting temperature (T_m) to be greater in a double-stranded DNA (dsDNA) segment with more C-G pairs than a segment with more A-T pairs. In all dsDNA molecules, the number of purines (A+G) equals the number of pyrimidines (C+T).

33.

B. Pulsed field gel electrophoresis (PFGE) is used to separate extremely large DNA molecules by placing them in an electric field that is charged periodically, which forces the molecule to reorient before moving through the gel. Larger molecules take more time to reorient, thus they move more slowly. Bacterial DNA is digested by restriction enzymes in agarose plugs. The PFGE of the digested fragments provides a distinctive pattern of 5 to 20 bands ranging from 10 to 800 kilobases. DNA sequencing determines the exact nucleotide sequence base by base of any organism; however, it would be too laborious for epidemiological purposes. Ribotyping is a Southern blot type of analysis using rRNA probes to detect ribosomal operons (i.e., sequences coding for 16S rRNA, 25S rRNA, and one or more tRNAs) of individual bacterial species. Its discriminatory power is less than PFGE. Reverse transcription–polymerase chain reaction (RT-PCR) is a method that determines whether a gene is being expressed. The starting material for RT-PCR is single-stranded RNA.

34.

B. PCR requires a thermocycler because cycling at three different temperatures is the basis for this technique. First, template DNA (i.e., which may contain the target sequence) is denatured at 94 °C. Next, the temperature is lowered to allow specific primers to anneal to the single-stranded target, generally at temperatures near 55 °C. In the third portion of the cycle, primers are extended using deoxynucleotide triphosphate molecules to form a complementary copy of DNA under the direction of a thermostable DNA polymerase enzyme, such as *Taq* polymerase. The optimal temperature at which *Taq* polymerase acts to extend the primers is 72 °C. Thus, at the end of one cycle, one molecule of dsDNA has now become two molecules of dsDNA. Cycles are generally repeated about 30 times to theoretically yield 2^{30} DNA molecules. The three steps of each cycle are termed *denaturation* (94 °C), *annealing* of primers (~55 °C), and *extension* of primers to form the PCR product (72 °C). The other methods listed, nucleic acid sequence-based amplification (NASBA), strand displacement amplification (SDA), and transcription mediated amplification (TMA), are also amplification methods; however, they have been modified so all reactions take place at a single temperature (isothermal).

35.

D. Applications of molecular biological techniques affect all areas of the clinical laboratory. Molecular biology techniques are used in virology (HIV, HCV, CMV, to name a few), mutational analyses of genetic diseases, oncology, histocompatibility testing, bone marrow engraftment, and forensic medicine. Detection of microorganisms in patient samples, culture confirmation, and detection of resistance genes are a few examples from the microbiology laboratory. Commercial kits and automated systems are now available for the diagnosis of sexually transmitted diseases, such as *Chlamydia trachomatis, Neisseria gonorrhoeae,* and *Mycobacterium tuberculosis.*

36.

C. The central dogma describes the flow of genetic information from DNA to RNA to protein. Individual DNA molecules serve as templates for ei-

ther complementary DNA strands during replication or complementary RNA molecules during transcription. In turn, RNA molecules serve as templates for ordering of amino acids by ribosomes to form polypeptides during protein synthesis, also known as translation.

37.

D. DNA in human somatic cells is compartmentalized into 22 pairs of chromosomes, referred to as autosome. They are numbered 1 through 22. In addition they have two sex chromosomes, *both* an X and Y (in males) or two X chromosomes (in females). Thus, the total number of chromosomes is 46 in a normal *diploid* cell. The genetic information of one set of chromosomes comes from the mother of the individual and the other set from the father. Gametes (i.e., eggs and sperm) are haploid and contain only one set of chromosomes, so that upon fertilization, a diploid zygote is formed.

38.

B. Most of the lifetime of a cell is spent in G1 phase, during which the cells can produce their specialized proteins and accomplish their essential functions. However, when the signal is received for cell division, the cell enters S phase. In S phase the DNA in all chromosomes is duplicated. At the end of S phase, the duplicated chromosomes remain attached at the centromere. A time delay, G2, separates events of the actual separation of individual chromosomes from their duplicated pairs. Next, the M phase or mitosis is when the two members of each pair of chromosomes go to opposite ends of the original cell. This separates 46 chromosomes into two sets of 23 in each cell. Finally, a cleavage furrow is formed and separates the original cell into two daughter cells. Each cell contains a copy of all the genetic information from each parent.

39.

C. Purified DNA is relatively stable provided it is reconstituted in buffer that does not contain DNases. Therefore, high-quality reagents and Type I sterile water should be used in preparing buffers used for this purpose. Experiments have shown that purified DNA is stable as long as three years at refrigerated temperature (4 °C). However, long-term storage of purified DNA is best accomplished at −20 to −70 °C in ways that avoid freeze-thaw cycles that may potentially damage DNA (i.e., dividing the original DNA sample into multiple aliquots for storage).

40.

C. Refer to Color Plate 57. Given that the probe used will recognize the trinucleotide repeat found in the Fragile X gene, *FMR-1,* the location of positive signals will give information about the size of the repeat sequence within each person's DNA. The normal allele for *FMR-1* has 6–50 trinucleotide repeats (found in normal individuals), the premutation for *FMR-1* contains 50–200 trinucleotide repeats (found in unaffected individuals), and the disease allele (found in affected individuals) has > 200 repeats. Since electrophoresis separates DNA by size such that the larger fragments travel shorter distances than smaller fragments, then the larger fragment in the affected individual caused by the expansion of the trinucleotide repeat would be represented in Color Plate 57 by lane 4 of the diagram.

41.

A. Amplification methods can be automated and standardized, which is proven by the variety of test systems presently on the market. Amplification methods are exquisitely sensitive and theoretically can detect one target DNA molecule in a sample. However, increased sensitivity raises the likelihood of "false-positive" results due to contamination of testing areas with PCR amplicons. In addition, most amplification methods can be completed within 4 to 6 hours and can detect microorganisms that do not grow readily by standard culture techniques. At this time, test reagents are still quite expensive, although if decreased turnaround time would translate into shorter hospital stays, then resultant health care costs could be reduced by use of these methods in the clinical laboratory. A disadvantage of amplification technologies is that they require a unique set of primers for each target DNA being sought. Thus, amplification techniques may be replaced by use of DNA microarrays because thousands of genes can be assessed at one time, rather than a limited number of molecules of interest being assayed.

42.

A. Reverse transcription–polymerase chain reaction (RT-PCR) is used to look for gene expression; genes are expressed by transcription into mRNA. The starting material for RT-PCR is mRNA. The only method listed whose target sequence is found in mRNA is RT-PCR. Transcription mediated amplification (TMA) targets are usually ribosomal RNA. In ribotyping, rRNA probes detect ribosomal RNA genes present in total bacterial DNA; bacteria can be grouped on the basis of banding patterns that result. Multiplex PCR describes a method in which DNA is the target or template, and several different primer sets are included in the reaction mix. An example of multiplex PCR would include methods that detect *Chlamydia trachomatis* and *Neisseria gonorrhoeae* in one reaction mix.

43.

D. Both human immunodeficiency virus (HIV) and hepatitis C virus (HCV) have RNA genomes and thus must include a reverse transcriptase step to convert RNA into a complementary DNA for use in the subsequent PCR that makes multiple copies of the target sequence. RT-PCR is both highly specific and sensitive. Viral load testing requires that the methodology be quantitative, also. One way quantification can be accomplished is by inclusion of a known amount of a synthetic nucleic acid, known as a quantitation standard (QS), in the sample. The QS binds the same primers as the viral target and so the kinetics of amplification for both may be assumed to be approximately equal. The viral target and QS are coamplified in the same reaction, and the raw data manipulated mathematically to determine the viral load present in the specimen. To detect the presence of bacteria, gene mutations, and remaining malignant cells in the circulation, the starting material generally used is DNA.

44.

A. The exquisite sensitivity of amplification techniques can be viewed as a double-edged sword. On one hand, the techniques have allowed detection of genetic sequences that are found in limited numbers within a sample. However, since the method creates large amounts of target sequence, the areas within the laboratory can become contaminated with amplicons. Amplicon contamination produces "false-positive" results and must be avoided. The use of dUTP in the reaction mix results in PCR products (i.e., amplicons) containing uracil in place of thymidine. The enzyme used to decrease contamination of previously generated dU-containing amplicons is Uracil-*N*-glycosylase (UNG). Samples are pretreated with this enzyme before their use in subsequent PCR reactions to remove contaminating dU-containing amplicons if present. It has no effect on sample DNA containing thymidine residues. Other procedures that are necessary to avoid contamination include: impeccable technique, dedicated areas for reagent preparation, specimen preparation, amplification and postamplification analysis, and use of aerosol-barrier pipette tips. Treatment of work surfaces, equipment, and pipettors with UV light can also be used to prevent contamination.

45–47.

(45:D, 46:B, 47:C)

Questions 45–47 are associated with Color Plate 58. The reaction shown in Color Plate 58 is the Ligase Chain Reaction (LCR). This procedure has been developed and marketed by Abbott Diagnostics and is classified as a probe amplification method. Other probe amplification methods include cycling probe technology and Q-beta replicase. Other nucleic acid amplification assay methods are classified as either target amplification (e.g., PCR, TMA, SDA, and NASBA) or signal amplification (e.g., branched chain DNA) methods. Some manufacturers have combined target amplification methods with detection systems that also amplify signal (e.g., hybrid capture systems) to increase sensitivity of their protocols. LCR is frequently used for detection of sexually transmitted organisms, such as *Chlamydia trachomatis* and *Neisseria gonorrhoeae*. It can also be used to detect gene mutations.

Color Plate 58 illustrates the steps of a generic LCR reaction. LCR involves mixing target (patient) DNA, a thermostable enzyme DNA ligase, four DNA probes that are complementary to the target sequence (in Color Plate 58 labeled primers 1–4) and other ingredients. In Step 1, double-stranded, target DNA is denatured (i.e., made single-stranded) by heating to 94–95 °C. In Step 2, the four primer oligonucleotide probes anneal or hybridize to their complementary DNA sequence on each sister strand of the target DNA. The two probes that bind to each strand are designed so a small gap exists between them. In Step 3, DNA ligase then binds (ligates) the two probes together (primer 1-primer 2 and primer 3-primer 4), thereby doubling the amount of target DNA. Annealing and ligation occur at 65 °C. Through additional cycles (10–20 cycles) an exponential amplification occurs because the new amplicons

can serve as templates for probes. *Note:* The generic LCR is modified slightly in the Abbott LCX® probe systems for the detection of *C. trachomatis* and *N. gonorrhoeae*. When the pairs of oligonucleotide primers bind to a target sequence on a single-strand DNA template, there is a gap of a few nucleotides between the probes. DNA polymerase acts to fill in the gap with the deoxynucleotides provided in the LCR mix. Once the gap is filled, DNA ligase covalently joins the pair of probes to form an amplification product that is complementary to the original target sequence. The ligated probe pairs (i.e., amplification products) can serve as a target in subsequent rounds of amplification. Forty thermal cycles can achieve up to a billion-fold amplification. In this system the DNA polymerase is found at low concentrations (> 1 Unit) and is present simply to fill in the gap between primer pairs, not to act as the enzyme responsible for amplification. In contrast, high concentrations of DNA ligase (> 10,000 Units) and primer pairs are supplied in the amplification mixture and are largely responsible for the exponential increase in target sequences (i.e., ligated primer pairs) produced in this reaction.

48.

C. Refer to Color Plate 59. Factor V Leiden mutation (A506G) causes activated protein C resistance that results in increased risk of hypercoagulability. The mutation destroys an *MnlI* restriction enzyme site in an amplified 223 bp PCR product from patient DNA. From the electrophoretic pattern, wild-type or normal factor V will show three bands after *MnlI* digestion (104 bp, 82 bp, 37 bp), as in patients 1, 4, and 5. The pattern seen with patient 2 is that of a homozygous mutant with two bands (141 bp and 82 bp). In the heterozygous patient 3, one allele is normal and the other is mutant. Thus, the banding pattern results in four bands (141 bp, 104 bp, 82 bp, and 37 bp). Sometimes the 37 bp fragment band is not seen because it is below detectable levels.

49.

D. The translocation resulting in the Philadelphia chromosome can be detected by reverse transcriptase–polymerase chain reaction (RT-PCR), Southern blot, and cytogenetic analysis. The presence of a Philadelphia (Ph[1]) chromosome confirms the diagnosis of chronic myelogenous leukemia (CML). The Ph[1] chromosome is a shortened chromosome 22 that arises from a reciprocal translocation involving the long arms of chromosomes 9 and 22. This translocation involves the c-*abl* proto-oncogene, normally present on chromosome 9q34, and the BCR gene on chromosome 22q11. The juxtaposition of *abl* with BCR results in the formation of a BCR/*abl* fusion gene, which is subsequently transcribed into a chimeric BCR/*abl* mRNA that is ultimately translated into a chimeric BCR/*abl* protein product. Traditionally, this rearrangement can be seen cytogenetically by visualization of the patient's karyotype (i.e., metaphase spread of patient's chromosomes). Recent techniques have been developed in which fluorescently labeled probes for this gene rearrangement can be used to probe the patient's metaphase or interphase spread, called fluorescence *in situ* hybridization (FISH). Molecular methods to check for this gene rearrangement include Southern blotting and RT-PCR. PCR cannot be used for this particular gene rearrangement because BCR/*abl* breakpoints span large segments of DNA, which prevents direct PCR testing. Instead, RT-PCR is used. The BCR/*abl* chimeric mRNA is used as a template because primer annealing sites in the breakpoint region of the mRNA are a smaller size, suitable for amplification.

50.

A. DNA chips (i.e., DNA microarrays) allow detection and discrimination of multiple genetic sequences at the same time. DNA chips have thousands of oligonucleotide probes arranged on glass or silicon surfaces in an ordered manner. Target sequences within the patient sample are fluorescently labeled in solution. The labeled sequences in solution are then incubated with the DNA chips containing the oligonucleotide probes attached to the silicon or glass surface. Hybridization will occur between labeled complementary sequences within the patient samples and their corresponding probe on the chip. The DNA chip is placed in an instrument that scans the surface with a laser beam. The intensity of the signal and its location are analyzed by computer and provide a quantitative description of the genes present. Since placement of the oligonucleotides is known, identification of the gene or organism may be determined.

REFERENCES

Alberts, B., et al (ed.) (1998). *Essential Cell Biology.* New York: Garland Publishing.

Coleman, W., and Tsongalis, G. (eds.) (1997). *Molecular Diagnostics for the Clinical Laboratorian.* Totowa, NJ: Humana Press.

Current Protocols in Molecular Biology (1994–1999). New York: John Wiley & Sons.

Farkas, D. H. (1999). *DNA Simplified II.* Chicago, IL: American Association for Clinical Chemistry.

Sack, G. H. (1999). *Medical Genetics.* New York: McGraw-Hill.

INTERNET REFERENCES

Included here is a listing of the techniques followed by the manufacturer that presently owns the technology. This information is included so you can search their Websites to obtain the most current information regarding technologies now being used and/or developed.

PCR (developed by Kary Mullis, Cetus Corp.) The rights to the PCR (Polymerase Chain Reaction) biochemical reaction were purchased by Hoffman-LaRoche and are now marketed by Roche Diagnostics as the AMPLICOR® product line *(http://us.labsystems. roche.com/pcr/mainpage.htm)*.

TMA (Transcription Mediated Amplification) and HPA (Hybridization Protection Assay) has been developed by Gen-Probe, Inc. *(http://www.gen-probe. com/)*.

SDA (Strand Displacement Amplification) is a product of Becton-Dickinson Biosciences under the product name BDProbeTec™ *(http://www.bd.com/diagnostics/ microservices/innovations/sda/index.html)*.

NASBA (Nucleic Acid Sequence Based Analysis), now called NucliSens®, is being developed and distributed by Organon Teknika *(http://www.nuclisens. com/frameset_ns.html)*.

The reaction shown is the Ligase Chain Reaction (LCR). This procedure has been developed by Abbott Diagnostics *(http://www.abbottdiagnostics. com/)*.

Branched chain DNA is a technology developed by Chiron Diagnostics, recently acquired by Bayer Corporation. *(http://www.bayerdiag.com/about/ innovation/bdna_schematic.html)*.

Hybrid capture® assays are developed and marketed through Digene Corporation *(http://www.digene. com/bvirus/bvframe.html)*.

9 Laboratory Calculations

contents

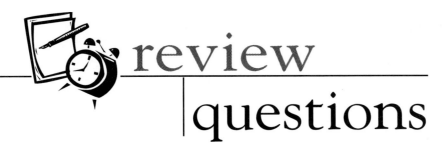

review questions

INSTRUCTIONS Each of the questions or incomplete statements that follow comprises four suggested responses. Select the *best* answer or completion statement in each case.*

1. What is the molarity of a solution that contains 18.7 g of KCl in 500 mL?
   A. 0.1
   B. 0.5
   C. 1.0
   D. 5.0

2. A calcium standard solution contains 10 mg/dL of calcium. What is its concentration in millimoles per liter?
   A. 2.5 mmol/L
   B. 5.0 mmol/L
   C. 7.5 mmol/L
   D. 10.0 mmol/L

3. How much NaCl is needed to prepare 100 mL of a standard solution of concentration 135 mEq/L of Na?
   A. 0.31 g
   B. 0.79 g
   C. 1.2 g
   D. 1.8 g

4. How much 95% alcohol is required to prepare 5 L of 70% alcohol?
   A. 2.4 L
   B. 3.5 L

*Note: A periodic chart of the elements is located on p. 448.

C. 3.7 L
D. 4.4 L

5. A solution of NaOH is standardized by titration with 0.100 N HCl. A total of 10.0 mL of NaOH requires 11.25 mL of HCl. What is the normality of the NaOH solution?
   A. 0.100
   B. 0.112
   C. 0.113
   D. 1.125

6. How many milliliters of concentrated H_2SO_4 (sp gr = 1.84 g/mL; assay = 97%) are required to prepare 10 L of 0.1 N H_2SO_4?
   A. 1.84
   B. 9.20
   C. 27.5
   D. 54.4

7. How many grams of $CaCl_2 \cdot 2H_2O$ must be used to prepare 500 mL of 10% anhydrous $CaCl_2$?
   A. 33.1
   B. 41.3
   C. 50.0
   D. 66.2

8. What is the osmolality of a solution containing 5.85 g NaCl and 18 g glucose in 1 kg water?
   A. 0.2
   B. 0.3
   C. 0.6
   D. 0.9

9. Physiologic saline solution is 0.85% NaCl. What is its osmolarity?
   A. 0.15
   B. 0.29
   C. 0.85
   D. 8.5

10. Convert 70 °F to degrees Celsius.
    A. 7 °C
    B. 12 °C
    C. 20 °C
    D. 21 °C

11. A 5 N solution is diluted 1:4. The resulting solution is diluted 4:15. What is the concentration in normality of the final solution?
    A. 0.25
    B. 0.33
    C. 2.5
    D. 3.0

12. A colorimetric method calls for the use of 0.1 mL of serum, 5 mL of reagents, and 4.9 mL of water. What is the dilution of the serum in the final solution?
    A. 1 to 5
    B. 1 to 10
    C. 1 to 50
    D. 1 to 100

13. A solution of a colored substance that is known to follow Beer's law has an absorbance of 0.085 when measured in a cell 1 cm in length. Calculate the absorbance for a solution of twice the concentration measured in the same cell.

A. 0.042
B. 0.085
C. 0.170
D. 5.90

14. In a spectrophotometric procedure that follows Beer's law, the absorbance of a standard solution of concentration 15 mg/dL is 0.50 in a 1 cm cell. The absorbance of the sample solution is 0.62. What is the concentration?
    A. 0.62 mg/mL
    B. 6.2 mol/L
    C. 12.1 mg/dL
    D. 18.6 mg/dL

15. A stock standard solution of urea contains 10 mg/mL of urea nitrogen. How much stock (in milliliters) is needed to prepare 200 mL of a working standard containing 20 mg/dL of urea nitrogen?
    A. 1
    B. 2
    C. 4
    D. 8

16. How many milliliters of a 50%$^{v/v}$ acetic acid solution are required to prepare 1 L of 5%$^{v/v}$ acetic acid?
    A. 0.01
    B. 0.10
    C. 10
    D. 100

17. How many grams of sulfosalicylic acid (mol wt = 254) are required to prepare 1 L of a 3%$^{w/v}$ solution?
    A. 3.0
    B. 7.6
    C. 30
    D. 254

18. A quantitative protein analysis is performed on an aliquot of a 24-hour urine specimen.

The test indicates the presence of 1.2% protein. If a total urine volume of 2155 mL is collected, how many grams of protein are excreted in the 24-hour specimen?

A. 0.056

B. 2.6

C. 25.9

D. 258.6

19. How many grams of H_2SO_4 are required to prepare 750 mL of a 2 M solution?

A. 36.8

B. 73.5

C. 98

D. 147

20. How many grams of NaOH are required to prepare 4 L of a 2 N solution?

A. 40

B. 80

C. 160

D. 320

21. How many milliliters of glacial acetic acid (mol wt = 60; assay = 99.7%) are required to prepare 2 L of a 5%$^{v/v}$ solution?

A. 6

B. 10

C. 50

D. 100

22. How many grams of H_2SO_4 are required to prepare 6 L of a 5 N solution?

A. 245

B. 294

C. 490

D. 1470

23. How many grams of NaOH are required to prepare 2500 mL of a 4 M solution?

A. 40

B. 100

C. 160

D. 400

24. An isotonic saline solution contains 0.85%$^{w/v}$ NaCl. How many grams of NaCl are needed to prepare 5 L of this solution?

A. 4.25

B. 8.5

C. 42.5

D. 170

25. How many grams of NaOH are required to prepare 500 mL of a 0.02 N solution?

A. 0.4

B. 0.8

C. 4.0

D. 8.0

26. What is the normality of a 30%$^{w/v}$ H_2SO_4 solution?

A. 0.31

B. 0.61

C. 3.06

D. 6.12

27. A serum chloride concentration is 369 mg/dL. What is the concentration in milliequivalents per liter?

A. 5

B. 10

C. 36

D. 104

28. A serum calcium level is 8.6 mg/dL. What is the concentration in millimoles per liter?

A. 2.2

B. 2.5

C. 4.3

D. 8.6

29. How many milliliters of concentrated HNO_3 (sp gr = 1.42 g/mL; assay = 70%) are required to prepare 2 L of 0.15 N HNO_3?

A. 13.3

B. 19.0

C. 38.0

D. 189.9

30. With the use of concentrated HCl (sp gr = 1.19 g/mL; assay = 37.5%), 3 L of 0.50 N HCl are prepared. A total of 16 mL of 0.20 N NaOH is required to titrate 7 mL of the HCl solution, indicating a lower normality of the acid solution than desired. How many milliliters of concentrated HCl must be added to the acid solution to attain an accurate 0.50 N HCl solution?

    A. 6.40

    B. 10.53

    C. 101.03

    D. 105.33

31. A serum chloride concentration is 369 mg/dL. What is the concentration in millimoles per liter?

    A. 5

    B. 10

    C. 36

    D. 104

32. How many milliliters of a stock solution of 20% $^{w/v}$ NaOH are required to prepare 800 mL of a 2.5% $^{v/v}$ solution?

    A. 20

    B. 50

    C. 100

    D. 125

33. How many milliliters of a 40% $^{w/v}$ NaOH solution are required to prepare 1.5 L of 2 N NaOH?

    A. 0.3

    B. 3.0

    C. 30

    D. 300

34. How many grams of anhydrous sodium sulfate (mol wt = 142) are required to prepare 750 mL of a 23% $^{w/v}$ solution?

    A. 2.3

    B. 106.5

    C. 172.5

    D. 230

35. With the use of concentrated HCl, 2 L of 0.20 N HCl are prepared. On titration, it is determined that the normality is actually 0.208. To correct this error, how many milliliters of deionized water must be added to the solution (10 mL used in titration process) to make an accurate 0.20 N HCl solution?

    A. 10.4

    B. 76.5

    C. 79.6

    D. 80.0

36. A serum calcium level is 8.6 mg/dL. What is the concentration in milliequivalents per liter?

    A. 2.2

    B. 2.5

    C. 4.3

    D. 8.6

37. How many milliliters of a 5 N HCl solution are required to prepare 4 L of 10% $^{w/v}$ HCl?

    A. 219

    B. 292

    C. 1460

    D. 2192

38. A serum potassium level is 19.5 mg/dL. What is the concentration in milliequivalents per liter?

    A. 0.5

    B. 5.0

    C. 10.0

    D. 19.5

39. An analysis for sodium is performed on an aliquot of a 24-hour urine specimen. A sodium value of 122.5 mmol/L is read from the instrument. What is the amount of sodium in the 24-hour urine specimen if 1540 mL of urine are collected?

    A. 79.5

    B. 188.6

C. 1886.5

D. 18,865

40. With the use of concentrated HNO_3, 4 L of 0.50 N HNO_3 are prepared. On titration, it is determined that the normality is actually 0.513. To correct this error, how many milliliters of deionized water must be added to the remaining 3.975 L of solution to make an accurate 0.50 N HNO_3 solution?

   A. 25.6

   B. 100.7

   C. 103.4

   D. 104.0

41. What is the pH of a 0.2 N acetic acid solution that is 1% ionized?

   A. 0.703

   B. 1.699

   C. 1.703

   D. 2.699

42. What is the ionic strength of a 0.2 M Na_2SO_4 solution?

   A. 0.4

   B. 0.5

   C. 0.6

   D. 1.2

43. A 1.0 mg/dL bilirubin standard (purity = 99.0%; mol wt = 584) is prepared by dissolving it in chloroform at 25 °C. Under these conditions, the molar absorptivity at 453 nm is 60,700. What is the expected absorbance of this standard solution?

   A. 0.104

   B. 0.607

   C. 0.962

   D. 1.039

44. An enzyme assay is performed at 37 °C, and absorbance readings are taken each minute for a total of 4 minutes. Given the following information, what is the enzyme activity in units per liter at 37 °C?

Absorbance Readings	Method Information
0.204 A at 1 minute	Reagent volume = 3.0 mL
0.406 A at 2 minutes	Sample volume = 200 μL
0.610 A at 3 minutes	Light path = 1 cm
0.813 A at 4 minutes	$\varepsilon_{340\ nm}$ of NADH = 6.22×10^3

   A. 490

   B. 522

   C. 525

   D. 1307

45. A patient weighs 175.5 pounds. What is the patient's weight expressed in kilograms?

   A. 8.0

   B. 38.6

   C. 79.8

   D. 87.8

46. Convert 30 °C to degrees Fahrenheit.

   A. 4 °F

   B. 10 °F

   C. 49 °F

   D. 86 °F

47. A curie (Ci) is the quantity of radioactive material that exhibits

   A. 3.7×10^4 dps

   B. 3.7×10^7 dps

   C. 3.7×10^{10} dps

   D. 3.7×10^{10} dpm

48. Each radionuclide has a unique half-life associated with it. Assuming an initial activity of 100%, through how many half-life periods must a nuclide pass to bring its activity down to less than 1%?

   A. 3

   B. 7

   C. 10

   D. 100

49. ^{125}I has a half-life of 60 days. At the end of 180 days, what percent of activity would remain?
    A. 12.5
    B. 25.0
    C. 33.3
    D. 50.0

50. How many grams of NaOH are required to prepare 500 mL of a NaOH solution with a pH of 12?
    A. 0.02
    B. 0.2
    C. 0.4
    D. 2.0

51. What is the relative centrifugal force ($\times g$) of a centrifuge operating at 2500 rpm with a radius of 10 cm?
    A. 625
    B. 699
    C. 1250
    D. 6988

52. A 10 mL class A volumetric flask has an accuracy of $\pm0.2\%$. Express the $\pm0.2\%$ tolerance in terms of milliliters.
    A. ±0.002
    B. ±0.01
    C. ±0.02
    D. ±0.04

53. A sample of deionized water is found to contain a lead concentration of 0.01 ppm. What is the equivalent concentration expressed as milligrams per deciliter?
    A. 0.01
    B. 0.001
    C. 0.0001
    D. 0.00001

54. Because of a malfunction, a spectrophotometer is able to show only the percent transmittance (%T) readings on its digital display. Convert 68.0%T to its corresponding absorbance.
    A. 0.109
    B. 0.168
    C. 0.320
    D. 0.495

55. Which of the following correctly states the conditions required in using a colorimetric method based on Beer's law?
    A. Incident radiation should be monochromatic
    B. Absorption of light by the solvent must be insignificant in comparison with absorption by the solute (the analyte)
    C. The solution must be sufficiently dilute to provide a linear relation between absorption and concentration
    D. All the above

56. When one of two variable quantities changes as a result of a change in the other, the result is frequently presented in the form of a graph. Which of the following descriptions of a graph is correct?
    A. The x-axis is usually used to plot the independent variable
    B. Different scales may be used for each of the two axes
    C. Semilog paper uses a logarithmic scale for one axis and a linear, or Cartesian, scale for the other axis
    D. All the above

57. Primary standards used for analytical work should have what property?
    A. The substance must be available in a form not less than 99.95% pure
    B. It should not be hygroscopic
    C. It must be a stable substance that can be dried, preferably at 104–110 °C
    D. All the above

58. Which of the following weighs the least?
    A. 0.1 ng
    B. 0.01 g
    C. 1.0 mg
    D. 1000 pg

59. The OH^- concentration of a solution is 1×10^{-6}. What is the pH of this solution?
    A. 0.6
    B. 6
    C. 8
    D. 14

60. What amount of NaCl (mol wt = 58.5) is needed to obtain 50 mg Cl?
    A. 19.6 mg
    B. 30.3 mg
    C. 50.0 mg
    D. 82.4 mg

Main groups

Periodic Table of the Elements

1A[a] 1	2A 2	3B 3	4B 4	5B 5	6B 6	7B 7	8B 8	8B 9	8B 10	1B 11	2B 12	3A 13	4A 14	5A 15	6A 16	7A 17	8A 18
1 **H** 1.00794																	2 **He** 4.002602
3 **Li** 6.941	4 **Be** 9.012182											5 **B** 10.811	6 **C** 12.0107	7 **N** 14.00674	8 **O** 15.9994	9 **F** 18.998403	10 **Ne** 20.1797
11 **Na** 22.989770	12 **Mg** 24.3050											13 **Al** 26.981538	14 **Si** 28.0855	15 **P** 30.973762	16 **S** 32.066	17 **Cl** 35.4527	18 **Ar** 39.948
19 **K** 39.0983	20 **Ca** 40.078	21 **Sc** 44.95591	22 **Ti** 47.867	23 **V** 50.9415	24 **Cr** 51.9961	25 **Mn** 54.938049	26 **Fe** 55.845	27 **Co** 58.933200	28 **Ni** 58.6934	29 **Cu** 63.546	30 **Zn** 65.39	31 **Ga** 69.723	32 **Ge** 72.61	33 **As** 74.92160	34 **Se** 78.96	35 **Br** 79.904	36 **Kr** 83.80
37 **Rb** 85.4678	38 **Sr** 87.62	39 **Y** 88.90585	40 **Zr** 91.224	41 **Nb** 92.90638	42 **Mo** 95.94	43 **Tc** [98]	44 **Ru** 101.07	45 **Rh** 102.90550	46 **Pd** 106.42	47 **Ag** 107.8682	48 **Cd** 112.411	49 **In** 114.818	50 **Sn** 118.710	51 **Sb** 121.760	52 **Te** 127.60	53 **I** 126.90447	54 **Xe** 131.29
55 **Cs** 132.90545	56 **Ba** 137.327	57 ***La** 138.9055	72 **Hf** 178.49	73 **Ta** 180.9479	74 **W** 183.84	75 **Re** 186.207	76 **Os** 190.23	77 **Ir** 192.217	78 **Pt** 195.078	79 **Au** 196.96655	80 **Hg** 200.59	81 **Tl** 204.3833	82 **Pb** 207.2	83 **Bi** 208.98038	84 **Po** [210]	85 **At** [210]	86 **Rn** [222]
87 **Fr** [223]	88 **Ra** [226]	89 **†Ac** [227]	104 **Rf** [261]	105 **Db** [262]	106 **Sg** [266]	107 **Bh** [264]	108 **Hs** [265]	109 **Mt** [268]	110 [269]	111 [272]	112 [277]	113	114 [285]	115	116 [289]	117	118 [293]

Transition metals

*Lanthanide series

58 **Ce** 140.116	59 **Pr** 140.90765	60 **Nd** 144.24	61 **Pm** [145]	62 **Sm** 150.36	63 **Eu** 151.964	64 **Gd** 157.25	65 **Tb** 158.92534	66 **Dy** 162.50	67 **Ho** 164.93032	68 **Er** 167.26	69 **Tm** 168.93421	70 **Yb** 173.04	71 **Lu** 174.967

†Actinide series

90 **Th** 232.0381	91 **Pa** 231.03588	92 **U** 238.0289	93 **Np** [237]	94 **Pu** [244]	95 **Am** [243]	96 **Cm** [247]	97 **Bk** [247]	98 **Cf** [251]	99 **Es** [252]	100 **Fm** [257]	101 **Md** [258]	102 **No** [259]	103 **Lr** [262]

[a]The labels on top (1A, 2A, etc.) are common American usage. The labels below these (1, 2, etc.) are those recommended by the International Union of Pure and Applied Chemistry.
The names and symbols for elements 110 and above have not yet been decided.
Atomic weights in brackets are the masses of the longest-lived or most important isotope of radioactive elements.
Further information is available at http://www.shef.ac.uk/chemistry/web-elements/
The production of elements 116 and 118 was reported in May 1999 by scientists at Lawrence Berkeley National Laboratory.

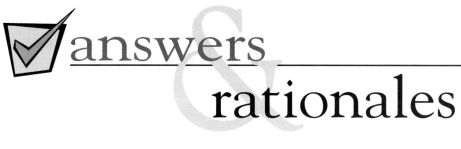
answers & rationales

1.

B. A simple and universally applicable method for solving laboratory calculation problems is to read the problem with three questions in mind:

1. What am I given?
2. What do I want?
3. What is the relation between no. 1 and no. 2?

Given: the concentration of a solution in terms of grams per 500 mL

Want: the concentration in terms of molarity (M)

Relation: molarity = moles per liter

Calculation: A molar solution is one that contains 1 gram molecular weight (usually called 1 mol) of solute per liter of solution. The gram molecular weight is the sum of the atomic weights. A table of atomic weights is used to determine that the gram molecular weight of KCl = 39 + 35.5 = 74.5 g. Express the concentration of the given solution (18.7 g/500 mL) in terms of grams per liter for easy comparison with molarity (moles per liter).

$$18.7 \text{ g/500 mL} = 18.7 \text{ g/0.5 L} = 37.4 \text{ g/L}$$

$$\text{moles} = \frac{\text{grams}}{\text{gram molecular weight}} = \frac{37.4}{74.5} = 0.50$$

$$0.50 \text{ mol/L} = 0.50 \text{ M}$$

A solution that contains 18.7 g KCl/500 mL is 0.50 M KCl.

2.

A. To convert 10 mg of calcium per deciliter to millimoles per liter, proceed as follows. Calculate the milligrams of calcium per liter.

$$10 \text{ mg Ca/dL} = 10 \text{ mg/dL} \times 10 \text{ dL/L}$$
$$= 100 \text{ mg Ca/L}$$

Calculate the weight of 1 mmol of calcium.

Mol wt of Ca = 40 g/mol = 40,000 mg/mol

Thus, 1 mmol Ca = 40 mg Ca.

Then convert 100 mg Ca to mmol Ca:

$$\frac{100 \text{ mg/L}}{40 \text{ mg/mmol}} = 2.5 \text{ mmol Ca/L}$$

Therefore, a concentration of 10 mg Ca/dL = 2.5 mmol Ca/L.

3.

B. To calculate how much NaCl is needed to prepare 100 mL of a standard solution of concentration 135 mEq/L of Na, first consider how many equivalents of Na are present in a mole of NaCl. Find the molecular weight of NaCl. Note that the concentration is expressed in milliequivalents *per liter* (mEq/L), but the desired volume is 100 mL.

Calculation: Since sodium has a valence of 1, one mole of NaCl contains 1 Eq of Na. Molecular weight of NaCl = 23 + 35.5 = 58.5 g. It follows that if 1 Eq of Na is present in 58.5 g NaCl, then 1 mEq of Na is present in 0.0585 g NaCl. There are 135 mEq of Na present in 135 × 0.0585 = 7.90 g NaCl. Therefore a concentration of 135 mEq/L = 7.90 g NaCl/L.

Let *X* equal the weight of NaCl in 100 mL of the desired solution. Then

$$\frac{X}{100 \text{ mL}} = \frac{7.90 \text{ g}}{1000 \text{ mL}}$$

$$X = \frac{7.90 \text{ g} \times 100 \text{ mL}}{1000 \text{ mL}} = 0.790 \text{ g NaCl}$$

4.

C. Problems requiring the conversion of one concentration to another are conveniently solved by applying the formula

$$C_1 \times V_1 = C_2 \times V_2$$

where C_1 and V_1 are the concentration and volume of the starting solution; C_2 and V_2 are the concentration and volume of the final solution. Thus to prepare 5 L of 70% alcohol from 95% alcohol, let C_1 and V_1 refer to the 95% alcohol, and let C_2 and V_2 refer to the 70% alcohol.

$$95\% \times V_1 = 70\% \times 5 \text{ L}$$
$$V_1 = \frac{70 \times 5 \text{ L}}{95} = 3.7 \text{ L}$$

5.

B. To solve questions involving standardization of an acid or a base by titration, bear in mind the fact that at the end point of the titration, the number of equivalents of acid used will be the same as the number of equivalents of base used. Therefore the following formula applies,

$$C_1 \times V_1 = C_2 \times V_2$$

where C_1 and V_1 are the concentration and volume of HCl needed to neutralize the NaOH solution. The equation is set up below.

$$(0.100 \text{ N HCl}) (11.25 \text{ mL}) = C_2 (10.0 \text{ mL})$$
$$C_2 = \frac{11.25 \times 0.100 \text{ N}}{10.0} = 0.112 \text{ N}$$

6.

C. To calculate how many milliliters of concentrated H_2SO_4 (sp gr = 1.84 g/mL, assay = 97%) are required to prepare 10 L of 0.1 N H_2SO_4, first calculate the concentration of the concentrated sulfuric acid in terms of normality. Since the specific gravity is the weight of 1 mL, it follows that 1 mL of concentrated sulfuric acid weighs 1.84 grams. The assay is 97%; that is, 97% of the 1.84 g is H_2SO_4. Therefore, 1 mL of concentrated sulfuric acid contains

$$\frac{97}{100} \times 1.84 \text{ g } H_2SO_4 = 1.78 \text{ g } H_2SO_4$$

and 1 L of concentrated sulfuric acid contains 1780 g H_2SO_4. To convert this concentration (1780 g/L) to normality, recall that a normal solution contains 1 gram equivalent weight per liter. A gram equivalent weight (g Eq wt) is the weight that will combine with or replace 1 g of hydrogen. Since H_2SO_4 has two replaceable hydrogens, the

$$\text{g Eq wt of } H_2SO_4 = \frac{\text{mol wt}}{2} = \frac{98}{2} = 49 \text{ g}$$

Therefore, the concentrated sulfuric acid, which is 1780 g/L, contains

$$\frac{1780 \text{ g/L}}{49 \text{ Eq/L}} = 36.3 \text{ Eq/L}$$

Hence its concentration is 36.3 N.

Now the question becomes: How many milliliters of 36.3 N H_2SO_4 are required to prepare 10 L of 0.1 N H_2SO_4? Using the relation $N_1 \times V_1 = N_2 \times V_2$, let N_1 and V_1 be the concentration and volume of the concentrated H_2SO_4 and let N_2 and V_2 be the concentration and volume of the 0.1 N H_2SO_4.

$$N_1 \times V_1 = N_2 \times V_2$$
$$36.3 \text{ N} \times V_1 = 0.1 \text{ N} \times 10 \text{ L}$$
$$V_1 = \frac{0.1 \times 10 \text{ L}}{36.3} = 0.0275 \text{ L} = 27.5 \text{ mL}$$

Therefore, 27.5 mL of concentrated H_2SO_4 are required to prepare 10 L of 0.1 N H_2SO_4.

7.

D. The problem requires the preparation of 500 mL of 10%$^{w/v}$ $CaCl_2$ with the use of the hydrate $CaCl_2 \cdot 2H_2O$. First calculate how much $CaCl_2$ is needed: 500 mL of 10%$^{w/v}$ $CaCl_2$ contains

$$500 \text{ mL} \times \frac{10 \text{ g}}{100 \text{ mL}} = 50 \text{ g } CaCl_2$$

Then calculate how much $CaCl_2$ is present in $CaCl_2 \cdot 2H_2O$ by comparing molecular weights:

mol wt of $CaCl_2$ = 40 + 71 = 111 g
mol wt of $CaCl_2 \cdot 2H_2O$ = 40 + 71 + 4 + 32 = 147 g

There are 111 g of $CaCl_2$ present in 147 g $CaCl_2 \cdot 2H_2O$; 50 g of $CaCl_2$ are present in

$$\frac{147}{111} \times 50 = 66.2 \text{ g } CaCl_2 \cdot 2H_2O$$

As an alternate method, let X = grams $CaCl_2 \cdot 2H_2O$ needed.

$$\frac{111}{147} = \frac{50}{X}$$

$$X = \frac{147 \times 50}{111} = 66.2 \text{ g}$$

Therefore, a total of 66.2 g $CaCl_2 \cdot 2H_2O$ are needed to prepare 500 mL of 10% w/v $CaCl_2$.

8.

B.

Given: weights of NaCl and glucose dissolved in 1 kg of water

Want: osmolality of solution

Relation: osmolality = moles per kilogram of solvent times the number of particles into which solute molecules dissociate

Calculation: Express the amount of each solute in terms of moles (grams per molecular weight)

$$5.85 \text{ g NaCl} = \frac{5.85 \text{ g}}{58.5 \text{ g/mol}} = 0.1 \text{ mol NaCl}$$

$$18 \text{ g glucose} = \frac{18 \text{ g}}{180 \text{ g/mol}} = 0.1 \text{ mol glucose}$$

Consider the dissociation of each solute.

$$0.1 \text{ mol NaCl} \rightarrow 0.1 \text{ mol Na}^+ + 0.1 \text{ mol Cl}^-$$

Glucose does not dissociate appreciably.

Number of Osmols =

$$0.1 \times 2 = 0.2 \text{ Osmol NaCl}$$
$$+ \, 0.1 \text{ Osmol glucose}$$
$$\text{Total} \quad 0.3 \text{ Osmol in 1 kg H}_2\text{O} = 0.3 \text{ Osmolal}$$

9.

B.

Given: concentration in grams per deciliter: 0.85% NaCl = 0.85 g/dL

Want: concentration in osmolarity

Relation: osmolarity = moles per liter times the number of particles into which the solute dissociates

Calculation: molecular weight of NaCl = 23 + 35.5 = 58.5 g/mol

In dilute solution, NaCl is assumed to be fully dissociated; therefore, each molecule of NaCl will produce two particles, a sodium ion and a chloride ion.

Osmolarity =

mol/L × No. of particles/dissociate molecule

$$= \frac{\text{g}}{\text{mol wt}}/\text{L} \times \text{No. of particles/dissociate molecule}$$

Convert to grams per liter:

$$0.85 \text{ g/dL} \times 10 \text{ dL/L} = 8.5 \text{ g/L}$$

$$\text{Osmolarity} = \frac{8.5 \text{ g/L}}{58.5 \text{ g/mol}} \times 2 = 0.29 \text{ Osmol/L}$$

10.

D. To convert 70 °F to degrees Celsius, compare the size of Fahrenheit and Celsius degrees. There are $212 - 32 = 180$ Fahrenheit degrees between the boiling point and the freezing point of water, respectively. There are $100 - 0 = 100$ Celsius degrees between the boiling point and the freezing point of water, respectively. Therefore, 180 Fahrenheit degrees equal 100 Celsius degrees. From the relationship

$$\frac{°C - 0}{°F - 32} = \frac{100}{180} = \frac{5}{9}$$

two formulas may be derived:

$$°F = \left(°C \times \frac{9}{5}\right) + 32$$

and

$$°C = (°F - 32) \times \frac{5}{9}$$

Thus using the relationship

$$1 \, °F = \frac{100}{180} = \frac{5 \, °C}{9}$$

it follows that:

$$70 \, °F = 70 - 32 = 38 \, °F \text{ degrees above freezing}$$
$$= 38 \times \frac{5 \, °C}{9} \text{ degrees above freezing}$$
$$= 21 \, °C$$

11.

B. When more than one dilution is carried out on a sample, the final concentration is the initial concentration multiplied by each dilution expressed as a fraction. If a 5 N solution is diluted 1:4 and then further 4:15, the final concentration is:

$$5 \text{ N} \times \frac{1}{4} \times \frac{4}{15} = 0.33 \text{ N}$$

The same principle applies in testing a specimen that is too concentrated to fall within the range of the test procedure. The specimen is diluted, the test repeated, and the result multiplied by the reciprocal of the dilution. Thus, if the specimen had to be diluted 1:10 (1/10) to fall within the range of the test procedure, the result would be multiplied by 10 (10/1) to give the correct value.

12.

D. To find the dilution of serum in a mixture, calculate the total volume. The total volume equals 0.1 mL serum + 5 mL reagents + 4.9 mL water = 10 mL. Therefore, the dilution of serum is 0.1 mL to 10 mL, or 0.1:10. Since dilutions are usually expressed as 1 to some number, multiply both the serum volume (0.1) and the total volume (10) by a common factor of 10. Thus, the 0.1:10 serum dilution may be expressed as 1:100.

13.

C. Beer's law states that $A = abc$; where A = absorbance, a = absorptivity, b = light path in cm, and c = concentration of the absorbing compound. If a and b are constant, then A is directly proportional to c. Therefore, if c is doubled, then A also is doubled:

$$0.085\ A \times 2 = 0.170\ A$$

14.

D. In any given photometric procedure, the length of the light path (= width of the cuvet) and the absorptivity of the analyte are constant. Hence, if the procedure follows Beer's law, absorbance (A) is proportional to the concentration (C). This can be expressed as a ratio:

$$C_{unknown}/C_{standard} = A_{unknown}/A_{standard}$$

$$C_u = \frac{A_u}{A_s} \times C_s$$

$$\frac{0.62}{0.50} \times 15\ \text{mg/dL} = 18.6\ \text{mg/dL}$$

15.

C. Problems requiring the conversion of one concentration to another can use the following formula:

$$C_1 \times V_1 = C_2 \times V_2$$

where C_1 and V_1 are the concentration and volume of the stock solution. C_2 and V_2 are the concentration and volume of the final solution. The units of concentration must be the same; therefore, first convert 20 mg/dL to 0.2 mg/mL before solving the equation.

$$(10\ \text{mg/mL})\ V_1 = (0.2\ \text{mg/mL})\ (200\ \text{mL})$$

$$V_1 = \frac{0.2 \times 200\ \text{mL}}{10} = 4\ \text{mL}$$

16.

D. When starting with a percent solution, one may prepare a percent solution of a lesser concentration by using the following formula:

$$V_1 \times \%_1 = V_2 \times \%_2$$

Substitute the given information of the problem in the preceding formula:

$$1000\ \text{mL} \times 5\% = V_2 \times 50\%$$

$$\frac{1000\ \text{mL} \times 5}{50} = V_2$$

$$100\ \text{mL} = V_2$$

Therefore, 100 mL of a 50%$^{v/v}$ acetic acid solution are required to prepare 1 L of 5% $^{v/v}$ acetic acid. Add 100 mL of 50% acetic acid to the solvent, diluting with solvent to a final volume of 1 L.

17.

C. Percent solution refers to a specific number of parts per hundred. The term *parts* refers to the weight of a solute in grams or the volume of liquid in milliliters. The term *hundred* refers to the final volume of 100 mL of solution or 100 g of solution. Thus percent solutions may be expressed as weight per volume (w/v), weight per weight (w/w), or volume per volume (v/v). Preparation of a weight per volume solution may be done as follows: 3%$^{w/v}$ sulfosalicylic acid = 3 g/dL (remember that 100 mL is equivalent to 1 dL). To find the number of grams needed to prepare 1 L, multiply by the required volume in deciliters as follows: 3 g/dL × 10 dL/L × 1 L = 30 g. To prepare 1 L of a 3% $^{w/v}$ sulfosalicylic acid solution, dissolve 30 g of sulfosalicylic acid in deionized water (solvent) and dilute to a final volume of 1 L using a volumetric flask.

18.

C. The urine sample contained 1.2% protein, which is equivalent to 1.2 g of protein per deciliter. Since the total urine volume is given in milliliters, it is necessary to express the volume in deciliters so that the units of measurement correspond. This may be done by dividing the 24-hour volume in milliliters by 100, since there are 100 mL in each deciliter. The amount of protein excreted in the 24-hour urine specimen may now be calculated.

$$\frac{\text{Protein conc. in g/dL} \times \text{urine volume in mL/24 hr}}{100\ \text{mL/dL}} = \text{g/24 hr}$$

$$\frac{1.2 \text{ g/dL} \times 2155 \text{ mL/24 hr}}{100 \text{ mL/dL}} = 25.9 \text{ g/24 hr}$$

19.

D. A 1 molar solution contains 1 mole or 1 g molecular weight of a solute in 1 L of solution. One gram molecular weight of H_2SO_4 consists of 98 g. Thus 1 L of a 1 M solution contains 98 g of H_2SO_4, and a 2 M solution contains twice this amount or 196 g of H_2SO_4 per liter.

> 1 M H_2SO_4 = 98 g/L
> 2 M H_2SO_4 = 2 × 98 g/L = 196 g/L

Thus to find the number of grams needed to prepare only 750 mL of a 2 M H_2SO_4 solution, multiply by the required volume expressed in liters as follows:

$$196 \text{ g/L} \times \frac{750 \text{ mL}}{1000 \text{ mL/L}} = 147 \text{ g}$$

Therefore, 147 g of H_2SO_4 are needed to prepare 750 mL of a 2 M H_2SO_4 solution.

20.

D. A one normal (1 N) solution contains 1 g equivalent weight of a solute in 1 L of solution. For a base, the equivalent weight is defined as that weight which combines with 1.008 g of replaceable hydrogen. One gram equivalent weight of NaOH consists of 40 g. Thus 1 L of a 1 N solution contains 40 g of NaOH, and a 2 N solution contains twice this amount or 80 g of NaOH per liter.

> 1 N NaOH = 40 g/L
> 2 N NaOH = 2 × 40 g/L = 80 g/L

Thus to find the number of grams needed to prepare 4 L of a 2 N NaOH solution, multiply by the required volume as follows: 80 g/L × 4 L = 320 g. Therefore, 320 g of NaOH are needed to prepare 4 L of a 2 N NaOH solution. Prepare this solution by dissolving the 320 g of solute in solvent and bring to a final volume of 4 L.

21.

D. Percent solution refers to a specific number of *parts per hundred*. For a volume per volume solution, measure the volume of liquid solute required in milliliters and add solvent to a final volume of 100 mL of solution. Preparation of a 5%$^{v/v}$ CH_3COOH solution may be done as follows: 5% glacial acetic acid = 5 mL/dL (remember, 100 mL is equivalent to 1 dL). Thus to find the number of

milliliters needed to prepare 2 L of 5% CH_3COOH, multiply by the required volume in deciliters as follows: 5 mL/dL × 10 dL/L × 2 L = 100 mL. Thus to prepare 2 L of a 5% acetic acid solution, add 100 mL of glacial acetic acid to deionized water (remember—always add acid to water) and dilute using a volumetric flask to a final volume of 2 L.

22.

D. A 1 normal (1 N) solution contains 1 g equivalent weight of a solute in 1 L of solution. For an acid, the equivalent weight is defined as that weight which is equivalent to 1.008 g of replaceable hydrogen. The gram equivalent weight may be determined by dividing the gram molecular weight by the positive valence. One equivalent weight of H_2SO_4 equals 49 g, since the molecular weight of 98 g divided by the positive valence 2 is 49 g. Thus 1 L of a 1 N solution contains 49 g of H_2SO_4, and a 5 N solution contains five times this amount or 245 g of H_2SO_4 per liter.

> 1 N H_2SO_4 = 49 g/L
> 5 N H_2SO_4 = 5 × 49 g/L = 245 g/L

Thus to find the number of grams needed to prepare 6 L of a 5 N H_2SO_4 solution, multiply by the required volume as follows: 245 g/L × 6 L = 1470 g. Therefore, 1470 g of H_2SO_4 are needed to prepare 6 L of a 5 N H_2SO_4 solution.

23.

D. A 1 molar solution contains 1 mol or 1 gram molecular weight of a solute in 1 L of solution. One gram molecular weight of NaOH consists of 40 g. Thus 1 L of a 1 M solution contains 40 g of NaOH, and a 4 M solution contains four times this amount or 160 g of NaOH per liter.

> 1 M NaOH = 40 g/L
> 4 M NaOH = 4 × 40 g/L = 160 g/L

Thus to find the number of grams needed to prepare 2500 mL of a 4 M NaOH solution, multiply by the required volume expressed in liters as follows:

$$160 \text{ g/L} \times \frac{2500 \text{ mL}}{1000 \text{ mL/L}} = 400 \text{ g}$$

Therefore, 400 g of NaOH are needed to prepare 2500 mL (2.5 L) of a 4 M NaOH solution.

24.

C. A weight per volume percent solution contains a specific number of grams (equivalent to the per-

cent indicated) of solute per 100 mL (equivalent to 1 dL) of solution. An 0.85%$^{w/v}$ isotonic saline solution contains 0.85 g of NaCl per 100 mL of solution. To find the number of grams needed to prepare 5 L of solution, multiply by the required volume in deciliters as follows:
0.85 g/dL × 5 L × 10 dL/L = 42.5 g NaCl. Using a volumetric flask, prepare 5 L of an 0.85%$^{w/v}$ NaCl solution by dissolving 42.5 g of NaCl in deionized water and diluting to a final volume of 5 L.

25.

A. A 1 normal solution contains 1 g equivalent weight of a solute in 1 L of solution. One equivalent weight of NaOH contains 40 g; thus, a 0.02 N solution contains one fiftieth of this amount, or 0.8 g of NaOH per liter.

> 1 N NaOH = 40 g/L
> 0.02 N NaOH = 0.02 × 40 g/L = 0.8 g/L

Thus to find the number of grams needed to prepare 500 mL (0.5 L) of a 0.02 N NaOH solution, multiply by the required volume as follows: 0.8 g/L × 0.5 L = 0.4 g or 400 mg. Therefore, 0.4 g (or 400 mg) of NaOH are needed to prepare 500 mL of a 0.02 N NaOH solution.

26.

D. When starting with a 30% $^{w/v}$ H_2SO_4 solution, the normality of the solution may be calculated by employing the following steps:

1. Determine the molecular weight of H_2SO_4: mol wt = 98 g.
2. Find the g/Eq in 1 L of 1 N H_2SO_4 solution: 98 g/L ÷ 2 Eq/L = 49 g/Eq = 49 g/L.
3. Find the corresponding percent of a 1 N H_2SO_4 solution: 49 g/L ÷ 10 dL/L = 4.9 g/dL = 4.9%$^{w/v}$ H_2SO_4.
4. Find the normality of the 30% H_2SO_4 solution. Divide the stated percent by the percent of the 1 N H_2SO_4 solution: 30% ÷ 4.9% = 6.12 N H_2SO_4.

27.

D. To convert 369 mg/dL of chloride to milliequivalents per liter, use the following formula:

$$\frac{mg/dL \times 10 \times valence}{atomic\ mass} = mEq/L$$

For the problem presented, let 10 represent the number of deciliters per liter, 35.5 is the atomic mass of chloride, and 1 is the valence of chloride:

$$\frac{369\ mg/dL \times 10 \times 1}{35.5} = 104\ mEq/L$$

28.

A. To convert 8.6 mg/dL of calcium to millimoles per liter, the following formula may be used:

$$\frac{mg/L}{molecular\ mass} = mmol/L$$

For the problem presented:

$$\frac{8.6\ mg/dL \times 10\ dL/L}{40} = 2.15\ mmol/L$$

The calculated value of 2.15 mmol/L rounded to the nearest tenth gives the answer 2.2 mmol/L.

29.

B. When starting with a concentrated HNO_3 solution, a 0.15 normal solution may be prepared by employing the following steps:

A. Calculate the normality of the concentrated HNO_3 solution.
1. Multiply the specific gravity (expressed as grams per milliliter) by the assay (expressed as percent by weight) to find the number of grams per milliliter:
   1.42 g/mL × 0.70 = 0.994 g/mL
2. To find the number of grams per liter, multiply by 1000 mL/L:
   0.994 g/mL × 1000 mL/L = 994 g/L
3. To find the normality (equivalents per liter) of the concentrated HNO_3, divide the grams per liter by the equivalent weight of HNO_3:
   > 1 N HNO_3 = 63 g/Eq
   > 994 g/L ÷ 63 g/Eq = 15.8 Eq/L
   > = 15.8 N HNO_3
B. Calculate the number of milliliters of concentrated HNO_3 needed to prepare 2 L of 0.15 N HNO_3 using the formula $V_1 \times N_1 = V_2 \times N_2$.

> 2000 mL × 0.15 N = V_2 × 15.8 N
> $$\frac{2000\ mL \times 0.15}{15.8} = V_2$$
> 19.0 mL = V_2

Thus 2 L of 0.15 N HNO_3 are prepared by diluting 19.0 mL of concentrated HNO_3 to a final volume of 2000 mL.

30.

B. Since titration reveals that the normality of the HCl solution is lower than the desired normality of 0.50 N, it is apparent that concentrated HCl must be added. Use the following formula to determine the actual normality of the acid solution:

$$V_1 \times N_1 = V_2 \times N_2$$

where V_1 = 7 mL of the HCl solution, N_1 = actual normality of the HCl solution, V_2 = 16 mL of the 0.20 N NaOH solution, and N_2 = 0.20 N NaOH solution.

1. Find the actual normality of the acid solution:
   7 mL $\times N_1$ = 16 mL $\times$ 0.20 N
   $$N_1 = \frac{16 \text{ mL} \times 0.20}{7 \text{ mL}}$$
   N_1 = 0.457 actual N of HCl solution
2. Find the number of milliequivalents per milliliter lacking in the initial HCl solution: 0.500 mEq/mL − 0.457 mEq/mL = 0.043 mEq/mL lacking.
3. Find the number of milliliters of the initial HCl solution remaining: 3000 mL − 7 mL = 2993 mL remaining.
4. Find the number of milliequivalents of HCl that must be added to the remaining solution: 2993 mL $\times$ 0.043 mEq/mL = 128.7 mEq required.
5. Find the number of grams per milliliter of HCl in concentrated HCl: 1.19 g/mL (sp gr) $\times$ 0.375 (assay) = 0.446 g HCl/mL of concentrated acid. It follows that there are 446 g HCl/L.
6. Find the normality of concentrated HCl (Eq wt = 36.5 g): 446 g/L ÷ 36.5 g/Eq = 12.22 Eq/L, or 12.22 N, or 12.22 mEq/mL.
7. Find the number of milliliters of concentrated HCl that must be added:
   $$\frac{128.7 \text{ (mEq required)}}{12.22 \text{ (mEq/mL in conc. HCl)}} = 10.53 \text{ mL}$$

Thus, 10.53 mL of concentrated HCl must be added to the remaining volume of 2993 mL for a total volume of 3003.53 mL to prepare an accurate 0.50 N HCl solution.

31.

D. When the concentrations of the four serum electrolytes—sodium, potassium, chloride, and carbon dioxide—are expressed, the preferred terminology is an expression of the unit designation as millimoles per liter (mmol/L). To convert from milligrams per deciliter to millimoles per liter, the following formula may be used:

$$\frac{mg/L}{\text{molecular mass}} = mmol/L$$
$$\frac{369 \text{ mg/dL} \times 10 \text{ dL/L}}{35.5} = 104 \text{ mmol/L}$$

32.

C. When a dilute solution is prepared from a concentrated solution, the following equation may be used:

$$V_1 \times C_1(\%) = V_2 \times C_2(\%)$$

For the stated problem let V_1 = milliliters of the 20% NaOH solution, C_1 = the 20% NaOH solution, V_2 = 800 mL of the desired 2.5% solution, and C_2 = the 2.5% NaOH solution. Using this information in the above equation:

$$V_1 \times 20\% = 800 \text{ mL} \times 2.5\%$$
$$V_1 = \frac{800 \text{ mL} \times 2.5\%}{20\%}$$
$$V_1 = 100 \text{ mL}$$

Thus, 100 mL of the 20%$^{w/v}$ NaOH solution are required to prepare a total volume of 800 mL of 2.5%$^{v/v}$ NaOH. This may be done by diluting 100 mL of 20% NaOH to a final volume of 800 mL.

33.

D. When one starts with a percent solution, a normal solution may be prepared by employing the following steps.

A. Calculate the normality of the 40%$^{w/v}$ NaOH solution.
   1. Find the number of grams in 1 equivalent weight of a 1 N NaOH solution:
      1 N NaOH = 40 g/Eq = 40 g/L
   2. Find the grams per liter in the 40%$^{w/v}$ NaOH solution:
      40 g/100 mL $\times$ 1000 mL/L = 400 g/L
   3. Find the normality of the 40% NaOH solution by dividing the number of grams per liter in the 40% NaOH solution by the equivalent weight of NaOH:

$$400 \text{ g/L} \div 40 \text{ g/Eq} = 10 \text{ Eq/L}$$
$$= 10 \text{ N NaOH}$$

B. Calculate the number of milliliters of 40%$^{w/v}$ NaOH needed to prepare 1.5 L of 2 N NaOH using the formula:

$$V_1 \times N_1 = V_2 \times N_2$$
$$1500 \text{ mL} \times 2 \text{ N} = V_2 \times 10 \text{ N}$$
$$\frac{1500 \text{ mL} \times 2}{10} = V_2$$
$$300 \text{ mL} = V_2$$

Therefore, 300 mL of 40%$^{w/v}$ NaOH are required to prepare 1.5 L of 2 N NaOH. Add 300 mL of 40% NaOH to the solvent, diluting with solvent to a final volume of 1.5 L.

34.

C. A weight per volume percent solution contains a specific number of grams of solute per 100 mL of solution. Preparation of a 23%$^{w/v}$ Na$_2$SO$_4$ solution may be done as follows: 23%$^{w/v}$ Na$_2$SO$_4$ = 23 g/dL. Thus to find the number of grams needed to prepare 750 mL, multiply by the required volume in deciliters, as follows:

$$23 \text{ g/dL} \times 10 \text{ dL/L} \times \frac{750 \text{ mL}}{1000 \text{ mL/L}} = 172.5 \text{ g}$$

To prepare 750 mL of a 23%$^{w/v}$ Na$_2$SO$_4$ solution, dissolve 172.5 g of Na$_2$SO$_4$ in solvent and dilute to a final volume of 750 mL.

35.

C. Since the normality of the HCl solution is greater than the desired normality, this problem can be considered similar to that of preparing a dilute solution from a concentrated solution. Thus the following equation may be used to determine the new total volume required, and indirectly the amount of deionized water that must be added to the remaining volume, to achieve the desired normality:

$$V_1 \times N_1 = V_2 \times N_2$$

where V_1 = mL of the desired 0.20 N HCl solution, N_1 = 0.20 N HCl solution, V_2 = 1990 mL remaining of the 0.208 N HCl solution, and N_2 = 0.208 N HCl solution. Using this information in the above equation:

$$V_1 \times 0.20 \text{ N} = 1990 \text{ mL} \times 0.208 \text{ N}$$
$$V_1 = \frac{1990 \text{ mL} \times 0.208 \text{ N}}{0.20 \text{ N}}$$
$$V_1 = 2069.6 \text{ mL}$$

Thus a new total volume of 2069.6 mL is required to make an accurate 0.20 N HCl solution. To determine the amount of deionized water that must be added to the remaining 1990 mL volume, find the difference between the new total volume and the remaining volume: 2069.6 mL − 1990 mL = 79.6 mL of deionized water that must be added to the remaining volume of solution.

36.

C. To convert milligrams per deciliter to milliequivalents per liter, use the following formula:

$$\frac{\text{mg/dL} \times 10 \times \text{valence}}{\text{atomic mass}} = \text{mEq/L}$$

For the problem presented, let 10 represent the number of deciliters per liter, 40 is the atomic mass of calcium, and 2 is the valence of calcium.

$$\frac{8.6 \text{ mg/dL} \times 10 \times 2}{40} = 4.3 \text{ mEq/L}$$

37.

D. When one starts with a 5 N HCl solution, 4 L of a 10%$^{w/v}$ HCl solution may be prepared by employing the following steps:

A. Calculate the normality of the 10%$^{w/v}$ HCl solution.
1. Find the number of grams in 1 equivalent weight of a 1 N HCl solution: 1 N HCl = 36.5 g/Eq.
2. Find the number of grams per liter in the 10%$^{w/v}$ HCl solution: 10%$^{w/v}$ HCl = 10 g/dL = 100 g/L.
3. Find the normality of the 10%$^{w/v}$ HCl solution. Divide the number of grams per liter in the 10% solution by the equivalent weight of HCl: 100 g/L ÷ 36.5 g/Eq = 2.74 N HCl.

B. Calculate the number of milliliters of 5 N HCl needed to prepare 4 L of 10%$^{w/v}$ HCl using the following formula:

$$V_1 \times N_1 = V_2 \times N_2$$
$$4000 \text{ mL} \times 2.74 \text{ N} = V_2 \times 5 \text{ N}$$
$$\frac{4000 \text{ mL} \times 2.74 \text{ N}}{5 \text{ N}} = V_2$$
$$2192 \text{ mL} = V_2$$

Therefore, 2192 mL of 5 N HCl are required to prepare 4 L of 10% $^{w/v}$ HCl. Add 2192 mL of 5 N

HCl to the solvent, diluting with solvent to a final volume of 4 L.

38.

B. To convert milligrams per deciliter to milliequivalents per liter, use the following formula:

$$\frac{mg/dL \times 10 \times valence}{atomic\ mass} = mEq/L$$

For the problem presented, let 10 represent the number of deciliters per liter, 39 is the atomic mass of potassium, and 1 is the valence of potassium.

$$\frac{19.5\ mg/dL \times 10 \times 1}{39} = 5.0\ mEq/L$$

39.

B. The urine sample contained 122.5 mmol/L of sodium. Since the total urine volume is given in milliliters, it is necessary to express the volume in liters so that the units of measurement correspond. This may be done by dividing the 24-hour volume in milliliters by 1000, since each liter has 1000 mL. The amount of sodium excreted in the 24-hour urine specimen may now be calculated.

$$\frac{\frac{Sodium\ conc.}{mmol/L} \times \frac{urine\ volume}{mL/24\ hr}}{1000\ mL/L} = mmol/24\ hr$$

$$\frac{122.5\ mmol/L \times 1540\ mL/24\ hr}{1000\ mL/L} = 188.6\ mmol/24\ hr$$

40.

C. Since titration reveals that the normality of the HNO_3 solution is higher than the desired normality, it is apparent that the solution needs to be diluted. The following equation may be used to determine the new total volume required, and indirectly the amount of deionized water that must be added to the remaining volume to make the desired normality:

$$V_1 \times N_1 = V_2 \times N_2$$

where V_1 = milliliters of the desired 0.50 N HNO_3 solution, N_1 = 0.50 N HNO_3 solution, V_2 = 3975 mL remaining of the 0.513 N HNO_3 solution, and N_2 = 0.513 N HNO_3 solution. Using this information in the above equation:

$$V_1 \times 0.50\ N = 3975\ mL \times 0.513\ N$$
$$V_1 = \frac{3975\ mL \times 0.513\ N}{0.50\ N}$$
$$V_1 = 4078.4\ mL$$

Thus, a new total volume of 4078.4 mL is required to make an accurate 0.50 N HNO_3 solution. To determine the amount of deionized water that must be added to the remaining 3975 mL volume, find the difference between the new total volume and the remaining volume:

4078.4 mL − 3975 mL = 103.4 mL of deionized water that must be added to the remaining volume of solution.

41.

D. The degree to which an acid solution dissociates determines the hydrogen ion concentration and thus the strength of the acid solution. Since the dissociation of acetic acid is only 1%, it is considered a weak acid. To calculate the pH of a 0.2 N acetic acid solution that is 1% ionized, proceed as follows:

1. Find the hydrogen ion concentration with the following formula:
$$[H^+] = N \times \%\ ionized$$
$$[H^+] = 0.2 \times 0.01 = 0.002\ g\ H^+/L$$
2. Find the pH of this solution with the following formula:

$$pH = \log \frac{1}{[H^+]}$$
$$pH = \log \frac{1}{0.002}$$
$$pH = 2.699$$

42.

C. A solution of Na_2SO_4 dissociates into two Na^+ ions and one SO_4^{2-} ion. The ionic strength is governed by the concentration (moles per liter) of each ion present in solution and the ionic charges associated with each ion. To calculate the ionic strength, derive half the sum for all ions present when the concentration of each ion present is multiplied by its valence squared. For a 0.2 M Na_2SO_4 solution, proceed as follows:

$$Ionic\ strength = \frac{[0.2 \times 2 \times (1)^2] + [0.2 \times (2)^2]}{2}$$

$$Ionic\ strength = 0.6$$

43.

D. The equation $A = abc$, where A represents the absorbance of a substance at a specified wavelength, a represents the absorptivity, b represents the length of the light path in centimeters, and c represents the concentration of the absorbing compound, is commonly referred to as Beer's law. When a 1 cm light path is used and the concentration is expressed in moles per liter, the constant a is replaced by the symbol ε (epsilon), which is referred to as the molar absorptivity. The molar absorptivity is generally defined as the absorbance determined, at a specified wavelength using a 1 cm light path, for a 1 M solution of a pure substance. The equation becomes $A = \varepsilon bc$. Use this formula to determine the absorbance of the 1.0 mg/dL (0.01 g/L) bilirubin standard solution. The molecular weight of bilirubin is 584 and ε is 60,700 at 453 nm using a 1 cm light path.

$$A = \varepsilon bc$$
$$A = (60{,}700)\,(1)\,(0.01 \div 584)$$
$$A = 1.039$$

Thus, a 1 mg/dL bilirubin standard solution should have an absorbance reading of 1.039.

44.

B. Over the years, numerous units have been used to express enzyme activity, including the Bodansky unit, the Gutman-Gutman unit, and the Bowers-McComb unit. The introduction of the International Unit (U) brought a common unit of comparison to enzyme assays. The International Unit is defined as the amount of enzyme activity that converts 1 μmol of substrate in 1 minute under standard conditions. The following formula is used to calculate enzyme activity.

$$\frac{\Delta A/\text{min} \times 1000 \times TV \times 1000 \times Tf}{6.22 \times 10^3 \times LP \times SV} = \text{U/L}$$

where ΔA/min is the average absorbance change per minute and 1000 converts milliliters to liters. TV is the total reaction volume and 1000 converts millimoles to micromoles. Tf is the temperature factor (1.0 at 37 °C), 6.22×10^3 is the molar absorptivity of reduced nicotinamide-adenine dinucleotide (NADH) at 340 nm, LP is the light path in centimeters, and SV is the sample volume. For the problem presented, determine the average ΔA/min and then substitute the given information into the above equation.

Absorbance Readings	ΔA/min	Average ΔA/min
0.204 A at 1 min		
0.406 A at 2 min	0.202	
0.610 A at 3 min	0.204	0.203
0.813 A at 4 min	0.203	

$$\frac{0.203\ \Delta A/\text{min} \times 1000 \times 3.2\ \text{mL} \times 1000 \times 1}{6.22 \times 10^3 \times 1.0 \times 0.2\ \text{mL}}$$
$$= 522\ \text{U/L}$$

45.

C. A kilogram is approximately equal to 2.2 pounds. A weight expressed in pounds may be converted to kilograms by dividing the weight in pounds by the conversion factor 2.2 as follows:

$$175.5\ \text{lb} \div 2.2\ \text{lb/kg} = 79.8\ \text{kg}$$

46.

D. When converting Celsius to Fahrenheit degrees, remember that 1 °C equals 9/5 °F. Thus multiplying the temperature in degrees Celsius by 9/5 is necessary to express the temperature in the degrees Fahrenheit unit, and the addition of 32 allows for adjustment to the Fahrenheit scale's zero point. To convert 30 °C to degrees Fahrenheit, the following formula may be used:

$$°F = (°C \times 9/5) + 32$$
$$°F = (30 \times 9/5) + 32$$
$$°F = 86$$

47.

C. Unlike most units of measurement used in chemistry, the curie (Ci) is a unit of measure for radioactivity that is independent of weight. The curie is defined as the quantity of radioactive material that exhibits 3.7×10^{10} disintegrations per second (dps). Other terms frequently used refer to units of radioactivity of smaller dimensions than the curie. These are the millicurie (mCi), which exhibits 3.7×10^7 dps, and the microcurie (μCi), which exhibits 3.7×10^4 dps.

48.

B. Each radionuclide has a unique half-life associated with it: ^{14}C = 5730 years; ^{3}H = 12.3 years; ^{125}I = 60 days; and ^{131}I = 8.1 days. Since half-life refers to the percent of activity remaining after a specified time, it will be necessary for all radionuclides to pass through seven half-life periods in order to reduce the initial activity of 100% to less than 1%. The following example expresses this phenomenon:

$$A_n = A_0(\tfrac{1}{2})^7$$
$$A_7 = 100(\tfrac{1}{2})^7$$
$$A_7 = 0.78\%$$

49.

A. The term *half-life* refers to the time required for the activity of a known amount of radioactive material to decrease to half of the initial activity. In a radioimmunoassay (RIA), this loss of activity is critical to the sensitivity of the assay. As activity decreases with time, the sensitivity of the assay will also decrease. In the problem presented, assume 100% activity originally. Since ^{125}I has a half-life of 60 days, the lapse of 180 days represents three half-life periods (3 $t_{\frac{1}{2}}$), 180 days ÷ 60 days/$t_{\frac{1}{2}}$ = 3 $t_{\frac{1}{2}}$. Use the following formula where A_n is the activity at the specified number of half-life periods. A_0 is the initial activity, and n is the number of half-life periods.

$$A_n = A_0(\tfrac{1}{2})^n$$
$$A_3 = 100(\tfrac{1}{2})^3$$
$$A_3 = 12.5\%$$

Therefore, 12.5% of the initial activity remains at the end of 3 $t_{\frac{1}{2}}$.

50.

B. For a strong base such as NaOH, dissociation into Na^+ and OH^- is complete. Thus in terms of molarity, the concentration of sodium ions equals the concentration of hydroxyl ions, which in turn equals the molar concentration of NaOH originally present. Proceed with the problem for a solution of NaOH with a pH of 12 by finding the molar concentration of the hydroxyl ions.

$$pH + pOH = 14$$
$$12 + pOH = 14$$
$$pOH = 2$$
$$pOH = -\log[OH^-]$$
$$2 = -\log[OH^-]$$
$$[OH^-] = 1 \times 10^{-2} = 0.01 \text{ mol/L}$$

Since 0.01 mol/L is the molar concentration of hydroxyl ions, it follows that the molar concentration of NaOH is 0.01 mol/L. The following formula is used to find the number of grams required to pre-

pare a 0.01 M NaOH solution (molecular weight of NaOH = 40).

$$\frac{g/L}{mol\ wt} = M$$
$$\frac{X}{40} = 0.01$$
$$X = 0.4 \text{ g/L} = 0.2 \text{ g/500 mL}$$

Thus, 0.2 g of NaOH is required to prepare 500 mL of a solution of NaOH with a pH of 12.

51.

B. By use of centrifugal force, a centrifuge effects the separation of substances of different densities. The most common use of a centrifuge in the clinical laboratory is the separation of serum or plasma from the blood cells. The use of the proper amount of centrifugal force with serum separator tubes is especially important. In order for a thixotropic, silicone gel to form a barrier between the serum and the cell clot, it is critical that the tube be centrifuged for a specified time and with the specified centrifugal force. The following formula is used to calculate the relative centrifugal force (RCF) in terms of gravities (*g*) where 1.118×10^{-5} represents a constant, r represents the rotating radius in centimeters, and rpm represents the rotating speed in revolutions per minute:

$$RCF = 1.118 \times 10^{-5} \times r \times (rpm)^2$$
$$= 1.118 \times 10^{-5} \times 10 \times (2500)^2$$
$$= 698.75$$
$$RCF = 699 \times g$$

52.

C. Class A volumetric flasks are calibrated at 20 °C. Glassware that is designated as class A must meet the requirements of the National Institute of Standards and Technology. The College of American Pathologists (CAP) requires that CAP-approved clinical laboratories use only class A glassware. A 10 mL class A volumetric flask that is accurate to ±0.2% has a tolerance of ±0.02 mL; 10 mL × 0.2% = 0.02 mL = ±0.02 mL. Thus the capacity of a 10 mL flask is within the range of 9.98 to 10.02 mL.

53.

B. The term *parts per million* (ppm) is a unit of concentration that describes the number of parts of a substance that are contained in 1 million parts of the solution. *Parts per million* refers to the number of grams of a substance in 1 million grams of solution. To convert from parts per million to concentration, the following formula is used:

$$\frac{g}{X\,mL} \times 1{,}000{,}000 = ppm$$

In referring to parts per million it is important to remember that the unit of measure may vary (e.g., milligrams, micrograms, or nanograms), provided that the relationship of some number of parts in 1 million parts is maintained. Therefore it follows that to convert 0.01 ppm to mg/dL:

$$\frac{mg}{X\,mL} \times 1000 = ppm$$

$$\frac{mg}{100} \times 1000 = 0.01$$

$$mg = \frac{0.01}{1000} \times 100$$

$$mg = 0.001$$

Thus 0.01 ppm of lead is equivalent to 0.001 mg/dL or 0.001 mg/100mL.

54.

B. To convert 68.0 %T to absorbance (A), use the following formula:

$$A = -\log T = \log \frac{1}{T} = \log \frac{100\%}{\%T}$$

$$A = \log 100 - \log \%T$$
$$A = 2 - \log \%T$$
$$A = 2 - \log 68$$
$$A = 2 - 1.832 = 0.168$$

After determining absorbance values, they may be used in the Beer's law equation, $A = abc$, to determine concentration values. Absorbance and percent transmittance values may both be used to construct standard curves to determine concentration values of unknown samples.

55.

D. Spectrophotometric analysis is based on Beer's law, which states that under appropriate conditions the concentration of a colored substance in solution is directly proportional to the amount of light absorbed and inversely proportional to the logarithm of the transmitted light. The narrower the band of wavelengths of light used, the more closely is Beer's law followed. Since Beer's law applies only to absorption of light by the analyte,

absorption by any other substance, such as the solvent, would make the law inapplicable. Beer's law is applicable only to dilute solutions. Fluorescing compounds would add light to the system. A chemical reaction would change the concentration of the analyte. In either case, Beer's law would be inapplicable.

56.

D. When one of the two variable quantities changes as a result of changing the other, the result is frequently presented in the form of a graph. It is essential that the scale chosen for each axis of the graph be used consistently. For example, when using Cartesian graph paper where both axes are linear to plot spectrophotometric data (concentration *vs.* absorbance), if 1 cm represents a concentration of 10 mg/dL on the ordinate or horizontal x-axis, 1 cm cannot represent 100 mg/dL toward the end of the scale. Similarly, for the abscissa or vertical y-axis a uniform scale must be used (e.g., 1 cm represents 0.1 absorbance units), but it need not be, and generally it is not, the same as the scale used for the horizontal axis, as illustrated by this example.

57.

D. Primary standards are substances that react quantitatively with other analytes. The caliber of the analysis depends on the caliber of the primary standard. It is therefore essential that the primary standard available be at least 99.95% pure. The primary standard must not be hygroscopic to avoid errors in weighing caused by absorption of water. For accurate weighing, the primary standard must be dry. Dryness is obtained in an oven at a temperature slightly above the boiling point of water. Hence the primary standard must be stable at 110 °C. Since the primary standard should have a large equivalent weight and hence a large molecular weight, a relatively large amount will be needed to react with the analyte. The error inherent in weighing out very small quantities is thereby avoided.

58.

A. To solve this problem all the values must be converted to a common unit. In metric measurement the gram is the primary unit for weight. The value 0.1 ng is equal to 1×10^{-10} g, which is the lightest weight given. The gram relationships for the other values stated are $0.01 \text{g} = 1 \times 10^{-2}$ g, 1.0 mg $= 1 \times 10^{-3}$ g, and 1000 pg $= 1 \times 10^{-9}$ g.

59.

C. A solution with an OH^- concentration of 1×10^{-6} has a pOH of 6. The pH + pOH = 14; therefore the pH is 8. The H^+ concentration of pure water is 10^{-7} and has a pH of 7.

60.

D. The molecular weight of NaCl is 58.5 and the atomic weight of Cl is 35.5. To change 50 mg Cl into an equivalent amount of NaCl, the answer must be greater than the amount of Cl. The solution follows:

$$50 \text{ mg Cl} \times \frac{58.5 \text{ mg NaCl}}{35.5 \text{ mg Cl}} = 82.4 \text{ mg NaCl}$$

REFERENCES

Burtis, C. A., and Ashwood, E. R. (Eds.) (2000). *Tietz Fundamentals of Clinical Chemistry,* 5th ed. Philadelphia: W. B. Saunders.

Campbell, J. B., and Campbell, J. M. (1997). *Laboratory Mathematics Medical and Biological Applications,* 5th ed. St. Louis: Mosby-Year Book.

Doucette, L. J. (1997). *Mathematics for the Clinical Laboratory.* Philadelphia: W. B. Saunders.

Henry, J. B. (Ed.) (2001). *Clinical Diagnosis and Management by Laboratory Methods*, 20th ed. Philadelphia: W. B. Saunders.

10

General Laboratory Principles and Safety

contents

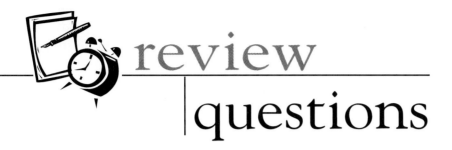

review questions

INSTRUCTIONS Each of the questions or incomplete statements that follow comprises four suggested responses. Select the *best* answer or completion statement in each case.

---

1. Which of the following are reactive chemicals that have the potential to become shock sensitive if stored for a prolonged period of time?
   A. Xylene and methanol
   B. Ethyl ether and picric acid
   C. Chloroform and phenol
   D. Ethidium bromide and scintillation fluid

2. A fire extinguisher used in the event of an electrical fire should include which of the following classifications?
   A. Type A
   B. Type B
   C. Type C
   D. Type D

3. In the Hazards Identification System, four color-coded, diamond-shaped symbols are arranged to form a larger diamond shape. What type of hazard does the blue diamond positioned to the left identify?
   A. Flammable
   B. Health
   C. Reactivity
   D. Contact

4. Xylene, ethanol, methanol, and acetone would be in which hazard class?
   A. Corrosive
   B. Flammable
   C. Oxidizer
   D. All the above

5. Which of the following is an aluminum-silicate glass that is at least six times stronger than borosilicate and is resistant to alkaline etching and scratching?
   A. Kimax
   B. Pyrex
   C. Corning boron free
   D. Corex

6. Which of the following terms is used to identify a chemical that causes cancer?
   A. Mutagen
   B. Teratogen
   C. Carcinogen
   D. Reactive

7. A Biosafety Level 2 (BSL-2) laboratory is designed to work with microorganisms that are

A. Not associated with disease in healthy adult humans

B. Associated with serious or lethal human disease for which preventative or therapeutic interventions may be available

C. Likely to cause serious or lethal human disease for which preventive or therapeutic interventions are not usually available

D. Associated with human disease that is rarely serious and for which preventive or therapeutic interventions are often available

8. The College of American Pathologists (CAP) requires that volumetric pipets and flasks be certified as

A. Class A
B. Class B
C. Class C
D. Class D

9. Which of the following desiccants is the most hygroscopic?

A. Silica gel
B. Alumina
C. Barium oxide
D. Magnesium perchlorate

10. Which of the following may be safely pipetted by mouth?

A. Serum
B. Urine
C. Saline solution
D. None of the above

11. The flash point of a liquid may be defined as the

A. Minimum temperature at which self-sustained ignition will occur

B. Maximum vapor pressure at which spontaneous ignition will occur

C. Temperature at which an adequate amount of vapor is produced, forming an ignitable mixture with air at the liquid's surface

D. Temperature that is 20 °F greater than the liquid's boiling point

12. A corrosive material was spilled onto the hand of a laboratorian. After diluting the material under running cold water, what should be done next?

A. Consult the MSDS (Material Safety Data Sheet)

B. Wipe up the spill with paper towels

C. Dilute the spill with water and remove it in a biohazard bag

D. Go to the Emergency Room

13. SI units are the designated units employed by the International System of Units. The unit class that encompasses the seven fundamental quantities of measurement is

A. Base
B. Primary
C. Derived
D. Elemental

14. A laboratory professional was asked to send a blood specimen from an HIV-positive patient to a laboratory for special tests. This specimen must be properly packaged and shipped as a(n)

A. Infectious substance
B. Diagnostic specimen
C. Biological product
D. Clinical specimen

15. In a microscope with a fixed tube length of 160 mm, the magnification obtained with a 43× objective and a 10× ocular would be

A. 160
B. 430
C. 1600
D. 68,800

16. What is the most appropriate term to describe water that is used as a solvent in the clinical laboratory?
    A. Distilled water
    B. Deionized water
    C. Reagent grade water
    D. Tap water

17. A substance that resists changes in the pH of a system is termed a(n)
    A. Acid
    B. Base
    C. Buffer
    D. Filter

18. The accuracy of thermometers used to monitor heating baths should be verified
    A. Weekly
    B. Monthly
    C. Every 6 months to 1 year
    D. Not at all

19. The air from a chemical fume hood is
    A. Recirculated through a HEPA filter
    B. 30% is recirculated through a HEPA filter and 70% is exhausted to the outside
    C. Totally exhausted from the building
    D. Totally exhausted from the building through a HEPA filter

20. "To deliver" (TD) pipettes are identified by
    A. Two etched bands near the mouthpiece
    B. Self-draining capacity
    C. Dual-purpose pipette labels
    D. Blue graduation levels

21. Which of the following is true of a volumetric pipette?
    A. Blow out the last drop
    B. Is labeled "to contain" (TC)
    C. Is used for diluting control material
    D. Is rinsed out

22. If a laboratory needs to keep certain chemical materials dry, the apparatus used will be a
    A. Buret
    B. Desiccator
    C. Separatory funnel
    D. Vacuum

23. Which of the following steps should be incorporated into a wash routine for pipettes?
    A. Rinse with tap water before returning to appropriate drawer
    B. Soak in 10% sodium hypochlorite immediately after use
    C. Soak in strong sulfuric acid immediately after use
    D. Put in glassware washer as soon as possible after use

24. The type of water desired for use in test methods requiring maximum accuracy and precision is
    A. Distilled
    B. Pure grade
    C. Type I
    D. Type II

25. The speed of a centrifuge should be checked at least once every 3 months with a(n)
    A. Tachometer
    B. Wiper
    C. Potentiometer
    D. Ergometer

26. The type of balance that uses an electromagnetic force to counterbalance the load placed on the pan is a(n)
    A. Trip balance
    B. Class A balance
    C. Class S balance
    D. Electronic balance

27. The air-handling system for a microbiology laboratory should
    A. Maintain negative pressure with respect to the administrative areas
    B. Maintain positive pressure with respect to the administrative areas
    C. Have a HEPA filter
    D. Have no particular requirement

28. Which of the following precautions should be followed when radioactive materials are used for radioimmunoassays?
    A. Any refrigerators and cabinets can be used for storage
    B. Assays may be performed in any high-bench laboratory
    C. Personnel must wear film badges when working
    D. Solid waste material may be incinerated for disposal

29. Precautions such as using a fume hood, wearing rubber gloves, donning a respirator, and cleaning glassware with a strong acid or organic solvent are consistent with working with
    A. Corrosives
    B. Carcinogens
    C. Azides
    D. All reagents

30. A laboratorian, properly dressed in white pants, labcoat, and shoes, prepares to leave the lab for lunch. In addition to washing down the bench with disinfectant and washing one's hands, for safety's sake one should also
    A. Put on safety goggles
    B. Remove labcoat
    C. Sip from coffee cup on the bench
    D. Remove polyvinyl gloves and place them into labcoat pocket for future use

31. Which of the following may be a potentially hazardous biologic situation?
    A. Handling specimens collected from patients in isolation according to standard precautions
    B. Keeping the centrifuge lid closed until the system has stopped completely
    C. Discarding sharp objects, including broken glass, in a puncture-proof container
    D. Discarding disposable blood collection needles in the patient's wastebasket

32. Which of the following is associated with proper storage of chemicals?
    A. All chemicals should be stored in alphabetical order for ease of handling
    B. Flammable chemicals should be stored in a fume hood
    C. Large containers of liquid chemicals should be stored on a top shelf to allow easy visibility from below
    D. Volatile solvents should be stored in small amounts in an explosion-proof refrigerator

33. A laboratorian spills a bottle of concentrated sulfuric acid and slips in the fluid, exposing the lower length of his/her body to the burning fluid. To help, what would be the best thing another tech could do?
    A. Take the injured person to the Emergency Room
    B. Put the person under the safety shower
    C. Call security
    D. Pour concentrated base on the person to neutralize the acid

34. A stat procedure requiring a corrosive reagent (organic acid) is requested. To transport this reagent to the work area under the hood a laboratorian should
    A. Carry the brown bottle by the loop with one hand under the bottom of the container
    B. Employ a rubber carrier with handles

C. Pour an amount near the storage site and transport it

D. Pipette the required volume and carry the pipette to the work area

35. Which of the following statements pertains to the safe handling of compressed gases?
    A. Large cylinders should be loosely placed on a hand cart when being transported
    B. Cylinders must be secured to a wall or bench when in use
    C. Cylinders should be stored along with flammable liquids because both are combustible
    D. Large cylinders should be ordered to avoid frequent movement in and out of stock

36. The major job-related disease hazard in clinical laboratories produces symptoms of malaise, anorexia, nausea, vomiting, fatigue, diarrhea, and abdominal tenderness. What is it?
    A. AIDS
    B. Salmonella
    C. Tuberculosis
    D. Hepatitis

37. Which of the following is an example of an engineering control?
    A. Latex gloves
    B. Biological safety cabinet
    C. Pipette
    D. Glasses

38. Based on the chemical properties of azides, which of the following factors has motivated laboratories to monitor their use?
    A. The buildup of salts can lead to explosions
    B. They are corrosive to pipes even when diluted

C. They are extremely volatile

D. They are flammable and dangerous near an open flame

39. Which of the operating procedures listed should be followed for safe operation of an autoclave?
    A. Any type of plastic container may be used because all plastics are autoclavable
    B. Insulated gloves should never be worn when removing materials for fear of contamination
    C. All caps must be tightened before autoclaving to ensure sterility
    D. Before opening the door, check that the temperature and pressure are down to safe levels

40. Solvents that are extremely volatile and produce vapors that can accumulate and ignite should be
    A. Stored uncapped to release pressure
    B. Kept in a walk-in refrigerator with dry ice
    C. Frozen until needed
    D. Stored in an explosion-proof refrigerator

41. The term "Standard Precautions" refers to a concept of bloodborne disease control, which requires that all human blood and other potentially infectious materials:
    A. Be treated as if known to be infectious for HIV or HBV or other bloodborne pathogens regardless of the perceived "low risk" of a patient population
    B. Be treated as if it is not infectious unless it is known to be infectious
    C. Must be handled using a respirator (for aerosol exposure)
    D. Need not be treated with caution unless there is a cut on your hand

42. A laboratory professional was instructed to draw blood from a patient in the outpatient clinic. After the blood was drawn, the laboratorian did not see a sharps container in the area. What should the laboratorian do?
   A. Put the cap on the needle very carefully to avoid getting stuck
   B. Set the needle down, without capping it, until a sharps container can be found
   C. Recap the needle using the one-handed technique
   D. Try to remove the needle from the syringe, cap the needle, and dispose of it in a biohazard red bag

43. The Biological Safety Cabinet is the single most useful safety device in the microbiology laboratory. Of the three classes of cabinets, which one is the most used in the clinical laboratory?
   A. Class I
   B. Class II
   C. Class III
   D. Clean Bench

44. Chlorine is most often used in the form of sodium hypochlorite (NaOCl), found in household bleach, for a disinfectant. What percentage does the Centers for Disease Control and Prevention (CDCP) recommend using to clean up blood spills?
   A. 2%
   B. 10%
   C. 20%
   D. Full strength

45. The clinical hematology laboratory just received a new disinfectant to use in place of the one normally used. Never having used this particular disinfectant before, how should the lab professional proceed?
   A. Use it full strength; you can always be sure if you do this
   B. Read the manufacturer's package insert and prepare the product according to directions

C. Make the concentration 10% higher than the manufacturer's recommendations
D. Put the new disinfectant under the sink for storage

46. What written plan of specific measures does your laboratory have in place to minimize the risk of exposure to bloodborne pathogens?
   A. Chemical Hygiene Plan
   B. Exposure Control Plan
   C. MSDS
   D. Infection Control Plan

47. Which of the following information is found on a Material Safety Data Sheet (MSDS)?
   A. Health hazard data
   B. Fire and explosion hazard data
   C. First Aid measures
   D. All the above

48. Work is being done with *Mycobacterium tuberculosis* in the microbiology laboratory. It is important that you enter this lab while work is being done with positive samples. What is the most important personal protective equipment you should don before entering this laboratory?
   A. Carbon cartridge respirator
   B. Mask
   C. Gloves
   D. N95 HEPA filter respirator

49. When working with chemicals, the selection of your gloves depends on
   A. The chemical hazard and the tasks involved
   B. How far you must transport the chemical
   C. Whether you use a fume hood or not
   D. Whatever is available in the laboratory

50. As Sally was performing an experiment, something splashed into her eye. What should she do immediately?

    A. Wipe her eye with a tissue and continue working

    B. Find the eyewash and flush the eye for 15 minutes

    C. Find the eyewash and rinse eyes for several minutes

    D. Finish her experiment and then flush her eye with water

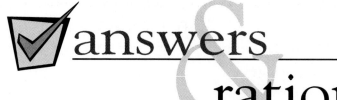

answers & rationales

1.

B. Ethyl ether and picric acid have the potential to form peroxides if stored for a period of time and not used. If this happens, the bottle can become shock sensitive with the potential to explode if knocked. All others given do not pose this risk.

2.

C. A fire extinguisher is classified and labeled for the type of fire on which it should be used. An ABC fire extinguisher is commonly found in laboratories. Type A extinguishers are used on fires of ordinary combustibles such as paper, cloth, wood, rubber, and plastics. Type B extinguishers are used on fires of flammable liquids including oils, gasoline, and solvents. Type C extinguishers are used on electrical equipment fires. Type D extinguishers are used on fires involving combustible metals (e.g., magnesium, sodium).

3.

B. The National Fire Protection Association developed the Hazards Identification System to provide common, recognizable warning signals for chemical hazards. The system consists of four color-coded, diamond-shaped symbols arranged to form a larger diamond shape. The diamond symbol located at the top of the larger diamond is color-coded red, indicating a flammability hazard. The yellow diamond symbol to the right represents reactivity-stability hazards. The white diamond symbol located at the bottom provides information on special precautions. The blue diamond symbol located to the left identifies potential health hazards. Contained within each color-coded diamond is a number ranging from 0 to 4, indicating the severity of the respective hazard (0 = none and 4 = extreme). It should be noted that a number of chemical manufacturers have adopted this warning system for their labels.

4.

B. All hazardous chemicals in the workplace must be identified and clearly marked with a National Fire Protection Association label. All these chemicals are flammable. Corrosive chemicals are harmful to mucous membranes, skin, eyes, or tissues.

5.

D. Several types of glassware are commonly used in the laboratory, each having its specific purpose. Corex glass is used in the manufacture of centrifuge tubes and thermometers. Pipettes, beakers, and flasks are generally made from Pyrex or Kimax borosilicate glass.

6.

C. A carcinogen is defined as a substance or agent producing or inciting cancer. Mutagens cause changes in DNA or RNA. Teratogens cause birth defects.

7.

D. The NIH guidelines describe Biosafety Level 2 laboratories as those laboratories that work with microorganisms associated with human disease that is rarely serious and for which preventive or therapeutic interventions are often available. Biosafety Level 1 laboratories handle agents that have no known potential for infecting healthy

470

people. Biosafety Level 3 is recommended for materials that may contain viruses not normally encountered in a clinical laboratory.

8.

A. The inspection requirements of the College of American Pathologists (CAP) state that volumetric pipettes and flasks must be of certified accuracy. Class A glassware meets federal guidelines and fulfills the CAP requirements. All non–class A glassware must be recalibrated periodically by an acceptable verification procedure.

9.

D. Desiccants are drying agents employed to keep some chemicals, thin-layer chromatography (TLC) plates, and gases used in gas chromatography from combining with water and becoming hydrated. The most effective desiccant is magnesium perchlorate; one of the least hygroscopic is silica gel. Some desiccants can be regenerated for repeated use by heating them at a high temperature for several hours.

10.

D. Pipetting by mouth should be totally forbidden in the clinical laboratory. Since biological specimens may be infected, and since most reagents are either corrosive, poisonous, or both, a pipetting device should be used. Although it may not seem harmful to pipette saline solution by mouth, it is good laboratory practice to use a pipetting device always.

11.

C. Both flammable and combustible liquids are commonly used in the laboratory. These two categories are differentiated on the basis of their flash points—that is, the temperature at which a liquid forms an adequate amount of vapor to produce an ignitable mixture with the air at the liquid's surface. The flash point of flammables is designated as less than 100 °F and that of combustibles as greater than 100 °F.

12.

A. Manufacturers of chemicals, reagents, and kits provide Material Safety Data Sheets (MSDSs) for all products. These sheets must be available to all technologists in case of emergency. Even before a technologist goes to the emergency room, she/he must have the MSDS to give to the ER physician in order to get prompt, correct treatment. A laboratory professional must be confident to report any accident and take appropriate measures to clean it up.

13.

A. The International System of Units was established to facilitate a uniform system of measurement. SI units may be classified as base, derived, or supplemental units. Base units were established for each of the seven fundamental quantities of measurement: length (meter), mass (kilogram), time (second), electric current (ampere), amount of substance (mole), temperature (kelvin), catalytic amount (katal), and luminous intensity (candela). Derived units are mathematically calculated from more than one base unit.

14.

A. An infectious substance, according to the definition by the International Air and Transportation Association (IATA), is a substance known to contain or reasonably expected to contain, pathogens. Pathogens are microorganisms or recombinant microorganisms that are known or reasonably expected to cause infectious disease in humans or animals. Special shipping devices for infectious substances less than 50 mL are available that wrap tubes in a treated sponge placed in a biohazard bag and then in a labeled red plastic container. If spills should occur, the sponge absorbs and disinfects so that the package is noninfectious when handled.

15.

B. When the tube length is fixed, magnification is equal to the magnification of the objective times the magnification of the ocular. In this case, $43 \times 10 = 430$. Only if the tube length is adjustable is length taken into account.

16.

C. Both deionized and distilled reflect procedures to achieve reagent grade water or water that is used as a solvent. These terms, therefore, are not accurate. The National Committee for Clinical Laboratory Standards has published specifications for reagent grade water, which is independent of the method of preparation. There are three types: Type I, Type II, and Type III.

17.

C. Buffers are defined as substances that resist changes in the pH of a system. All weak acids or bases form buffer systems in the presence of their salts. The action of buffers and their role in maintaining the pH of a solution can best be explained by the Henderson-Hasselbalch equation.

18.

C. The primary types of thermometers used in clinical laboratories are liquid (mercury) in glass and thermistor probe. Mercury-in-glass thermometers should be checked periodically for breaks in the mercury column. They should be calibrated at the recommended interval of 6 months to 1 year, using a thermometer certified by the National Institute of Standards and Technology (NIST). The accuracy range of a thermometer should be such that it is able to measure within half of the temperature accuracy desired of a particular instrument; for example, if the required accuracy of a heating bath is $\pm$ 1.0 °C, the minimum accuracy of the thermometer would be $\pm$ 0.5 °C.

19.

C. A chemical fume hood is an engineering control to provide protection from chemicals. Correct airflow is critical in containing fumes. All air in a chemical fume hood is exhausted out of the building. Chemicals should not be used in a Biological Safety Cabinet unless a Class II, B2 cabinet can be used, in which case all the air is also exhausted to the outside but through a HEPA filter.

20.

A. Serologic pipettes are "to deliver" (TD) types and are not rinsed out. These pipettes are not self-draining but must be blown out to deliver their entire contents, as is indicated by the two etched rings at the mouthpiece. "To contain" (TC) pipettes, such as Sahli pipettes, must be rinsed out to deliver their entire contents.

21.

C. Volumetric pipettes are a type of transfer pipette designed to deliver (TD) their stated volume. These pipettes are self-draining and should not be blown out. Because of their high degree of accuracy and precision, volumetric pipettes are often used to dilute control materials, standards, and calibrators.

22.

B. Desiccators provide a dry environment for chemical materials. A shelf is placed on top of the desiccant on which the material to be stored can be set. A heavy glass cover closes the system. An airtight seal is pro-

vided by placing stopcock grease around the ground glass joints between the desiccator and the lid.

23.

B. Although a variety of methods may be followed to ensure the cleanliness of glassware, there are several basic steps that should be incorporated into a good wash routine. Pipettes should be initially soaked in a 10% bleach solution (sodium hypochlorite) to eliminate any clinging protein. The soak should be followed by a detergent wash and thorough tap water rinse. The pipettes should then be soaked in an acid solution such as acid dichromate, nitric acid, or sulfuric acid for 30 minutes to remove stubborn materials. Rinse the pipettes in tap water for 30 minutes, followed by three rinses with deionized water. Finally, dry pipettes in an oven set at 100 °C for approximately 30 minutes.

24.

C. Type I water should be used when a high degree of accuracy is desired, as in quantitative chemistry assays and in the preparation of standards and buffers. Type I water requires deionization through acidic and basic ion-exchange columns, removal of organic materials by activated charcoal adsorption, and semipermeable membrane filtration for the removal of microorganisms and other particulate material. Distillation, although recommended before the deionization process, is not mandatory.

25.

A. Centrifugal force may be determined by knowing the mass of the solution and the speed and radius of the centrifuge. With aqueous solutions having a specific gravity near 1.000, the specific mass need not be known. To determine the speed, use either a strobe light, positioned over the revolving centrifuge head, or a tachometer to establish the revolutions per minute (rpm).

26.

D. An electronic balance is a single-pan balance that uses an electromagnetic force to counterbalance the load placed on the pan. These balances are top-loading in design and permit weighings to be made in 5 seconds or less. The Mettler Instrument Corporation makes a representative electronic balance.

27.

A. Laboratory areas should maintain negative pressure with respect to the administrative areas to prevent toxic or pathogenic materials used in laboratory work areas from escaping and injuring humans or contaminating the environment. The amount of air provided to the negative pressure laboratory should be equal to 85% of the air exhausted from the area. Positive pressure is maintained in the office areas.

28.
C. The Nuclear Regulatory Commission (NRC) regulations must be followed by users of radioisotopes. Radioactive materials, waste containers, storage facilities, and the door leading into the room must all be properly labeled. Disposal of radioimmunoassay (RIA) waste products must be according to regulations. Under no circumstances should radioactive materials be incinerated. The radioactivity is so small that it can be harmlessly flushed down the sewer. In addition to precautions such as not eating, drinking, or smoking when working with radioisotopes, personnel must wear a film badge to monitor their radiation exposure.

29.
B. Occasionally there may be need to work with carcinogenic chemicals. Some of the precautions that should be followed include performing the procedure in a fume hood, wearing rubber gloves and proper protective clothing, never pipetting by mouth, and wearing a respirator when working with organic vapors and dust-producing materials. If possible, use disposable glassware, and all other glassware should be washed with a strong acid before being processed in the general wash cycle.

30.
B. Safe practices in the laboratory are essential to the well-being of all employees. Each laboratorian should disinfect his/her work area daily. Pens and pencils placed on laboratory bench tops may be contaminated and should never be placed near one's mouth. Laboratory coats should never be worn in the cafeteria because they may be contaminated. Laboratory personnel should never smoke, eat, or drink in the laboratory, nor should food be placed in a refrigerator used for storage of reagents or biologic specimens. Cosmetics should not be applied in the laboratory because contamination is always a potential problem. Personnel should always wash their hands before leaving the laboratory, discarding their used polyvinyl gloves in a biohazard receptacle.

31.
D. It should be remembered that all body fluids from patients are potentially hazardous to one's health. Specimens collected from infectious patients in isolation should be handled according to universal precautions. Blood specimens need to be centrifuged, and inhalation of aerosols is prevented by never raising centrifuge lids prematurely. All sharp objects, including broken glass and needles, should be disposed of in a puncture-proof container. The blood collection needles should never be discarded in a wastebasket in a patient's room, since housekeeping personnel or others may easily be injured and infected.

32.
D. Chemicals should not be stored in alphabetical order because some chemicals are incompatible with others and will react adversely. Large containers of chemicals should always be stored on a shelf as close to the floor as possible to avoid severe injury in the event of breakage. Flammable chemicals should be stored in a fire-safety cabinet. Although flammables should be used in a fume hood, the hood is not a proper storage area.

33.
B. Emergency showers must be available to anyone working with corrosive materials. The victim should be removed from the area as rapidly as possible and showered with water. No attempt should be made to neutralize the acid on the person's skin.

34.
B. Bottles of chemicals and solutions should be handled carefully. Chemical containers made of glass should be transported in rubber or plastic holders that will protect them from breakage. In the event of breakage, the plastic holders will contain the spill.

35.
B. Compressed gas cylinders should be stored in a vertical position in a ventilated, fire-resistant location. Gas cylinders must never be stored in the same area as flammable liquids, since both are highly combustible. Because of their shape, gas cylinders may easily fall, causing the regulator valve to rupture. To prevent such an occurrence, cylinders must always be fastened when stored, transported, and used in the laboratory.

36.

D. Viral hepatitis is the major job-related disease hazard in all clinical laboratories. No technologist who handles blood or body fluids is immune to this risk. The modes of transmission include ingestion and injection. Thus it is crucial that the laboratorian follows proper safety practices at all times.

37.

B. A biological safety cabinet is an engineering control used to eliminate or minimize the potential for exposure to infectious materials. Latex gloves and other personal protective equipment may also be used. Cabinets are designed according to the degree of containment they provide. Class II biological safety cabinets are commonly used in clinical microbiology laboratories.

38.

A. Although now considered a carcinogen, sodium azide has been used previously as a preservative of some laboratory reagents. When disposal of these reagents is made in the sewer, a build-up of copper and iron salts of azide may occur. These metallic salts are explosive, especially when subjected to mechanical shock.

39.

D. Because of the elevated temperature and increased pressure required for proper operation of an autoclave, it is important that safety procedures be followed. The temperature and pressure must be down to safe levels before the autoclave door is opened. Heat-resistant gloves must be worn when one is removing materials that have not cooled completely. Caps should be left loose during the autoclave process to prevent explosions and boiling over. Care must be exercised in the use of plastic containers because some plastics cannot withstand autoclaving.

40.

D. The primary characteristic of an explosion-proof refrigerator is that all the electrical components are housed outside the unit and sealed in a conduit to eliminate sparks and arcs. In addition, compressors and controls are mounted on top of the refrigerator to eliminate a potential hazard from spills. The absence of internal lights and blowers, as well as the use of magnetic gaskets for door closure, is to ensure a sparkfree environment. It is the best location for volatile chemicals requiring refrigeration.

41.

A. In 1987, the Centers for Disease Control and Prevention (CDCP) established guidelines for universal precautions. These guidelines were established to lower the risk of HBV, and HIV transmission in clinical laboratories and blood banks. In 1996, CDCP published new guidelines, standard precautions, for isolation precautions in hospitals. Standard precautions synthesize the major features of Body Substance Isolation (BSI) and universal precautions to prevent transmission of a variety of organisms.

42.

C. Contaminated needles and other contaminated sharps shall not be bent, recapped, or removed unless there is no alternative feasible. Recapping or needle removal must be accomplished through the use of a mechanical device or one-handed technique. Discard all sharps in an appropriate puncture-resistant container.

43.

B. The single most useful safety device used in a clinical microbiology laboratory is the Class II biological safety cabinet. This engineering device is designed with inward airflow at a velocity to protect personnel. In addition, it is constructed with HEPA-filtered vertical laminar flow for product protection and HEPA-filtered exhaust air for environmental protection.

44.

B. Halogens, especially chlorine and iodine, are frequently used as disinfectants. Chlorine is most often used in the form of sodium hypochlorite (NaOCl), the compound known as household bleach. The CDCP recommends that tabletops be cleaned following blood spills with a 1:10 dilution of bleach.

45.

B. The most important point to remember when working with biocides or disinfectants is to prepare a working solution of the compound exactly according to the manufacturer's package insert. Many people think that if the manufacturer says to dilute to 1:200, they will be getting a stronger product if they dilute it 1:10. The ratio of water to active ingredient may be critical, and if sufficient water is not added, the free chemical for surface disinfection may not be released.

46.

B. Each employer having an employee with occupational exposure to human blood or any other infectious materials including bloodborne pathogens must establish a written Exposure Control Plan designed to eliminate or minimize employee exposure. The plan identifies tasks that are hazardous and promotes employee safety. The plan incorporates education, proper disposal of hazardous waste, engineering controls, use of personal protective equipment, and a postexposure plan.

47.

D. Material Safety Data Sheets (MSDSs) will specifically include: chemical identity as it appears on the label; chemical name and common name; physical and chemical characteristics; signs and symptoms of exposure; routes of entry; exposure limits; carcinogenic potential; safe handling procedures; spill cleanup procedures; and emergency first-aid. MSDSs are provided by the manufacturers for every hazardous chemical. MSDSs contain information on the nature of the chemical, precautions if spilled, and disposal recommendations.

48.

D. *Mycobacterium tuberculosis* is spread by the aerosol route. The risk of inhalation of infectious materials can occur in the laboratory environment and poses a significant potential health hazard to the employee. The proper personal protective equipment is extremely important when working with particular infectious materials. The N95 HEPA filter respirator is a high-energy particulate air filter and is used for microorganisms spread via the aerosol route.

49.

A. Hands are more likely to contact chemicals than any other part of the body. Gloves made of appropriate materials can effectively protect the hands from exposure if they are worn during routine handling of chemicals. Selection of protective gloves is based on chemical hazard and the tasks involved. The glove fabric must have an acceptably slow breakthrough time and permeation rate for the chemical of interest.

50.

B. Eyewash facilities should be readily accessible, marked as to their location, and tested at least weekly by running water to clear the pipes. It is recommended to flush the eyes for 15 continuous minutes. Eyewash stations should be located within 10 seconds and 100 feet of each work area.

REFERENCES

Bishop, M. L., Duben-Engelkirk, J. L., and Fody, E. P. (Eds.) (2000). *Clinical Chemistry Principles, Procedures, Correlations,* 4th ed. Philadelphia: Lippincott Williams & Wilkins.

Bolyard, E. A., Tablan, O. C., Williams, W. W., Pearson, M. L., Shapiro, C. N., Deitchman, S. D., and The Hospital Infection Control Practices Advisory Committee. *Guidelines for Infection Control in Health Care Personnel, 1998.* American Journal of Infection Control, 1998; 26: 289-354.

Brown, B. A. (1993). *Hematology Principles and Procedures,* 6th ed. Philadelphia: Lea & Febiger.

Burtis, C. A., and Ashwood, E. R. (Eds.) (2001). *Tietz Fundamentals of Clinical Chemistry,* 5th ed. Philadelphia: W. B. Saunders.

Fleming, D. O., Richardson, J. H., Tulis, J. J., and Vesley, D. (1995). *Laboratory Safety, Principles and Practices,* 2nd ed. Washington, DC: ASM Press.

Forbes, B. A., Sahm, D. F., & Weissfeld, A. S. (1998). *Bailey and Scott's Diagnostic Microbiology,* 10th ed. St. Louis: Mosby.

Jamison, R., Noble, M. A., Proctor, E. M., and Smith, J. A. (1996). *Cumitech 29, Laboratory Safety in Clinical Microbiology.* Washington, DC: American Society for Microbiology.

Kaplan, L. A., and Pesce, A. J. (1996). *Clinical Chemistry Theory, Analysis, and Correlation,* 3rd ed. St. Louis: Mosby-Year Book.

Sewel, D. L. (1995). "Laboratory-Associated Infections and Biosafety." *Clin. Microbiol. Rev. 8:389.*

United States Department of Health and Human Services. (1993). *Biosafety in Microbiological and Biomedical Laboratories.* Washington, DC: U.S. Government Printing Office HHS publication (CDC) 93–8395.

11

Laboratory Management

contents

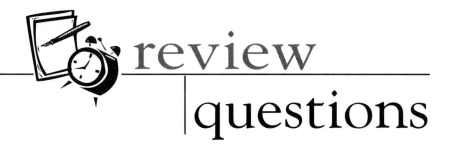
review questions

INSTRUCTIONS Each of the questions or incomplete statements that follow comprises four suggested responses. Select the *best* answer or completion statement in each case.

---

1. What is the Laboratory Management Index Program?
   A. A system to measure productivity and assess laboratory staffing needs
   B. A peer comparison of productivity, use, and financial operation
   C. A method of evaluating equipment, consumables, and labor for equipment selection
   D. A program to develop staffing levels appropriate to numbers of tests performed

2. What section of the clinical laboratory is regulated by the Food and Drug Administration?
   A. Chemistry
   B. Immunohematology
   C. Serology
   D. Hematology

3. The abbreviation MBO stands for which of the following?
   A. Means by objectives
   B. Management by objectives
   C. Management by order
   D. Measurement by objectives

4. A number of management styles are used by supervisors in laboratories. Which of the following is *not* a management style?

   A. Autocratic
   B. Consultative
   C. Formal
   D. Democratic

5. What is the meaning of the abbreviation FTE?
   A. Full-time equivalent
   B. Full-time expenditure
   C. Fixed total expenditure
   D. Fixed-timely equivalency

6. Most laboratories have a definite structure that establishes the formal setup of the various departments and levels. Which of the following refers to this structure?
   A. Administration table
   B. Laboratory directory
   C. Report of contact
   D. Organizational chart

7. In a budget, what terminology is used to describe money spent for a nonexpendable item that has a life expectancy greater than 1 fiscal year?
   A. Expenditure
   B. Annual cost
   C. Capital expenditure
   D. Depreciable item

8. Which governmental legislation has had the greatest impact on the health care industry?
   A. Clinical Laboratory Improvement Act
   B. Medicare and Medicaid
   C. Fair Labor Standards Act
   D. Occupational Safety

9. Which of the following is the process by which a competent public authority grants permission to an organization or an individual to engage in a specific professional practice, occupation, or activity?
   A. Accreditation
   B. Certification
   C. Licensure
   D. Credentialing

10. Scheduling is a responsibility of most laboratory supervisors. Which factor is *not* a consideration in scheduling?
    A. Herzberg guidelines
    B. Laboratory hours
    C. Work load trends
    D. Leave patterns

11. A proper understanding of why a laboratory may become liable for the actions of its personnel requires a basic knowledge of the laws involved. This area is known as tort law and involves three types of wrongful conduct. Which of the following is *not* considered wrongful conduct?
    A. Causation
    B. Intentional acts
    C. Strict liability
    D. Negligence

12. DRG is a commonly used abbreviation. Which of the following statements is *not* associated with DRGs?
    A. Related to Medicare patients
    B. Deals with hospital reimbursement
    C. Used in budgeting and planning
    D. Same system used in every state

13. Which of the following is associated with the outpatient PPS system of reimbursement?
    A. DRG
    B. Capitated rate
    C. APC
    D. PPO

14. Which of the following factors is *not* needed for an effective employee performance appraisal?
    A. Job description
    B. Organization standards
    C. Written evaluation
    D. Employer-employee discussion

15. The College of American Pathologists (CAP) workload recording method is an effective management tool. Which of the following is *not* associated with it?
    A. Measurement of labor-hours with worked and paid productivity
    B. Quality-control device
    C. Capital expenditures
    D. Common rating system used by supervisors

16. Which of the following is invaluable in the budget-making process as related to laboratories?
    A. Comment analysis
    B. Coordinating
    C. Determination of fixed and variable costs
    D. Boost-even analysis

17. Which area of questioning in the interview process is inappropriate or illegal?
    A. References
    B. Age
    C. Organizations
    D. Experience

18. Which of the following should *not* be included in a job description?
    A. Job duties
    B. Position title
    C. Qualifications
    D. Job securities

19. Disciplinary action is a responsibility of supervision. Which of the following characteristics should be included for discipline to be effective and positive?
    A. Public
    B. Casual
    C. Timely
    D. Written

20. What voluntary agency is developing and implementing Blood Bank practices for the clinical laboratory?
    A. OSHA
    B. FDA
    C. AABB
    D. PPS

21. Which of the following is *not* associated with the goals of a laboratory continuing education program?
    A. Staff development
    B. Improvement of laboratory functioning
    C. Compliance with accreditation requirements
    D. Prevention of boredom

22. Which of the following is *not* considered a line item of the laboratory budget?
    A. Labor union dues
    B. Supplies
    C. Maintenance and repair of instruments
    D. Fixed expenses

23. Which of the following agencies is generally responsible for the inspection and accreditation of clinical laboratories in the United States?
    A. JCAHO
    B. NCA
    C. CDC
    D. ASCP

24. What is the strategic process of attracting and maintaining a customer base called?
    A. Marketing
    B. Discretionary factors
    C. Market environment
    D. Product differentiation factors

25. For marketing purposes, which term best describes the laboratory customer?
    A. Captive market
    B. Patient-physician as partners
    C. Discretionary buyer
    D. Person or organization paying the bill

26. Assume that the chemistry analyzer in the laboratory of a 500-bed hospital yields 60,000 profiles per year made up of ten results each. The number of quality-control (QC) tests performed per year numbers 2400, and the total direct labor cost is $1.50 per test. The cost for a year's supply of QC reagents is $3,000. What are the QC direct labor cost per profile and the QC consumable cost per profile respectively?
    A. $0.05, $0.06
    B. $0.06, $0.05
    C. $0.08, $0.05
    D. $0.60, $1.25

27. Your lab has added a new test. It is important that you determine what the break-even point is in the number of tests. The revenue per unit has been $10.00, whereas your fixed cost is $400.00 and your variable cost is $2.00. What is the break-even point, if you expect your net income to be zero (no profit and no loss)?
    A. 45
    B. 48
    C. 50
    D. 52

28. A laboratory has 14,159 total hours paid. Of the total hours paid, 1263 hours are nonproductive hours. Assuming that a full-time employee works 2080 hours annually, what is the total number of FTEs needed to run the laboratory and the number of productive FTEs respectively?
   A. 6.2, 5.8
   B. 6.8, 6.2
   C. 7.4, 6.8
   D. 11.2, 10.2

29. As a result of fraud and abuse identified by the Office of the Inspector General (OIG), what are laboratories required to develop?
   A. Chemical hygiene plan
   B. Compliance plan
   C. PPE plan
   D. Life safety plan

30. Which of the following refers to the portion (percentage) of the cost of an item or service that the Medicare beneficiary must pay?
   A. Deductible
   B. Balance bill
   C. Coinsurance
   D. Reasonable charges

31. Which of the following established the Equal Employment Opportunity Commission (EEOC)?
   A. Title VII of the Civil Rights Act of 1964
   B. Age Discrimination Employment Act of 1967
   C. Rehabilitation Act of 1973
   D. The Equal Pay Act of 1963

32. Which of the following refers to a program where the overall activities conducted by the institution are directed toward assuring the quality of the products and services provided?
   A. Quality control
   B. Quality assurance

C. Total quality management
D. Continuous quality improvement

33. Who introduced the use of statistical tools in decision making, in problem solving, and for troubleshooting the production process?
   A. Philip Crosby
   B. Joseph Juran
   C. James Westgard
   D. Edward Deming

34. Your laboratory is considering expansion. You will have to buy land and build a new lab. One of the financial aspects to consider is the annual depreciation of the project. The total cost of the project is $800,000 ($200,000 for the land and $600,000 for the building). At current estimates, the building is expected to be used for 20 years, with a salvage value of $40,000. What is the annual depreciation of the project?
   A. $38,000/year
   B. $30,000/year
   C. $28,000/year
   D. $10,000/year

35. What process is designed to measure the value (level of success) of performing diagnostic tests and other services related to the improvement of a patient's disease or condition?
   A. Clinical pathways
   B. Outcomes assessment
   C. Clinical practice guidelines
   D. Quality assurance

36. Which category of personnel is required in laboratories performing tests using high-complexity methodology?
   A. General supervisor
   B. Clinical consultant
   C. Technical consultant
   D. Director

37. The standard operating procedure manual (SOPM) contains all the following *except*
    A. Literature references
    B. Control procedures
    C. Reference ranges
    D. Personnel requirements

38. When a manager does not possess the expertise or knowledge to implement change and the resisters have significant power to impede the efforts, which strategy for change will be used?
    A. Facilitation and support
    B. Participation and involvement
    C. Negotiation and agreement
    D. Manipulation and co-optation

39. The struggle is underway, and the behavior of the participants makes the existence of the conflict apparent to others who are not directly involved. What is this stage of conflict known as?
    A. Perceived
    B. Felt
    C. Manifest
    D. Latent

40. Influence exerted through the control of support services, such as a safety officer or quality assurance coordinator, which provide recommendations to the manager and set policies, is a type of authority known as
    A. Staff
    B. Line
    C. Formal
    D. Functional

41. What is horizontal communication?
    A. The official communication message generated by the business activities of the organization
    B. The formal messages that are channeled through the hierarchical network of the organization
    C. The activity that occurs during the normal conduct of business among departments, managers, and staff
    D. Live discourse in which all parties exchange ideas and information and receive spontaneous feedback

42. Which agency develops and monitors engineering and work practice controls?
    A. CDC
    B. OSHA
    C. JCAHO
    D. CAP

43. Which of the following refers to the continuum of care under one common computerized communication channel that links hospitals, labs, pharmacies, physicians, employers, payers, and medical information systems?
    A. Common Healthcare Integrated Network
    B. Continuum Health Internal Network
    C. Community Health Information Network
    D. Computerized Health Information Network

44. Which budgeting process attempts to set expenditures on a variable workload volume?
    A. Operational
    B. Capital
    C. Zero-based
    D. Flexible

45. In addition to preparing a capital budget for the institution's own use, federal and state regulations require health care facilities to submit capital plans on certain projects for approval and to obtain a
    A. Certificate of Approval
    B. Certificate of Need
    C. Capital Budget Appropriation
    D. Capital Need Assessment

46. What will be the payback period for a new chemistry analyzer, costing $150,000 and producing an annual income of $420,000?
    A. 2.3 months
    B. 2.8 months
    C. 4.3 months
    D. 33.6 months

47. The total cost per test can be determined by adding together all the following *except*
    A. Direct and indirect labor
    B. Direct and indirect materials
    C. Equipment and overhead costs
    D. Depreciation and equipment costs

48. All the following are roles of a team leader *except*
    A. Leading all team activities
    B. Teaching problem-solving techniques to team members
    C. Keeping records of team activities and progress
    D. Providing guidance for group activities

49. What is the primary coding system that is used by the federal government to determine levels of reimbursement for Medicare services?
    A. CPT codes
    B. HCPCS codes
    C. Modifiers
    D. ICD–9 codes

50. Your laboratory wants to buy a new hematology analyzer. In determining the total cost per test analysis, you need to know what the cost will be for equipment per test. The analyzer costs $55,000 and has a useful life of 7 years. After the one-year warranty expires the annual maintenance contract will cost $8,000. You estimate that you will perform 3500 tests per year on this analyzer. What is the equipment cost for each test performed?
    A. $1.38
    B. $2.10
    C. $2.81
    D. $4.53

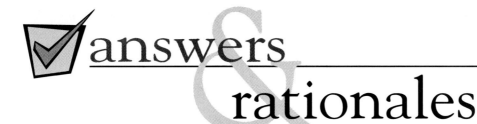

answers & rationales

1.

B. The Laboratory Management Index Program is a peer comparison program of productivity, use, and financial operation. It is a structured approach to laboratory management using a series of ratios derived from daily operational data. The program was to step past the traditional workload unit and look to a broader approach for evaluating management performance. The program was to integrate use and cost-effectiveness programs, be simple to collect, and generate only essential data with clear target monitors that permit continuous quality improvement (CQI) of management decisions.

2.

B. Immunohematology (blood bank) is the only laboratory section that is regulated by the Food and Drug Administration (FDA). The FDA enforces the Food, Drug, and Cosmetic Act. This act regulates the preparation of blood and blood products as well as the facilities, including hospital laboratories and transfusion services, where preparation occurs.

3.

B. Management by objectives (MBO) is a management system developed in the 1950s and widely used by many organizations, laboratories, and businesses. MBO uses various management concepts of planning, participation, motivation, and controlling. This system uses performance objectives as a means of accomplishing management goals.

4.

C. The word formal is not descriptive of the type of leadership style used by laboratory managers. Au-

tocratic, consultative, persuasive, and democratic are words that describe the styles routinely used, although rarely as purely one style; instead, a combination of various styles is used generally. Managers who are autocratic hold Theory X philosophies and allow for little input from their staff. Managers who are democratic are Theory Y managers and are participatory in their leadership style, actively seek advice and counsel from their coworkers, and allow employees to share in the decision-making process. Various factors such as the situation, the individuals concerned, and the complexity of concepts involved will determine what is appropriate.

5.

A. Full-time equivalent (FTE) is a term routinely used by every laboratory, particularly during the budget process. An FTE equals 2080 person-hours paid in 1 year's time. An FTE combines productive hours and nonproductive hours, i.e., vacation, holiday, and sick time. The FTE is based on a 40-hour workweek and is more easily used in a discussion of personnel and hours worked. In one FTE, one full-time person or two or more part-time persons may occupy the 40-hour position.

6.

D. The organizational chart shows the lines of supervision, relationships of various staff members, and interrelationships of the various departments. There are generally three types of organizational charts: vertical, horizontal, and circular. Most hospital administrations use the vertical chart, which is a summary or a snapshot of the structure of the organization. It is also used by many levels of laboratory management.

7.

C. The term capital expenditure refers to the money spent for nonexpendable items having a life expectancy of more than 1 fiscal year. Capital expenditures are generally for permanent items of equipment and laboratory improvements in the physical setup of the laboratory. Very often such equipment items are high-cost items and require the approval of the institution's budgetary administration.

8.

B. Although the other items have had an impact on health care today, the Medicare and Medicaid legislation of 1966 has had the greatest influence on the industry because it determines the reimbursement of health care services. This legislation provides a mechanism for financing the health care of elderly persons and poor persons. In 1960, the federal government financed 9.3% of health care. In 1984, 29.6% of all health care expenditures was paid by the federal government through Medicare and Medicaid, and this figure continues to rise.

9.

C. Requiring a license is the most restrictive form of government regulation of professional practice. Licensure makes it illegal for an unlicensed organization or individual to provide a professional service within a scope of practice that is defined by statute. Licensing is designed to protect the public from inadequate manufacturing practice and incompetent practitioners.

10.

A. Laboratory hours, procedures offered, workload trends, and leave patterns are important factors to consider in the scheduling process. In addition, the physical design of the facility, financial considerations, the abilities and qualifications of personnel involved, and the ratio of urgent procedures to routine work should be considered. Herzberg, a psychologist, dealt with job satisfaction and motivation, which are not pertinent to scheduling.

11.

A. Causation is the act or process of causing that which is needed in order for a lawsuit to be initiated. Wrongful conduct is cause for a lawsuit. Intentional acts are those that a person intends to commit and intends to result in harm to someone else. Negligent acts are defined as the failure to do something that a reasonable person, guided by the considerations that ordinarily regulate human affairs, would do or not do. Strict liability applies to product liability and to the performance of a service.

12.

D. DRG stands for diagnostic related group. These groups of diagnoses were developed by the federal government in the 1970s and adopted in the 1980s. The groupings provide a method of determining reimbursement for Medicare patient care by the federal government and have been used by hospital management for budgeting and planning. Several states (e.g., New Jersey, Maryland) are using a slightly different or modified version.

13.

C. On August 1, 2000, HCFA and the OIG (Office of Inspector General) instituted the use of an outpatient prospective payment system (PPS) known as APC (Ambulatory Payment Classification). Mandated by the Omnibus Budget Reconciliation Act (OBRA) of 1990, APCs comprise an outpatient PPS that parallels the inpatient DRGs. PPS rates are established for each group of services provided in hospital outpatient departments for the diagnosis and treatment of Medicare beneficiaries. Services are grouped by the APC groups, which categorize services according to similarity of clinical diagnosis and resource use. The capitated rate is a fixed rate of reimbursement for health care organizations to a minimum amount per covered life. This is a process used by managed care organizations and insurers. Under capitation, a payer pays a provider a fixed amount for each member of the plan who is assigned to receive services (laboratory, radiology, cardiology, etc.) during any given month.

14.

B. A good performance appraisal should include a complete job description, performance standards based on the job description, and a regularly scheduled evaluation using the first two factors. The performance appraisal system as a whole should combine the evaluation process with a thorough discussion with the employee once he/she has had time to review the written evaluation. The appraisal should occur on a regular basis, usually once a year.

15.

C. The College of American Pathologists (CAP) workload recording method is a tool used to provide a database that will assist in cost accounting and in projecting future needs. The system measures the productive time expended by technical and clerical staff members as they perform laboratory procedures. It measures both worked and paid productivity.

16.

C. Cost analysis, forecasting, determination of fixed and variable costs, and break-even analysis are all parts of the budget-making process. These tools must be used in the determination of all costs before any intelligent forecast or budget can be made. All have become increasingly important in today's climate of stringent reimbursement methods.

17.

B. Questions regarding race, age, and child care needs are all inappropriate in an interview; only the applicant's experience is relevant. There are many other areas, such as marital status, arrests, credit history, religious affiliation, and spouse's occupation, that also should not be discussed. Education and past employment experience, as well as interests and short- and long-range plans, are appropriate areas in which to concentrate.

18.

D. Job descriptions will vary from one institution to another. However, the position title, job responsibilities, necessary qualifications, and job relationships should be part of any job description. Some other aspects that may also be covered include immediate supervisor, limitations or hazards, training, working conditions, skills, shift worked, and section or division assigned.

19.

C. Positive discipline should involve privacy, be timely, and be progressive, although it is not necessary that it be in a written format. Discipline can be informal and oral in the early stages, and it should always be private. Disciplinary action may progress through the following stages: oral, informal talk; oral warning or reprimand; written warn-

ing; disciplinary layoff or similar penalty; demotional downgrading; and discharge.

20.

C. The Food and Drug Administration (FDA) is the only compulsory agency that currently develops and implements standards and practices for blood banks. The American Association of Blood Banks (AABB) is also an agency that performs these functions but it is a voluntary, not compulsory, program. The Occupational Safety and Health Administration addresses safety practices in the laboratory overall, but does not develop specific practices for blood banks. The Prospective Payment System has to do with Medicare reimbursement and is not an agency dealing with blood banks.

21.

D. Staff development that generally improves the capabilities of the laboratory worker, improvement of laboratory functioning through in-service programs, and the meeting of accreditation requirements are important goals of a continuing education program. These goals may be accomplished by means of seminars, journal clubs, lectures, workshops, and so forth. Participation in continuing education programs is the responsibility of every laboratory professional and should be maintained throughout the career.

22.

A. Employee salaries, supplies, repair and maintenance of instruments, and fixed expenses are line items in a laboratory budget. Also considered as line items are employee benefits, purchased services, allocations, and miscellaneous expenses. The aforementioned items can be further broken down into smaller, more specific components; for example, employee benefits include such items as life and health insurance, vacations, holidays, sick leave, and pensions.

23.

A. The Joint Commission on Accreditation of Health Care Organizations (JCAHO) and the College of American Pathologists (CAP) are two nongovernmental agencies that accredit hospitals and associated laboratories. The JCAHO oversees the entire hospital facility, whereas the CAP accredits only clinical laboratories. These accreditation systems consist of their own set of predetermined qualifications or standards that each laboratory must meet to receive accreditation. CAP inspects clinical laboratories every 2 years, and JCAHO inspects hospital and clinical laboratories every 3 years.

24.

A. Marketing, as a specific function of management, may be defined as the strategic process of attracting and maintaining a customer base. Without success in this area, the very survival of the organization may be placed in jeopardy. Marketing has to do with how the laboratory deals with the new reimbursement and the restructuring of the laboratory delivery system.

25.

C. There is no question that the person toward whom the laboratory directs its professional concerns is the patient. However, the laboratory must also identify the customer—the entity that sends the patient to the laboratory. The discretionary buyer is the entity that decides where a service is performed. The discretionary buyer may be the patient, a physician, a third-party payer, or even another institution. Market research shows that the mother is usually the one who decides where the family receives medical care. For this reason much of health care's promotional focus is on the mother and on women in general and associated family issues.

26.

B. Product costs are an integral part of cost accounting. Labor and consumables are product costs. To calculate the cost per test of a particular assay you must include quality control (QC) material as part of the total cost to perform a particular assay. When calculating the QC direct labor cost per test you need to know the total number of QC tests performed each year, the total profiles performed per year, and the total direct labor cost. Therefore, the QC direct labor cost per profile would be:

$$\frac{(2{,}400 \times \$1.50)}{60{,}000} = \$0.06/\text{profile}$$

To calculate the QC consumable costs you need to know the cost for a year's supply of QC reagents and the total profiles performed per year. Therefore, the QC consumable cost per profile would be:

$$\frac{\$3{,}000}{60{,}000} = \$0.05/\text{profile}$$

27.

C. Break-even analysis is used to determine how many units or in this case tests must run to recoup your costs (both fixed and variable) and make your net income (in this case, zero). A laboratory might use this to see how much a new test would cost them to implement. The formula to calculate the break-even point is as follows:

$$rx = vx + f + c$$

where

r = revenue per unit
x = break-even point
v = variable costs
f = fixed costs
c = net income

For this particular problem, the values are

x = break-even point—this is the unknown that you are trying to determine
r = $10.00 per test
v = $2.00
f = $400.00
c = 0 (net income with no profit and no loss)

So

$$10(x) = 2(x) + 400 + 0$$
$$10x - 2x = 400$$
$$8x = 400$$
$$x = 50$$

The laboratory would have to perform a minimum of 50 tests to reach the break-even point and meet both the fixed and variable costs. Once the lab determines that the test should be included in its menu, the next step might be to determine what net income is necessary to maintain the test.

28.

B. An important concept in salary and wage management is the calculation of full-time equivalents (FTEs), which can be used for setting and measuring budgeting and staffing goals. To calculate FTEs, divide the number of hours (total = productive and nonproductive) by 2080, the number of hours a full-time person works in 1 year (40 hours per week × 52 weeks = 2080). In this example in order to calculate the total FTE needed you need to know the total hours paid and the number of hours an FTE works in a year.

$$\frac{14{,}159 \text{ total hours paid}}{2080 \text{ hours/person}} = 6.8 \text{ total FTEs}$$

To calculate the productive FTE you need to know the productive hours worked. This is determined by

14,159 total hours paid − 1263 nonproductive hours
= 12,896 productive hours

The number of productive FTEs equals:

$$\frac{12{,}896 \text{ productive hours}}{2080 \text{ hours/person}} = 6.2 \text{ productive FTEs}$$

29.
B. The Office of the Inspector General (OIG) and other federal agencies charged with responsibility for enforcement of federal law have emphasized the importance of voluntarily developed and implemented compliance plans. In recent years, the OIG has been asked to supply guidance as to the elements of a model compliance plan. The purpose of this issuance, therefore, is to respond to those requests by providing some guidance to health care providers that supply clinical laboratory testing services for Medicare and Medicaid beneficiaries.

30.
C. Coinsurance is the portion of the cost of an item or service that the Medicare beneficiary must pay. Currently, the Medicare Part B coinsurance is generally 20% of the reasonable charge for the item or service. Typically, if the Medicare reasonable charge for a Part B item or service is $100, the Medicare beneficiary (who has met the deductible) must pay $20 of the physician's bill and Medicare will pay $80.

31.
A. The Equal Employment Opportunity Commission (EEOC) was established by Title VII of the Civil Rights Act of 1964 and began operating on July 2, 1965. The EEOC enforces the principal federal statutes prohibiting employment discrimination, including Title VII of the Civil Rights Act of 1964, the Age Discrimination in Employment Act of 1967, the Equal Pay Act of 1963, Title I of the Americans with Disabilities Act (ADA) of 1990, and Section 501 of the Rehabilitation Act of 1973.

32.
B. Quality assurance (QA) developed out of the limitations of the QC approach and defined quality in health care institutions by the success of the total organization, not just individual components of the system, in achieving the goals of patient care. When introduced by the JCAHO in 1980, quality assurance was defined as the overall activities conducted by the institution that are directed toward assuring the quality of services provided. QA focuses on the recipient—namely, the patient.

33.
D. Edward Deming is often credited with providing the Japanese with the information and training that brought them to their position as the world's leader in the production of quality products. A statistician who worked with Walter Shewhart, he introduced the use of statistical tools in decision making, problem solving, and troubleshooting the production process. Deming is also frequently cited as the source of most of the concepts and methods contained in the Total Quality Management (TQM) model.

34.
C. Straight-line depreciation is a method based on the time element. As a product grows older, its value decreases and maintenance costs increase. This method can be used for all capital items, but it is usually used to establish depreciation rates for buildings and other structures with an extended life expectancy (i.e., greater than 10 years). Land is considered to last forever and is never depreciated. Therefore:

$$\text{Annual depreciation} = \frac{\text{cost of project} - \text{salvage value}}{\text{Life expectancy}}$$

$$\text{Annual depreciation} = \frac{\$800{,}000 - (\$200{,}000 + \$40{,}000)}{20 \text{ years}}$$
$$= \frac{\$800{,}000 - \$240{,}000}{20 \text{ years}}$$
$$= \$28{,}000/\text{year}$$

35.
B. Clinical practice guidelines are published by professional medical groups, insurers, federal agencies and departments, and other groups that

recommend when a selected medical procedure, test, or practice should be used. Clinical pathways are developed by hospitals for specific diseases or conditions (e.g., pneumonia, hip replacement) by the medical staff and other health care personnel. They may include some of those practice guidelines determining what test, procedure, or practice should be used when treating a patient with that disease or condition, so that quality treatment is consistent from patient to patient. Quality assurance is a program in which the overall activities conducted by the hospital are directed toward assuring the quality of the products and services provided. The outcomes assessment is used to measure the value of the clinical practice guidelines, clinical pathways, and quality assurance program that the hospital has decided to put in place.

36.

A. A general supervisor, who must be responsible for day-to-day supervision, is stipulated for laboratories doing high-complexity testing. This is a laboratorian with an associate's degree or higher in medical laboratory technology and two years of training and experience in a high-complexity laboratory. The director and technical consultant must be a doctoral-level scientist with an appropriate laboratory specialty or a physician with training or experience in laboratory medicine. A physician or doctoral-level clinical scientist may provide the services of a clinical consultant.

37.

D. Personnel requirements are not required to be part of the Standard Operating Procedure Manual (SOPM). Tests are categorized by waived, moderate-complexity, and high-complexity. The type of personnel allowed to perform testing is determined by these categories as described by the Clinical Laboratory Improvement Act (CLIA) of 1988.

38.

B. Participation and involvement allow subordinates to be part of the planning or implementation of change. It is an excellent method when the manager does not possess the expertise or knowledge to implement change himself and the resisters have significant power to impede his efforts. Participation often generates commitment by the participants to the change process. This approach can also result in time-consuming compromise that does not fit the organizational needs. It must be handled carefully, because once a decision has been made by the group it is difficult for the manager to push it aside.

39.

C. Conflict does not usually appear overnight. It often festers without the knowledge of the recipient party. Conflict usually passes through several progressive stages before it manifests itself to others. The parties may be at different stages of the conflict cycle, which complicates management of conflict. The manager must have a keen sensitivity to and understanding of his/her work environment to deal effectively with conflict at all stages.

40.

A. Staff authority is exercised through such positions as the lab safety officer or quality assurance coordinator—those areas that provide supportive services in a more indirect fashion, where ability to implement change depends on the action of the section supervisors. They exercise their influence by making recommendations, providing specific support services, giving assistance and advice in technical areas, facilitating paperwork and other procedures, and developing general lab policies. Line authority is supervisory responsibility assigned through the formal delegation of authority—in the lab this is from administration to department head to supervisor to staff. Functional authority is the power to enforce directives, such as physician's medical orders, within the context and boundaries of a clearly defined specialty and span of control. Formal authority is the official, sanctioned lines of authority assigned by the owners of the organization.

41.

C. Members of organizations receive communications from two sources, formal and informal. Formal comes from two directions in a company—from above or below. Vertical communications take the form of memos and other directives that come down through the bureaucratic hierarchy and the responses and other information that make their way back up through the same network. Horizontal communication occurs in the course of the normal exchange of services, information, and work orders, when managers and staff talk to each other as peers.

42.

B. Engineering and work practice controls involve taking physical steps to isolate or remove any possible pathogen hazards from the workplace. The Occupational Safety and Health Administration (OSHA) requires specific engineering action by employers. Some primary areas where these actions are required include hand-washing facilities, needles and sharps, and procedures that minimize splashing, spraying, and generating aerosols. Although work practice controls are developed by OSHA, the Joint Commission on Accreditation of Health Care Organizations (JCAHO) and the College of American Pathologists (CAP) also require that these work practice controls be in place to become accredited. The Centers for Disease Control (CDC), just like any other lab, is required to follow the same work practice controls.

43.

C. The Community Health Information Network (CHIN) links all health care participants involved in the continuum of care under one computerized communication channel. This channel, or electronic highway, serves as the information's translation medium. It enables members of the health care community to talk to one another without leaving their computer terminals, learning another computer language, or buying another computer system. A sophisticated security system allows only authorized users to access information contained in various databases at its members' systems.

44.

D. At a certain patient census, the hospital should have a specific number of employees. When the number of patients increases, more staff is hired; when the census drops, employees are laid off. In practice this has been difficult to implement because of recruitment and retention problems. Even supplies must be ordered in advance to ensure adequate levels. For this reason, a flexible budget similar to the forecast method is prepared and then closely monitored to ensure that projections are on target.

45.

B. The process of submitting capital plans for governmental approval is required for projects, equipment, or buildings above an established monetary level. Most states have set this limit at $150,000, following federal guidelines. A Certificate of Need (CON) must also be obtained before new services such as oncology or obstetrics can be offered. This program was established in an attempt to control medical costs and to avoid duplication of services and the overbuilding of hospital beds.

46.

C. Payback period = *P/I,* where *P* = purchase price of project and *I* = annual income generated. Many investors and lenders perform this calculation to determine the length of time needed to recover their investment. Businesses use this same formula to assist in determining the affordability of a project. By the nature of the business, laboratory instruments need a relatively shorter payback period because of the rapid technological obsolescence in the field.

$$\text{Payback period} = \frac{\$150,000}{\$420,000/\text{year}}$$
$$= 0.36 \text{ year} \times \frac{12 \text{ months}}{1 \text{ year}}$$
$$= 4.3 \text{ months}$$

47.

D. Depreciation is not part of the total cost per test but is part of the overall budget. The way depreciation is determined and recorded has a direct impact on the financial status of the company as a whole. The total cost per test can be determined by adding together direct and indirect labor, direct and indirect materials, and equipment and overhead costs. Direct labor cost includes the cost of technical personnel who actually perform the testing. Indirect labor cost represents the cost of all other laboratory support and supervisory personnel. Direct material includes reagents, sample cups, and pipette tips. Indirect material cost encompasses the cost of shared equipment and supplies that cannot be directly allocated to individual tests, such as the cost of the LIS, centrifuge, or refrigerator. Overhead cost includes the hospital's allocation for utilities, housekeeping, administration, and other costs.

48.

C. The team leader, to be successful, must be knowledgeable of the project area and possess the skills for getting cooperation from multiskilled and multidisciplinary team members. It is helpful if the team leader comes from the unit most impacted by the problem to be solved. Keeping records of team activities and progress is the role of the facilitator. The facilitator is an internal consultant, specializing in the quality process, who works with several team leaders.

49.

B. The HCPCS codes (HCFA Common Procedural Coding System) are broken down into three levels: Level I, II, and III. The CPT is actually Level I of the HCPCS codes. CPT is authored by the American Medical Association and, therefore, most codes are historically identified physician provided procedures. To supplement these codes, the HCFA established Level II HCPCS codes. Level II codes are alphanumeric, five-digit codes that are nationally recognized. Level III codes are assigned by local carriers to fill voids in CPT and Level II codes. They are also alphanumeric, five-digit codes and may only be used when billing the carrier that assigned them. ICD-9 codes, which are numeric codes, identify diagnoses. They relate to signs, symptoms, and conditions; their use is important in substantiating procedural orders. Modifiers are attached to CPT codes to further describe a procedure. They can be alpha or numeric in nature. An example used in lab procedures is modifier "91," indicating that the same procedure was performed more than once on the same date of service.

50.

D. Equipment cost is an essential part of determining the total cost per test. In order to determine the equipment cost per test, you need to know the cost of the equipment, the useful life of the equipment, the annual maintenance cost, and the estimated number of tests to be performed by the equipment you want to purchase.

$$\text{Equipment cost} = \frac{[(E/L) + M]}{A}$$

where

E = Cost of equipment

L = Useful life

M = Maintenance costs

A = Annual tests performed

Equipment cost =

$$\frac{[(\$55,000/7) + \$8000]}{3500} = \$4.53$$

REFERENCES

Nigon, D. L. (2000). *Clinical Laboratory Management: Leadership Principles for the 21st Century.* New York: McGraw-Hill.

O'Brien, J. A. (2000). *Common Problems in Clinical Laboratory Management.* New York: McGraw-Hill.

Snyder, J. R., and Wilkinson, D. S. (1998). *Management in Laboratory Medicine,* 3rd ed. Philadelphia: Lippincott-Raven.

Varnadoe, L. A. (1996). *Medical Laboratory Management and Supervision: Operations, Review, and Study Guide.* Philadelphia: F. A. Davis.

CHAPTER

12

Education

contents

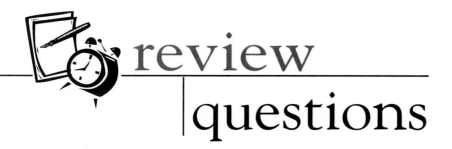

review
questions

INSTRUCTIONS Each of the questions or incomplete statements that follow comprises four suggested responses. Select the *best* answer or completion statement in each case.

---

1. In studies of effective teachers, what personal quality is consistently rated the highest by students?
   A. Enthusiasm
   B. Sense of humor
   C. Self-confidence
   D. Friendliness

2. The statement, "The curriculum is designed to prepare graduates to develop procedures for the analysis of biological specimens," is an example of a(n)
   A. Course description
   B. Goal
   C. Task analysis
   D. Objective

3. The statement, "Given a hemacytometer, the student will perform manual red cell counts with 90% accuracy," is an example of a(n)
   A. Course description
   B. Goal
   C. Task analysis
   D. Objective

4. Which of the following represents an action verb?
   A. Appreciate
   B. Diagram

C. Know
D. Realize

5. Of the major domains for behavioral objectives, which domain contains objectives involving values and attitudes?
   A. Affective
   B. Analytical
   C. Cognitive
   D. Psychomotor

6. Which of the taxonomic levels in the cognitive domain is represented by the following objective?
   Objective: Given the glucose control values for a month, the student will calculate the mean and standard deviation.
   A. Knowledge
   B. Comprehension
   C. Application
   D. Analysis

7. What part of the following statement represents the conditions of the objective?
   Objective: Given the appropriate tools and written procedure, the student will perform daily maintenance on the chemistry analyzer without error.

A. Given the appropriate tools and written procedure

B. The student will perform daily maintenance on the chemistry analyzer

C. The student will

D. Without error

8. A name tag reads: "Jane Smith, MT(ASCP), CLS(NCA)." What does this tell us about Jane Smith's professional credentials? She is
   A. Accredited
   B. Certified
   C. Licensed
   D. Registered

9. Which of the following terms refers to the voluntary process by which an agency evaluates a medical technology program and recognizes that it has met certain preset standards?
   A. Accreditation
   B. Certification
   C. Licensure
   D. Registration

10. An instructor observes a medical technology student cheating on an examination. What is the best action to take?
    A. Ignore the behavior because the student is hurting only himself/herself
    B. Stop the examination and collect all the papers
    C. Document the incident, but do not report it unless it is repeated
    D. Document the incident and report it to the appropriate authority

11. Which of the following activities is associated with Problem-Based Learning (PBL)?
    A. The learner determines what information needs to be learned
    B. The instructor serves as a facilitator

C. The learner identifies the appropriate educational resources

D. All the above

12. Which of the following is an advantage of the lecture method?
    A. Useful for teaching technical skills
    B. Student is an active participant
    C. Pace is controlled by the learner
    D. Disseminates large amounts of information

13. What is one of the most common problems encountered with use of overhead transparencies?
    A. Classroom kept dark when they are used
    B. Contain too much information
    C. Take long time to prepare
    D. Difficult to design

14. Why are computer-projected visual aids a benefit to the instructor?
    A. Classroom is not dark or dim when they are used
    B. Do not require special projection equipment
    C. Motion, color, and sound can be incorporated
    D. Inexpensive to produce

15. Role-playing is designed to strengthen skills in which educational domain?
    A. Affective
    B. Psychomotor
    C. Aesthetic
    D. Cognitive

16. What is the key to teaching more and having it remembered better?
    A. Frequent testing
    B. Organization
    C. Small class size
    D. Distance education

17. Which of the following tests assesses a student's performance on an examination independent of peer performance?
    A. Norm-referenced
    B. Objective-referenced
    C. Criterion-referenced
    D. Standard-referenced

18. The ASCP Board of Registry certification examination is an example of which of the following types of tests?
    A. Placement
    B. Formative
    C. Summative
    D. Diagnostic

19. Which of the following refers to the contract between an academic institution and a clinical education site that describes the responsibilities of the institutions and the rights of students?
    A. Accreditation agreement
    B. Affiliation agreement
    C. Education contract
    D. Clinical policy statement

20. The evaluation tool that monitors the steps comprising a technical procedure is called a
    A. Checklist
    B. Rating scale
    C. List of objectives
    D. Practical exam

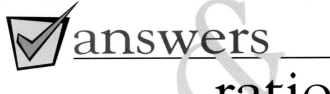

answers & rationales

1.

A. The personal quality of an effective teacher that is rated the highest is enthusiasm. Teachers who are enthusiastic about teaching and about the material presented are able to stimulate students' interest in the subject being taught. Other characteristics of effective teachers include knowledge and organization of the subject matter and skills in instruction and evaluation.

2.

B. Goals describe what a learner will be able to do and are written in general terms and do not describe behaviors. An objective is a statement that describes what a learner will be able to do at the end of a unit of instruction. A task analysis is a description of the knowledge and skills needed for competence in the work setting. Course descriptions differ from objectives in that the former do not describe what the learner is expected to achieve but give information about course content.

3.

D. An objective is a statement that describes what a learner will be able to do at the end of a unit of instruction. Goals also describe what the learner will be able to do; however, they are written in general terms and do not describe behaviors. A task analysis is a description of the knowledge and skills needed for competence in the work setting. Course descriptions differ from objectives in that the former do not describe what the learner is expected to achieve but give information about course content.

4.

B. Action verbs describe an activity that is observable and measurable. Using action verbs in writing objectives clearly conveys the instructor's expectations of students. Verbs that are more general, such as appreciate, know, and realize do not describe performances that are measurable; they may be used for goals.

5.

A. Objectives have been classified into three major domains: cognitive, affective, and psychomotor. The cognitive domain includes those objectives that emphasize the intellect. Cognitive behavior includes the recall of information, the comprehension of that information, and the processes of application, analysis, synthesis, and evaluation. The affective domain includes those objectives that emphasize values and attitudes, such as the importance of maintaining patient confidentiality and the desire to follow laboratory safety procedures. The psychomotor domain deals with those behavior outcomes that require neuromuscular function, such as the actual performance of a laboratory procedure.

6.

C. At the application level, the student is taking previously learned material and using it to resolve a problem such as a calculation. Knowledge is the lowest level of cognitive learning and involves simply recalling learned material. At the comprehension level, the student grasps the meaning of the material but does not see the fullest implication of that material. Analysis represents higher

answers & rationales

495

levels of learning in which the student understands the organization of the material and can reorganize the component parts so that they form a new pattern or structure.

7.

A. The conditions in an objective ("Given the appropriate tools and written procedure") describe what will be provided or denied to the student in order to accomplish the objective. Other parts of an objective include the terminal behavior required by the learner ("the student will perform daily maintenance on the chemistry analyzer") and the standards of performance ("without error"). The terminal behavior addresses what the learner must be able to do after completing the instructional unit. The standards of performance indicate how well the learner must perform for an acceptable behavior.

8.

B. The initials MT(ASCP), CLS(NCA) indicate that Jane Smith is certified by the American Society of Clinical Pathologists as a medical technologist and by the National Credentialing Agency for Laboratory Personnel, Inc., as a clinical laboratory scientist. Certification is the process by which an individual's qualifications are recognized by a nongovernmental organization or agency. It is a voluntary process and usually involves meeting specific academic requirements and passing an examination.

9.

A. The National Accrediting Agency for Clinical Laboratory Sciences (NAACLS) is responsible for the evaluation and recommendation of accreditation of medical technology programs after self-study and the site visit. The term certification refers to the process by which an individual's competence is recognized by a nongovernmental agency or association. Licensure is the process by which a governmental agency grants an individual the permission to work in a certain field after successful completion of an examination. The term registration refers to the process by which individuals are identified by an agency as being certified.

10.

D. An instructor should be familiar with the institution's procedure for handling cheating and should follow established guidelines when cheating is de-

tected. Ignoring the problem or assigning a failing grade does not help the student. Ignoring the problem will also damage the morale of the other students, who are often aware when an individual is cheating.

11.

D. Problem-based learning is designed for the instructor to serve as a facilitator in the learning process. The goal for students is to resolve problems, develop critical thinking skills, and learn team communication skills. The students determine what information is needed to solve the problems posed and select the appropriate resources.

12.

D. The lecture format is good for disseminating large amounts of information to the learner. It is the most popular learning format and is useful for bringing together information from a variety of sources. It can be limiting, however, due to the lack of involvement of the learner.

13.

B. Overhead transparencies represent a very useful and versatile audiovisual teaching aid. They are easy to prepare and can be used in a lighted room while the instructor faces the audience. A common problem with overhead transparencies is that they contain too much information. Overhead transparencies should be designed with brief, concise highpoints and simple graphics.

14.

C. The addition of motion, color, and sound to visual media facilitates the learning process by stimulating interest, and they are attention grabbing. Grab a student's interest and attention, and the motivation to learn will follow. Classrooms are typically darkened when computer projected visual aids are used. They require special projection equipment and that equipment is usually costly.

15.

A. Role-playing represents a learning format that is specifically designed to promote cooperative problem solving and communication skills. For these reasons, role-playing is useful for developing learning outcomes in the affective domain. Role-playing is especially effective when it represents a situation that the student will be likely to encounter in the future.

16.

B. Students can learn more when educational sessions are organized. The communication of volumes of facts without organization is unlikely to be effective. In an ideally organized lesson, the students will be one step ahead of the instructor.

17.

C. Criterion-referenced examinations test a student for mastery of a skill or body of knowledge with the use of predetermined minimal standards. Unlike a traditional norm-referenced test, in which students compete with one another on test performance, it is possible and even desirable for all students to do well on a criterion-referenced test. Examples of criterion-referenced examinations are the certification examinations of the Board of Registry of ASCP (American Society of Clinical Pathologists) and the National Credentialing Agency for Laboratory Personnel, Inc. (NCA).

18.

C. The certification examination of the Board of Registry of ASCP is an example of a summative test, because it is comprehensive and designed to assess the mastery of a body of material. Placement tests are designed to test for prerequisite skills necessary for a course of study. Formative tests are administered during a course of study and allow the student to assess his knowledge at that time. Diagnostic tests are administered to aid in defining learning disabilities.

19.

B. The National Accrediting Agency for Clinical Laboratory Sciences (NAACLS) essentials require affiliation agreements between academic institutions and clinical education sites. The affiliation agreement describes the responsibilities between the two institutions. Its purpose is to ensure a quality learning experience for the students.

20.

A. A checklist is a list of statements describing the student behaviors that comprise a particular task or procedure. The behaviors are checked to indicate whether or not they occurred. A checklist is differentiated from a rating scale by its "all or none" format.

REFERENCES

Beck, S. J., and LeGrys, V. L. (1996). *Clinical Laboratory Education,* 2nd ed. Dubuque, Iowa: Kendall/ Hunt Publishing Co.

McKeachie, W. J. (1994). *Teaching Tips: Strategies, Research, and Theory for College and University Teachers,* 9th ed. Lexington, MA: D. C. Heath.

Wallace, M. A., and Klosinski, D. D. (1998). *Clinical Laboratory Science Education & Management.* Philadelphia: W. B. Saunders.

Wilkinson, I. (1998). *Super Seminars, Legendary Lectures, and Perfect Posters, The Science of Presenting Well.* Washington, DC: AACC Press.

13 Computers and Laboratory Informatics

contents

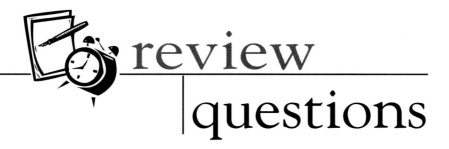
review questions

INSTRUCTIONS Each of the questions or incomplete statements that follow comprises
four suggested responses. Select the *best* answer or completion statement in each case.

1. How many bits are in a byte?
   A. 2
   B. 4
   C. 8
   D. 16

2. A computer's processor is regulated by the system clock and is measured in megahertz. What is the clock speed?
   A. Number of intervals or cycles per second
   B. Memory storage capacity on the microprocessor
   C. Memory storage capacity of the hard drive
   D. Communication speed between the microprocessor and the motherboard

3. An open laboratory information system is a system with
   A. Terminals located outside the laboratory
   B. Software able to run on servers from different vendors
   C. A graphical user interface
   D. Minimal security

4. What type of file will provide the best conservation of memory space for the storage of patient demographic data?
   A. Random-access
   B. Sequential
   C. Hard
   D. ROM

5. In the event that electrical power to a computer with microchip memory is interrupted, all data, language, or programs in the random access memory (RAM) would be
   A. Conserved
   B. Lost
   C. Conserved or lost, depending on the length of the interruption
   D. Conserved or lost, depending on the electronic activity at the time of interruption

6. In networked computer systems, what does the term client refer to?
   A. Manufacturer of the software
   B. Software that allows the connected hardware to communicate
   C. Computer that provides software to user terminals
   D. Workstation from which the user requests services from the server

7. Laboratory instruments may output data in different types of signals. If one is considering the possibility of interfacing the instrument with a computer, which type of signal would be the best to have an instrument output?
   A. Digital
   B. Analog
   C. Parallel
   D. Serial

8. When comparing monitors, it is important to consider the dot pitch. What is dot pitch?
   A. Total number of pixels on the screen
   B. Distance between pixels
   C. Number of different colors the monitor can display
   D. Angle of the screen

9. Computers may communicate by telephone with other computers in order to access large databases or to exchange data. What hardware device allows the computer to translate its output to telephone line signals as well as translate incoming telephone line signals derived from another computer?
   A. RS-232
   B. CPU
   C. Modem
   D. DCE

10. Most computers use a standard code to represent the individual characters, and this standard code is the main reason that computer-computer intercommunication may be easily accomplished. What is the accepted standard code for microcomputers?
   A. ASCII
   B. EBCDIC
   C. COBOL
   D. ADA

11. Which of the following may be used as a pointing device by a graphical user interface?
   A. Mouse
   B. Trackball
   C. Touch-sensitive pad
   D. All the above

12. If you frequently perform a series of operations within a program, what may you want to create to perform these operations automatically?

A. Device driver
B. Style sheet
C. Macro
D. Theme

13. Which of the following is a powerful computer language allowing access to data in a database?
   A. SQL
   B. COBOL
   C. ALGOL
   D. TWAIN

14. Which of the following is not an important part of laboratory information systems?
   A. Specimen tracking
   B. Data retrieval
   C. Transportation
   D. Order entry

15. Windows and Apple operating systems allow users to switch back and forth between programs; this was not possible with DOS. What is the capability to switch between programs called?
   A. Short cutting
   B. Task swapping
   C. Multithreading
   D. Multitasking

16. Most Web browsers support images in which file formats?
   A. jpg and bmp
   B. jpg and gif
   C. tif and gif
   D. bmp and tif

17. The speed of Internet access is partly determined by the carrying capacity of the communication line. What is this called?
   A. Bandwidth
   B. Interface

C. Internet protocol

D. Uniform resource locator

18. Many laboratory information systems allow users the option to define actions in response to certain patient results, such as performing additional tests or sending test results to public health authorities. What is this feature called?

A. Flagging

B. Hot key inquiry

C. Host query

D. Reflexing

19. Communication among laboratory information systems in different hospitals is becoming more common. File transfers can be facilitated if hospitals use which standardized communication interface?

A. Health level 7

B. RS-232C

C. Hypertext transfer protocol

D. Unix

20. Some Web sites you visit create small text files on your computer's hard drive containing log-in information for that Web site. What are these files called?

A. WANs

B. Cookies

C. Spiders

D. Robots

21. When files are attached to e-mail messages or uploaded to Web servers, special software is used. This software uses standards called _____ that ensure error-free transmission.

A. File transfer protocol (FTP)

B. Hypertext markup language (HTML)

C. Hypertext transfer protocol (HTTP)

D. Serial line Internet protocol (SLIP)

22. After a hospital has decided to purchase a laboratory information system, what does it issue to solicit bids from vendors?

A. Ancillary report

B. Good manufacturing practice request

C. Request for proposal

D. Hot key inquiry

23. What feature of a laboratory information system compares a patient's test value to a previous value?

A. Prompt

B. Delta check

C. System validation

D. Archiving

24. Of the following hardware, which one is normally *not* an input device?

A. Bar-code reader

B. Keyboard

C. Modem

D. Cathode ray tube

25. What does telemedicine include?

A. Physician-patient consultation via videoconference

B. Transmitting patient data (e.g., laboratory tests and X-rays)

C. Physician-physician consultation via interactive two-way video

D. All the above

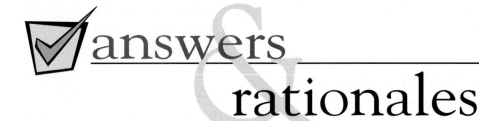

answers & rationales

1.

C. There are eight bits in a byte. A byte represents a character or symbol. A bit (<u>bi</u>nary dig<u>it</u>) is the basic unit of information in the binary system.

2.

A. A computer's clock speed is the number of intervals or cycles per second. Most computers perform one operation per second. Newer microprocessing chips, since the Pentium, can execute more than one instruction per cycle by a process known as superscalar architecture.

3.

B. An open laboratory information system is an operating system able to run on servers from different vendors. An open system is normally a better option, allowing the purchaser freedom to choose any hardware vendor, which may result in getting a better price. A closed system is an operating system that will run only on one brand of server.

4.

B. Since sequential files store data end to end, each file may have a different length with no spaces between data or files. Random-access files have a set length, or number of bytes, that must be filled for each file. If the number of data bytes does not fill the length allotted for each random-access file, blank spaces are appended. Therefore, the use of sequential files is the most efficient way to store patient data. As these files use only the space for the actual data, there would be no blanks.

5.

B. When a computer loses power, either accidentally or intentionally by turning it off, anything in the random access memory (RAM) will be lost or erased. In contrast, everything in the read-only memory (ROM) remains at all times. Both the length of interruption and the electronic activity in which the computer is involved at the time of power interruption are irrelevant. Any power interruption to the computer causes all data in RAM to be erased.

6.

D. The client is the workstation or terminal requesting data from the server. In other words, the server provides information to the client or user. The client can be a stand-alone desktop computer or a thin client that is only a terminal (monitor and keyboard).

7.

A. Digital is the type of electronic signal that computers receive and transmit, making it the easiest signal to interface to a computer. Analog signals must be converted first to digital signals before they can be accepted by the computer. The terms parallel and serial refer to the modes of transmission rather than the type of signal. Serial transmission is bit behind bit, or one bit at a time, and is slower than parallel transmission, which is in multiples of eight bits (1 byte) at a time.

8.

B. Pixels are the smallest picture elements that a device can display, or in other words, points of light on a monitor. Dot pitch is measured in millimeters, and the smaller the dot pitch, the sharper the image. A dot pitch of 0.28 mm is standard.

9.

C. The digital output from computers has to be translated to analog form for telephone transmission, and the receiving computer must translate the telephone analog form back to digital form in order to understand the transmission. A modem is a <u>mo</u>dulation-<u>dem</u>odulation device that translates digital to analog and analog to digital. The abbreviation CPU stands for central processing unit, which is the primary functioning chip, the "brain," of a computer. The RS-232 is a popular type of serial interface with 25 pins. DCE, data communications equipment, is another type of connection.

10.

A. The ASCII code (American Standard Code for Informational Interchange) is the numerical, standard code used in most microcomputers. The abbreviation EBCDIC stands for Extended Binary-Coded Decimal Interchange Code, which is the standard code for the IBM mainframe computers. COBOL and ADA are high-level languages designed for business.

11.

D. Pointer devices control the movement of a movable icon, usually an arrow, on the monitor. A mouse is the most common type of pointing device. Trackballs are like an upside-down mouse. Trackballs and touch-sensitive pads are generally found on laptop computers.

12.

C. A macro is a recorded series of commands executed within a software application. Most applications allow users to create their own macros. A device driver is a set of commands that allow a computer to communicate with hardware such as monitors, mouse, and printers. A style sheet is most often used in word processing programs to save commonly used settings such as font type, font style, margin settings, etc. The style sheet can then be applied to any text document. A theme is part of the Windows user environment that controls the appearance of the desktop, icon, pointer, screen saver, etc. Themes can also be applied to Microsoft Office documents.

13.

A. The value of a database is the ability to do queries to retrieve information in different ways. Standard or structured query language (SQL) is an American National Standards Institute (ANSI) standardized language allowing access to data in a database. COBOL is a high-level programming language designed for accounting information such as billing and payroll. Algorithmic language (ALGOL) is a language used for efficient handling of arithmetic and logical processes. TWAIN is an acronym for technology without an interesting name; it refers to connections for downloading images from digital cameras to computers.

14.

C. Laboratory information systems (LISs) can increase the efficiency of clinical laboratories by allowing for specimen tracking, data (e.g., patient results) retrieval, and order entry. The LIS does not transport specimens; a robotics system would be necessary to handle this function. Features of LISs vary considerably among the different vendors and can be customized to the needs of individual hospitals.

15.

D. With multitasking, more than one program can be loaded into random access memory (RAM) at one time. As computers have become more powerful and equipped with more RAM, multitasking has become a time saver for users. It is easy to move from one program to another without having to close the first program. Task swapping was a feature of DOS that allowed users to work in a file of one program and quickly leave that program to go to another one. When the user returned to the first program, the file with which the user was working would be open at the same location. With task swapping, only one program is actually in RAM at a time. Multithreading is performing multiple functions within an application, such as performing spell check while adding more text.

16.

B. Most Web browsers support images in jpg (Joint Photographic Experts Group: JPEG) and gif (Graphical Interchange Format) formats. Bitmap (bmp) and tagged image file (tif) are other formats in which images can be saved, but Web browsers do not recognize these formats. A new image format, that newer versions of Web browsers can recognize, is called portable network graphics (PNG). Ultimately, this format may become the preferred format for Web browsers.

17.

A. Bandwidth is measured in bits per second (bps). It is the amount of information that can be transmitted through a channel or communication line. Other factors affecting the speed of Internet access is the microprocessor speed and amount of random access memory (RAM) of the computer and the number of users on the local network accessing the Internet at the time. Internet protocols (IPs) are the standards allowing computers to exchange data via the Internet. Uniform resource locators (URLs) are the addresses used to find Web sites.

18.

D. Most laboratory information systems (LISs) allow users to program additional operations to be performed based on specified patient results. If a patient result for a particular test falls within certain parameters, an additional test may be suggested. These reflexes should automatically include billing codes. Flagging is simply marking high or low critical (panic) values. Hot key inquiries are keys on the computer keyboard programmed to provide the user with additional information, such as reference ranges during data entry. A host query is a type of bidirectional interface between an instrument and the LIS.

19.

A. Hospitals, health maintenance organizations (HMOs), and physician offices in an area may want to share patient information. In order for the computer information systems to communicate with each other and to exchange data, they must use a standardized transfer protocol. The most widely used interface for this purpose is Health Level 7 (HL7). The RS-232C is a popular type of serial interface with 25 pins. Hypertext transfer protocol (HTTP) is the protocol followed for the exchange of information on the Web. Unix is a text-based operating system for servers.

20.

B. Some Web sites require visitors to log-in to access certain Web pages. Cookies are text files some of these Web sites create to keep track of this information so the user only has to log-in once. With each additional visit, the Web site will retrieve the log-in information from the cookie. Wide area networks (WANs) are computers connected over a large distance. Spiders or robots are computer programs that search the Worldwide Web to create a database of web pages. Spiders are used by Internet search engines.

21.

A. In order for computer files to be accurately transferred on the Internet, standard protocols must be used. These protocols are called file transfer protocols (FTPs). Hypertext markup language (HTML) is the language used to create Web pages. Hypertext transfer protocol (HTTP) is the protocol followed for the exchange of information on the Worldwide Web, and serial line Internet protocol (SLIP) are standards providing for direct Internet connections via a phone line.

22.

C. In order to get the best price and solutions to a laboratory's computer needs, a request for proposal (RFP) is issued. The laboratory's needs are described, and companies submit proposals describing how the needs would be addressed and what the cost would be. Good manufacturing practice (GMP) are regulations issued by the Food and Drug Administration (FDA). Hot key inquiries are keys on the computer keyboard programmed to provide the user with additional information.

23.

B. A laboratory information system (LIS) may be programmed to compare a patient's test value to a previous value of the same assay. This is called a delta check. A prompt is the user interface of a text based operating system such as DOS or Unix. System validation is a tool within the LIS allowing the user to set up and monitor testing, regulatory compliance, and quality control. Archiving refers to storing patient data that is no longer needed onto a backup system to free storage space on the LIS.

24.

D. Input devices are those that send data to the computer. The cathode ray tube (CRT) is the monitor that displays information; however, touch screen monitors can be an input device. Both disk drives and modems can be either input or output devices. The keyboard and bar-code reader are always input devices.

25.

D. Telecommunication can be applied to public health in two main areas: telemedicine and teleprevention. Telemedicine was developed to provide health care to residents in rural areas by allowing laboratory and nursing personnel to exchange data and expertise with physicians at major medical centers. Telemedicine can include a variety of activities in health care such as physician-physician and physician-patient consultations.

REFERENCES

Cooper, S. D. (1998). Laboratory Information Systems. In C. A. Lehmann (Ed.), *Saunders Manual of Clinical Laboratory Science* (pp. 1163–1209). Philadelphia: W. B. Saunders.

Elevitch, F. R., and Spackman, K. A. (2000). Clinical Laboratory Informatics. In C. A. Burtis and E. R. Ashwood (Eds.), *Tietz Fundamentals of Clinical Chemistry,* 5th ed. (pp. 262–271). Philadelphia: W. B. Saunders.

Meyer, M., and Baber, R. (1997). *Computers in Your Future,* 2nd ed. Indianapolis: Que Education & Training, Macmillan Publishing.

CHAPTER

14 Self-Assessment Test

contents

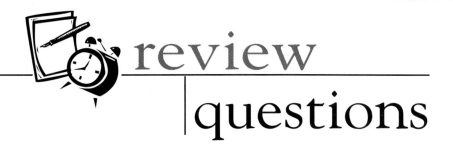

review questions

INSTRUCTIONS Each of the questions or incomplete statements that follow comprises four suggested responses. Select the *best* answer or completion statement in each case.

1. Given that a method mean is 25 mg/dL and the standard deviation is 1.2 mg/dL, what would be the coefficient of variation?
   A. 2.1%
   B. 2.4%
   C. 4.8%
   D. 9.6%

2. Which quality control chart is a graphic representation of the acceptable limits of variation in the results of an analytical method?
   A. Gaussian
   B. Youden
   C. Levey-Jennings
   D. Cusum

3. In a quality control program the confidence interval has been set at 95%. How many test results are expected to fall beyond the established limits?
   A. 1 in 5
   B. 1 in 10
   C. 1 in 20
   D. 1 in 95

4. What is the composition of the packing of a column in gas-liquid chromatography?

   A. An inert material
   B. A stationary phase
   C. An inert material and a mobile phase
   D. An inert material and a stationary phase

5. The absorbance of a 6 mg/L standard is 0.50. An unknown has an absorbance of 0.38. What is the value of the unknown?
   A. 7.9 mg/L
   B. 6.3 mg/L
   C. 4.6 mg/L
   D. 2.3 mg/L

6. If 30 grams of H_2SO_4 (mol wt = 98) are dissolved in 500 mL of water, what is the normality of the solution?
   A. 0.82
   B. 1.22
   C. 2.94
   D. 3.40

7. What is the principal estrogen produced during pregnancy?
   A. Estrone
   B. 17β-Estradiol
   C. Estriol
   D. 6β-Hydroxyestrone

8. Insecticides that are organic phosphorus compounds, such as parathion and tetraethyl pyrophosphate, may cause insecticide poisoning by inhibiting
   A. Lactate dehydrogenase
   B. Acid phosphatase
   C. Cholinesterase
   D. Glucose-6-phosphate dehydrogenase

9. Which of the following is a water-soluble vitamin?
   A. A
   B. C
   C. D
   D. E

10. Which of the following is a laboratory assay used for detecting cystic fibrosis?
    A. Serum lipase
    B. Serum amylase
    C. Serum trypsin
    D. Sweat chloride

11. In primary hypothyroidism one would expect the serum FT_4 level to be _____, the TSH level to be _____, and the TBG level to be _____.
    A. Decreased, increased, slightly increased
    B. Decreased, decreased, slightly increased
    C. Increased, decreased, slightly increased
    D. Decreased, increased, slightly decreased

12. A serum sample is moderately hemolyzed. Which of the following analyses would be most significantly affected by the hemolysis?
    A. Sodium
    B. Potassium
    C. Glucose
    D. Urea

13. A black male 62 years of age is admitted in a semiconscious state experiencing shortness of breath and a temperature of 100 °F. His

skin is pale and cool, and he has been experiencing severe pain in his back and jaw for approximately 75 minutes. He experienced these same symptoms two days earlier. The laboratory data shows the following:

    Total CK—elevated
    CK-MB—elevated
    Myoglobin—elevated
    cTnI—elevated

Utilizing this information, what is the most likely diagnosis for this patient?
    A. Pulmonary infarction
    B. Acute myocardial infarction
    C. Muscular dystrophy
    D. Angina pectoris

14. A blood specimen is drawn in the morning, and the serum is removed from the clot and left standing at room temperature till late in the afternoon. Which of the following parameters would be most severely affected by delayed analysis?
    A. Urea
    B. Potassium
    C. Alanine aminotransferase
    D. Bilirubin

15. In ketoacidosis, the anion gap would most likely be affected in what way?
    A. Unchanged from normal
    B. Increased
    C. Decreased
    D. Balanced

16. If the aspartate aminotransferase (AST) and the alanine aminotransferase (ALT) serum levels are increased 50-fold over the reference range, what would be the most consistent diagnosis?
    A. Extrahepatic cholestasis
    B. Cirrhosis
    C. Carcinoma of the liver
    D. Viral hepatitis

17. A decreased bicarbonate level in the blood without a change in P_{CO_2} will result in what acid/base imbalance?
    A. Respiratory acidosis
    B. Respiratory alkalosis
    C. Metabolic acidosis
    D. Metabolic alkalosis

18. Elevated serum levels of urea, creatinine, and uric acid would be suggestive of what disorder?
    A. Gout
    B. Chronic renal failure
    C. Cirrhosis
    D. Malnutrition

19. The following results were obtained on a patient following the ingestion of 75 grams of glucose as part of an oral glucose tolerance test.

Time Specimen Collected	Serum Glucose (mg/dL)
Fasting	124
½ hour	185
1 hour	220
1½ hours	195
2 hours	170

Based on the preceding information, how would this patient be classified?
    A. Normal
    B. Diabetic
    C. Gestational diabetic
    D. Hypoglycemic

20. Which of the following methods may be used to quantify total protein in serum, urine, or cerebrospinal fluid?
    A. Coomassie brilliant blue
    B. Sulfosalicylic acid
    C. Bromcresol green
    D. Ponceau S

21. A patient who received a blood transfusion experienced a moderate transfusion reaction. Due to the presence of free hemoglobin in the plasma, which serum protein will exhibit a decreased level?
    A. Ceruloplasmin
    B. Transferrin
    C. Alpha$_2$-macroglobulin
    D. Haptoglobin

22. When employing a diazo method to quantify serum bilirubin, which of the following blood constituents when present in an elevated amount will cause a falsely depressed bilirubin result?
    A. Ammonia
    B. Creatinine
    C. Hemoglobin
    D. Uric acid

23. What quality incorporated into a spectrophotometer can sometimes improve the linearity of a chemistry procedure?
    A. Flow-through cuvette
    B. Wider bandwidth
    C. Narrower bandwidth
    D. Chopper

24. What hormone plays a primary role in controlling the reabsorption of sodium in the tubules?
    A. Cortisol
    B. Cortisone
    C. Estriol
    D. Aldosterone

25. Individuals with Addison's disease tend to exhibit which of the following?
    A. Hyperglycemia
    B. Hypoglycemia
    C. Normal blood glucose levels
    D. Increased 2-hour postprandial glucose levels

26. Which of the following tests when used together are helpful in monitoring treatment and identifying recurrence of testicular cancer?
   A. AFP and CEA
   B. AFP and CG
   C. CEA and CG
   D. CA 125 and CA 19-9

27. To detect respiratory distress syndrome, what specimen is used for measuring the surfactant/ albumin ratio by fluorescence polarization?
   A. Serum
   B. Plasma
   C. Urine
   D. Amniotic fluid

28. High levels of cholesterol leading to increased risk of coronary artery disease would be associated with which lipoprotein fraction?
   A. LDL
   B. VLDL
   C. HDL
   D. Chylomicrons

29. A female patient upon hospital admission exhibits a serum osmolality level of 350 mOsm/kg. A possible cause of this result may be all the following *except*
   A. Elevated serum potassium level
   B. Elevated serum sodium level
   C. Elevated serum glucose level
   D. Dehydration

30. If the ratio of bicarbonate to carbonic acid is 30:1, what would the blood pH be?
   A. Increased
   B. Decreased
   C. Stable
   D. Normal

31. Upon what principle is nephelometric measurement based?
   A. Fluorescence produced
   B. Phosphorescence produced
   C. Light transmitted
   D. Light scattered

32. Which of the following would be considered acceptable specimens for PCR?
   A. Blood and body fluids
   B. Solid and paraffin-embedded tissues
   C. Hair, skin, and nails
   D. All the above

33. Stringency can be decreased by increasing
   A. Time and/or temperature
   B. Ionic strength (i.e., NaCl)
   C. pH
   D. All the above

34. In their correct order, what are the steps involved in the polymerase chain reaction?
   A. Denaturation of dsDNA, annealing of primers, synthesis of complementary DNA strand
   B. Annealing of primers, denaturation of dsDNA, synthesis of complementary DNA strand
   C. Synthesis of complementary DNA strand, denaturation of dsDNA, annealing of primers
   D. Denaturation of dsDNA, synthesis of complementary DNA strand, annealing of primers

35. Sickle-cell anemia is a genetic disease caused by a single base mutation in the beta-globin gene. The single change abolishes a *Cvn*I restriction site. Using specific primers that target a portion of beta-globin gene a 726 base pair PCR product is generated. After enzyme digestion of PCR products from normal individuals with *Cvn*I, fragments of the following sizes are produced: 256 bp, 201 bp, 181 bp, and 88 bp. Which of the following restriction fragment patterns represent the results you would see in a patient homozygous for the sickle cell gene?
   A. Two bands—457 bp and 269 bp

B. Three bands—382 bp, 256 bp, and 88 bp

C. Four bands—382 bp, 201 bp, 181 bp, and 88 bp

D. Five bands—382 bp, 256 bp, 201 bp, 181 bp, and 88 bp

36. What should dedicated work areas within a molecular diagnostics laboratory include?
    A. Reagent preparation and postamplification areas
    B. Specimen preparation and preamplification areas
    C. Specimen preparation, reagent preparation, and pre- and postamplification procedure areas
    D. Reagent preparation and pre- and postamplification areas

37. Amplification techniques make molecular methods highly sensitive. For viral load testing quantitative results are needed. An internal quantification standard is included in these tests. Which of the following methodologies is (are) currently being used for HIV and HCV viral quantification?
    A. Reverse transcriptase–polymerase chain reaction (RT-PCR), such as Amplicor®
    B. Branched chain DNA (bDNA), such as Quantiplex®
    C. Nucleic acid sequence based amplification (NASBA), such as NucliSens®
    D. All the above

38. Which of the following causes thalassemia?
    A. Amino acid substitution in a globin chain
    B. Deficiency in an enzyme for heme synthesis
    C. Abnormal gene for globin production
    D. Presence of an unstable hemoglobin

39. What tissue is the primary producer of erythropoietin?

A. Liver
B. Kidneys
C. Bone marrow
D. Red blood cells

40. Red blood cell distribution width (RDW) is an indication or measure of
    A. Poikilocytosis
    B. Macrocytosis
    C. Anisocytosis
    D. Microcytosis

41. Aminolevulinic acid (ALA) synthase is an enzyme involved in the
    A. Early stages of heme synthesis in the mitochondria
    B. Intermediate stages of heme synthesis in the cytoplasm
    C. Late stages of heme synthesis in the mitochondria
    D. Embden-Meyerhof glycolytic pathway

42. Hemoglobin A_2 consists of
    A. Two alpha-globin and two beta-globin chains
    B. Two alpha-globin and two gammaglobin chains
    C. Four beta-globin chains
    D. Two alpha-globin and two delta-globin chains

43. Increased osmotic fragility could be expected in which of the following disorders?
    A. Sickle cell anemia
    B. Iron deficiency anemia
    C. Thalassemia
    D. Hereditary spherocytosis

44. Color Plate 9 represents red blood cells that can be described as
    A. Having slight anisocytosis
    B. Containing Pappenheimer bodies
    C. Having marked poikilocytosis
    D. Macrocytic hypochromic

45. Erythrocytes that show increased lysis in the presence of complement and acidified serum are seen in which disorder?
    A. Glucose-6-phosphate dehydrogenase deficiency
    B. Hereditary spherocytosis
    C. Paroxysmal nocturnal hemoglobinuria
    D. Paroxysmal cold hemoglobinuria

46. Primary polycythemia (polycythemia vera) will show an increase in all the following laboratory results *except*
    A. Erythrocyte sedimentation rate
    B. Leukocyte alkaline phosphatase
    C. Blood volume
    D. White blood cell count

47. Which of the following stains is used to visualize reticulocytes?
    A. Wright's
    B. Crystal violet
    C. Prussian blue
    D. New methylene blue

48. In the red blood cell, what is the function of the hexose monophosphate shunt?
    A. Produces adenosine triphosphate (ATP)
    B. Produces 2,3-bisphosphoglycerate (2,3-BPG)
    C. Helps prevent oxidation of hemoglobin
    D. Participates in heme synthesis

49. Hemoglobin is measured spectrophotometrically at what wavelength?
    A. 410 nm
    B. 472 nm
    C. 540 nm
    D. 610 nm

50. Color Plate 8 would most likely be associated with which of the following conditions?
    A. Basophilic stippling
    B. Reticulocytosis
    C. Iron deficiency
    D. Bone marrow failure

51. Blockage or deactivation of an enzyme in the heme synthesis pathway results in what disorder?
    A. Thalassemia
    B. Hemoglobinopathy
    C. Unstable hemoglobins
    D. Porphyria

52. What structures in neutrophils and macrophages are responsible for microbial digestion?
    A. Ribosomes
    B. Golgi complexes
    C. Lysosomes
    D. Nucleoli

53. What plasma protein is increased in Waldenström's macroglobulinemia?
    A. IgM
    B. IgE
    C. IgA
    D. Fibrinogen

54. Which of the following serum chemistry values is often elevated in chronic myelogenous leukemia and other malignancies?
    A. Glucose
    B. Uric acid
    C. Bilirubin
    D. Lactic acid

55. Which type of cell is normally the most numerous in the bone marrow?
    A. Lymphocytic
    B. Monocytic
    C. Erythrocytic
    D. Granulocytic

56. Which FAB type of myelodysplastic syndrome is *least* likely to progress to acute myelogenous leukemia?
    A. Refractory anemia (RA)
    B. Chronic myelomonocytic leukemia (CMML)

C. Refractory anemia with excess blasts (RAEB)

D. Refractory anemia with excess blasts in transformation (RAEBIT)

57. The blood and bone marrow smears shown in Color Plates 20 and 14 are from a 5-year-old girl recently diagnosed with acute lymphocytic leukemia. Which of the following is *not typical* of this diagnosis?

A. Her age

B. CALLA positive type has a poor prognosis

C. Presence of anemia, neutropenia, and thrombocytopenia

D. Leukemic cells show PAS positivity

58. For which of the following is tartrate resistant acid phosphatase (TRAP) positivity characteristic?

A. Sézary cells

B. Reactive lymphocytes

C. Hairy cells

D. Large granular lymphocytes

59. A patient is evaluated for severe thrombocytopenia and severe absolute neutropenia. What test is likely to provide the most useful information about this patient?

A. Bleeding time

B. Bone marrow aspirate and biopsy

C. Sedimentation rate

D. Test for heterophile antibodies

60. The Philadelphia chromosome is seen in patients with what disorder?

A. Chronic myelogenous leukemia

B. Acute myelogenous leukemia

C. Myelodysplastic syndrome

D. Myelofibrosis with myeloid metaplasia

61. Which of the following is characteristic of true Pelger-Huët anomaly?

A. Associated with acute leukemia

B. Presence of large metachromatic granules in all leukocytes

C. Abnormality of neutrophilic phagocytosis

D. Morphologically immature but normally functioning neutrophils

62. Plasma cells are found in large numbers in the bone marrow and occasionally in the peripheral blood of patients with what disorder?

A. Multiple myeloma

B. Myeloid metaplasia

C. Acute lymphocytic leukemia

D. Viral infection

63. The blood smear shown in Color Plate 11 is from a 16-year-old male with complaints of extreme fatigue and sore throat. His WBC, hemoglobin, and platelet values are normal. Based on the clinical and laboratory information, which of the following is the most likely cause of his condition?

A. Staphylococcal pneumonia

B. Hookworm infection

C. Infectious mononucleosis

D. Chronic lymphocytic leukemia

64. In which of the following conditions is pancytosis often present?

A. Primary polycythemia

B. Primary thrombocythemia

C. Refractory anemia

D. Aplastic anemia

65. Inability to obtain a bone marrow sample by needle aspiration is frequently encountered in patients with which of the following disorders?

A. Acute monocytic leukemia

B. Myelofibrosis

C. Polycythemia vera

D. Erythroleukemia

66. The cytoplasmic inclusion present in the cell shown in Color Plate 15 excludes a diagnosis of
   A. Acute myelocytic leukemia
   B. Acute promyelocytic leukemia
   C. Acute myelomonocytic leukemia
   D. Acute lymphocytic leukemia

67. Which one of the following cells is considered diagnostic of Hodgkin's disease?
   A. Rappaport cell
   B. Niemann-Pick cell
   C. Reed-Sternberg cell
   D. Kupffer cell

68. What is the test of choice to detect abnormalities in the intrinsic system?
   A. Bleeding time
   B. Thrombin time
   C. Activated partial thromboplastin time
   D. Prothrombin time

69. A patient has a prothrombin time of 23 seconds (control = 12.0 seconds) and activated partial thromboplastin time of 61 seconds (control = 33.0 seconds). Of the following, which one is probably *not* deficient in this patient?
   A. Factor II
   B. Factor V
   C. Factor IX
   D. Factor X

70. Which of the following describes plasmin?
   A. Substance that can digest cross-linked fibrin into D-dimers
   B. Activator of plasminogen
   C. Circulates in the plasma ready to immediately digest fibrin clots
   D. Forms a complex with tissue plasminogen activators to digest fibrinogen

71. By what mechanism does aspirin ingestion impair platelet function?

   A. Blocks glycoprotein receptors on the surface of the platelet
   B. Interferes with liver synthesis of a number of the coagulation factors
   C. Interferes with the ability of platelets to adhere to subendothelial collagen
   D. Decreases thromboxane A_2 formation by inhibiting cyclooxygenase

72. Which of the following describes idiopathic thrombocytopenic purpura?
   A. Occurs only in a chronic form
   B. Disorder where a platelet autoantibody is responsible for platelet destruction
   C. Develops in the majority of cases after recovery from a bacterial infection
   D. Usually causes decreased bone marrow synthesis of platelet precursors

73. What is the most important naturally occurring inhibitor to clotting?
   A. Antithrombin III
   B. Heparin
   C. Protein C
   D. α_2-Antiplasmin

74. The prothrombin time is usually *not* prolonged in patients with which of the following disorders?
   A. Hemophilia A
   B. Obstructive liver disease
   C. Congenital factor VII deficiency
   D. Venous thrombosis treated with coumadin®

75. An 18-year-old male was seen in the emergency room following a motorcycle accident. The patient was not wearing his helmet at the time of the accident. He was comatose and was admitted to the hospital with a diagnosis of severe closed head injury. The next day the patient was noted to have increased bleeding from venipuncture

sites. Given the following results, what was the most likely diagnosis for this patient?

Tests	Patient Results	Reference Ranges
PT	25.0 seconds	11.0–13.0 seconds
APTT	89.0 seconds	22.0–38.0 seconds
Fibrinogen	65 mg/dL	150–400 mg/dL
Thrombin time	45 seconds	15–20 seconds
Platelet count	32×10^9/L	$150–440 \times 10^9$/L
FDP test	>20 μg/mL	<5 μg/mL
D-Dimer	>1.0 μg/mL	<0.5 μg/mL

A. Hemophilia A
B. von Willebrand's disease
C. Thrombotic thrombocytopenic purpura
D. Disseminated intravascular coagulation

76. Of the following hemostatic abnormalities, which is the most common?
A. Hemophilia A
B. Thrombocytopenia
C. von Willebrand's disease
D. Hemophilia B

77. Patients with classic von Willebrand's disease may have all the following *except*
A. Easy bruising
B. Decreased platelet aggregation in the presence of ristocetin
C. Prolonged prothrombin time
D. Prolonged bleeding time

78. How are individuals with cellular immune deficiencies best identified?
A. Determining serum complement concentration
B. HLA typing
C. Serum electrophoresis
D. Skin testing

79. Which of the following is characteristic of DiGeorge's syndrome?
A. Defective T lymphocyte production
B. Depressed thymus development
C. Normal antibody levels
D. All the above

80. The interaction between antigen presenting cells and T-helper cells is mediated by surface expressed antigen and
A. Interferon gamma
B. Interleukin 2
C. Interleukin 3
D. MHC class II molecules

81. Which of the following cell types is the primary mediator of antibody-dependent cellular cytotoxicity (ADCC) reactions?
A. B cells
B. Cytotoxic T cells
C. Natural killer cells
D. Suppressor T cells

82. What is the portion of an antigen that binds specifically to the binding site of an antibody called?
A. Epitope
B. Hapten
C. Idiotope
D. Paratope

83. Which of the following is *not* true of the alternate complement pathway?
A. Activated by bacterial polysaccharide
B. C4 is not involved
C. Primarily activated by antibody
D. Properdin protein may activate C3

84. What is the type of hypersensitivity reaction mediated by IgE and mast cells?
A. Anaphylactic
B. Cytotoxic
C. Delayed hypersensitivity
D. Immune complex

85. Which of the following lymphokines is involved in tumor immunology?
    A. Interleukin 2 (IL-2)
    B. Macrophage-activating factor (MAF)
    C. Interferon gamma
    D. All the above

86. The B cell surface receptor for antigen is
    A. Immunoglobulin
    B. Interleukin 1
    C. Interleukin 2
    D. MHC I antigen

87. Which of the following frequently functions as an antigen presenting cell?
    A. B cell
    B. Macrophage
    C. Natural killer cell
    D. T cell

88. Which of the following cell types contains class II human leukocyte antigens?
    A. All nucleated cells
    B. B cells
    C. Platelets
    D. All the above

89. What disease is associated with the possession of HLA-B27?
    A. Ankylosing spondylitis
    B. Goodpasture's syndrome
    C. Hashimoto's disease
    D. Lupus erythematosus

90. In the radial immunodiffusion assay (RID), to what is the concentration of antigen directly proportional?
    A. Diameter of the precipitin ring squared
    B. Four times the diameter of the precipitin ring
    C. Four times the radius of the precipitin ring
    D. Twice the diameter of the precipitin ring

91. Which of the following leukocyte antigens is found on mature helper T cells?
    A. CD4
    B. CD8
    C. CD10
    D. CD25

92. Which of the following is an example of a double diffusion assay?
    A. Immunofixation electrophoresis
    B. Ouchterlony
    C. Radial immunodiffusion (RID)
    D. Rocket electrophoresis

93. Which of the following is true of counter-immunoelectrophoresis (CIE)?
    A. Antigen migrates toward the cathode
    B. Electric current is applied to move antibody and antigen together
    C. Example of an agglutination reaction
    D. System buffered to pH 4.4

94. Which of the following is a nonphagocytic cytotoxic cell able to rapidly kill cells without having been previously exposed to that cell?
    A. Cytotoxic T cell
    B. Helper T cell
    C. Natural killer cell
    D. Suppressor T cell

95. Which of the following is a granulocytic cell with IgE receptors?
    A. Cytotoxic T cell
    B. Mast cell
    C. Natural killer cell
    D. Plasma cell

96. Which of the following is an oncofetal antigen whose presence in adult serum is suggestive of carcinoma?
    A. Alpha-fetoprotein (AFP)
    B. C reactive protein (CRP)
    C. Lymphocyte function-associated antigen 1 (LFA-1)
    D. Nuclear antigens

97. In the competitive radioimmunosorbent test (RIST) for serum IgE, what do low level counts per minute (cpm) indicate?
    A. High levels of interfering IgG
    B. High concentration of IgE
    C. Antibody-antigen complexes precipitated
    D. Radioisotope is weak

98. Information obtained from a volunteer blood donor at the time of registration is designed to protect the health of both donor and recipient. Of the responses below, which would cause the donor to be deferred from the collection process?
    A. Received his last injection in a vaccine series for hepatitis B three weeks ago
    B. Had a tooth filled one week ago
    C. Took aspirin yesterday for a headache
    D. Taking Tegison

99. Which of the following describes the principle by which separation of plasma, platelets, and granulocytes by apheresis is accomplished?
    A. Centrifugal force allows separation based on different density of blood components
    B. Centrifugal force allows separation based on different viscosity of blood components
    C. Intermittent flow rate allows separation of components
    D. Continuous flow rate allows separation of components

100. The inlet port on a closed unit of red blood cells is defective, preventing the addition of Adsol®. What will be the resulting shelf life of the red blood cells?
    A. 24 hours
    B. 21 days
    C. 35 days
    D. 42 days

101. What is the FDA licensed confirmatory test for anti-HIV1?
    A. Competitive binding EIA for p24 (core) and gp41 (envelope)
    B. Southern blotting
    C. Western blotting
    D. Radioimmunoprecipitation assay (RIPA)

102. What is the expiration date for fresh frozen plasma (FFP) that is stored at −65 °C or colder?
    A. 12 months
    B. 3 years
    C. 5 years
    D. 7 years

103. Which of the following is *not* concentrated in cryoprecipitate?
    A. Fibrinogen
    B. Factor V
    C. Factor VIII
    D. Factor XIII

104. Which of the following donors would most likely be allowed to donate autologous blood for elective surgery if all other criteria are acceptable?
    A. 15-year-old girl with a hemoglobin of 12 g/dL
    B. 17-year-old boy with intermittent bacteremia
    C. 30-year-old man with aortic stenosis
    D. 25-year-old woman who had a baby 4 weeks ago

105. The intravascular volume deficit of a cytopheresis donor shall *not* exceed _____ mL/kg of the donor's weight.
    A. 8.0
    B. 10.5
    C. 12.0
    D. 14.5

106. Hemophilia A and B (Christmas disease) both provide a classic example of which pattern of inheritance?
    A. X-linked recessive
    B. X-linked dominant
    C. Autosomal recessive
    D. Autosomal dominant

107. A and B blood group antigens are derived when glycosyltransferases add specific sugars to precursor H. What is the terminal sugar for the B antigen?
    A. Fucose
    B. *N*-acetylglucosamine
    C. *N*-acetylgalactosamine
    D. D-Galactose

108. Which of the following does *not* characterize Rh_{null} individuals?
    A. Red blood cells lack all antigens in the Rh system
    B. Red blood cell morphology shows stomatocytes
    C. Red blood cell survival is shortened with compensated anemia
    D. Condition may be inherited or acquired

109. Which of the following antigens is the most immunogenic after A, B, and D antigens?
    A. C
    B. E
    C. Fy^a
    D. K

110. All the following HLA antigens are defined by the serologic lymphocytotoxicity test *except*
    A. HLA-A
    B. HLA-B
    C. HLA-D
    D. HLA-DR

111. Following compatibility testing, for how long must the patient's blood sample and the donor's red blood cells be retained?
    A. 7 days after crossmatching
    B. 7 days after transfusion
    C. 9 days after crossmatching
    D. 10 days after transfusion

112. Which reagent red blood cells are used for antibody screening during pretransfusion testing?
    A. Group A
    B. Group B
    C. Group AB
    D. Group O

113. The use of an autocontrol during antibody screening for pretransfusion testing
    A. Is required
    B. Is optional
    C. May be eliminated if a DAT is performed
    D. May aid in detecting alloantibody

114. A "type and screen" established that a premature infant is group A, D-positive with a negative antibody screening test. Numerous small volume transfusions are predicted. If only group O RBC are to be transfused, how often must the infant be crossmatched?
    A. Before transfusion and whenever three days have elapsed before the next transfusion
    B. Before transfusion and whenever seven days have elapsed before the next transfusion
    C. If during the same admission, not until he reaches two months of age
    D. If during the same admission, not until he reaches four months of age

115. A blood sample from a patient with warm autoimmune hemolytic anemia is likely to demonstrate all the following serological characteristics *except*
    A. Serum reacts with all enzyme-treated panel cells
    B. Red cells have a positive DAT
    C. Eluate reacts with all panel cells
    D. Serum antibody appears to be directed against a high-incidence Lu system antigen

116. Following removal of plasma from a whole blood unit, the red blood cells (RBCs) may be resuspended in an additive solution. Which of the following does *not* describe these solutions?
    A. Must be added within 72 hours after plasma separation
    B. Contain inosine and pyruvate
    C. Maintain increased levels of ATP in stored cells
    D. Extend the shelf life of red blood cells to 42 days

117. Platelets prepared in polyolefin (PL-732) differ from platelets prepared in polyvinylchloride (PVC) because bags without plasticizers
    A. Increase platelet shelf life to 7 days
    B. Allow platelet storage at 1–6 °C
    C. Promote improved gas exchange with environmental air
    D. Promote accelerated lactic acid production

118. What is the pore size (in microns) of a standard blood transfusion filter?
    A. 20–40
    B. 60–80
    C. 100–120
    D. 170–260

119. Which of the following statements about blood warming devices is *true*?

    A. Are useful to prevent cardiac arrest when extended flow rates are high
    B. May not allow blood to exceed a temperature of 37 °C
    C. Must be quality controlled by the blood bank
    D. Are required if the donor has a cold-reacting autoantibody

120. What is the most common cause of anemia leading to transfusion in sick neonates?
    A. Bleeding from the umbilicus
    B. Red blood cell destruction because of HDN
    C. Blood drawn for laboratory testing
    D. Immature bone marrow response

121. What is the initial step to perform when a patient is suspected of having a transfusion reaction?
    A. Perform a DAT on a posttransfusion specimen
    B. Compare the pretransfusion and post-transfusion serum for evidence of hemolysis
    C. Check identification of the patient and donor blood
    D. Stop the transfusion

122. Hemolytic transfusion reactions result in all the following laboratory findings *except*
    A. Hemoglobinuria
    B. Haptoglobinemia
    C. Hemoglobinemia
    D. Bilirubinemia

123. To which organization must the hospital transfusion service laboratory report all cases of transfusion-associated disease?
    A. Blood collecting facility
    B. Center for Disease Control (CDC)
    C. Food and Drug Administration (FDA)
    D. State Health Department

124. To comply with the requirements of AABB *Standards*, which of the following tests must be performed on each unit before blood bank personnel may issue autologous units of blood drawn in their facility?
    A. ABO and Rh typing
    B. HBsAg
    C. Anti-HIV1
    D. DAT

125. The CDC recommends that "standard precautions" be exercised by all health care workers to prevent transmission of hepatitis B virus, HIV, and other bloodborne pathogens. What do these precautions include?
    A. Wearing protective clothing when testing blood specimens from patients in specific areas
    B. Using special precautionary methods when testing blood specimens with a biohazard label
    C. Handling every patient blood specimen as if it were infectious
    D. Carefully recapping needles before discarding

126. To ensure proper reactivity, how frequently must all blood bank reagents be quality controlled?
    A. With each test
    B. Daily
    C. Each day of use
    D. Weekly

127. What should one do to validate the reaction obtained in the antiglobulin test?
    A. Use green antiglobulin reagent
    B. Add IgG-coated red cells to each test tube
    C. Add IgG-coated red cells to each positive reaction
    D. Add IgG-coated red cells to each negative reaction

128. The outdate rate of blood in inventory can be minimized by all the following *except*
    A. Providing transfusion guidelines
    B. Implementing a first-in, last-out (FILO) policy
    C. Monitoring crossmatch to transfusion (CT) ratios
    D. Instituting a maximum surgical blood order schedule (MSBOS)

129. Clotting may be incomplete in blood specimens from patients treated with heparin. All the following are alternatives for providing an acceptable specimen for pretransfusion testing *except*
    A. Adding protamine sulfate
    B. Adding thrombin
    C. Adding chloroquine diphosphate
    D. Using an EDTA specimen for testing

130. A person with the genotype: *AO, HH, Sese, Lele* will have which of the following combination of substances in her secretions?
    A. A, H, Se, Le^a
    B. Le^a, Le^b
    C. A, H, Le^a, Le^b
    D. A, O, Le^b

131. An immediate spin (IS) crossmatch or a computer crossmatch (if the computer system is validated for this use) may be used as the sole compatibility test when a patient has a confirmed blood type and
    A. A negative DAT result
    B. A negative antibody screening test result
    C. No record of previous transfusion
    D. The same ABO and Rh type as the donor

132. Within how many hours after pooling must pooled platelet concentrates be transfused?

A. 4

B. 6

C. 8

D. 12

133. Pus with a blue-green color was aspirated from an empyema. A Gram stain of the aspirated material showed many WBCs and numerous gram-negative bacilli. What would be the most likely etiologic agent?

A. *Legionella pneumophila*

B. *Pseudomonas aeruginosa*

C. *Morganella morganii*

D. *Serratia marcescens*

134. In the early stages of the disease typhoid fever, *Salmonella typhi* is most likely to be recovered from which of the following specimen types?

A. Feces

B. Urine

C. Blood

D. Skin lesions

135. Symptoms of gastritis and peptic ulceration are most closely associated with which of the following specimen types?

A. *Campylobacter jejuni*

B. Enterotoxigenic *Escherichia coli*

C. *Helicobacter pylori*

D. *Vibrio cholerae*

136. A patient with impaired cell-mediated immunity presents with evidence of a pulmonary abscess and neurological involvement. A brain abscess was detected by MRI. Draining from the abscess grew an aerobic, filamentous, branching gram-positive organism, which stained weakly acid-fast. What is the most likely etiologic agent?

A. *Propionibacterium acnes*

B. *Nocardia asteroides*

C. *Actinobacillus israelii*

D. *Bacillus cereus*

137. The organism *Leptospira interrogans* serovar *icterohaemorrhagiae* is the etiologic agent of

A. Lyme disease

B. Relapsing fever

C. Weil's disease

D. Undulant fever

138. Which of the following is considered to be an endogenous infection?

A. Nocardiosis

B. Tuberculosis

C. Actinomycosis

D. Histoplasmosis

139. Which of the following is *not* recommended to maximize detection of methicillin-resistant staphylococci?

A. Oxacillin is the best drug to use for testing

B. Decrease concentration of salt in the media

C. Incubate the test plate at a temperature below 37 °C

D. Incubate the test plate for a full 24 hours

140. Which of the following statements is true regarding anaerobic infections?

A. Anaerobic pulmonary infections are rare because lung tissue is well ventilated

B. Because of the inaccessibility of organs such as the liver and brain to indigenous flora, they are seldom infected with anaerobes

C. Bacteremia due to anaerobes is benign because anaerobes do not possess endotoxin

D. Intraabdominal abscesses, peritonitis, and wound infections can occur postoperatively when devitalized tissue is contaminated with bowel contents

141. Foul-smelling pus aspirated from a crepitous postsurgical cholecystectomy patient grew a gram-positive bacillus. When cultured on an anaerobically incubated blood agar plate, it grew colonies surrounded by an inner zone of complete red cell lysis and an outer zone of incomplete cell lysis and caused a "stormy fermentation" reaction in litmus milk. What would be the most likely identification of this isolate?

    A. *Fusobacterium nucleatum*

    B. *Clostridium perfringens*

    C. *Clostridium tetani*

    D. *Bacteroides fragilis*

142. Which of the following is associated with *Legionella pneumophila*?

    A. Produces beta-lactamase

    B. Affects mostly a younger age group (5–19 years of age)

    C. Is unaffected by chlorination

    D. Has a role in asymptomatic or subclinical infections that is easy to assess

143. Antibodies to specific treponemal antigens

    A. Are never found unless a person has active syphilis

    B. Are nonspecific in that persons with chronic inflammatory diseases may possess these antibodies

    C. Are the basis for such tests as the RPR and VDRL tests

    D. Decline after successful treatment

144. Which of the following is associated with *Streptococcus agalactiae*?

    A. Is implicated in dental caries

    B. Can cause neonatal sepsis and meningitis

    C. Does not possess a group-specific polysaccharide

    D. Is also called viridans streptococcus

145. Which of the following is associated with *Streptococcus pyogenes*?

    A. Resistant to penicillin are being isolated in increasing numbers in the hospital setting

    B. Contain a group-specific polypeptide

    C. Only rarely cause acute infections

    D. Produce copious amounts of endotoxin (LPS)

146. Which of the following is associated with *Vibrio cholerae*?

    A. Is a component of the normal flora of the human intestine

    B. Needs a plasmid to produce its toxin

    C. Is not found in the United States

    D. Produces a toxin that causes increased secretion of water and electrolytes from the gut

147. A blood culture grew a small, pleomorphic, vacuolated, anaerobic gram-negative rod. It grew on KVLB agar, grew in the presence of 20% bile, and was esculin positive. This organism is most likely

    A. *Clostridium perfringens*

    B. *Bacteroides fragilis*

    C. *Fusobacterium nucleatum*

    D. *Eubacterium lentum*

148. A coagulase-negative staphylococcus was isolated from a urine culture. It was identified as *Staphylococcus saprophyticus* on the basis of its being

    A. Catalase positive

    B. Resistant to novobiocin

    C. DNase positive

    D. Mannitol positive

149. A nonhemolytic streptococcus isolated from a urine culture gave the following reactions: bile esculin positive, no growth in 6.5% NaCl. This streptococcus should be identified as

    A. *Streptococcus agalactiae*

    B. *Enterococcus faecalis*

    C. *Streptococcus mutans*

    D. *Streptococcus bovis*

150. Refer to Color Plate 26. The organism seen on this Gram stain was isolated from the spinal fluid of an infant. It grew on blood agar with faint beta-hemolysis. It was catalase positive and demonstrated active motility at 25 °C, but not at 37 °C. What should one immediately suspect?

    A. *Bacillus anthracis*

    B. *Lactobacillus* species

    C. *Bifidobacterium dentium*

    D. *Listeria monocytogenes*

151. You isolate a small pleomorphic gram-negative rod from the spinal fluid of a 6-month-old infant. It fails to grow on sheep blood agar or MacConkey agar, but grows well on chocolate agar incubated in 5% CO_2. What bacterium would you suspect as the etiologic agent?

    A. *Escherichia coli*

    B. *Streptococcus agalactiae*

    C. *Haemophilus influenzae*

    D. *Listeria monocytogenes*

152. An oxidase-positive slender gram-negative bacillus was isolated from a burn patient. It gave the following reactions: OF glucose open-acid; OF glucose closed-alkaline; OF maltose open-alkaline; negative for pyocyanin production; positive for fluorescein production; good growth at 42 °C. Select the organism that has been identified.

    A. *Alcaligenes faecalis*

    B. *Pseudomonas aeruginosa*

    C. *Xanthamonas maltophilia*

    D. *Acinetobacter anitratus*

153. What is the etiologic agent of pseudomembranous colitis?

    A. *Clostridium difficile*

    B. *Vibrio parahemolyticus*

    C. *Helicobacter pyloris*

    D. *Streptococcus pyogenes*

154. A gram-negative bacillus was isolated on MacConkey agar and appeared as a non-lactose fermenter. It tested oxidase negative and gave the following reactions: TSI-K/A with H_2S, motile, urease positive, and lysine negative. Which of the following would be characterized by the reactions?

    A. *Salmonella enteriditis*

    B. *Shigella sonnei*

    C. *Proteus mirabilis*

    D. *Edwardsiella tarda*

155. A patient with severe abdominal pain and diarrhea was admitted to the hospital. When the stool was cultured, no suspicious colonies were seen on Hektoen or XLD. However, on the MacConkey plate several non-lactose-fermenting colonies were observed. These colonies were picked and biochemicals were inoculated that gave the following reactions:

    TSI-A/A, no gas, no H_2S
    Urease negative
    Motility negative at 35 °C; positive at 24 °C
    Oxidase negative

    The most likely organism would be

    A. *Shigella sonnei*

    B. *Vibrio cholerae*

    C. *Salmonella typhi*

    D. *Yersinia enterocolytica*

156. The stool from a patient with severe gastroenteritis was cultured for enteric pathogens and was also submitted for parasitologic examination. No parasites were found and the routine culture was negative for salmonella and shigella. However, a small oxidase-positive gram-negative rod was isolated on enriched blood agar that had been incubated in a microaerophilic atmosphere of 5% O_2, 10% CO_2, and 85% N_2. The most likely organism would be

    A. *Yersinia enterocolitica*

    B. *Vibrio parahaemolyticus*

    C. *Vibrio cholerae*

    D. *Campylobacter jejuni*

157. A 45-year-old woman came to the emergency room after being bitten on the hand by her cat. The wound was extremely painful and produced a large amount of pus. The pus was cultured on blood agar and MacConkey agar. After 24 hours, growth was observed on the blood agar plate as tiny colonies that produced a slight greening on the underlying media. A Gram stain showed tiny gram-negative rods. There was no growth on the MacConkey agar. Biochemical tests gave the following reactions:

    TSI-A/A
    Oxidase positive
    Nonmotile
    Urease negative

    The most likely organism would be
    A. *Pasturella multocida*
    B. *Corynebacterium diphtheriae*
    C. *Brucella abortus*
    D. *Bordetella pertussis*

158. Buffered charcoal yeast extract agar with added l-cysteine (BCYE) is the primary medium for the isolation of
    A. *Bartonella bacilliformis*
    B. *Chlamydia pneumoniae*
    C. *Legionella pneumophila*
    D. *Mycoplasma pneumoniae*

159. Of the two common *Cladosporium* species that cause subcutaneous mycoses, the one containing longer, less-branched chains of blastoconidia causes
    A. Phaeohyphomycosis
    B. Mycetoma
    C. Sporotrichosis
    D. Chromoblastomycosis

160. *Coccidioides immitis* and *Geotrichum candidum* both produce arthroconidia, and both can produce systemic disease. Which of the following characteristics would *not* differentiate between these two organisms?
    A. Colony texture
    B. Dimorphism
    C. Disjunctor cells
    D. Colony color

161. In regard to the true systemic dimorphic pathogens, the phase of growth that is most infectious is the
    A. Phase seen in tissue
    B. Phase that grows at 25–30 °C
    C. Phase that grows at 37 °C
    D. All phases are equally infectious

162. Which of the following is the definitive host for *Plasmodium* sp.?
    A. Mosquitoes
    B. Ticks
    C. Lice
    D. Humans

163. What is the source of most human infections caused by *Toxoplasma gondii*?
    A. Dogs
    B. Cats
    C. Fleas
    D. Humans

164. Refer to Color Plate 43. What is the infective form of this parasite?
    A. Ova
    B. Oocysts
    C. Rhabditiform larvae
    D. Filariform larvae

165. In what way are HBV and HIV similar?
    A. Ability to survive in the environment
    B. Having cross-reacting antigens
    C. Nucleic acid composition
    D. Requiring reverse transcriptase for replication

166. When should a pregnant woman be most concerned about avoiding rubella infection?
    A. During birthing process
    B. First trimester
    C. Last 4 months of pregnancy
    D. Throughout pregnancy

167. Which of the following is *not* a vector for the transmission of rickettsial disease?
    A. Body louse
    B. Flea
    C. Mosquito
    D. Tick

168. In what form does the reclamation of filtered bicarbonate ion in the proximal tubular cells occur?
    A. Carbonic acid
    B. Carbon dioxide
    C. Sodium carbonate
    D. Sodium bicarbonate

169. In what area of the nephron does approximately 65% of renal reabsorption occur?
    A. Proximal tubule
    B. Distal tubule
    C. Bowman capsule
    D. Glomerulus

170. What is the renal blood flow for a 70-kg male/female?
    A. 12 mL/min
    B. 120 mL/min
    C. 1200 mL/min
    D. 12 L/min

171. The concentration of a solute in plasma at which no additional amount of the solute will be absorbed from the proximal tubule is known as the
    A. Plasma threshold
    B. Tubular threshold
    C. Renal threshold
    D. Blood threshold

172. Which biochemical component would be present in an increased amount in a dark yellow-amber-colored urine?
    A. Biliverdin
    B. Bilirubin
    C. Urobilin
    D. Blood

173. When should a 2-hour postprandial urine be collected?
    A. 2 hours after fluid ingestion
    B. 2 hours after a renal drug ingestion
    C. 2 hours after eating
    D. 2 hours after voiding a fasting specimen

174. Which of the following terms is another name for peritoneal fluid?
    A. Ascitic
    B. Synovial
    C. Pelvic
    D. Abdominal

175. Which of the following formed elements is *not* present in the high power field seen in Color Plate 53?
    A. Renal tubular epithelial cells
    B. Squamous epithelial cells
    C. Bacteria
    D. Calcium oxalate

176. Which of the following is true about Tamm-Horsfall protein?
    A. Measured using the conventional reagent test strips
    B. Appears only in abnormal urine
    C. Matrix of hyaline casts but not granular casts
    D. Excreted by renal tubules in small quantities

177. Which of the following procedures is used to assess glomerular permeability?
    A. Clearance test
    B. Osmolality
    C. 24-hour urine total protein
    D. Renal blood flow

178. With which crystals are urinary uric acid crystals often confused?
    A. Calcium pyrophosphate
    B. Cystine
    C. Cholesterol
    D. Calcium oxalate

179. In what sequence does urine formation occur?
    A. Proximal convoluted tubule, loop of Henle, distal convoluted tubule, collecting duct, Bowman's space
    B. Glomerulus, Bowman's space, proximal convoluted tubule, loop of Henle, distal convoluted tubule, collecting duct
    C. Bowman's space, glomerulus, proximal convoluted tubule, loop of Henle, distal convoluted tubule, collecting duct
    D. Bowman's space, glomerulus, distal convoluted tubule, proximal convoluted tubule, collecting duct

180. Renal clearance tests are used to evaluate which of the following parameters?
    A. Concentrating ability
    B. Glomerular filtration rate
    C. Glomerular permeability
    D. Tubular reabsorption

181. The formed elements present in the high power field in Color Plate 54 could suggest all the following *except*
    A. Glomerulonephritis
    B. Pyelonephritis
    C. Excessive exercise
    D. Diabetic nephropathy

182. The formed elements present in the high power field in Color Plate 55 can be detected by the appropriate reagent strip pad reacting with their
    A. Pseudoperoxidase
    B. Esterase
    C. Glucose oxidase
    D. Acetoacetate

183. When using polarized light microscopy, which urinary sediment component exhibits Maltese cross formation?
    A. RBCs
    B. WBCs
    C. Yeasts
    D. Oval fat bodies

184. Which urinary sediment component is frequently confused with the components in Color Plate 50?
    A. Yeasts
    B. WBCs
    C. Parasites
    D. Casts

185. Which of the following is a urinary ketone body that is measured using the acetest?
    A. Acetyl CoA
    B. Acetoacetate
    C. β-Hydroxybutyrate
    D. α-Hydroxybutyrate

186. What type of microscopy may also be used to observe the urinary components in Color Plate 51?
    A. Polarized
    B. Dark-field
    C. Phase contrast
    D. Electron

187. Which of the following urine biochemical results would be obtained in hemolytic anemia?
    A. Positive bilirubin
    B. Negative blood

C. Positive nitrite

D. Positive urobilinogen

188. Which of the following is a correct method for storing chemicals?

A. Acids and bases should be separated

B. Flammables must be stored in the refrigerator

C. Acids must be stored under the sink

D. Chemicals can be stored in the chemical fume hood

189. Which of the following statements describes Standard Precautions?

A. Everyone should be careful before entering a patient room

B. Treat all human blood and other potentially infectious materials as though they are infected with HIV, HBV, or any other bloodborne pathogen

C. Treat human blood as infectious only if it is known to be

D. All human blood and other infectious material must be handled using a respirator

190. Which of the following is attributed with being the most frequent cause of laboratory-acquired infections?

A. Human contact

B. Antiseptic conditions

C. Injection of infectious microorganisms

D. Inhalation of infectious microorganisms

191. Which type of fire extinguisher should be used to deal with a laboratory fire consisting of ordinary combustibles, flammable liquids, gases, and electrical equipment?

A. Water

B. Triplex dry chemical

C. Loaded stream

D. Foam

192. Which coding system is a systematized series of numbers corresponding to all diseases, op-

erations, procedures, diagnostic tests, and other medical, surgical, and mental health conditions, published annually by the American Medical Association (AMA) for the purpose of standardizing and coding for statistical and billing activities in health care?

A. CPT

B. HCPCS

C. ICD-9-CM

D. DRG

193. When pricing new tests a laboratory must use a factor to calculate the allowance for the hospital's cost for utilities, housekeeping, administration, and other services. What are these costs known as?

A. Direct

B. Overhead

C. Depreciation

D. Indirect labor

194. What is the authority relationship from administration to department head to supervisor to staff known as?

A. Line authority

B. Staff authority

C. Formal authority

D. Job-related authority

195. The verbs "comply with" and "support" would most likely be used in writing an objective in which of the following domains?

A. Affective

B. Cognitive

C. Psychomotor

D. Technical

196. Classify the following *objective:* "The student will calibrate a spectrophotometer according to the procedure manual."

A. Cognitive domain

B. Psychomotor domain

C. Psychosocial domain

D. Affective domain

197. Which of the following testing items is easy to develop but difficult to grade?
    A. True/false
    B. Multiple choice
    C. Matching
    D. Essay

198. Which of the following requires a continuous electrical supply to the computer for data retention?
    A. Hard disk
    B. CD ROM
    C. ROM
    D. RAM

199. What type of laboratory information system is designed to run only on one vendor's server?
    A. Closed system
    B. Sequential system
    C. Validation system
    D. Intranet system

200. What are the programs called that Internet search engines use to explore the Worldwide Web and collect information to create a database users can query?
    A. WANs
    B. TWAINs
    C. Spiders
    D. Cookies

answers & rationales

1.
C.

2.
C.

3.
C.

4.
D.

5.
C.

6.
B.

7.
C.

8.
C.

9.
B.

10.
D.

11.
A.

12.
B.

13.
B.

14.
D.

15.
B.

16.
D.

17.
C.

18.
B.

19.
B.

20.
A.

21.
D.

22.
C.

23.
C.

24.
D.

25.
B.

26.
B.

27.
D.

28.
A.

29.
A.

30.
A.

31.
D.

32.
D.

33.
B.

34.
A.

35.
B.

36.
C.

37.
D.

38.
C.

39.
B.

40.
C.

41.
A.

42.
D.

43.
D.

44.
A.

45.
C.

46.
A.

47.
D.

48.
C.

49.
C.

50.
B.

51.
D.

52.
C.

53.
A.

54.
B.

55.
D.

56.
A.

57.
B.

58.
C.

59.
B.

60.
A.

61.
D.

62.
A.

63.
C.

64.
A.

65.
B.

66.
D.

67.
C.

68.
C.

69.
C.

70.
A.

71.
D.

72.
B.

73.
A.

74.
A.

75.
D.

76.
B.

77.
C.

78.
D.

79.
D.

80.
D.

81.
C.

82.
A.

83.
C.

84.
A.

85.
D.

86.
A.

87.
B.

88.
B.

89.
A.

90.
A.

91.
A.

92.
B.

93. _____
B.

94. _____
C.

95. _____
B.

96. _____
A.

97. _____
B.

98. _____
D.

99. _____
A.

100. _____
B.

101. _____
C.

102. _____
D.

103. _____
B.

104. _____
A.

105. _____
B.

106. _____
A.

107. _____
D.

108. _____
D.

109. _____
D.

110. _____
C.

111. _____
B.

112. _____
D.

113. _____
B.

114. _____
D.

115. _____
D.

116. _____
B.

117. _____
C.

118. _____
D.

119. _____
A.

120. _____
C.

121. _____
D.

122. _____
B.

123. _____
A.

124. _____
A.

125. _____
C.

126. _____
C.

127.
D.

128.
B.

129.
C.

130.
C.

131.
B.

132.
A.

133.
B.

134.
C.

135.
C.

136.
B.

137.
C.

138.
C.

139.
B.

140.
D.

141.
B.

142.
A.

143.
D.

144.
B.

145.
A.

146.
D.

147.
B.

148.
B.

149.
D.

150.
D.

151.
C.

152.
B.

153.
A.

154.
C.

155.
D.

156.
D.

157.
A.

158.
C.

159.
A.

160.
D.

161.
B.

162.
A.

163.
B.

164.
D.

165.
D.

166.
B.

167.
C.

168.
B.

169.
A.

170.
C.

171.
C.

172.
B.

173.
C.

174.
A.

175.
A.

176.
D.

177.
C.

178.
B.

179.
B.

180.
B.

181.
C.

182.
B.

183.
D.

184.
A.

185.
B.

186.
C.

187.
D.

188.
A.

189.
B.

190.
D.

191.
B.

192.
C.

193.
B.

194.
A.

195.
A.

196.
B.

197.
D.

198.
D.

199.
A.

200.
C.

Index